Handbook of Medical Imaging

Handbook of Medical Imaging

Edited by Kenneth Washington

hayle
medical

New York

Hayle Medical,
750 Third Avenue, 9th Floor,
New York, NY 10017, USA

Visit us on the World Wide Web at:
www.haylemedical.com

ISBN: 978-1-63241-813-5

Cataloging-in-Publication Data

Handbook of medical imaging / edited by Kenneth Washington.
   p. cm.
Includes bibliographical references and index.
ISBN 978-1-63241-813-5
1. Diagnostic imaging. 2. Imaging systems in medicine. 3. Radiography, Medical.
4. Diagnosis, Radioscopic. I. Washington, Kenneth.
RC78.7.D53 H36 2019
616.075 4--dc23

Table of Contents

Preface

This book has been a concerted effort by a group of academicians, researchers and scientists, who have contributed their research works for the realization of the book. This book has materialized in the wake of emerging advancements and innovations in this field. Therefore, the need of the hour was to compile all the required researches and disseminate the knowledge to a broad spectrum of people comprising of students, researchers and specialists of the field.

Medical imaging is the technique that allows the creation of visual representations of the interior of the body for the visualization of the function of the tissues and organs. This is vital for the purpose of clinical analysis and development of medical intervention. Its purpose is to assess the condition of the internal structures hidden by the skin and bones, and to diagnose and treat diseases. Some of the common imaging techniques include X-ray radiography, medical ultrasonography, magnetic resonance imaging, X-ray computed tomography, endoscopy and positron emission tomography. The advancements in volume rendering techniques have resulted in the production of 3D images. This book outlines the processes and applications of medical imaging in detail. It elucidates the concepts and innovative models around prospective developments with respect to medical imaging. The book is appropriate for students seeking detailed information in this area as well as for doctors, pathologists, researchers and experts.

At the end of the preface, I would like to thank the authors for their brilliant chapters and the publisher for guiding us all-through the making of the book till its final stage. Also, I would like to thank my family for providing the support and encouragement throughout my academic career and research projects.

Editor

The use of matrigel has no influence on tumor development or PET imaging in FaDu human head and neck cancer xenografts

Frederikke P. Fliedner[1], Anders E. Hansen[1,2], Jesper T. Jørgensen[1] and Andreas Kjær[1*]

Abstract

Background: In preclinical research Matrixgel™ Basement Membrane Matrix (MG) is used frequently for the establishment of syngeneic and xenograft cancer models. Limited information on its influence on parameters including; tumor growth, vascularization, hypoxia and imaging characteristics is currently available. This study evaluates the potential effect of matrigel use in a human head and neck cancer xenograft model (FaDu; hypopharyngeal carcinoma) in NMRI nude mice. The FaDu cell line was chosen based on its frequent use in studies of cancer imaging and tumor microenvironment.

Methods: NMRI nude mice ($n = 34$) were divided into two groups and subcutaneously injected with FaDu cells in medium either including (+MG) or excluding matrigel (−MG). In sub study I seven mice from each group (+MG, $n = 7$; −MG, $n = 7$) were ^{18}F- fluorodeoxyglucose (^{18}F-FDG) PET/CT scanned on Day 5, 8, 12, 15, and 19. In sub study II ten mice from each group (+MG, $n = 10$; −MG, $n = 10$) were included and tumors collected for immunohistochemistry (IHC) analysis of tumor microenvironment including; proliferation ratio, micro vessel density, average vessel area, hypoxia, nuclear density, and necrosis. Tumors for IHC were collected according to size (200–400 mm^3, 500–700 mm^3, 800–1100 mm^3).

Results: FDG uptake and tumor growth was statistically compatible for the tumors established with or without MG. The IHC analysis on all parameters only identified a significantly higher micro vessel density for tumor size 500–700 mm^3 and 800–1100 mm^3 and average vessel area for tumor size 500–700 mm^3 in the −MG group. Comparable variations were observed for tumors of both the +MG and −MG groups. No difference in tumor take rate was observed between groups in study.

Conclusions: Matrigel did not affect tumor growth or tumor take for the FaDu xenograft model evaluated. Tumors in the -MG group displayed increased angiogenesis compared to the +MG tumors. No difference in ^{18}F-FDG PET uptake for tumors of different groups was found. Based on these observations the influence of matrigel on tumor imaging and tumor microenvironment seems minor for this particular xenograft model.

Keywords: Matrigel, FaDu, Xenograft, PET imaging, Tumor development, Hypoxia, MVD, Cancer, FDG-PET, Molecular imaging

* Correspondence: akjaer@sund.ku.dk
[1]Department of Clinical Physiology, Nuclear Medicine & PET and Cluster for Molecular Imaging, Rigshospitalet and University of Copenhagen, Blegdamsvej 9, 2100 Copenhagen, Denmark
Full list of author information is available at the end of the article

Background

Human cancer xenografts in immunodeficient mice are widely used in cancer research and provide vital models for the study of tumor growth, tumor development, and the response to therapy in preclinical research. Several human cancer cell linescan be succesfully implanted onto immune deficient mouse models, but variations in take rate and growth of solid tumors makes their use challenging. Matrixgel^{TM} Basement Membrane Matrix (Matrigel or MG) is commonly used to improve tumor take and growth [1]. Matrigel was originally extracted from connective tissue and research from the last century has shown that the extracts form matrix structures, and provide surrounding cells with substrates for growth promotion and development [1–3]. The reconstructed basement membrane complex includes; laminin, growth factors, entactin, and type IV collagen [3–5]. Studies have evaluated the advantages of MG for various cell lines [6–9] and generally it has been found to improve tumor take and growth. No change in tumor development and microenvironment is stated in these studies and reviews [4, 8, 9]. Isolated constituents from MG have been tested for impact on cell growth. However, no single substance was identified as the main mediator of effects [1, 10]. MG hereby lacks a fully defined impact on tumor growth, which could be a possible source of error in translation. By legislation the number of animals in preclinical research must be kept as low as possible while maintaining adequate power of studies. Enhancement of tumor growth by including MG can be used to decrease the number of animals in a study, but could also be a potential source of error from a translational perspective. ^{18}F-FDG PET/CT is clinically used for head and neck cancer in relation to staging, therapy planning and response to therapy [11]. FaDu head and neck cancer xenograft models are widely used for studies of PET imaging, tumor microenvironment, and radiation therapy in preclinical research [12–14]. The description of MG use for tumor inoculation in studies is not always specified. Accordingly, an understanding of possible impact of MG use is of great importance. The aim of this study was to investigate the influence of MG use, on tumor and imaging characteristics of FaDu hypopharyngeal carcinoma cells inoculated subcutaneously on NMRI nude mice.

Methods

Tumor model

All experimental procedures were approved by the Danish Animal Welfare Council, the Danish Ministry of Justice. Dulbecco's Modified Eagle Medium were supplemented with 10 % Fetal Calf Serum (FCS) and 1 % penicillin-streptomycin for growth of FaDu cells in culture flaks until confluency, retained in 5 % CO_2 incubator at 37 ° C. Six weeks old female NMRI nude (Naval Medical Research

Institute) mice were purchased from Taconic Europe (Borup, Denmark). After one week of adaptation, 34 animals were inoculated with FaDu tumor cells subcutaneously on both left and right flank. Half of the mice ($n = 17$) were injected with a suspension for each tumor consisting of 2.5×10^6 FaDu cells in 50 μL Dulbecco's Modified Eagle Medium (Life Technologies, Carlsbad, CA, USA) (–MG group; $n = 17$). For +MG group ($n = 17$) 50 μL Matrixgel™ Basement Membrane Matrix (BD Biosciences, San Jose, CA, USA) was added and a total volume of 100 μL containing 2.5×10^6 FaDu cells injected. Tumor size and weight were measured continuously from day 5 post implant to follow the development of tumors and monitor the health of the mice. Mice were housed in IVC rack from Techniplast in Type III SPF cages with 8 mice in each cage. Purified water and chow food was available ad libitum for mice unless anything else is described.

Group determination

Of the 34 mice included in study; 14 mice (+MG, $n = 7$; –MG, $n = 7$) were randomized to sub study I where all mice were ^{18}F- fluorodeoxyglucose (^{18}F-FDG) PET/CT scanned on Day 5, 8, 12, 15, and 19. In sub study II that included ten mice from the +MG group ($n = 10$) and ten mice from the -MG group ($n = 10$), tumors were collected when reaching predetermined sizes (200–400 mm^3, 500–700 mm^3, 800–1100 mm^3) for immunohistochemistry (IHC) analysis of tumor characteristics.

Volume determination

Tumor volume determination with external caliper was made by measuring the greatest longitudinal diameter and transverse diameter. Tumor volume was then calculated by following ellipsoid equation [15, 16]:

$$Tumor\ Volume = \pi \cdot \left(\frac{longitudinal\ diameter + transverse\ diameter}{2} \right)^3 \cdot \frac{1}{6}$$

Tumor volumes determined from ^{18}F-FDG PET/CT were generated by manually drawing regions of interest (ROIs) to cover the entire tumor by numerous tomographic voxels, and summation of these defined the 3D tumor volume.

^{18}F-FDG PET/CT imaging – sub study I

Mice were injected via the tail vein with a mean activity of 8.90 ± 1.55 MBq (Mean $\pm$ SD) ^{18}F-FDG in 0.2 mL 0.9 % isotonic saline solution. Prior to injection all mice were fasted for approximately 12 h to minimize the variation in ^{18}F-FDG uptake [17]. For injection, distribution, and scanning, all mice were kept anaesthetized with 3 % sevoflurane (Abbott Scandinavia AB, Solna, Sweden) mixed with 35 % O_2 and 65 % N_2. Body temperature was kept stable by external heating device when anaesthetized, and positioned on a heating pad during scan. ^{18}F-FDG PET/CT imaging was performed on Siemens Inveon® Small Animal Scanner (Siemens Medical Systems, PA, USA). The protocol included a five minute PET scan followed by a CT scan with attenuation correction to be used for reconstruction. Reconstruction of PET scans were performed using maximum a posteriori (MAP) reconstruction algorithm (voxel size: 0.815 × 0.815 × 0.796 mm; resolution (FWHM) 1.2 mm). Reconstructed images were analyzed with Inveon Research Workspace software (Siemens Medical Systems, PA, USA). Tracer uptake was determined as mean and maximum % injected dose pr. gram of tumor (%ID/g) (1 gram per cm^3), and mean and maximum standardized uptake value (SUV), corrected for decay.

Tumor microenvironment – sub study II

Tumors were collected when reaching a size of 200–400 mm^3 (+MG; $n = 6$, –MG; $n = 5$), 500–700 mm^3 (+MG; $n = 7$, –MG; $n = 6$), and 800–1100 mm^3 (+MG; $n = 6$, –MG; $n = 4$). Collection of tumors for IHC staining was initiated two weeks post injection of FaDu cells and the collection periods lasted for two weeks. Two hours prior to euthanasia 0.06 mg/g pimonidazole was injected i.p.. Tumors were fixed in 4 % formalin for 24 h, hereafter transferred to 70 % ethanol, and finally embedded in paraffin and cut into 4 μm slices. Each tumor was stained with the following antibodies; pimonidazole (PIMO; hypoxia) (HypoxyProbe-Omni Kit, HypoxyProbe Inc., Burlington, USA), Ki-67 (proliferation) (Dako; M7240), and CD31 (endothelial cell marker) (Abcam; ab28364). In addition haematoxylin eosin (HE) staining was performed.

Antibody concentrations were optimized on tumor samples from mice included in this study for optimal binding specificity. The following concentrations were used for analysis; PIMO 1:400, Ki-67 1:400, and CD31 1:50.

Deparaffination was performed by heating slides for 1 h at 40 ° C, increasing temperature to 60 °C and incubating for one additional hour. Slides were subsequently treated with xylene and rehydrated in descending concentrations of ethanol (99, 96, 70 %). Slides for Ki-67 antibody staining were furthermore exposed to microwave heating after rehydration to retrieve optimal binding. Endogenous peroxidase was blocked by Peroxidase Blocking Reagent (Dako, Glostrup, Denmark) for 8 min followed by Bovine Serum Albumin (BSA) blocking with 2 % BSA for 10 min to avoid unspecific binding of antibodies. Primary antibody incubated for 1 h followed by secondary biotinylated EnVision FLEX™ (Dako, Glostrup, Denmark) incubation for 40 min. Finally antibody staining was evoked by 3,3′-Diaminobenzidine (DAB) (Dako, Glostrup, Denmark) incubation for 10 min and counterstained with haematoxylin. Between all steps slides were rinsed in phosphate buffered saline (PBS, 0.2 M, pH = 7.4). After dehydration in increasing alcohol concentrations cover slides were mounted and slides scanned on an Axio scanner (Axio scan, Carl Zeiss, Germany). The Following parameters were analyzed; cell density, hypoxia percentages, micro vessel density (MVD), average vessel area, non-viable cell percentages, and proliferation percentages. Cell density and hypoxia was determined using the publicly available software Fiji (ImageJ). For nuclear density a nuclei count threshold of 50 $pixels^2$ to infinity was used (pixel size 0.022 × 0.022 μm). The percentage of tumor hypoxia was evaluated using Color Deconvolution based on pimonidazole DAB-H staining. Based on constructed binary images (threshold between 210 and 220 RGB values of intensity) the percentage of hypoxia positive stained area in tumor slides was determined. MVD and average vessel area was determined using online image segmentation and endothelial cell analysis software CAIMAN (CAncer IMage ANalysis: http://www.caiman.org.uk) [18] in 5 selected ROIs. ROIs, excluding necrotic regions and artifacts, were manually drawn to represent entire slide (pixel size 0.088 × 0.088 μm). Non-viable cell counts were determined in Fiji using the Advanced Weka Segmentation plug-in. Regions of viable cells, non-viable cells, and background in slide were marked to train the classifier and determine final segmentation. Calculation was made from the result image constructed by classifier. Proliferation in tumors was calculated using the online automated image analysis application ImmunoRatio (http://jvsmicroscope.uta.fi/sites/default/files/software/immunoratio-plugin/index.html) [19]. Five defined ROIs representing entire slide, excluding necrosis and artifacts, were manually drawn and uploaded to define percentage of

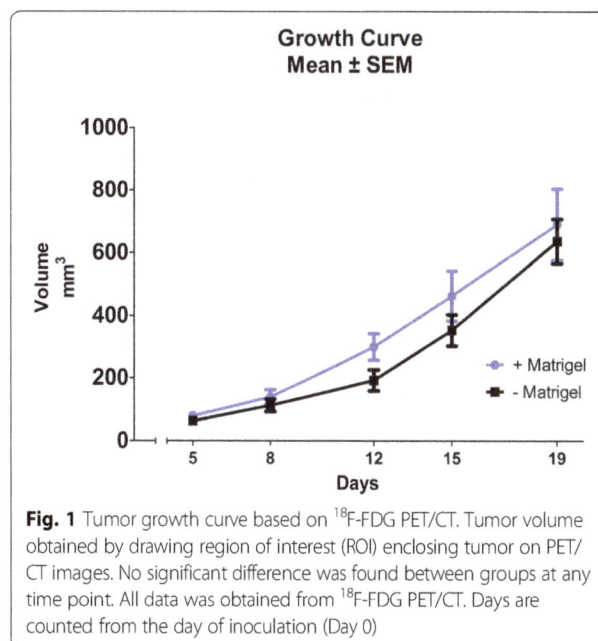

Fig. 1 Tumor growth curve based on ^{18}F-FDG PET/CT. Tumor volume obtained by drawing region of interest (ROI) enclosing tumor on PET/CT images. No significant difference was found between groups at any time point. All data was obtained from ^{18}F-FDG PET/CT. Days are counted from the day of inoculation (Day 0)

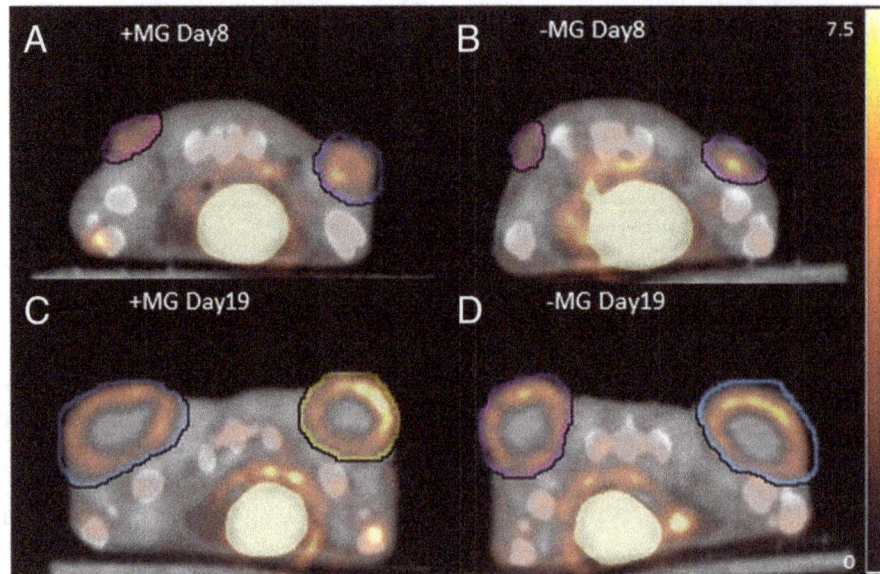

Fig. 2 Transverse section of an ^{18}F-FDG PET/CT image of mice with subcutaneous FaDu tumors. ^{18}F-FDG PET/CT scans 1 h after ^{18}F-FDG injection. Region of interests encapsulate tumor on each side of the flank. **a** and **c** +MG mouse at scan day 8 and 19, respectively. **b** and **d** −MG mouse scan day 8 and 19, respectively. Scale bar is indicated in %ID/g for all images calculated from a specific mass of 1 g/cm^3. Scan day represents number of days after inoculation

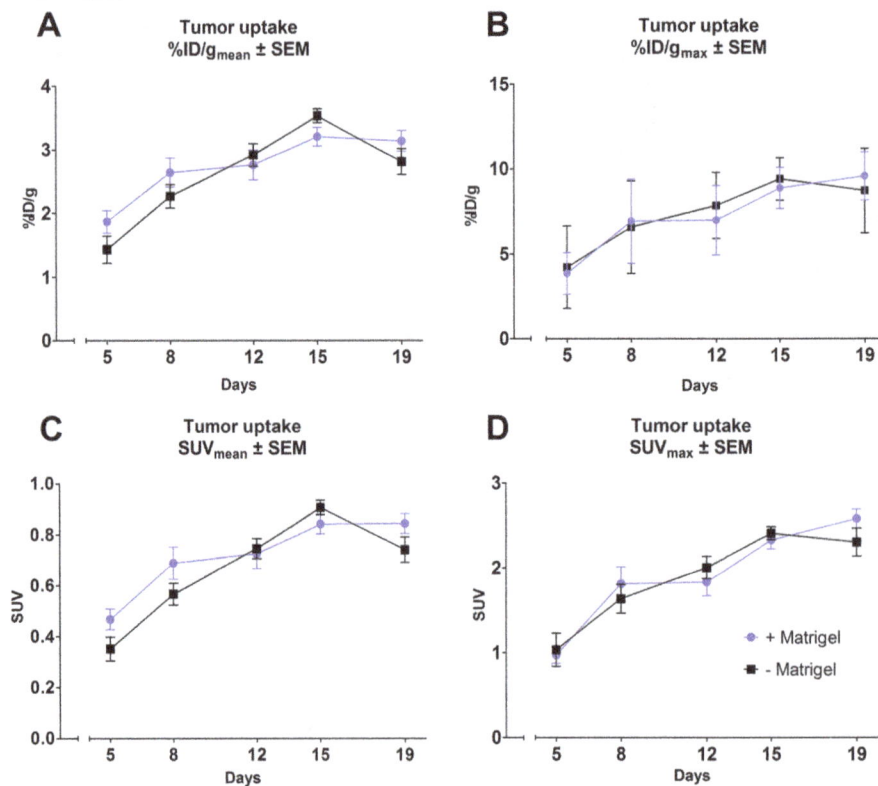

Fig. 3 Graphic presentation of tumor uptake results obtained from ^{18}F-FDG PET/CT scan data. Uptake obtained from ROIs drawn on tumor areas calculated as mean (**a**) and maximum (**b**) %ID/g from a specific mass of 1 g/cm^3 and also as mean (**c**) and maximum (**d**) standardized uptake value (SUV). All data in plots obtained from ^{18}F-FDG PET/CT scans on Siemens Inveon Small Animal scanner 1 h post injection of tracer

proliferating cells in total nuclei area (pixel size 0.088 × 0.088 μm).

Statistical analysis

Statistical analysis was performed in GraphPad 6 (Graph-Pad Software, CA, USA). Comparison between groups of data from PET/CT scan was performed using Student's T-test. Results are presented as Mean ± SEM (Standard Error of Mean). Analysis of data from histological staining's was performed using One-Way ANOVA variance analysis with Holm-Sidak's post hoc test for multiple comparisons test to evaluate differences between groups of different tumor sizes. A p-value < 0.05 was considered statistically significant in all tests.

Results and discussion

Tracer uptake and tumor volume determined by ^{18}F-FDG PET/CT scan

Data obtained from ^{18}F-FDG PET/CT identified no significant difference in FDG tumor uptake or tumor size between the +MG and -MG groups on each scan day, shown in Figs. 1 and 3. A tendency for increased growth rate of the tumors in the +MG group was observed between day 8 and 12 (Fig. 1), but growth was very

compatible at later time points. Figure 2 illustrate ^{18}F-FDG PET/CT images of mice from the different groups, and the compatible ^{18}F-FDG uptake can be readily appreciated at both time points. The observed compatibility of FDG uptake in tumors +/- MG indicates that ^{18}F-FDG PET/CT results are not influenced by the addition of MG for this tumor model (Fig. 3). SUV_{max} is often used clinically for classification of tumors in relation to staging, treatment, and response, and was therefore included in study to identify and evaluate maximum uptake in tumors [20]. No difference between SUV_{max} in tumors with or without MG was found, indicating that MG, in this setup, does not influence maximum FDG uptake (Fig. 3d).

Previous studies have shown that tumor take in models are increased using MG [21]. In this study the take rate of tumors inoculated without MG was approximately 95 % (32 out of 34 inoculated) and 100 % (34 out of 34 inoculated) with MG, which indicates that MG does not influence tumor take for the investigated model.

The doubling in injection volume between groups might lead to a falsely determined tumor volume for the +MG group at early and intermediate time points, where a distinct part is mostly due to MG volume and not division of tumor cells. However, as seen in Fig. 1, tumor volume at

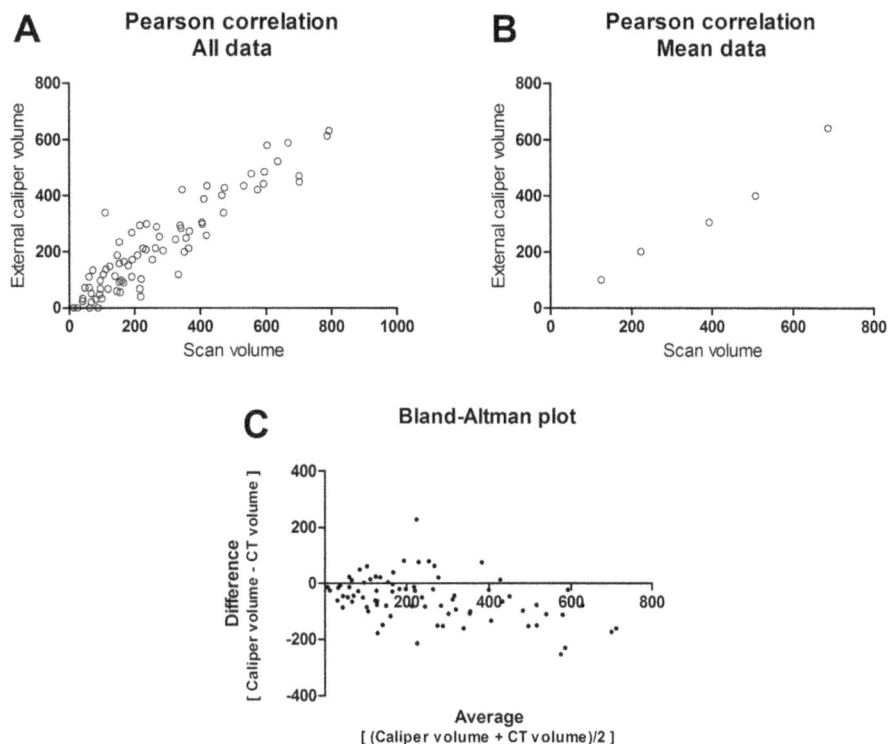

Fig. 4 Pearson correlation model for ^{18}F-FDG PET/CT determined tumor volume and external caliper determined tumor volume. Correlation between external caliper determined volumes and volumes determined from PET/CT scans. Pearson correlation model was used for the plotted values. **a** All scans. Correlation coefficient was 0.85 (p-value < 0.0001). **b** Same regression model with mean value at each time point (5, 8, 12, 15, and 19). Correlation coefficient was 0.98 (p-value = 0.0017). **c** Bland-Altman plot showing the difference between measurements against the average to visualize bias between methods

day 5 and 8 are virtually similar and the growth rates between these days follow the same development curve. Difference in growth rate was detected between day 8 and 12 (increase in rate for +MG). Grounds for injecting larger suspension volumes for the MG suspension was based on keeping the injected number of cells and concentration in media fixed, and from the results the difference in injection volume did not seem to have a distinct effect. Based on Figs. 1 and 3, it seems that the variation in size and tracer uptake is smaller in the –MG group compared to the +MG group. PET/CT scan data indicate that no significant advantage or drawback can be stated regarding MG use for tumor growth or tumor uptake in this model, but a decrease in group variation is observed for the –MG group. Based on this, there is little reason for using MG in FaDu xenograft models.

Tumor development from IHC data

IHC staining was made on tumors collected at different size groups in order to compare tumor microenvironment characteristics on different development stages. Size of collected tumors was defined using external caliper as described in the method section. To connect the two parts of the study in regard to tumor growth, Pearson correlation was performed between volumes determined from ^{18}F-FDG PET/CT scan and volumes determined from the external caliper (Fig. 4). A correlation coefficient of 0.85 (p-value < 0.0001) was found for the correlation including all data points (Fig. 4a). Pearson correlation analysis based on mean values at each time point identified a correlation coefficient of 0.98 (p-value = 0.0017) (Fig. 4b). Additionally, the validity of comaring tumor sizes between groups was found acceptable using Bland-Altman analysis (Fig. 4c).

Results obtained from IHC are presented in Fig. 5. One-way ANOVA test was used for the comparisons of characteristics between different size groups. IHC data showed that vascularization differed between the groups of the same tumor size. Statistical differences between micro vessel densities were found for tumor sizes; 500–700 mm^3 (p-value = 0.0457) and 800–1100 mm^3 (p-value = 0.0214), and for average vessel area at 500–700 mm^3 (p-value = 0.0237) with the highest numbers for the -MG group (Fig. 5a and b). Angiogenesis was found to

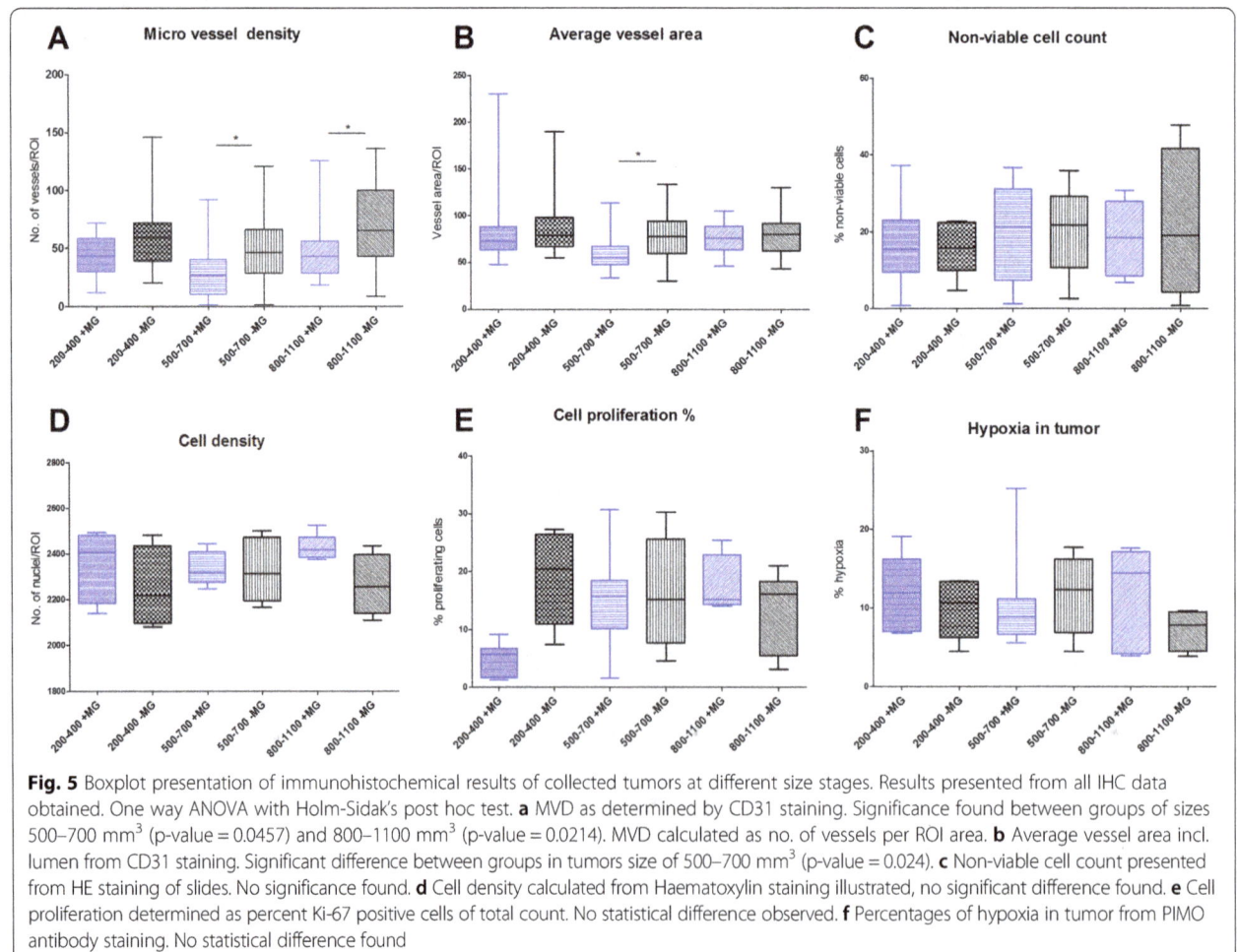

Fig. 5 Boxplot presentation of immunohistochemical results of collected tumors at different size stages. Results presented from all IHC data obtained. One way ANOVA with Holm-Sidak's post hoc test. **a** MVD as determined by CD31 staining. Significance found between groups of sizes 500–700 mm^3 (p-value = 0.0457) and 800–1100 mm^3 (p-value = 0.0214). MVD calculated as no. of vessels per ROI area. **b** Average vessel area incl. lumen from CD31 staining. Significant difference between groups in tumors size of 500–700 mm^3 (p-value = 0.024). **c** Non-viable cell count presented from HE staining of slides. No significance found. **d** Cell density calculated from Haematoxylin staining illustrated, no significant difference found. **e** Cell proliferation determined as percent Ki-67 positive cells of total count. No statistical difference observed. **f** Percentages of hypoxia in tumor from PIMO antibody staining. No statistical difference found

be significantly higher in tumors without MG. When comparing to the results of cell density, a tendency to a lower median in cell density for tumors without MG was observed. As discussed previously, tumor growth data obtained from PET/CT scans showed a tendency of increased tumor size for the +MG group at day 12–15 where tumors size was 200–400 mm^3. Tumor cell proliferation showed a distinct difference for the small tumor size group (200–400 mm^3) with a higher percentage of proliferating cells in the –MG group (Fig. 5e). These two observations are conflicting since the increased growth rate of the tumors in the +MG groups does not correlate with the proliferation percentage in collected tumors at same size. The tumor volume in the +MG group could, according to the proliferation percentages, hereby partly consist of MG volume but IHC results on other parameters contradicts this theory. Cell density in tumors of all sizes seemed to be rather similar, but as described previously, a lower median is observed for tumors in the –MG group. This hereby conversely describes the tumor area in +MG to be denser in cell concentration than the –MG group. For the larger sized tumor groups proliferating cells in slides

were compatible. In Fig. 6 examples of pre- and post-analysis images of IHC slides stained with CD31 (Fig. 6a + b), Ki-67 (Fig. 6c + d), and HE (Fig. 6e + f) are shown. From the IHC results MG seems to be without major influence on tumor development and the preclinical outcome in our model.

Conclusions

Our data indicate that using MG in cell suspension for inoculation induces no major impact on imaging and microenvironment characteristics of the FaDu hypopharyngeal carcinoma xenografts. Less variation is seen when no MG is used, which is in favor of not including MG in FaDu xenograft inoculation. Following the extensive use of the FaDu head and neck cancer xenograft model for PET imaging and tumor microenvironment characteristics, this study indicates that studies with and without MG use are comparable. Importantly, the observation in this study cannot be generally applied. Important differences potentially exist for human xenograft models other than FaDu in NMRI nude mice, which must be considered before comparing results between studies.

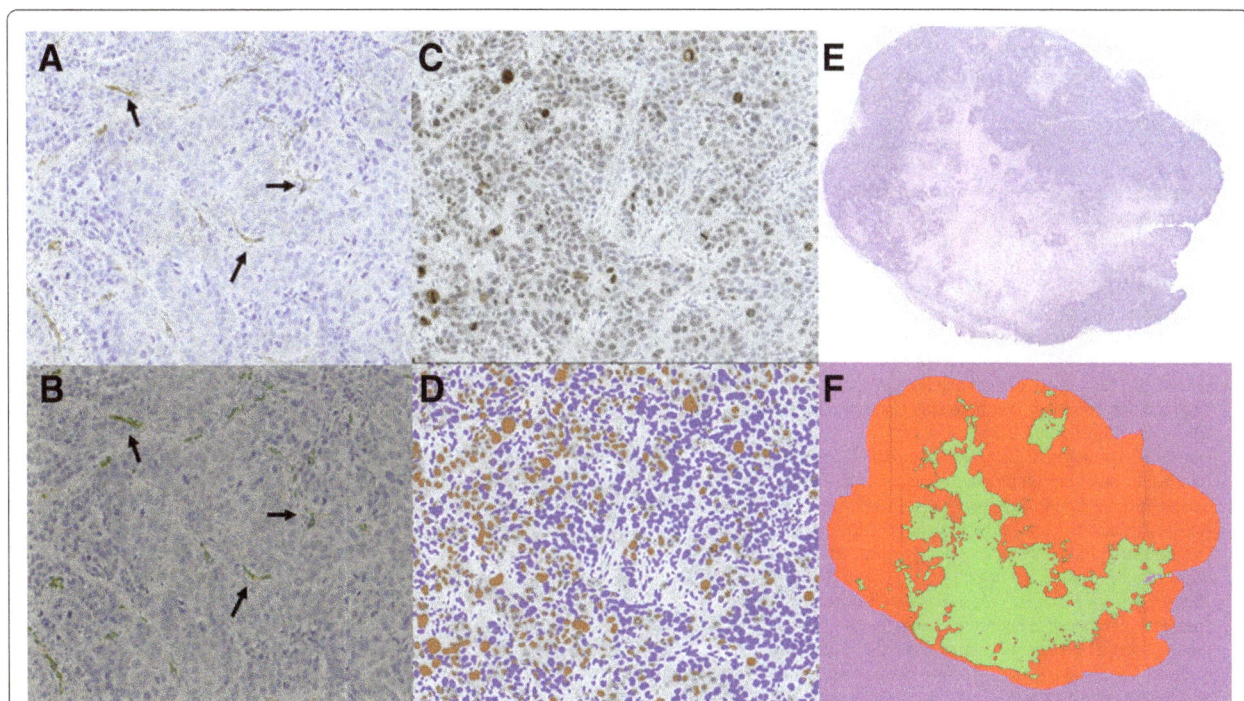

Fig. 6 Immunohistochemistry (IHC) sections of micro vessel density (CD31 staining), proliferating cells (Ki-67 staining), and non-viable cell count (HE staining). Selection of IHC results presented to illustrate collected tissue samples and analyzed tissue. a CD31 staining visualizing endothelial cells in vessels of tumor slide. Staining made with antibody concentration of 1:50. Picture originates from mouse in the –MG group. Arrows indicate positive staining of vessels in slide. b Edited version of picture A after using the CAIMAN segmentation algorithm to detect antibody stained areas. Arrows indicate vessels identified by the CAIMAN algorithm (marked by thin green contouring line). c Ki-67 staining for proliferating cells in tumor section from a mouse in the +MG group. Staining made using antibody concentration of 1:400. d Review of image C after using the ImmunoRatio application for selecting proliferating cell percentage. Cells marked in brown are considered as positive Ki-67 and blue cells negative. e Haematoxylin eosin staining for non-viable cell count in tumor slide from mouse in the +MG group. f Image E after separation of viable cells (red), non-viable cells (green), and background (purple) with the Advanced Weka Segmentation tool in FiJi (ImageJ)

Competing Interests
The authors declare that they have no competing interests.

Authors' contributions
Frederikke P. Fliedner (FPF), Anders E. Hansen (AEH) and Andreas Kjaer (AK) designed the study. FPF, AEH and Jesper T. Jørgensen (JTJ) performed the experiments. All authors contributed to data analysis and interpretations. FPF drafted the manuscript and all authors provided input to revision of the manuscript and approved the final version.

Acknowledgements
Generous support from the Danish Cancer Society, the Lundbeck foundation, the Novo Nordisk Foundation, the Svend Andersen Foundation, the Innovation Fund Denmark, the Danish Research Council for Independent Research, Rigshospitalets Research Foundation, the Research Foundation of the Capital Region, the AP Møller Foundation, and the John and Birthe Meyer Foundation.

Author details
[1]Department of Clinical Physiology, Nuclear Medicine & PET and Cluster for Molecular Imaging, Rigshospitalet and University of Copenhagen, Blegdamsvej 9, 2100 Copenhagen, Denmark. [2]Department of Micro- and Nanotechnology, Center for Nanomedicine and Theranostics, DTU Nanotech, Technical University of Denmark, Building 423, 2800 Lyngby, Denmark.

References
1. Vukicevic S, Kleinman HK, Luyten FP, Roberts AB, Roche NS, Reddi AH. Identification of multiple active growth factors in basement membrane Matrigel suggests caution in interpretation of cellular activity related to extracellular matrix components. Exp Cell Res. 1992;202(1):1–8.
2. Kleinman HK, McGarvey ML, Hassell JR, Star VL, Cannon FB, Laurie GW, et al. Basement membrane complexes with biological activity. Biochemistry. 1986;25(2):312–8.
3. Fridman R, Benton G, Aranoutova I, Kleinman HK, Bonfil RD. Increased initiation and growth of tumor cell lines, cancer stem cells and biopsy material in mice using basement membrane matrix protein (Cultrex or Matrigel) co-injection. Nat Protoc. 2012;7(6):1138–44.
4. Benton G, Arnaoutova I, George J, Kleinman HK, Koblinski J. Matrigel: from discovery and ECM mimicry to assays and models for cancer research. Adv Drug Deliv Rev. 2014;79–80:3–18. doi:10.1016/j.addr.2014.06.005.
5. Arnaoutova I, George J, Kleinman HK, Benton G. Basement membrane matrix (BME) has multiple uses with stem cells. Stem Cell Rev. 2012;8(1):163–9.
6. Fridman R, Kibbey MC, Royce LS, Zain M, Sweeney M, Jicha DL, et al. Enhanced tumor growth of both primary and established human and murine tumor cells in athymic mice after coinjection with Matrigel. J Natl Cancer Inst. 1991;83(11):769–74.
7. Pretlow TG, Delmoro CM, Dilley GG, Spadafora CG, Pretlow TP. Transplantation of human prostatic carcinoma into nude mice in Matrigel. Cancer Res. 1991;51(14):3814–7.
8. Noel A, De Pauw-Gillet MC, Purnell G, Nusgens B, Lapiere CM, Foidart JM. Enhancement of tumorigenicity of human breast adenocarcinoma cells in nude mice by matrigel and fibroblasts. Br J Cancer. 1993;68(5):909–15.
9. Topley P, Jenkins DC, Jessup EA, Stables JN. Effect of reconstituted basement membrane components on the growth of a panel of human tumour cell lines in nude mice. Br J Cancer. 1993;67(5):953–8.
10. Hughes CS, Postovit LM, Lajoie GA. Matrigel: a complex protein mixture required for optimal growth of cell culture. Proteomics. 2010;10(9):1886–90.
11. Koshy M, Paulino AC, Howell R, Schuster D, Halkar R, Davis LW. F-18 FDG PET-CT fusion in radiotherapy treatment planning for head and neck cancer. Head Neck. 2005;27(6):494–502.
12. Baumann M, Liertz C, Baisch H, Wiegel T, Lorenzen J, Arps H. Impact of overall treatment time of fractionated irradiation on local control of human FaDu squamous cell carcinoma in nude mice. Radiother Oncol. 1994;32(2):137–43.
13. Menegakis A, Eicheler W, Yaromina A, Thames HD, Krause M, Baumann M. Residual DNA double strand breaks in perfused but not in unperfused areas determine different radiosensitivity of tumours. Radiother Oncol. 2011;100(1):137–44.
14. Schutze C, Bergmann R, Yaromina A, Hessel F, Kotzerke J, Steinbach J, et al. Effect of increase of radiation dose on local control relates to pre-treatment FDG uptake in FaDu tumours in nude mice. Radiother Oncol. 2007;83(3):311–5.
15. Tomayko MM, Reynolds CP. Determination of subcutaneous tumor size in athymic (nude) mice. Cancer Chemother Pharmacol. 1989;24(3):148–54.
16. Russell PJ, Raghavan D, Gregory P, Philips J, Wills EJ, Jelbart M, et al. Bladder cancer xenografts: a model of tumor cell heterogeneity. Cancer Res. 1986;46(4 Pt 2):2035–40.
17. Fueger BJ, Czernin J, Hildebrandt I, Tran C, Halpern BS, Stout D, et al. Impact of animal handling on the results of 18 F-FDG PET studies in mice. J Nucl Med. 2006;47(6):999–1006.
18. Reyes-Aldasoro CC, Griffiths MK, Savas D, Tozer GM. CAIMAN: an online algorithm repository for cancer image analysis. Comput Methods Programs Biomed. 2011;103(2):97–103.
19. Tuominen VJ, Ruotoistenmaki S, Viitanen A, Jumppanen M, Isola J. ImmunoRatio: a publicly available web application for quantitative image analysis of estrogen receptor (ER), progesterone receptor (PR), and Ki-67. Breast Cancer Res. 2010;12(4):R56.
20. Paidpally V, Chirindel A, Lam S, Agrawal N, Quon H, Subramaniam RM. FDG-PET/CT imaging biomarkers in head and neck squamous cell carcinoma. Imaging Med. 2012;4(6):633–47.
21. Mullen P, Ritchie A, Langdon SP, Miller WR. Effect of Matrigel on the tumorigenicity of human breast and ovarian carcinoma cell lines. Int J Cancer. 1996;67(6):816–20.

2

The assessment of accessory mental foramen in a selected polish population: a CBCT study

Ewa Zmysłowska-Polakowska[1†], Mateusz Radwański[1†], Michał Łęski[1], Sławomir Ledzion[1], Monika Łukomska-Szymańska[2] and Michał Polguj[3*]

Abstract

Background: Accessory mental foramen (AMF) is a rare anatomical variation. When accessory mental foramen is present, the nerves and vessels that go through the mental foramen (MF) must follow alternative courses and special care must be taken during dental treatment planning. The purpose of this study was to evaluate the occurrence and the location of AMF in a selected Polish population using cone-beam computed tomography (CBCT).

Methods: Two hundred CBCT (105 males and 95 females) examinations were evaluated for the presence of AMFs. The location and side of AMFs were reported. The mean distance between MF and AMF was also calculated. The vertical size of MF on the side with and without AMF was measured. The obtained variables were statistically analyzed.

Results: AMFs were observed in 7% of the patients. There was no statistically significant difference between the appearance of AMF and sex ($p > 0.05$). We found no significant difference in the vertical size of MF between individuals with and without AMFs ($p < 0.05$).

Conclusion: Twenty-eight AMFs (7%) were observed from 400 sides of 200 patients. AMFs occurred more often in males (18 AMFs) than in females (10 AMFs). Twenty AMFs (71.4%) were located anteriorly, and eight (28.6%) - posteriorly. Fifteen AMFs (53.6%) were on the right side and thirteen (46.4%) - on the left.

Keywords: Accessory mental foramen, Cone-beam computed tomography, CBCT, Dental surgery, Endodontics

Background

The mental foramen (MF) is a bilateral opening in the mandible through which nerve endings such as the mental nerve, a branch of the inferior alveolar nerve and corresponding arteries and veins emerge [1–4]. Once the nerve leaves the MF, it branches to innervate the anterior teeth and neighboring structures. The blood vessels supply the soft tissues of the lower jaw [5, 6]. The position of the mental foramen is used as a reference point in the anesthetic technique such as the incisive/mental nerve block. In dental practice, the importance of this structure is mainly related to the positioning of dental implants and to other surgical procedures in this region,

for example endodontic surgery. There are some reports on the anatomical variations of the MF such as the presence of accessory mental foramina (AMFs) [2, 5, 7–11]. When AMF is present, the nerves and vessels that go through the mental foramen must follow alternative courses and special care must be taken during dental treatment planning.

Accessory mental foramen has a different description in literature. Some authors described AMF as any additional foramina except the main MF [5, 12]. On the other hand, only those foramina that are integrated with mandibular canal are nominated as AMFs [13–15]. Conversely, the foramen which does not originate in the mandibular canal and its dimensions are relatively small is recognized as a nutrient foramen [16].

The presence of AMF can be evaluated with different methods including macroscopic investigations on dry skulls [14, 17, 18], plane radiographs (including periapical

---

* Correspondence: michal.polguj@umed.lodz.pl
†Equal contributors
[3]Department of Angiology, Interfaculty Chair of Anatomy and Histology, Medical University of Lodz, ul. Narutowicza 60, Łódź 90-136, Poland
Full list of author information is available at the end of the article

and panoramic views) [19] and computed tomography images (CT or CBCT) [19]. The crucial benefit of cone-beam computed tomography (CBCT) is overcoming the limitations of conventional radiography by producing three-dimensional (3D) images that allow comprehensive evaluation of the anatomy of the chosen region [20]. CBCT is an useful tool that provides detailed information on the structures of the maxillofacial complex, permitting the identification and the evaluation of anatomical variations [19, 20].

The purpose of this study was to evaluate the occurrence and location of the accessory mental foramen in a selected Polish population using CBCT.

Methods

This retrospective study consisted of 487 CBCTs obtained from 2011 to 2012 in the Radiology Department at the Central Teaching Hospital, Institute of Dentistry, of the Medical University of Lodz (Poland). Images were performed for different diagnostic reasons, such as bone absence for implant placement, assessment of tooth relationships with clinically relevant anatomical structures, dental surgery and diagnosis of radiolucent lesions. The CBCT scans were selected according to the following inclusion criteria: visibility of MF, no lesion observed in the apical area of premolars and MF, no bone resorption occurrence. Only images with availability of precise information about patient age and sex were selected. The exclusion criteria consist of CBCT images with large pathological lesions in mandible and bone fractures in region of examination. Also inadequate picture quality with artefacts caused by osteosynthesis plates/implants or patient movement during exposure were rejected. According to our inclusion and exclusion criteria, the final sample group included data from 200 patients (105 males and 95 females). This study has obtained a positive opinion of the Ethics Committee of Medical University of Lodz, Poland (No. RNN/322/15/KE).

Accessory mental foramen (AMF) in this cross-sectional study was defined as a buccal foramen smaller than the mental foramen and followed by the accessory branch of the mental canal before it exits from the mental foramen, regardless of its location.

All CBCT images were obtained using a GX CB-500 (Gendex, USA) at 120 kVp and 5.0 mA, with a voxel size 0.125–0.25 mm and an exposure time of 20 s. All images were analyzed using specialized computer software (iCATVision Q, ver. 1.9.3.13; Gendex, USA). The samples were manually evaluated by independent two observers and any disagreement between them was discussed until a consensus was reached. To test the reproducibility, the two observers re-examined 50 randomly selected CBCT scans 4 weeks after the first evaluation. For the final analysis, each measurement was performed twice. Finally, obtained data by both investigators were averaged and mean values were calculated. Data were assessed on axial, sagittal and coronal CBCT slices of 0,13 mm thickness. The CBCT scans were evaluated in terms of the presence of accessory mental foramen (Figs. 1 and 2). When the AMF was present, the location and side (right or left branch of the mandible) were recorded. With regard to location, AMFs were classified into two groups according to Naitoh et al. [14]: anterior or posterior to mental foramen. The distance between the accessory mental foramen and the mental foramen was measured by formula previously proposed by Naitoh et al. [14]: distance = $\sqrt{x^2 + y^2}$ (Fig. 3). The mean vertical size of MF on the side with and without AMF was also calculated. The obtained variables were statistically analyzed using Statistica 12.5 PL° software (StatSoft, Poland). The chi-square test was used to determine potential differences between the presence of AMFs and sex of the patients and the Mann–Whitney U test was used to evaluate the relationship between the vertical size of the MF and the presence of AMFs. The level of statistical significance was set at $p < 0.05$.

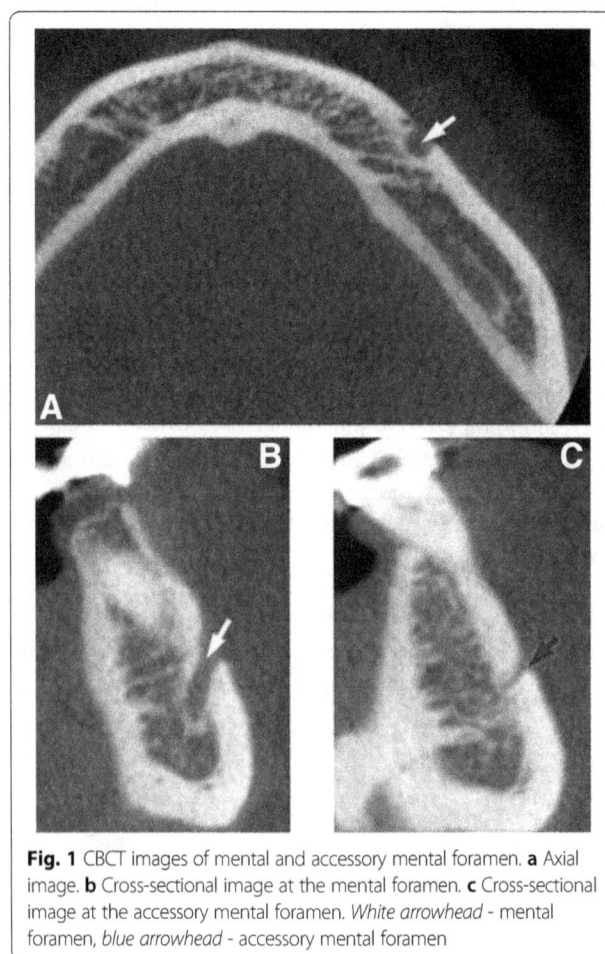

Fig. 1 CBCT images of mental and accessory mental foramen. **a** Axial image. **b** Cross-sectional image at the mental foramen. **c** Cross-sectional image at the accessory mental foramen. *White arrowhead* - mental foramen, *blue arrowhead* - accessory mental foramen

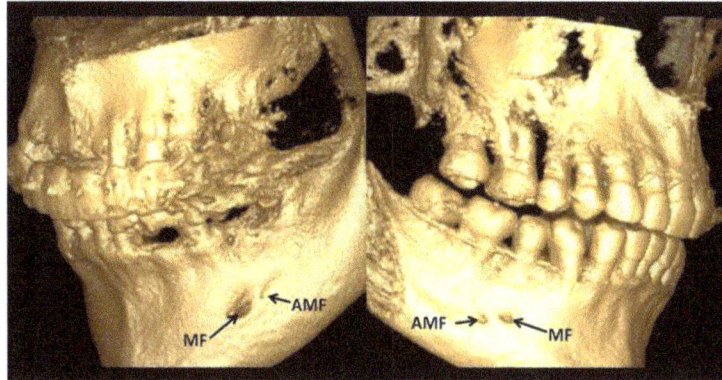

Fig. 2 Three-dimensional images (CBCT) of mental foramen and accessory mental foramen

Results

There were 105 males (52.5%) and 95 females (47.5%) in the study group. The average age of the 200 patients who were included in this study was 54.57 years (range: 29 to 76 years, SD: 10.26 years). The mean age of the males was 54.49 years (range: 29 – 76 years, SD: 10.79), while the mean age of the females was 54.66 years (range: 39 – 75 years, SD: 9.72).

Twenty-eight AMFs (7%) were observed from 400 sides of 200 patients. AMFs occurred more often in males (18 AMFs) than in females (10 AMFs). No statistical significant difference was found between the occurrence of AMF and sex ($p > 0.05$). The bilateral presence of AMF was not observed in the presented study. Twenty AMFs (71.4%) were located anteriorly, and eight (28.6%) - posteriorly. Fifteen AMFs (53.6%) were on the right side and thirteen (46.4%) were on the left. The

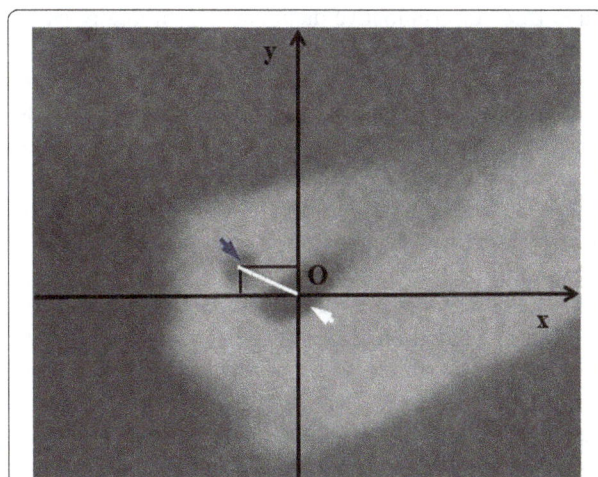

Fig. 3 Measurement of distance between MF and AMF. The origin (O) was defined as a centre of the mental foramen and x-axis was parallel to the occlusal plane. The distance (*white line*) was measured by formula previously proposed by Naitoh et al. [14]: distance $= \sqrt{x^2 + y^2}$. *White arrowhead*- mental foramen, *blue arrowhead*- accessory mental foramen

location (anterior/posterior) and side (right/left) of AMFs in respect to patient sex were presented in Fig. 4.

The distance between the AMF and the MF ranged from 0.64 to 6.5 mm with the mean of 2.86 mm (SD: 1.34 mm).

The mean values of vertical size of the MF with AMF (on the same side) and without AMF were presented in Table 1. The relationship between the mean vertical size of MF and the presence of AMF was not statistically significant ($p > 0.05$).

Discussion

The presence of an AMF has been suggested to result from the branching of the mental nerve before it exits the mental foramen. Ignoring the presence of AMF may cause unexpected damage to the neurovascular bundles or lead to the failure of a mental nerve block.

According to Balcioglu and Kocaelli [5], the presence of AMF is a rather rare anatomical variation with the prevalence ranging from 1.4 to 10%. The differences may be explained by different imaging techniques and race. Panoramic radiography provides a flat image of the curved structure and is not as accurate as CBCT in the horizontal localization of objects. Their report also revealed that non-Caucasians have a higher prevalence of AMF than Caucasians [5]. On the other hand, accessory mental foramen in comparison to very rare skeletal variations like double suprascapular foramen are a common anomaly [21].

The prevalence of AMF varies in different ethnic groups. The highest is reported in black and Maori males [22]. Kalender et al. [23] observed AMF in 6.5% of a Turkish population, and prevalence of 6.68 and 7% were found in Greek [24] and Japanese [15] populations, respectively. In adult Sri Lankan [25] and Indian [26] populations, the prevalence of AMF was found to be 3.92 and 8.9%, respectively. In the present study, the AMFs were detected in 7% of the selected Polish population.

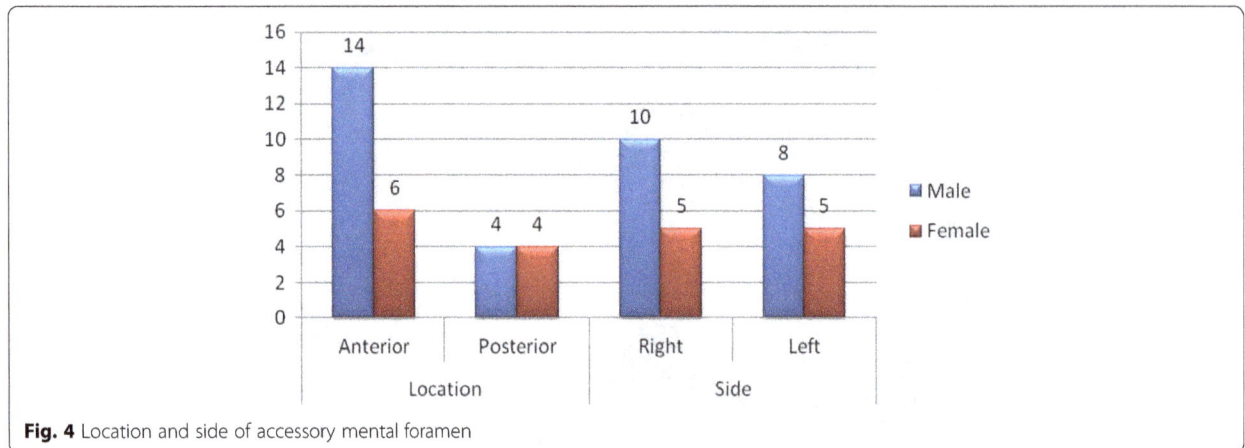

Fig. 4 Location and side of accessory mental foramen

In our study, AMFs occurred more often in males (18 AMFs) than in females (10 AMFs). However, the difference was no statistically significant ($p > 0{,}05$). Other studies also confirmed that AMFs were more commonly found in males [14, 15]. Göregen et al. [8] in their study observed the same number of AMFs in males and females with no statistical differences between these groups.

The location of AMF is also important and can directly affect the treatment plan since it might interfere with performed procedures. Katakami et al. [13] in the study of 150 patients, observed the presence of 17 accessory mental foramina by CBCT with 59% of which being posteriorly located to the mental foramen. Another study conducted on 157 patients demonstrated the presence of 15 accessory mental foramina, nine of which posteriorly located [15]. On the other hand, the study of 315 patients of a Turkish population revealed the occurrence of 22 AMFs, twelve of which (54,5%) anteriorly located [8]. In the present study, twenty (71.4%) of twenty-eight AMFs were anteriorly located.

The next measured parameter was the distance between the mental foramen and the accessory mental foramen. Göregen et al. [8] reported that the distance ranged from 1.6 to 4.9 mm, with the mean of 2.54 mm (SD: 1.1 mm). In the studies of Naitoh et al. [15] and Kalender et al. [23], the mean value ranged from 4.5 to 9.6 mm, with the mean of 6.3 mm (SD: 1.5 mm) and from 1.3 to 15.4 mm, with the mean of 5.2 mm (SD: 4.4 mm), respectively. In the present study, the distance between the AMF and the MF ranged from 0.64 to 6.5 mm with the mean of 2.86 mm (SD: 1.34 mm)

The mean vertical size of the MF on the same side as the AMF was 3.21 mm (range: 1.74 – 5.82 mm, SD: 0.98), and that of MF on the sides without AMF was 3.26 mm (range: 1.12 – 7.02 mm, SD: 0.97 mm). The relationship between the mean vertical size of the MF and the presence of the AMF was not statistically significant ($p > 0.05$). Similar results were reported by Naitoh et al. [15] and Göregen et al. [8].

In 2013, Chen et al. [27] described a new method of improvement of computed tomography images. They used fast dictionary learning-based processing. This method brings encouraging improvements in abdomen low-dose computed tomography images with tumours. In 2014, Chen et al. [28] used novel image-domain algorithm called "artefact-suppressed dictionary learning". In this method, orientation and scale information on artefacts is exploited to train artefact atoms. These artefact atoms are then combined with tissue feature atoms to build three discriminative dictionaries. Authors provided qualitative and quantitative evaluations of this method on a large set of abdominal and mediastinal computed tomography investigation. In 2016, Chen et al. [29] described new technique of minimal path propagation with backtracking for curve-like structure extraction. They found that the information in the process of backtracking from reached points can be well utilized to improve the extraction performance.

Preoperative imaging study is important prior to any surgical or anaesthetic procedure in mental regio. AMF is a relevant anatomic structure, which should be considered in treatment plan of procedure performed in mandible (i.e. root resection of mandibular premolars or molars, osteotomy, mandibular rehabilitation after trauma, placement of dental implants). The detection of AMF has a direct influence on therapeutic success. In patients with AMF, accessory mental nerve and vessels may be present. The presence of accessory innervations may explain failures to achieve adequate levels of anaesthesia during surgical and routine dental procedures

Table 1 Vertical sizes of MF and the presence of AMFs

Vertical size of MF (mm)				
	Mean	Range	SD	P-value
MF on the side with AMF	3.21	1.74–5.82	0.98	$p > 0.05$
MF on the side without AMF	3.26	1.12–7.02	0.97	

using conventional nerve block techniques. The detection of AMF can prevent nerve and vascular injury and reduce complications of dental treatment such as: paralysis, hemorrhage and post-operative pain.

Conclusion

In the present study, the occurrence of the accessory mental foramen in the study of the Polish population is similar to that described in Turkish, Greek and Japanese population. Awareness of anatomy and its variations are essential to ensure precise dental procedure execution. Moreover, it is crucial to better understand possible anatomical conditions that can promote neurosensory disturbance in treated area.

Abbreviations
AMF: Accessory mental foramen; CBCT: Cone-beam computed tomography; MF: Mental foramen

Acknowledgements
Not applicable.

Funding
Department of Endodontics, 503/2-044-02/503-01.

Authors' contributions
E Z-P: study design, data collection, data interpretation, manuscript preparation, figure preparation, fund collection; MR: study design, data collection, data interpretation, manuscript preparation, figure preparation, literature search; MŁ: data collection, manuscript preparation; SL: data collection, manuscript preparation, literature search; M Ł-Sz: manuscript preparation, fund collection; MP: study design, manuscript preparation. All authors read and approved the final manuscript.

Competing interests
The authors declare that they have no competing interests and no conflicts of interests to disclose.

Author details
[1]Department of Endodontics, Medical University of Lodz, ul. Pomorska 251, Łódź 92-213, Poland. [2]Department of General Dentistry, Medical University of Lodz, ul. Pomorska 251, Łódź 92-213, Poland. [3]Department of Angiology, Interfaculty Chair of Anatomy and Histology, Medical University of Lodz, ul. Narutowicza 60, Łódź 90-136, Poland.

References
1. Boopathi S, et al. Anthropometric analysis of the infraorbital foramen in a South Indian population. Singapore Med J. 2010;51(9):730–5.
2. Concepcion M, Rankow HJ. Accessory branch of the mental nerve. J Endod. 2000;26(10):619–20.
3. Iwanaga J, et al. The clinical anatomy of accessory mental nerves and foramina. Clin Anat. 2015;28(7):848–56.
4. Iwanaga J, et al. Accessory mental foramina and nerves: application to periodontal, periapical, and implant surgery. Clin Anat. 2016;29(4):493–501.
5. Balcioglu HA, Kocaelli H. Accessory mental foramen. North Am J Med Sci. 2009;1(6):314–5.
6. Roa I, Arriagada O. Anatomical variations of mandibular canal with clinical significance. Case report. Int J Morphol. 2015;33(3):971–4.
7. Al-Shayyab MH, et al. The mental foramen II: radiographic study of the superior-inferior position, appearance and accessory foramina in iraqi population. Int J Morphol. 2016;34(1):310–9.
8. Goregen M, et al. The assessment of accessory mental foramina using cone-beam computed tomography. Turk J Med Sci. 2013;43(3):479–83.
9. Neves FS, et al. Lingual accessory mental foramen: a report of an extremely rare anatomical variation. J Oral Sci. 2010;52(3):501–3.
10. Patil S, Matsuda Y, Okano T. Accessory mandibular foramina: a CT study of 300 cases. Surg Radiol Anat. 2013;35(4):323–30.
11. Trikeriotis D, et al. Anterior mandible canal communications: a potential portal of entry for tumour spread. Dentomaxillofac Radiol. 2008;37(3):125–9.
12. Singh R, Srivastav AK. Study of position, shape, size and incidence of mental foramen and accessory mental foramen in indian adult human skulls. Int J Morphol. 2010;28(4):1141–6.
13. Katakami K, et al. Characteristics of accessory mental foramina observed on limited cone-beam computed tomography images. J Endod. 2008;34(12):1441–5.
14. Khojastepour L, et al. Location of mental foramen in a selected iranian population: a CBCT assessment. Iran Endod J. 2015;10(2):117–21.
15. Naitoh M, et al. Accessory mental foramen assessment using cone-beam computed tomography. Oral Surg Oral Med Oral Pathol Oral Radiol Endod. 2009;107(2):289–94.
16. Torres MGG, et al. Accessory mental foramen: a rare anatomical variation detected by cone-beam computed tomography. Imaging Sci Dent. 2015;45(1):61–5. doi:10.5624/isd.2015.45.1.61.
17. Haktanir A, Ilgaz K, Turhan-Haktanir N. Evaluation of mental foramina in adult living crania with MDCT. Surg Radiol Anat. 2010;32(4):351–6.
18. Paraskevas G, Mavrodi A, Natsis K. Accessory mental foramen: an anatomical study on dry mandibles and review of the literature. Oral Maxillofac Surg. 2015;19(2):177–81.
19. Nozu Imada TS, et al. Accessory mental foramina: prevalence, position and diameter assessed by cone-beam computed tomography and digital panoramic radiographs. Clin Oral Implants Res. 2014;25(2):94–9.
20. Naitoh M, et al. Comparison between cone-beam and multislice computed tomography depicting mandibular neurovascular canal structures. Oral Surg Oral Med Oral Pathol Oral Radiol Endod. 2010;109(1):19–25.
21. Polguj M, Podgórski M, Jędrzejewski K, Topol M. The double suprascapular foramen: unique anatomical variation and the new hypothesis of its formation. Skeletal Radiol. 2012;41(12):1631–6.
22. Kieser J, et al. Patterns of emergence of the human mental nerve. Arch Oral Biol. 2002;47(10):743–7.
23. Kalender A, Orhan K, Aksoy U. Evaluation of the mental foramen and accessory mental foramen in Turkish patients using cone-beam computed tomography images reconstructed from a volumetric rendering program. Clin Anat. 2012;25(5):584–92.
24. Zografos J, Mutzuri A. Incidence of double mental foramen in a sample of Greek population. Odontostomatol Proodos. 1989;43(6):521–3.
25. Ilayperuma I, Nanayakkara G, Palahepitiya N. Morphometric analysis of the infraorbital foramen in adult Sri lankan skuls. Int J Morphol. 2010;28(3):777–82.
26. Sankar DK, Bhanu SP, Susan PJ. Morphometrical and morphological study of mental foramen in dry dentulous mandibles of south andhra population of india. Indian J Dent Res. 2011;22(4):542–6.
27. Chen Y, Yin X, Shi L, Shu H, Luo L, Coatrieux JL, Toumoulin C. Improving abdomen tumor low-dose CT images using a fast dictionary learning based processing. Phys Med Biol. 2013;58(16):5803–20.
28. Chen Y, Shi L, Feng Q, Yang J, Shu H, Luo L, Coatrieux JL, Chen W. Artifact suppressed dictionary learning for Low-dose CT image processing. IEEE Trans Med Imaging. 2014;33(12):2271–92.
29. Chen Y, Zhang Y, Yang J, Cao Q, Yang G, Chen J, Shu H, Luo L, Coatrieux JL, Feng Q. Curve-like structure extraction using minimal path propagation with backtracking. IEEE Trans Image Process. 2016;25(2):988–1003.

3

Radiation dosimetry of 18F-FDG PET/CT: incorporating exam-specific parameters in dose estimates

Brian Quinn[1*], Zak Dauer[1], Neeta Pandit-Taskar[2], Heiko Schoder[2] and Lawrence T. Dauer[1,2]

Abstract

Background: Whole body fluorine-18 fluorodeoxyglucose positron emission tomography/computed tomography (PET/CT) is the standard of care in oncologic diagnosis and staging, and patient radiation dose must be well understood to balance exam benefits with the risk from radiation exposure. Although reference PET/CT patient doses are available, the potential for widely varying total dose prompts evaluation of clinic-specific patient dose. The aims of this study were to use exam-specific information to characterize the radiation dosimetry of PET/CT exams that used two different CT techniques for adult oncology patients and evaluate the practicality of employing an exam-specific approach to dose estimation.

Methods: Whole body PET/CT scans from two sets of consecutive adult patients were retrospectively reviewed. One set received a PET scan with a standard registration CT and the other a PET scan with a diagnostic quality CT. PET dose was calculated by modifying the standard reference phantoms in OLINDA/EXM 1.1 with patient-specific organ mass. CT dose was calculated using patient-specific data in ImPACT. International Commission on Radiological Protection publication 103 tissue weighting coefficients were used for effective dose.

Results: One hundred eighty three adult scans were evaluated (95 men, 88 women). The mean patient-specific effective dose from a mean injected 18F-FDG activity of 450 ± 32 MBq was 9.0 ± 1.6 mSv. For all standard PET/CT patients, mean effective mAs was 39 ± 11 mAs, mean CT effective dose was 5.0 ± 1.0 mSv and mean total effective dose was 14 ± 1.3 mSv. For all diagnostic PET/CT patients, mean effective mAs was 120 ± 51 mAs, mean CT effective dose was 15.4 ± 5.0 mSv and mean total effective dose was 24.4 ± 4.3 mSv. The five organs receiving the highest organ equivalent doses in all exams were bladder, heart, brain, liver and lungs.

Conclusions: Patient-specific parameters optimize the patient dosimetry utilized in the medical justification of whole body PET/CT referrals and optimization of PET and CT acquisition parameters. Incorporating patient-specific data into dose estimates is a worthwhile effort for characterizing patient dose, and the specific dosimetric information assists in the justification of risk and optimization of PET/CT.

Keywords: PET/CT, CT, Radiation exposure, Effective dose, 18F-FDG

* Correspondence: quinnb@mskcc.org
Brian Quinn is the first author.
[1]Department of Medical Physics, Box 84, Memorial Sloan Kettering Cancer Center, 1275 York Avenue, New York, NY 10065, USA
Full list of author information is available at the end of the article

Background

Positron emission tomography/computed tomography (PET/CT) has become an indispensable imaging modality for the diagnosis, staging and monitoring of therapy response of a broad range of malignancies [1, 2]. PET/CT is a valuable tool in oncology due to the combined metabolic and morphological information provided. The PET emission scan provides physiological information using a set of detectors that are independent of CT transmission detection, and although two independent PET and CT images may be coregistered to form a single image, the two scans are most accurately coupled when both are acquired during the same exam using a combined PET and CT scanner. For this reason, and because a built-in CT provides other conveniences such as attenuation correction, most modern PET scanners are dual PET/CT units. Regardless of acquisition circumstances, the patient dose from PET and the patient dose from CT in PET/CT exams are first estimated separately in different ways, and then combined to give a total whole body radiation dose. Referral for PET/CT studies must be justified in each case as a first general principle of radiological protection [3]. Optimization, or ensuring that the diagnostic information is as high as reasonably achievable while maintaining radiation doses as low as reasonably achievable, is the second general principle in radiologic protection according to the International Committee on Radiological Protection (ICRP) [4]. Additionally, increased awareness of the risk of exposure to ionizing radiation has resulted in efforts to minimize radiation dose incurred during x-ray and nuclear medical imaging tests [5]. Implementation of any dose saving strategies depends critically on accurate dose measurement/dosimetry to maximize the benefit/risk ratio from imaging tests [6].

A reliable method of estimating patient dose, which includes appropriate units of dose measurement and appropriate calculation methods, is important for any exam involving ionizing radiation. As Stabin stated, the biokinetic model used to calculate the dose is one of the major uncertainties in the evaluation of radiation doses for radiopharmaceuticals [7]. If careful patient specific dosimetry is performed, with attention paid to accurate measurement of individual organ volumes, many of the biokinetic model uncertainties can be minimized, and the total uncertainty in the individual dose estimate can be reduced to perhaps ±10 %-20 %[7]. Effective dose is a parameter that allows a meaningful comparison of the radiation dose from the radiopharmaceutical and the x-ray portions of a PET/CT scan. Effective dose is not directly measured, rather it is calculated based on equivalent doses to organs and the radiosensitivities of the organs. Effective dose is commonly used when evaluating relative biologic risk (4), and the Monte Carlo–based

organ dose coefficients should not be used to calculate effective dose for individual patients [6, 8]. The International Organization for Medical Physics, ICRP, Health Physics Society and American Association of Physicists in Medicine (AAPM) all have issued policy statements that note the dangers of extrapolating biological risk estimates for radiation doses less than 100 mSv [6, 9–11]. The establishment and use of risk coefficients to estimate public health determinants from individual or population exposures must be considered in the context of uncertainties in the estimates [12]. These uncertainties include dosimetric uncertainties, epidemiological and methodological uncertainties, uncertainties from low statistical power and precision in epidemiology studies of radiation risk, uncertainties in modeling risk data, generalization of risk estimates across different populations and dose rates, as well as reliance on epidemiological studies on observational rather than experimental data [13]. Uncertainties in such risk estimates have been suggested as being up to a factor of 3 lower or higher than the value itself [14]. These rather large uncertainties cause predictions of radiation induced cancers or detriment to be susceptible to biases and confounding influences that are unidentifiable. With due recognition of the limitations imposed by the uncertainties inherent in correlating dose to risk, effective dose is a useful approximation for relating patient dose from internal and external sources, evaluating population characteristics and evaluating optimization efforts. Organ doses from PET are estimated based on the injected activity, while organ doses from CT are estimated based on scanner-specific monte carlo simulations or the dose parameter reported in the exam dose report. Both approaches can be made to more accurately reflect the actual patient dose by including scanner- and patient-specific factors.

Without specific information, risk evaluations may be based on reference or literature values that must be carefully chosen if used for risk evaluation. The International Atomic Energy Agency's "Radiation Protection of Patients" (RPOP) is a reputable online reference resource that provides information for health healthcare professionals, member states and the general public to achieve safer use of radiation [15]. In the absence of specifics, reference values can overgeneralize and can result in conservative overestimates of dose in an attempt to account for many variables. Such generalization is inherent in non-specific reference values for PET/CT exams because of the number of PET and CT variables contributing to overall dose. CT technique differs greatly if it is just for attenuation correction or if it is for diagnostic-quality images. Attenuation correction can be performed with CT currents as low as 10 mA but most institutions use CT currents of 40-80 mA [16]. Further, an oncology center, for example, may have an intermediate CT technique that provides images with better image quality than a technique only for attenuation correction but lower image quality than a diagnostic CT technique. PET dose varies primarily with injected activity, but like CT dose varies with patient size. The dependency of total dose on many factors warrants a critical review of general reference values and suggests the importance of specific data.

Several approaches to PET/CT dose estimation utilize exam-specific parameters. Dose Length Product (DLP) is a standardized CT dose parameter that is established for each CT scanner using a phantom, equal to CTDIvol multiplied by the length of the scan. DLP can be related to effective dose by multiplying DLP by a patient-specific factor, or scanner-specific monte carlo simulation data can be employed to estimate CT dose [17, 18]. ImPACT method calculates organ dose from CT and uses simplified stylized anatomic models that are anatomically crude but widely used for practical applications with the standard mathematic representations of the reference man and other representative phantoms in radiation protection, nuclear medicine, and medical imaging [19–21]. Radiopharmaceutical organ dose is estimated utilizing conversion coefficients and injected activity, such as those in ICRP 106. Effective dose is typically calculated from both PET and CT organ dose utilizing tissue-weighting factors, such as those in ICRP 103.

In these ways, effective dose from both PET and CT both are calculated and combined to represent a whole body burden. This combined whole body burden is useful in evaluating both the relative and absolute benefit of the combined scan. Although PET/CT is widely performed, published patient dose data is as varied as the parameters determining the dose and often focuses on a narrow patient population [22–31]. The potential for variation in PET scan practices and CT techniques is especially apparent when one considers the wide range of scanner makes & models, injected activity and patient populations in different countries. Many clinic-specific elements that influence radiation dose can be incorporated into the dose estimate to make the dose more specific to the patient.

The aim of the present study was to characterize the radiation dosimetry of two types of routine whole body PET/CT protocols at our institution using patient-specific data and commonly available dose estimation techniques. We compare the results of using patient-specific data with reference and published values and ascertain the utility of such data in the evaluation of risk/benefit for justification and protocol optimization in routine clinical utilization.

Methods
Study population
Institutional review board approval with waiver of patient informed consent was obtained to perform a retrospective study of clinically indicated whole body PET/

CT scans performed on consecutive adult oncology patients at Memorial Sloan Kettering Cancer Center from January 2010 through December 2011. Patient consent was not required.

Patient population data
Consecutive adult patients who had undergone PET/CT with either standard registration or full dose diagnostic quality CT techniques for a variety of oncological indications, were identified. Patient demographics are shown in Table 1.

Exam data
For each PET exam performed, the amount of 18F-FDG administered was obtained from the medical records. For each CT study, image data was reviewed to determine the body region that was being examined, and this was repeated for each CT series. The following parameters for each series were extracted from the DICOM headers, dose reports and scan scout images for later organ equivalent dose and effective dose calculation: (a) kVp, (b) mA, (c) beam collimation, (d) rotation time, (e) pitch, (f) volume CT dose index (CTDIvol) and (g) dose length product (DLP).

18F-FDG PET/CT exam
All whole-body PET/CT patients fast for at least 6 h, blood glucose concentration is determined before the injection of the radiopharmaceutical. A nominal injection activity of 12 mCi (444 MBq) is prescribed in our clinic, and +/- 10 % of the prescribed activity is actually injected intravenously into the patient. The actual injected activity is recorded for each patient. Following an approximately 60 min uptake time, PET/CT exams are performed on General Electric (GE) scanners. Data for this study were recorded from patients scanned on Discovery 690 DSTE PET/CT, which utilizes a GE Lightspeed 16 CT scanner (GE Healthcare, Milwaukee, Wis). Tube current modulation is utilized for all CT acquisitions except the "scout" scan, which uses a fixed technique of 120 kVp, 10 mA, pitch 3 and rotation time 0.5 s. The first part of the exam sequence is acquisition of a scout CT image used to select the desired anatomy to be scanned and establish bed positions for PET acquisition. The technologist selects from base of the skull to

Table 1 Patient demographics

	No. patients	Age Yrs	Body mass index
Male	95	53.7 ± 18.1 (18.8–90.2)	26.2 ± 4.8 (15.1–46.1)
Female	88	52.1 ± 20.3 (18.4–96.7)	26.6 ± 7.8 (15.6–71.5)
Male and female	183	52.3 ± 19.3 (18.4–96.7)	26.4 ± 6.4 (15.1–71.5)

All data are mean ± standard deviation (range)

mid thighs for body PET/CT scans. Next a CT scan is acquired using either the standard or the diagnostic CT technique, depending on the required patient specific protocols completed by the radiologist. The technique for all standard PET/CT exams in this study is 120 kVp, auto-mA, rotation time 0.8 sec, slice thickness 3.75 mm, collimator width 10 or 40 mm, pitch 1.75. The technique for all PET/CT exams with a diagnostic CT is 120 kVp, auto-mA, rotation time 0.6 s, slice thickness 5.00 mm, collimator width 20 or 40 mm, pitch 1.375. CT techniques are summarized in Table 2.

CT is followed immediately by PET acquisition with a 3-min emission acquisition time per bed position, a 15.3-cm axial field of view per bed position with a 23 % bed overlap.

Internal radiation-absorbed dose assessment

The OLINDA\EXM code (version 1.1, Vanderbilt University, Nashville, TN, USA) was used to determine the organ equivalent dose and effective dose from each PET series with patient-specific parameters [32]. The biokinetic model parameters as defined in Bolch et al (2009) and specifically identified in ICRP Publication 106 for 18F-FDG were used as input factors for OLINDA [33, 34]. The ICRP biokinetic model for 18F-FDG was derived from data in Hayes et al and Deloar et al [35, 36]. The OLINDA code also allows for the modification of standard reference phantoms to more closely represent patient-specific factors, such as patient weight and corresponding organ mass. We used the standard anthropomorphic models as well as models modified to represent patients weight and height (i.e., organ sizes of the phantom models used by OLINDA were modified to reflect the patient-specific mass of the organ as described by Marine et al and Clark et al [37–39]. Modified adult male, adult female models in OLINDA's phantom library were utilized to generate patient-specific organ equivalent dose, and then tissue weighting factors from ICRP Publication 103 were used to generate patient-specific effective dose conversion factor (mSv/MBq) [6]. These factors were multiplied by

injected activity (MBq) for each PET study to obtain an estimation of effective dose.

External radiation-absorbed dose assessment

Effective dose from CT examination was estimated using the CT-specific method using the ImPACT spreadsheet, employing ICRP 103 weighting factors [17].

Statistical analysis

Descriptive and summary statistics were performed with a spreadsheet application (Excel 2007, Microsoft, Redmond, WA). Statistical analysis included average, median, standard deviation, minimum, maximum and range.

Results

Study population

Of the total 183 PET/CT scans evaluated, 95 (52 %) were performed on male patients and 88 (48 %) were performed on female patients. Forty-six male patients and 39 female patients received the standard CT technique. Forty-nine male patients and 49 female patients received the diagnostic CT technique. Subjects ranged in age from 18 to 96 years (mean ± standard deviation (SD) 52.6 ± 18.2 years). The subjects' weight ranged (mean ± SD) from 42.0 to 182 kg (74.9 ± 17.7 kg), height ranged (mean ± SD) from 120 to 198 cm (168 ± 10.3 cm), and BMI ranged (mean ± SD) from 15.1 to 71.5 (26.4 ± 6.4).

18F-FDG

The mean ± SD (range) 18F-FDG injected activity for all patients was 454 ± 33.3 MBq (152 to 488 MBq).

CT techniques

The mean ± SD (range) effective mAs of the standard CT for all patients was 39.0 ± 11.2 mAs (27.4 to 69.4 mAs), 38.6 ± 10.0 mAs (27.4 to 69.4 mAs) for male patients and 39.4 ± 12.4 mAs (27.4 to 69.4 mAs) for female patients.

The mean ± SD (range) effective mAs of the diagnostic CT for all patients was 119 ± 50.6 mAs (27.4 to 231 mAs),

Table 2 CT technique summary

CT technique description	Tube potential	Tube current	Revolution time	Collimator width	Pitch	Effective mAs[a]	CTDIvol	DLP	Effective Dose	Effective dose per unit mAs
	(kVp)	(mA)	(s)	(mm)			(mGy)	(mGy cm)	(mSv)	(mSv/mAs)
Standard male	120	78 ± 8.2	0.8	10 or 40	1.75	38.6 ± 10.0	5.1 ± 0.6	464 ± 86	5.3 ± 1.0	0.142 ± 0.026
Standard female	120	72 ± 11	0.8	10 or 40	1.75	39.4 ± 12.4	4.8 ± 0.7	407 ± 73	4.6 ± 0.8	0.124 ± 0.028
Diagnostic male	120	236 ± 86	0.6	20 or 40	1.375	116 ± 40.5	12.1 ± 2.8	1185 ± 249	17.4 ± 3.7	0.164 ± 0.063
Diagnostic female	120	223 ± 109	0.6	20 or 40	1.375	122 ± 59.3	10.2 ± 3.9	912 ± 368	13.4 ± 5.5	0.121 ± 0.039

Data are the mean ± standard deviation
[a]Effective mAs is calculated as [(mA*tube rotation)/pitch]

116 ± 40.5 mAs (50.0 to 231 mAs) for male patients and 121.6 ± 59.3 mAs (27.1 to 231 mAs) for female patients.

CT techniques are summarized in Table 2.

Radiation doses – 18F-FDG

The five organs with the highest organ equivalent doses from 18F-FDG in all patients, in order of highest to lowest dose, were bladder, heart, brain, liver and lungs. 18F-FDG organ equivalent doses are summarized in Tables 3 and 4.

Mean ± SD (range) patient-specific effective dose from 18F-FDG calculated by OLINDA for all patients was 9.0 ± 1.6 mSv (3.4 to 13.6 mSv), 9.1 ± 1.7 mSv (5.4 to 12.8 mSv) for male and 10.0 ± 1.5 mSv (3.4 to 13.6 mSv) for female. Mean ± SD (range) effective dose per unit injected activity for all patients was 0.0199 ± 0.0032 mSv/MBq (0.0132 to 0.0291 mSv/MBq). 18F-FDG patient-specific effective doses are summarized in Table 5.

Radiation doses - CT

The mean ± SD (range) effective dose for all patients from the CT portion of scans employing the standard technique was 5.0 ± 1.0 mSv (2.9 to 7.2 mSv), while it was 15.4 ± 5.0 mSv (5.4 to 27.8 mSv) for the scans employing a diagnostic technique.

The mean ± SD (range) effective dose per unit effective mAs from all exams was 0.138 ± 0.046 mSv/mAs (0.036 to 0.445 mSv/mAs) for all patients, from standard CT was 0.134 ± 0.028 mSv/mAs (0.067 to 0.185 mSv/mAs), and from diagnostic CT was 0.142 ± 0.056 mSv/mAs (0.036 to 0.445 mSv/mAs).

The mean ± SD (range) effective dose per unit dose-length product (DLP) from all exams was 0.018 ± 0.046 mSv/mGy-cm (0.036 to 0.445 mSv/mGy-cm) for all patients.

CT radiation doses are summarized in Table 6.

The five organs with the highest organ equivalent doses from standard CT in all patients, in order of highest to lowest dose, were thyroid, osteogenic cells, thymus, lungs

Table 3 Organ equivalent dose and effective dose from 18F-FDG PET/CT with standard CT to adult male and female patients

Organ	Dose from 18F-FDG, mGy[a]		Dose from CT, mGy[b]		Total dose, mGy	
	Male (n = 46)	Female (n = 39)	Male (n = 46)	Female (n = 39)	Male (n = 46)	Female (n = 39)
Adrenals	5.1 ± 0.9	6.0 ± 1.0	5.3 ± 1.0	4.6 ± 0.8	10.4 ± 0.9	10.6 ± 0.9
Brain	15.9 ± 3.2	17.3 ± 3.2	6.0 ± 1.0	5.3 ± 0.9	21.9 ± 2.8	22.6 ± 2.9
Breasts	3.6 ± 0.7	4.3 ± 0.8	4.9 ± 0.9	4.2 ± 0.7	8.4 ± 0.8	8.5 ± 0.7
Gallbladder wall	5.4 ± 1.0	6.2 ± 1.8	5.6 ± 1.0	4.9 ± 0.9	11.1 ± 0.9	11.1 ± 1.0
Colon	4.9 ± 0.9	5.9 ± 1.0	5.2 ± 1.0	4.6 ± 0.8	10.2 ± 0.9	10.5 ± 0.9
Small intestine	5.1 ± 0.9	5.7 ± 1.0	5.2 ± 1.0	4.6 ± 0.8	10.3 ± 0.9	10.2 ± 0.9
Stomach wall	4.7 ± 0.9	5.6 ± 1.0	5.7 ± 1.0	4.9 ± 0.9	10.3 ± 0.9	10.5 ± 0.9
Heart wall	29.1 ± 6.2	35.4 ± 6.9	5.9 ± 1.1	5.2 ± 0.9	35.0 ± 5.6	40.6 ± 6.5
Kidneys	4.5 ± 0.8	5.3 ± 0.9	5.8 ± 1.1	5.1 ± 0.9	10.3 ± 0.9	10.3 ± 0.9
Liver	8.9 ± 1.7	11.0 ± 2.0	5.6 ± 1.0	4.8 ± 0.8	14.4 ± 1.4	15.8 ± 1.7
Lungs	8.3 ± 1.7	10.0 ± 1.8	6.3 ± 1.2	5.4 ± 1.0	14.6 ± 1.4	15.4 ± 1.5
Muscle	4.2 ± 0.8	5.0 ± 0.9	3.8 ± 0.7	3.3 ± 0.6	8.0 ± 0.7	8.3 ± 0.7
Ovaries/Testes[c]	4.6 ± 0.8	7.0 ± 1.2	1.1 ± 0.2	4.3 ± 0.8	5.6 ± 0.8	11.2 ± 1.0
Pancreas	5.2 ± 1.0	6.2 ± 1.0	5.2 ± 1.0	4.5 ± 0.8	10.4 ± 0.9	10.7 ± 0.9
Red marrow	4.2 ± 0.9	4.8 ± 1.0	4.4 ± 0.8	3.8 ± 0.7	8.5 ± 0.8	8.6 ± 0.9
Osteogenic cells	6.2 ± 1.8	67.4 ± 2.0	8.0 ± 1.6	6.9 ± 1.2	14.2 ± 1.5	14.3 ± 1.7
Skin	3.2 ± 0.6	3.7 ± 0.7	3.4 ± 0.6	3.0 ± 0.5	6.6 ± 0.6	6.7 ± 0.6
Spleen	4.4 ± 0.8	5.2 ± 0.9	5.4 ± 1.0	4.7 ± 0.8	9.8 ± 0.9	9.9 ± 0.9
Thymus	4.8 ± 0.9	5.7 ± 1.0	6.4 ± 1.2	5.6 ± 1.0	11.2 ± 1.0	11.3 ± 1.0
Thyroid	4.2 ± 0.8	4.4 ± 0.8	8.3 ± 1.4	7.3 ± 1.3	12.4 ± 1.2	11.7 ± 1.1
Urinary bladder wall	59.1 ± 5.2	79.5 ± 6.7	5.5 ± 1.0	4.8 ± 0.8	64.6 ± 4.8	84.3 ± 6.4
Uterus	–	8.8 ± 1.4	–	4.6 ± 0.8	–	13.4 ± 1.2
Effective dose[d]	8.1 ± 1.2	10.1 ± 1.4	5.3 ± 1.0	4.6 ± 0.8	13.4 ± 1.1	14.7 ± 1.2

[a]Patient specific average dose calculated by OLINDA
[b]Patient specific average dose calculated by ImPACT
[c]Ovaries for female patients/Testes for male patients
[d]Effective dose in mSv estimated by ICRP Publication 103

Table 4 Organ equivalent dose and effective dose from 18F-FDG PET/CT with diagnostic CT to adult male and female patients

Organ	Dose from 18F-FDG[a]		Dose from CT[b]		Total dose	
	Male (n = 49)	Female (n = 49)	Male (n = 49)	Female (n = 49)	Male (n = 49)	Female (n = 49)
Adrenals	5.0 ± 0.6	5.9 ± 1.1	17.6 ± 3.7	13.5 ± 5.5	22.6 ± 3.4	19.4 ± 5.0
Brain	15.9 ± 2.1	16.6 ± 3.6	21.0 ± 4.4	16.1 ± 6.5	36.9 ± 3.6	32.8 ± 5.5
Breasts	3.6 ± 0.5	4.2 ± 0.9	15.7 ± 3.3	12.0 ± 4.8	19.3 ± 3.0	16.2 ± 4.4
Gallbladder wall	5.4 ± 0.7	6.0 ± 1.2	18.7 ± 3.9	14.4 ± 5.8	24.1 ± 3.1	20.4 ± 5.2
Colon	4.9 ± 0.6	5.8 ± 1.1	17.5 ± 3.7	13.5 ± 5.5	22.4 ± 3.4	19.3 ± 5.0
Small intestine	5.1 ± 0.6	5.6 ± 1.1	17.5 ± 3.7	13.5 ± 5.5	22.6 ± 3.4	19.1 ± 5.0
Stomach wall	4.7 ± 0.6	5.4 ± 1.1	18.6 ± 3.9	14.4 ± 5.8	23.3 ± 3.6	19.8 ± 5.3
Heart wall	29.0 ± 4.1	34.4 ± 7.7	20.0 ± 4.2	15.3 ± 6.2	48.9 ± 3.8	49.7 ± 6.4
Kidneys	4.4 ± 0.5	5.2 ± 1.0	19.1 ± 4.0	14.7 ± 6.0	23.5 ± 3.8	19.9 ± 5.5
Liver	8.9 ± 1.2	10.7 ± 2.2	17.9 ± 3.8	13.8 ± 5.6	26.8 ± 3.3	24.5 ± 4.7
Lungs	8.3 ± 1.1	9.8 ± 2.1	20.0 ± 4.2	15.3 ± 6.2	28.3 ± 3.7	25.1 ± 5.2
Muscle	4.2 ± 0.5	4.8 ± 1.0	12.5 ± 2.7	9.6 ± 3.9	16.7 ± 2.4	14.4 ± 3.4
Ovaries/Testes[c]	4.6 ± 0.6	6.8 ± 1.3	3.5 ± 0.7	12.6 ± 5.1	8.1 ± 0.6	19.4 ± 4.5
Pancreas	5.2 ± 0.6	6.1 ± 1.2	17.2 ± 3.6	13.2 ± 5.3	22.4 ± 3.3	19.3 ± 4.8
Red marrow	4.1 ± 0.6	4.7 ± 1.1	14.6 ± 3.0	11.2 ± 4.5	18.7 ± 2.7	15.9 ± 3.9
Osteogenic cells	6.1 ± 1.2	7.1 ± 2.1	26.4 ± 5.5	20.3 ± 8.2	32.6 ± 4.8	27.5 ± 7.0
Skin	3.2 ± 0.4	3.6 ± 0.7	11.1 ± 2.3	8.6 ± 3.4	14.2 ± 2.1	12.2 ± 3.1
Spleen	5.2 ± 1.08	5.1 ± 1.0	17.4 ± 3.7	13.4 ± 5.4	21.7 ± 3.4	18.5 ± 4.9
Thymus	4.4 ± 0.5	5.5 ± 1.1	21.8 ± 4.6	16.9 ± 6.8	26.6 ± 4.3	22.5 ± 6.2
Thyroid	4.2 ± 0.5	4.3 ± 0.9	28.0 ± 5.8	21.6 ± 8.7	32.2 ± 5.6	25.9 ± 8.2
Urinary bladder wall	59.1 ± 3.7	78.9 ± 9.2	18.5 ± 3.9	14.2 ± 5.7	77.7 ± 4.8	93.1 ± 10.2
Uterus	-	8.6 ± 1.6	-	13.8 ± 5.8	-	22.4 ± 4.9
Effective dose[d]	8.1 ± 0.8	9.9 ± 1.6	17.4 ± 3.7	13.4 ± 5.5	25.5 ± 3.4	23.4 ± 4.9

[a]Patient specific average dose calculated by OLINDA
[b]Patient specific average dose calculated by ImPACT
[c]Ovaries for female patients/Testes for male patients
[d]Effective dose estimated by ICRP publication 103

and brain. CT organ equivalent doses are summarized in Tables 3 and 4.

The five organs with the highest organ equivalent doses from diagnostic CT in male patients, in order of highest to lowest dose, were thyroid, osteogenic cells, thymus, brain and lungs, and in female patients thyroid, osteogenic cells, thymus, brain and heart.

Radiation doses – total dose

The mean ± SD (range) effective dose from the combined PET and CT portions of all PET/CT exams was 19.6 ± 6.1 mSv (11.0 to 34.3 mSv) for all patients, 19.5 ± 2.3 mSv (11.0 to 31.1 mSv) for male patients and 19.1 ± 3.1 mSv (12.8 to 34.3 mSv) for female patients.

The mean ± SD (range) effective dose from the combined PET and CT portions of the exams using standard CT was 14.0 ± 1.3 mSv (11.0 to 17.6 mSv) for all patients, 13.4 ± 1.1 mSv (11.0 to 16.2 mSv) for male patients and 14.7 ± 1.2 mSv (12.8 to 17.6 mSv) for female patients.

The mean ± SD (range) total effective dose from the combined PET and CT portions of the exams using diagnostic CT technique was 24.4 ± 4.3 mSv (14.6 to

Table 5 18F-FDG Dose summary

CT technique description	Injection activity (MBq)		Effective dose (mSv)		Effective dose per unit activity (mSv/MBq)	
	Male	Female	Male	Female	Male	Female
Standard CT	455 ± 30	450 ± 26	8.1 ± 1.2	10.1 ± 1.4	0.018 ± 0.002	0.022 ± 0.002
Diagnostic CT	455 ± 25	454 ± 51	8.1 ± 0.8	9.9 ± 1.6	0.018 ± 0.002	0.022 ± 0.003

Data are the mean ± standard deviation. n, male standard CT=46. n, female standard CT = 39. n, male diagnostic CT = 49. n, female diagnostic CT = 49

Table 6 CT effective dose summary for all patients

CT technique description	DLP (mGy cm)	mAs (mAs)	Effective dose (mSv)	Effective dose per unit mAs (mSv/mAs)	Effective dose per unit DLP (mSv/mGy cm)
Standard	438 ± 84.8	39 ± 11	7.9 ± 1.5	0.134 ± 0.028	0.013 ± 0.002
Diagnostic	1050 ± 342	119 ± 51	15.4 ± 5.0	0.142 ± 0.056	0.015 ± 0.0002

Data are the mean ± standard deviation

34.3 mSv) for all patients, 25.5 ± 3.4 mSv (17.8 to 31.1 mSv) for male patients and 23.4 ± 4.9 mSv (14.6 to 34.3 mSv) for female patients. Total doses are summarized in Tables 7 and 8.

The five organs with the highest organ equivalent doses from PET/CT in all patients, in order of highest to lowest dose, were bladder, heart, brain, liver and lungs. PET/CT organ equivalent doses are summarized in Tables 3 and 4.

Discussion

Risk from radiation exposure to the individual patient is important for evaluation of risk/benefit for justification, and relevant to protocol optimization and personnel protection [40]. The doses themselves utilized in the risk estimation are useful for characterizing the patient population and image acquisition practices of a clinic. A dose estimation method can be based on a combination of reference values and patient- and scanner-specific data. Accurate estimation of patient dose, rather than a conservatively high estimate, is important for many oncology patients who can potentially have many scans and must track cumulative radiation exposure. The accuracy of the patient dose used in the estimation of risk depends on the dose estimation method employed: dose estimated based on reference values depends on the characteristics of the patient population in comparison with the reference population, while the accuracy of the dose estimated based on specific information depends on the extent to which specific information is utilized. Exam- and patient-specific factors are accounted for in an ideal approach to dose estimation. In the current study, we assessed radiation dosimetry of PET/CT for all organs using patient- and exam-specific data and commonly available dosimetry resources.

Effective dose is commonly used when evaluating relative biologic risk, and the Monte Carlo–based organ

dose coefficients should not be used to calculate effective dose for individual patients [6, 8]. The International Organization for Medical Physics, ICRP, Health Physics Society and American Association of Physicists in Medicine (AAPM) all have issued policy statements that note the dangers of extrapolating biological risk estimates for radiation doses less than 100 mSv [6, 9–11]. The establishment and use of risk coefficients to estimate public health determinants from individual or population exposures must be considered in the context of uncertainties in the estimates [12]. These uncertainties include dosimetric uncertainties, epidemiological and methodological uncertainties, uncertainties from low statistical power and precision in epidemiology studies of radiation risk, uncertainties in modeling risk data, generalization of risk estimates across different populations and dose rates, as well as reliance on epidemiological studies on observational rather than experimental data [13]. Uncertainties in such risk estimates have been suggested as being up to a factor of 3 lower or higher than the value itself [14]. These rather large uncertainties cause predictions of radiation induced cancers or detriment to be susceptible to biases and confounding influences that are unidentifiable. With due recognition of the limitations imposed by the uncertainties inherent in correlating dose with risk, effective dose is a useful approximation for relating patient population characteristics and evaluating optimization efforts in addition to the clinical benefits of exams.

For internal absorbed dose assessment, OLINDA\EXM was used to perform dosimetry calculations for the various body organs [32]. This code allows calculations for 814 radionuclides and a wide variety of adult, pediatric and pregnant female phantoms; furthermore, it also allows users to modify organ masses in the phantoms for more patient-specific dose calculations. Organ doses calculated by OLINDA\EXM based on reference phantoms

Table 7 Effective dose for male and female patients

CT Technique Description	18F-FDG PET (mSv)		CT (mSv)		Total (mSv)	
	Male	Female	Male	Female	Male	Female
Standard CT	8.1 ± 1.2	10.1 ± 1.4	5.3 ± 1.0	4.6 ± 0.8	13.4 ± 1.1	14.7 ± 1.2
Diagnostic CT	8.1 ± 0.8	9.9 ± 1.6	17.4. ± 3.7	13.4 ± 5.5	25.5 ± 3.4	23.4 ± 4.9

Data are the mean ± standard deviation

Table 8 Effective dose summary for all patients

CT technique description	18F-FDG PET	CT	Total
Standard CT	9.0 ± 1.6	5.0 ± 1.0	14.0 ± 1.3
Diagnostic CT	9.0 ± 1.6	15.4 ± 5.0	24.4 ± 4.3

Data are the mean ± standard deviation in mSv

representing the average patient were found to be in good agreement with patient specific Monte Carlo mean dose estimates [41]. Monte Carlo results suggest that the difference between the organ equivalent dose estimates in our calculations and those derived from the use of earlier stylized MIRD-type phantoms can be different by a margin as great as 277 %[42]. Patient-specific organ masses were derived from previous reports on variations in the mass of different body organs in relation to stature and BMI ([37–39]. Marine et al, and Clark et al described phantoms that model different body types in a series of percentile height phantoms to evaluate the variation of specific absorbed fractions with height and weight differences across the human population [37, 39]. With patient-specific data and a mean injected activity of 454 MBq, the mean effective dose of 9.0 mSv is consistent with dose per unit injected activity reported in the literature, and also with the dose estimates from ICRP publication 106 [23, 25–28, 34]. The relatively higher injected activity in our clinic at the time of the study results in a relatively higher whole body dose than is observed in other clinics with lower fixed standard injection activity or body mass adjusted injection activity. Despite a lack of 18F-FDG uptake in lung, this organ received the third-highest organ dose according to our methods, and this is most likely due to the proximity of the lung to the heart. Injected activity, patient body mass and height, all available from the patient record, were among the specific factors employed in our estimation of specific internal dose from 18F-FDG.

ImPACT Dose is a readily available CT organ dose calculation tool that reports organ doses based on modeled radiation transport data specific to the CT scanner and represents improved accuracy over previous methods [17]. Without using patient-specific inputs to ImPACT, organ dose was overestimated by 17 %. A contributing factor to this difference is likely the relatively larger size of our patient population. The mean BMI of our patient population was 26.4 while a reference BMI from ICRP Reference Man characteristics is 23.5. It should be noted that there is an opportunity to make the CT organ dose estimate more specific than in our study. Because the Dose Length Product (DLP) in the exam dose report is itself a general value based on a single phantom, the dose estimate may be made more specific by modifying CTDIvol to account for patient size [43]. Scanner-specific results such as the average scan length are useful for identifying opportunities for optimization and for evaluation against similar protocols and standards. For example, the scan length for a whole-body PET/CT can be compared to the scan length for a whole body CT at the same clinic or to a reference value. The average ± SD scan length of diagnostic whole body PET/CT in the present study is 89.5 ± 14.7 cm, while the combined scan length of chest + abdomen + pelvis CT scans is reported as 73 cm [29]. Knowledge of the relative scan lengths puts differences in dose and DLP in perspective. Further, the anatomy in a diagnostic PET/CT is fixed to PET anatomy selection, while the anatomy during the CT-only acquisition may be optimally adjusted. Anatomy selection, and avoidance, is an important aspect of CT protocol optimization that may be overlooked for incorporation into PET/CT scanners. Individual technologists may incorporate optimal anatomy selection in both CT and PET/CT scans, but this optimization measure is more likely to be routinely incorporated as a matter of policy for CT scanners than PET/CT scanners utilized for diagnostic PET/CT exams. In these ways, scanner-specific data are useful for characterizing the clinic's practices and identifying opportunities for optimization.

Although the average diagnostic PET/CT scan length in this study is greater than that reported in the literature, the dose from the CT portion of the diagnostic PET/CT exams we evaluated in this study is consistent with the average whole body CT dose reported in the literature. Table 9 summarizes doses reported in the literature for whole body CT and chest-abdomen-pelvis (CAP) CT exams, which have approximately the same length scans as whole body PET/CT scans [22, 24, 29–31].

The average value of the five included studies reporting whole-body or equivalent CT dose is 15.1 mSv and likely represents a conservative estimate of average dose from a whole body diagnostic CT. A clear advantage of a combined diagnostic PET/CT is the higher patient throughput relative to separate scheduling, along with a relatively shorter exam time than the lower-dose alternatives. From the patient's perspective, a single visit to the imaging clinic is easier than two separate visits. If the doses are the same, then a combined scan has the additional patient benefit convenience. Depending on the contributing factors at a given imaging clinic, the radiation dose from a standard PET/CT with separate

Table 9 Comparison of reported whole body diagnostic CT effective dose

CT study	1[a]	2[b]	3[c]	4[d]	5[e]	Average	This study
Effective dose (mSv)	19	9.25	12.5	22.5	16	15.1	15.4

Data are mean mSv
[a]CT-based transmission scan in high quality mode [31]
[b]73-cm CAP CT [29]
[c]Whole body CT, C3 to symphisis pubis [22]
[d]Complete whole body CT includes thyroid contribution [24]
[e]Based on UK survey of CAP CT [30]

diagnostic CT may be more or less than the radiation dose from a diagnostic PET/CT. Intuitively, a PET/CT with diagnostic technique compared to a standard PET/CT with separately acquired diagnostic CT may appear to be qualitatively equivalent but dosimetrically different because the PET/CT with diagnostic technique CT can also be used for attenuation correction. CT dose from the standard PET/CT appears to be in addition to the dose from the separate diagnostic CT. However, differences in PET/CT and CT scanner hardware and software can cause the dose to be higher or lower. For example, the number of slices is typically different between dual- and single-modality units, and adaptive filtering may not available on PET/CT machines. Both hardware and software factors can cause the patient dose from a combined scan to be higher or lower than separately acquired scans and must be considered when evaluating the dose at a given clinic with reference or literature doses. Less variation is observed in reported PET dose that is estimated from a single source, such as ICRP 106. Even the standards at an imaging clinic for uptake time and acquisition time can affect dose by influencing injected activity. A busy clinic with a fixed injected activity per patient, for example, may administer relatively more activity to account for the inevitable changes in scheduling that come with patient cancellations, delays and other impacts on timing. There is evidence, however, that weight- or BMI-adjusted injected activity reduces patient dose and staff exposure without compromising image quality [44]. A busy clinic may also benefit from a relatively higher injected activity to shorten the acquisition time, as PET acquisition is based on total counts in a bed field and more activity results in the total counts achieved relatively sooner.

The potential for variation in reported dose from PET is apparent in the variability in those PET exam parameters that depend on clinical setting. The patient dose in a clinic employing Germanium-based attenuation correction will differ from a clinic that uses CT-based attenuation correction. Germanium-based attenuation correction has been found to result in negligible patient dose, but it also results in lower diagnostic value in terms of anatomical delineation and longer scanning time than CT-based attenuation correction [31]. The additional challenge of coregistering separate image sets also accompanies this approach. Nonetheless, Germanium-based attenuation correction is sufficient for standard PET/CT exams and still finds routine usage amongst clinics that wish to add PET imaging, but already have a CT scanner. The possibility of different attenuation correction methods makes a one-size-fits-all estimate of expected radiation dose for PET/CT exams unrealistic, and promotes a specific approach to dose evaluation.

Brix et al evaluated total dose from PET/CT exams utilizing CT-based attenuation correction at different hospitals and demonstrated that regardless of whether the PET/CT protocol is standard or diagnostic, the dose from a PET/CT exam is about 23 mSv, due to different approaches, hardware, standards and clinical objectives [23]. RPOP reference doses are compared with the results of our study and with typical literature data in Table 10.

The range of doses observed in Table 10 demonstrates the importance of careful choice of data, characterizing the dose at one's own clinic and understanding the factors contributing to patient dose from PET/CT.

Dose estimated using reference values and standard body models requires the least amount of effort and results in a non-specific estimate that may not be consistent with the characteristics of the actual patient population. However, many exam-specific parameters are conveniently accessed with minimal effort. Reference DLP values are available, but in practice the actual DLP from the exam is readily available from the dose report and is easily used to estimate effective dose by employing either a standard or scanner-specific factor [18]. An approach employing all available patient-specific resources (i.e. patient-adjusted DLP and organ mass, scanner-specific factors) results in accurate estimation but requires moderate effort because this data must be retrieved from electronic records. A retrospective dose estimate requires accessing DICOM information and patient records for relevant information, while estimating dose from a present exam for an individual patient can utilize information at hand. Whether the risk estimate is made at the time of the exam or retrospectively, and whether it is for an individual or representative group, the effort involved in gathering the information must be weighed against the value of the information gained.

Conclusions

An ideal dose estimation method is convenient to employ and considers clinic- and patient-specific factors to an appropriate extent. Patient specific parameters (e.g., weight, and height) identified from patient data allow for more accurate estimate of organ equivalent doses and the effort involved in obtaining the data is worthwhile

Table 10 Comparison of reference dose with our results and literature

	RPOP	This study	Literature[a]
Injected activity (MBq)	400	454	370
PET dose	8	9	7
Standard CT dose	7	5	2.7
Diagnostic CT dose	30	15.4	16.1
Total dose, standard PET/CT	15	14	9.7
Total dose, Diagnostic PET/CT	38	24.4	23.1

Note: doses are in mSv. [a]Brix et al [23]

for a retrospective analysis of a representative patient sample and for some individual patients. Accurate estimation of patient dose, rather than a conservatively high estimate, is important for many oncology patients who can potentially have many scans and must track cumulative exposure. Considering actual patient-specific characteristics resulted in lower organ equivalent dose estimates than traditional reference phantoms and models, but the methods employed in this study resulted in organ doses and effective doses that are in agreement with alternative methods. Considering the substantial radiation dose of whole body PET/CT exams and the potential for wide variation in contributing factors, all aspects of the exam process should be considered for optimization. Radiopharmaceutical injection activity, CT technique, CT protocol optimization measures, anatomy selection, and convenience to both patient and imaging clinic are all factors which must be considered for comprehensive optimization and subsequent justification of the PET/CT exam. The effort involved in obtaining patient-specific data is reasonable to help justify the risk associated with the radiation exposure, optimize the image acquisition parameters to balance dose with the objectives of the exam, and characterize the patient population.

Clinic-specific patient dose for each type of PET/CT exam can reasonably be estimated for comparison with industry standards, reference values and literature values. Opportunities for optimization may also be apparent in better understanding how the clinic's doses compare with other sources of data.

Abbreviations
AAPM, American Association of Physicists in Medicine; BMI, Body mass index; ICRP, International Commission on Radiological Protection; PET/CT, Fluorine-18 positron emission tomography/computed tomography; RPOP, Radiation protection of patients

Acknowledgements
The authors wish to acknowledge the assistance of the department of Radiology and Molecular Imaging and Therapy Service for their support of the project. This work was supported by Memorial Sloan Kettering Cancer Center Support Grant/Core Grant (P30 CA008748).

Authors' contributions
BQ drafted the manuscript and analyzed data. ZD collected and analyzed data, participated in design of the study and helped draft the manuscript. NPT provided practical clinical input and technical review of imaging parameters and helped draft the manuscript. HS provided practical and technical clinical input and technical review of imaging procedures and helped draft the manuscript. LD conceived of and designed the study, provided technical oversight for dose calculation methods and results. All authors read and approved the manuscript.

Authors' information
BQ and ZD are Medical Health Physicists, NPT and HS are nuclear medicine physicians in the molecular imaging and therapy service with clinical expertise in positron emission tomography, LD is a Medical Health Physicist with expertise in dose and risk estimation methodology.

Competing interests
The authors declare that they have no competing interests.

Author details
[1]Department of Medical Physics, Box 84, Memorial Sloan Kettering Cancer Center, 1275 York Avenue, New York, NY 10065, USA. [2]Department of Radiology, Memorial Sloan Kettering Cancer Center, New York, USA.

References
1. Czernin J, Schelbert H. PET/CT Imaging: Facts, opinions, hopes, and questions. J Nucl Med. 2004;45(Suppl):1S–3S.
2. Czernin J, Allen-Auerbach M, Schelbert HR. Improvements in cancer staging with PET/CT: Literature-based evidence as of September 2006. J Nucl Med. 2007;48(1):78S–88S.
3. Bockisch A, Beyer T, Antoch G, et al. Positron emission tomography/computed tompgraphy–imaging protocols, artifacts, and pitfalls. Mol Imag Bio. 2004;6:188–89.
4. ICRP. Radiological Protection and Safety in Medicine. A Report of the International Commission on Radiological Protection. Ann ICRP. 1996;26:1–47.
5. Brink JA, Amis E. Image wisely: a campaign to increase awareness about adult radiation protection. Radiology. 2010;257(3):601–2.
6. ICRP. The 2007 Recommendations of the International Commission on Radiological Protection, ICRP Publication 103. Ann ICRP. 2007;37:1–332.
7. Stabin MG. Uncertainties in Internal Dose Calculations for Radiopharmaceuticals. J Nucl Med. 2008;119:853–60.
8. Shrimpton PC, Wall B, Yoshizumi TT, Hurwitz LM, Goodman PC. Effective Dose and Dose-Length Product in CT. Radiology. 2009;250(2):604–5.
9. Hendee WR, I.O.f.M.P. Policy Statement of the International Organization for Medical Physics. Radiology. 2013;267(2):326–7.
10. Health Physics Society. Radiation Risk in Perspective. Health Physics Society. https://hps.org/documents/radiationrisk.pdf.
11. AAPM. AAPM Position Statement on Radiation Risks from Medical Imaging Procedures. PP 25-A. American Association of Physicists in Medicine. http://www.aapm.org/org/policies/details.asp?id=318&type=PP. Accessed 7 Jun 2016.
12. Dauer LT, Branets I, Stabulas-Savage J, et al. Optimising Radiographic Bitewing Examination to Adult and Juvenile Patients Through the Use of Anthropomorphic Phantoms. Radiat Prot Dosimetry. 2013;158:51–8.
13. NCRP. Uncertainties in Internal Radiation Dose Assessment. NCRP Report 164. NCRP Publications, Bethesda, MD; 2009.
14. UNSCEAR. Report of the United Nations Scientific Committee on the Effects of Atomic Radiation. Fifty-ninth Session. General Assembly Official Records Sixty Seventh Session, Supplemental No. 46.A/67/46. United Nations Scientific Committee on the Effects of Atomic Radiation. http://www.unscear.org/docs/reports/2012/UNSCEAR2012Report_15-08936_eBook_website.pdf. Accessed 7 Jun 2016.
15. IAEA. Radiation Protection of Patients PET/CT scanning. https://rpop.iaea.org/RPOP/RPoP/Content/InformationFor/HealthProfessionals/6_OtherClinicalSpecialities/PETCTscan.htm. Accessed 7 Jun 2016.
16. Kamel E, Hany T, Burger C, et al. CT vs 68Ge Attenuation Correction in a Combined PET/CT System: Evaluation of the Effect of Lowering CT Tube Current. Eur J Nucl Med Mol Imaging. 2002;29(3):346–50.
17. Kalender WA, Schmidt B, Zankl M, Schmidt M. A PC Program for Estimating Organ Dose and Effective Dose Values in Computed Tomography. Eur Radiol. 1999;9(3):555–62.
18. Kalender W, Deak P, Smal Y. Multisection CT protocols: sex- and age-specific conversion factors used to determine effective dose from dose length product. Radiology. 2010;257(1):158–66.

19. ICRP. Report of the Task Group on Reference Man. ICRP Publication 23. Oxford: Pergamon Press; 1975.

20. Measurements, I.C.o.R.U.a. Measurement of Dose Equivalents from External Photon and Electron Radiations. ICRU Report 47. Bethesda, MD: ICRU; 1992.

21. ICRP. Radiation Dose to Patients from Radiopharmaceuticals: Addendum 2 to ICRP Publication 53, Also Includes Addendum 1 to ICRP Publication 72. ICRP Publication 80. Oxford, UK: Pergamon Press; 1998.

22. Brenner DJ, Elliston C. Estimated Radiation Risks Potentially Associated with Full-Body CT Screening. Radiology. 2012;232:735–8.

23. Brix G, Lechel U, Glatting G, Ziegler S, Munzig W, Muller S, Beyer T. Radiation Exposured of PAtients Undergoing Whole-Body Dual-Modality 18F-FDG PET/CT Examinations. J Nucl Med. 2005;46(4):608–13.

24. Groves AM, Owen K, Courtney HM, et al. 16-detector Multiclice CT: Dosimetry Estimation by TLD Measurement Compared with Monte Carlo Simulation. Br J Radiol. 2004;77:662–5.

25. Huang B, Law M, Khong PL. Whole-Body PET/CT Scanning: Estimation of Radiation Dose and Cancer Risk. Radiology. 2009;251(1):166–74.

26. Khamwan K, Krisanachinda A, Pasawang P. The Determination of Patient Dose From F-18-FDG PET/CT Examination. Radiat Prot Dosimetry. 2010;141:50–5.

27. Mahmud MH et al. Estimation of patient radiation dose from whole body18F- FDG PET/CT examination in cancer imaging: a preliminary study. Journal of Physics: Conference Series. 2014;546:012008.

28. Leide-Svegborn S. Radiation Exposure of Patients and Personnel from a PET/CT Procedure with 18F-FDG. Radiat Prot Dosimetry. 2010;139:208–13.

29. Theocharopoulos N, Damilakis J, Perisinakis K, et al. Effective Doses to Adult and Pediatric Patients from Multislice Computed Tomography: A Method Based on Energy Imparted. Med Phys. 2006;33(10):3846–56.

30. Tsalafoutas IA, Koukourakis G. Patient Dose Considerations in Computed Tomography Examinations. World J Radiol. 2004;2(7):262–8.

31. Wu TH, Huang Y, Lee JJ, et al. Radiation Exposure During Transmission Measurements: Comparison Between CT- and Germanium-based Techniques with a Current PET Scanner. Eur J Nucl Med Mol Imaging. 2004;77:662–5.

32. Stabin MG, Sparks R, Crowe E. OLINDA/EXM: The Second-Generation Personal computer Software for Internal Dose Assessment in Nuclear Medicine. J Nucl Med. 2005;46(6):1023–7.

33. Bolch WE, Eckerman K, Sgouros G, Thomas SR. MIRD Pamphlet No 21: A Generalized Schema for Radiopharmaceutical Dosimetry-Standardization of Nomenclature. J Nucl Med. 2009;50(3):477–84.

34. ICRP. Radiation Dose to Patients from Radiopharmaceuticals. Addendum 3 to ICRP Publication 53. ICRP Publication 106. Ann ICRP. 2008;38(1-2):1–197.

35. Hays MT, Watson E, Thomas SR, Stabin M. MIRD Dose Estimate Report No 19: Radiation Absorbed Dose Estimates from 18F-FDG. J Nucl Med. 2002; 43(2):210–4.

36. Deloar HM, Fujiwara T, Shidahara M, Nakamura T, Watabe H, Narita Y, Itoh M, Miyake M, Watanuki S. Estimation of Absorbed Dose for 2-[F-18]fluoro-2-deoxy-D-glucose Using Whole-Body Positron Emission Tomography and Magnetic Resonance Imaging. Eur J Nucl Med. 1998;25(6):585–74.

37. Clark LD, Stabin M, Fernald MJ, Brill AB. Changes in Radiation Dose with Variations in Human Anatomy: Moderately and Severely Obese Adults. J Nucl Med. 2010;51:929–32.

38. ICRP. Basic Anatomical and Physiological Data for Use in Radiological Protection: Reference Values. A Report of Age- and Gender-Related Differences in the Anatomical and Physiological Characteristics of Reference Individuals. Ann ICRP. 2002;32:5–265.

39. Marine PM, Stabin MG, Fernald MJ, Brill AB. Changes in Radiation Dose with Variations in Human Anatomy: Larger and Smaller Normal-Stature Adults. J Nucl Med. 2010;51(5):806–11.

40. ICRP. ICRP Publication 105. Radiation Protection in Medicine. Ann ICRP. 2007;37:1–63.

41. Grimes J, Celler A. Comparison of Internal Dose Estimates Obtained Using Organ-Level, Voxel 5 Value, and Monte Carlo Techniques. Med Phys. 2014;41(9):92501.

42. Ding A, Gu J, Liu H, Caracappa P, Xu XG. The Design of a New PC Software for Estimating Patient Doses from CT Scans. Health Phys. 2009;97(1):S56.

43. AAPM. Size-specific dose estimates (SSDE) in pediatric and adult body CT examinations: Report of AAPM Task Group 204. College Park, MD: American Association of Physicists in Medicine; 2011.

44. Saade C, H.M., Ammous A et al, Weight-based Protocols during Whole Body FDG PET/CT Significantly Reduces Radiation Dose without Compromising Image Quality, in RSNA 2015 Scientific Assembly and Annual Meeting. Chicago, IL.

4

Chemical shift MR imaging in the lumbar vertebra: the effect of field strength, scanner vendors and flip angles in repeatability of signal intensity index measurement

Zebin Xiao[1†], Jian Li[1†], Chengqi Li[2], Yuyang Zhang[1], Dejun She[1] and Dairong Cao[1*]

Abstract

Background: To evaluate the reproducibility of signal intensity index (SII) measurements with MRI systems from different vendors and with different field strengths, and to test the effectiveness of flip angle.

Methods: Thirty-two healthy volunteers (mean age 35.3 ± 9.3 years) were enrolled in this ethics committee-approved study. Chemical shift MR imaging was performed on 1.5- and 3.0-T MR systems from three vendors. Two independent observers measured SII values in five lumbar segments. Inter- and intraobserver agreement was assessed using the interclass correlation coefficients (ICCs). Differences of mean SII values between different field strengths and MR vendors as well as flip angles were compared by using repeated-measures analysis of variance. Differences of mean SII values between different flip angles were also compared by using paired-sample t test.

Results: Inter- and intra-observer correlation coefficients showed good agreement (all ICC > 0.75) when measuring SII values at different MR systems (ICCs ranging from 0.896 to 0.983) and flip angles (ICCs ranging from 0.824 to 0.983). There were no significant differences in mean SII values measured by different MR vendors with different field strengths (all $p > 0.05$ ranging from 0.337 to 0.824). The differences in the mean SII between the four different flip angles were statistically significant (all $p < 0.05$ ranging from < 0.001 to 0.004) except the group of flip angle 50° versus 70° ($p = 0.116$).

Conclusion: The SII measurement using chemical shift MR imaging may be comparable between different MR systems. Also high flip angles showed better stability to quantitate lumbar fat content.

Keywords: Chemical shift MRI, Repeatability, Bone marrow, In-phase and out-of-phase, Signal intensity index (SII)

Background

Chemical shift magnetic resonance (MR) imaging (also known as in-phase and out-of-phase imaging or opposed-phased imaging) is a simple technique that takes advantage of the fact that water and lipid hydrogen protons in a single voxel show slightly different precession frequencies [1]. Based on phase differences in

images acquired via different TEs, lipid and water signals are additive on in-phase images and subtracted on opposed-phase images [2]. This technique has been proved to be extremely useful for characterization of lesions and organs with fatty components and has gained widespread acceptance [3–6]. In clinical practice, it is widely used to diagnose lipid-poor adrenal adenomas [3, 7]. On the same bias, chemical shift MR imaging has been used to evaluate vertebral bone marrow fat content in osteoporosis or in distinguishing benign and malignant causes of vertebral bone marrow infiltration [2, 4, 7–16]. Furthermore, some

* Correspondence: dairongcao@163.com
†Equal contributors
[1]Department of Radiology, First Affiliated Hospital of Fujian Medical University, 20 Cha-Zhong Road, Fuzhou, Fujian 350005, China
Full list of author information is available at the end of the article

Table 1 Intra- and interobserver agreement for SII measurement with different field strengths and vendors (Flip angle = 70°)

Agreement	Siemens		GE		Toshiba	
	Reader 1/First time	Reader 2/Second time	Reader 1/First time	Reader 2/Second time	Reader 1/First time	Reader 2/Second time
Intraobserver	0.935 (0.912, 0.952)	0.896 (0.860, 0.923)	0.961 (0.947, 0.973)	0.930 (0.905, 0.948)	0.972 (0.962, 0.989)	0.906 (0.874, 0.930)
Interobserver	0.983 (0.954, 0.995)	0.916 (0.885, 0.938)	0.954 (0.893, 0.971)	0.952 (0.935, 0.965)	0.976 (0.967, 0.982)	0.932 (0.878, 0.964)

SII, Signal intensity index; Note. —Data in parentheses are 95% LOA

investigators measured the signal intensity index (SII) value to avoid the problem of signal intensity variability produced by the reference tissue, and found that it appeared to be the most reliable method for differentiating adenomas from non-adenomas [7, 17]. However, there exists a major difference if measurements are performed at the adrenal gland or the bone marrow as reproducibility errors always have to be considered in relation to the variance that is expected in a population.

In spite of great interest in and enthusiasm about chemical shift MR imaging, there is a clear need for standardization of both the acquisition and the interpretation of chemical shift MR images to resolve current difficulties in comparing SII values from different studies or from different sites to enable validation of this quantitative parameter as a qualified biomarker in the context of multicenter studies.

SII measurements can be influenced by many factors such as chemical shift effect, susceptibility effect (i.e. T2* decay) and T1 relaxation, etc. [8, 18, 19]. Chemical shift effect occurs due to the slightly different precession frequency of water and fat. Susceptibility effect results from field inhomogeneity which is obvious at 3.0 Tesla or from the composition of the lesion itself [19]. As for the T1 relaxation, it depends on imaging parameters such as repetition time (TR) and flip angle [20]. Overall, whether SII values measured by chemical shift MR imaging can be compared across MR systems from different vendors and across field strengths remains an open question.

Thus, the aims of this study were to evaluate the reproducibility of SII values in the lumbar segments measured with MRI systems from different vendors and at different field strengths, and to test the effect of flip angle on assessing bone marrow fat content with respect to measurement of the signal intensity index (SII).

Methods

This clinical study was approved by our Institutional Review Board (First Affiliated Hospital of Fujian Medical University) and written informed consent was obtained from all healthy volunteers enrolled in the study.

Study population

In this present study, 35 healthy volunteers were included for chemical shift MR imaging of the lumbar spine between March 2015 and May 2015. The inclusion criteria for this study were as follows: (1) no history of trauma or surgery in the lumbar spine; (2) no history of acute or chronic pain in lower back; (3) no history of diseases which could change the signal intensity of lumbar marrow. The exclusion criteria was performed after interviewing the volunteers and reviewing their medical records, which included: (a) a history of or findings related to marrow diseases such as osteoporotic/traumatic fracture, traumatic, myeloma, osteosarcoma, lymphoma, spondylitis, etc.; (b) contraindications to MR imaging; (c) failure to complete the chemical shift imaging procedure for any reason; and (d) poor image quality insufficient for image analysis.

MR imaging protocol

Data were acquired with 1.5 T MR systems (Vantage Altas, Toshiba Medical Systems, Otawara-shi, Japan) using phased-array spine coils with the following sequences: sagittal T1-weighted spin-echo sequence (500/10 [repetition time msec/echo time msec]), sagittal T2-weighted fast spin-echo sequence (4000/110 [repetition time msec/echo time msec]) and sagittal short inversion time inversion-recovery (STIR) fast spin-echo sequence (3500/65 [repetition time mse/echo time msec]). Chemical shift imaging data were acquired with 1.5 T MR

Table 2 Intra- and interobserver agreement for SII measurement with different flip angles

Agreement	Flip angle = 10°		Flip angle = 30°		Flip angle = 50°		Flip angle = 70°	
	Reader 1/First time	Reader 2/Second time	Reader 1/First time	Reader 2/Second time	Reader 1/First time	Reader 2/Second time	Reader 1/First time	Reader 2/Second time
Intra-	0.824	0.881	0.961	0.913	0.926	0.936	0.935	0.896
observer	(0.668, 0.907)	(0.796, 0.941)	(0.944, 0.983)	(0.902, 0.941)	(0.854, 0.963)	(0.879, 0.964)	(0.912, 0.952)	(0.860, 0.923)
Inter-	0.858	0.891	0.969	0.912	0.923	0.971	0.983	0.916
observer	(0.671, 0.914)	(0.815, 0.943)	(0.923, 0.985)	(0.897, 0.937)	(0.852, 0.958)	(0.933, 0.989)	(0.954, 0.995)	(0.885, 0.938)

Note. —Data in parentheses are 95% LOA
SII, Signal intensity index

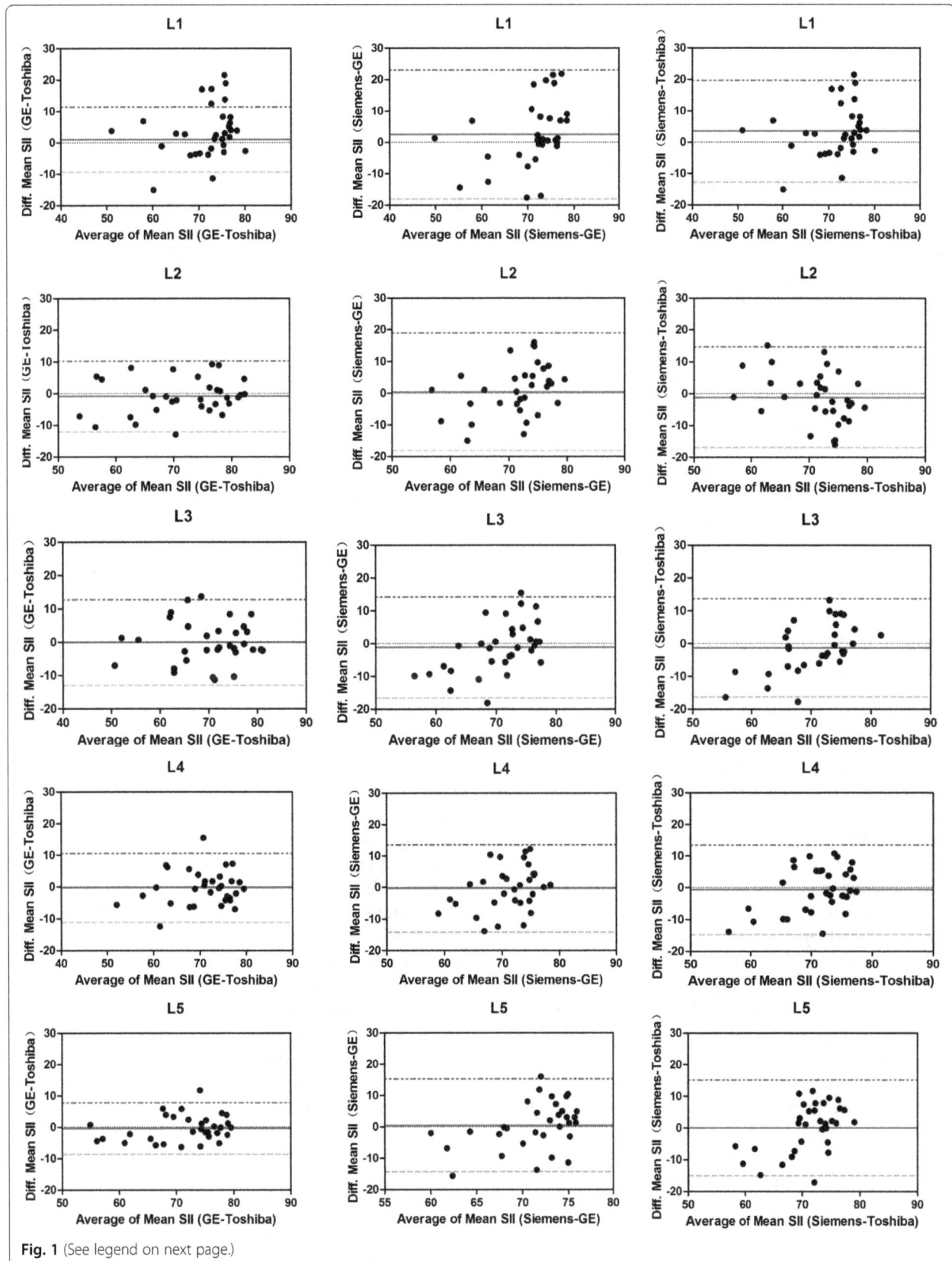

Fig. 1 (See legend on next page.)

(See figure on previous page.)
Fig. 1 Mutual agreement of signal intensity index (SII) measured from different MR systems. The Bland-Altman plots show SII difference versus SII mean in different MR systems. For each lumbar segment, the mean SII difference (the red solid line) and the limits of agreements (lower limit: the green interrupted horizontal line; upper limit: the blue interrupted horizontal line) are shown. For reference, zero SII difference is shown as a black dotted line

systems from two vendors (Vantage Altas, Toshiba Medical Systems, Otawara-shi, Japan; Signa Twinspeed, GE Healthcare, Milwaukee, WI) and 3.0 T MR system from one vendor (Magneton Verio, Siemens Medical Solutions, Erlangen, Germany) using phased-array spine coils in one week. The sequence parameters on 1.5 T MR systems were as follows: sagittal out-of-phase (OP) (2.4/192 [repetition time mse/echo time msec]) fast spoiled gradient echo MR imaging was first scanned, followed by sagittal in-phase (IP) (4.8/192 [repetition time mse/echo time msec]) MR imaging. And the sequence parameters on 3.0 T MR system were as follows: sagittal in-phase (IP) (2.4/192 [repetition time mse/echo time msec]) MR imaging was first scanned, followed by out-of-phase (OP) (5.8/192 [repetition time mse/echo time msec]) fast spoiled gradient echo MR imaging. In addition, chemical shift MR imaging was performed on 3.0 T MR scanners with four flip angles (10, 30, 50, 70°), whereas only one flip angle at 70° was used in 1.5 T scanner. For all sagittal sequences, the field of view was 24 cm × 24 cm. The matrix was 256 × 256, and the section thickness was 4.0 mm, with a skip of 1.0 mm.

Image analysis

All chemical shift MR imaging data were transferred to an independent workstation for evaluation. Two readers (Z.X. and Y.Z., radiologists with 2 and 4 years of clinical experience in musculoskeletal MR imaging, respectively) independently drew rectangular regions of interest (ROIs) with a specific size in the center of three representative sections of each vertebral body, including midsagittal sections and adjacent two sections. The ROI size was initially defined by two authors in consensus (D.C. and J.L., radiologists with 28 and 23 years of clinical experience in musculoskeletal MR imaging, respectively) in a test set of images. The ROI was defined based on the largest possible rectangular size measuring 1.0 cm × 1.5 cm for the respective sections, and size for each region was kept constant during placement of ROIs by using the function of copy and paste in our workstation. Thus, a total of 54 ROIs were collected for each volunteer (three sections per vertebral body, five vertebral body, three vendors with two field strength plus other three flip angles in three sections of one vertebral body in 3.0 T scanner, $3 \times 5 \times 3 + 3 \times 3 \times 1 = 54$). Care was taken to exclude areas with obvious artifacts from the ROIs.

The signal intensity index (SII) was measured independently by two radiologists blinded for patient data (C.L. and D.S. with 6 and 4 years of clinical experience in musculoskeletal MR imaging, respectively). SII was defined as the percentage of signal change on the OP sequence compared to the IP sequence according to previously described equation [21, 22]: $SII = (SI_{IP}-SI_{OP})/SI_{IP} \times 100\%$. SI_{IP} refers to mean signal intensity of the bone marrow on IP sequences and SI_{OP} refers to mean signal intensity of the bone marrow on OP sequences. For further analyses, the mean SII value of the two readers was calculated for each placed ROI.

Statistical analysis

SII values were expressed as mean ± standard deviation (SD) and were tested first with the Kolmogorov-Smirnov test for normality and then with the Levene test for variance homogeneity.

Intra- and inter-observer agreement of SII measurements were assessed using intra- and interclass correlation coefficients (ICCs). An ICC greater than 0.75 was indicative of good agreement [23]. The mean differences, SD, and 95% limits of agreement (LOA) were calculated using the Bland-Altman method [24, 25]. Measurement repeatability was assessed by the Bland-Altman analysis in order to define the agreement between replicate measurements. The repeatability coefficient, which represents the threshold value below which the absolute differences between two measurements on the same subject is expected to lie for 95% of the measurement pairs, was assessed using the formula $1.96 \times SD$ of the mean difference (dSD), and expressed as percentage of the mean SII value.

Differences of mean SII values between different field strengths and MR vendors as well as flip angles were compared by using repeated-measures analysis of variance. Next, differences of mean SII values between different flip angles were also compared by using paired-sample t test. The Bonferroni method was used to adjust for multiple comparisons when necessary.

All statistical calculations were performed using the commercially available software package (PASW, Version 18.0, SPSS Inc., Chicago, IL, USA). Differences were considered significant when p values were less than 0.05.

Results

Population demographics

Thirty-five volunteers were enrolled in this study. Three of them did not complete the study because of poor image quality (n = 2) or incomplete acquisition of all

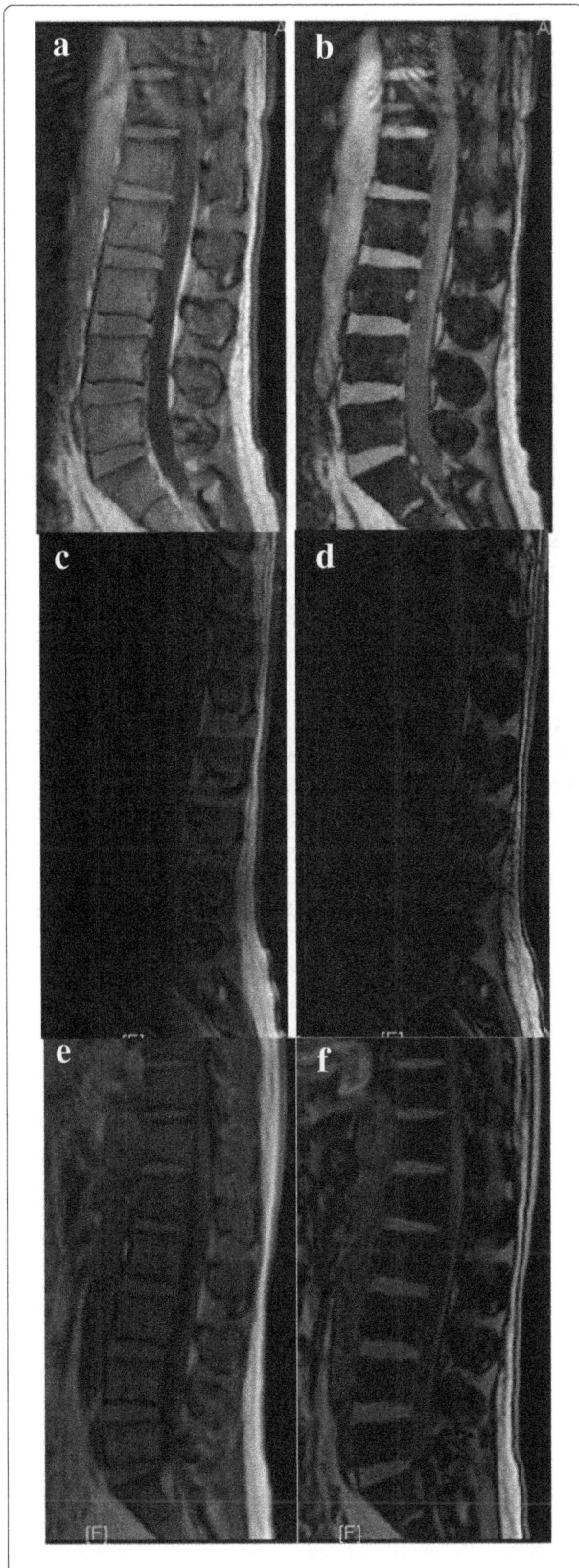

Fig. 2 Representative images of chemical shift MR imaging in different MR systems. (**a**) in-phase image acquired at 3.0 T Siemens MR system; (**b**) out-of-phase image acquired at 3.0 T Siemens MR system; (**c**) in-phase image acquired at 1.5 T GE MR system; (**d**) out-of-phase image acquired at 1.5 T GE MR system; (**e**) in-phase image acquired at 1.5 T Toshiba MR system; (**f**) out-of-phase image acquired at 1.5 T Toshiba MR system

sequences (n = 1). Thirty-two volunteers successfully completed the imaging examinations (22 men and 10 women; mean age 35.3 ± 9.3 years; age range 21–50 years), and all the MR data sets were eligible for evaluation.

Repeatability of SII measurements in different MR systems and flip angles

The SIIs measured in this study met the normal distribution ($p = 0.193$) and homogeneity of variance ($p = 0.128$). The intraobserver ICC calculated based on reader 1's two measurements of SII values in 3.0 T Siemens system ranged from 0.896 to 0.972, with the 95% LOA ranging from (0.860, 0.923) to (0.962, 0.989) (Table 1). Interobserver agreement between reader 1's first measurements and reader 2's measurements was good for the three MR systems, with ICC (95% LOA) ranging from 0.916 (0.885, 0.938) to 0.983 (0.954, 0.975). The intra- and interobserver ICC results show good agreement between MR systems (all ICC > 0.75).

As shown in Table 2, the intra- and inter-observer ICC (95% LOA) ranged from 0.824 (0.668, 0.907) to 0.983 (0.954, 0.995), showing good agreement in measuring SIIs in different flip angles (all ICC > 0.75).

Mutual agreement of mean SII measurements with different MR systems

The goal of this study was to assess agreement of mean SII values with different vendors at the same field strength (1.5 T Toshiba Vantage–1.5 T GE Signa), different field strengths and vendors (1.5 T GE Signa–3.0 T Siemens Verio; 1.5 T Toshiba Vantage-3.0 T Siemens Verio).

Overall, the agreement of above three conditions was desirable as the mean differences were very small (the mean differences ranged from –1. 324 to 3.462) and most of the data points lied within 95% LOA (Figs. 1, 2). As shown in Table 3, the bias was not systematic, but depended on the specific lumbar segments and on the different MR systems. For instance, there existed significant bias on the measurements of SII values in L1 with three different MR systems; some segments (for example L3) showed negligible bias in comparison within the same field strength (Toshiba-GE), but a little bias when combining 1.5 T and 3.0 T data (1.5 T GE–3.0 T Siemens and 1.5 T Toshiba–3.0 T Siemens).

Table 3 Reproducibility of Mean SII Measurements in Each of the Five Lumbar Segments with Three Vendors in Two Field Strengths

Lumbar Segment	1.5 T Toshiba– 1.5 T GE	1.5 T GE– 3.0 T Siemens	1.5 T Toshiba - 3.0 T Siemens
L1	1.002 (−9.384, 11.388)	2.460 (−18.067, 22.987)	3.462 (−12.770, 19.693)
L2	−0.906 (−12.100, 10.289)	−0.327 (−18.893, 18.239)	−1.233 (−17.012, 14.547)
L3	−0.094 (−12.940, 12.751)	−1.230 (−16.663, 14.203)	−1.324 (−16.319, 13.671)
L4	−0.303 (−11.095, 10.488)	−0.327 (−14.208, 13.554)	−0.631 (−14.787, 13.526)
L5	−0.452 (−8.683, 7.779)	0.456 (−14.329, 15.242)	0.004 (−15.133, 15.142)

Note. —Data in parentheses are 95% LOA

Comparison of mean SII values with three vendors in Two field strengths

The mean SII values of all lumbar vertebrae at 3.0 T Siemens, 1.5 T GE and 1.5 T Toshiba were $70.9 \pm 5.4\%$, $71.3 \pm 5.4\%$, and $71.5 \pm 8.2\%$, respectively. Table 4 and Fig. 3 summarized the comparison of mean SII values with 3 MR systems in different lumbar segments. From the aspect of different field strength of MR systems, there were no significant differences in mean SII values (3.0 T Siemens vs 1.5 T GE, $p = 0.337$; 3.0 T Siemens vs 1.5 T Toshiba, $p = 0.561$). From the aspect of the same field strength of different vendors (1.5 T GE vs 1.5 T Toshiba), there were no significant differences in mean SIIs ($p = 0.824$). Moreover, the mean SII values in the same lumbar segment had no significant differences among the measurement in the three different MR vendors (all $p > 0.05$, range from 0.26 to 0.95), and the mean SIIs for each MR vendor at different lumbar segments had no significant differences either (all $p > 0.05$, ranging from 0.17 to 0.88).

Comparison of mean SII values in different flip angles

The mean SII of lumbar vertebra at 3.0 T Siemens with different flip angles (flip angle = 10, 30, 50, 70°) was $63.7 \pm 7.4\%$, $67.7 \pm 7.5\%$, $69.7 \pm 6.0\%$ and $71.0 \pm 5.5\%$, respectively. The mean SII values showed a tendency of increasing with flip angles, and there were significant differences between different flip angles ($p < 0.001$) although there was no significant difference between the groups of flip angle 50° and 70° ($p = 0.116$) (Fig. 4, 5).

Table 4 Comparison of Mean SII Measurement in Each of the Five Lumbar Segments with Three Vendors in Two Field Strengths

	3.0 T Siemens	1.5 T GE	1.5 T Toshiba	P Value[*]
L1	70.124 ± 6.865	72.564 ± 10.121	73.505 ± 8.429	0.257
L2	70.711 ± 5.721	71.156 ± 9.278	71.987 ± 8.255	0.810
L3	71.223 ± 4.939	70.010 ± 8.401	69.917 ± 8.642	0.737
L4	71.344 ± 4.953	71.077 ± 6.925	71.015 ± 6.909	0.930
L5	71.225 ± 4.458	71.601 ± 6.882	71.658 ± 6.822	0.949
P Value[+]	0.882	0.171	0.643	

Note. —Data are mean SIIs (%) ± standard deviation
[*] Comparison of Mean SIIs in the left- right direction
[+] Comparison of Mean SIIs in the superior- inferior direction

Discussion

Chemical shift imaging is an useful technology in abdominal imaging by detecting lipid content [1, 3, 22, 26]. It was initially introduced for the assessment of bone marrow in 1985 by Wismer et al. [27], and also has been widely used in musculoskeletal imaging by measuring SII value for evaluation of bone marrow fat content or differentiation benign from malignant lesions [8, 9, 11–14]. But the lack of standardization in data analysis is a major challenge to the widespread and uniform use of chemical shift MR imaging in musculoskeletal imaging when comparing results of different studies. Furthermore, a reliable interpretation of the results contributed by different centers requires comparability of data acquired with MR systems at different institutions, which are often from different vendors and are operated at different field strengths. To the best of our knowledge, there are no previous reports describing the repeatability of SII measurements in different vendors, field strengths and flip angles.

In the present study, inter- and intraobserver correlation coefficients were good when measuring SII values with different MR systems (all ICC > 0.75), which indicates an excellent repeatability. Further study demonstrated that the mutual agreement of three MR systems was satisfying as the mean differences were very small and most of the data points lied within 95% LOA. Considering that imaging parameters are typically optimized for signal-to-noise ratio (SNR) and/or scan time, a given protocol may induce significant T1-weighting bias in the fat fraction estimate [18]. Our study has also shown that the bias was not systematic but depended on specific lumbar segments and on the different MR systems.

The mean SII values measured in our study for different lumbar segments lied within the previously reported range for all three vendors and for both field strength [15], but the mean SII values were slightly higher than the literature reported, which probably resulted from the effects of T1-weighting amplification induced by the high flip angle in our study. For the same field strength of different MR vendors, we did not find a significant difference in mean SII values in any of the evaluated lumbar segments. Furthermore, the agreement of mean SII values in the same field strength was better than different field strengths. All of these pointed to the

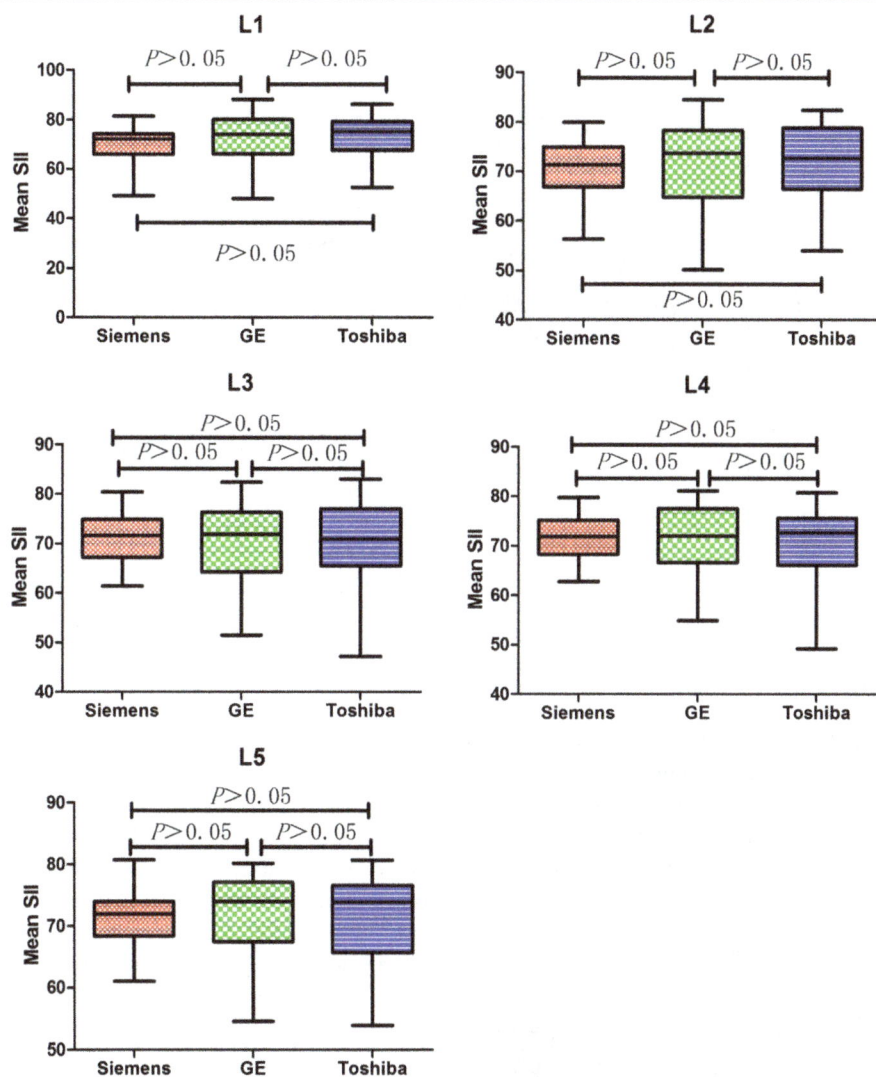

Fig. 3 Comparison of mean SII values between different MR systems. In each box, horizontal line is the median, boundaries are 25th and 75th percentiles, and whiskers are lowest and highest data points still within a 1.5 interquartile range of the lower and upper quartiles, respectively. The mean SII values in the same lumbar segment had no significant differences in three different MR vendors

conclusion that quantitative analysis for lumbar fat content with chemical shift imaging in different MR vendors of the same field strength is comparable.

With the improvements in MR technology, the theoretical advantage of an increased SNR provided by the higher field strength is paralleled by disadvantages and challenges [19, 22]. Moreover, there exists fundamental differences in the MR physics of 3.0- and 1.5-T MR systems. As a result, chemical shift MR imaging at 1.5 T cannot be applied to 3.0 T MR imaging [19]. Thus, the repeatability of different field strengths is necessary to be researched. In this context, we found no significant difference in mean SII values with 1.5- and 3.0-T MR systems, and the repeatability of mean SII values in different field strength were good. Although the literature had reported that there were two factors influencing SI

loss on OP images: chemical shift effect and susceptibility effect (i.e. T2* decay), and susceptibility effect occurred due to field strength inhomogeneity which was stronger at 3.0 T than at lower field strength [18, 19, 28], the results in our study indicated that quantitative analysis for lumbar fat content with chemical shift imaging in different field strengths MR systems may be comparable. Sebastian et al. had investigated the SII at 3.0- and 1.5-T MR imaging for prospectively quantitative analysis in a phantom study, and the result was similar to what we obtained.

In theory, the SI loss on OP images should be sensitive to differences in T1 relaxation, except for chemical shift effect and susceptibility effect [19]. With a poor choice of TE, susceptibility artifact on an OP image acquired later than an IP images can occur and may lead to the misinterpretation of a malignant adrenal lesion as a

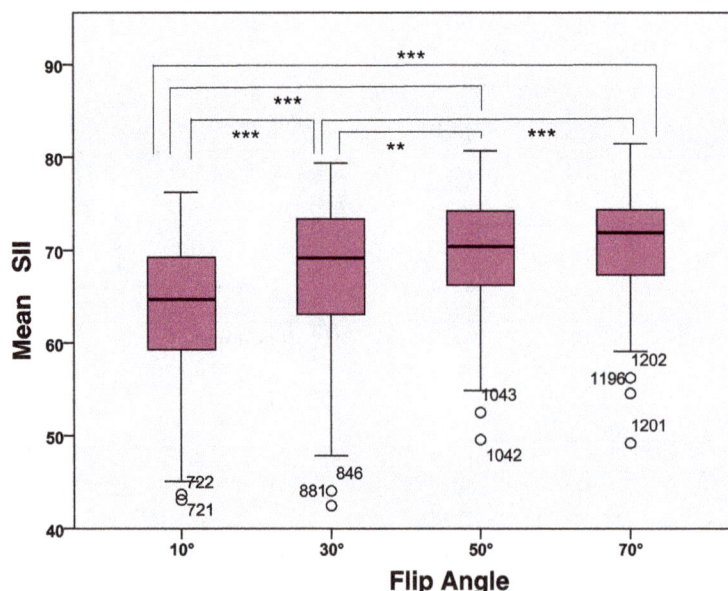

Fig. 4 Graph shows SII values for each flip angle at 3.0 T Siemens MR scanner. In each box, horizontal line is the median, boundaries are 25th and 75th percentiles, straight line (bar) on each box is the range of data distribution and empty circles represent outliers (value > 1.5 box length from the 75th and 25th percentile). **: $p < 0.01$; ***: $p < 0.001$

benign adenoma [22]. As a result, there were several studies focusing on effect of echo time in chemical shift MR imaging, but little or none literatures discuss the effects of T1 relaxation, which introduces a dependence on imaging parameters such as flip angle. In our current

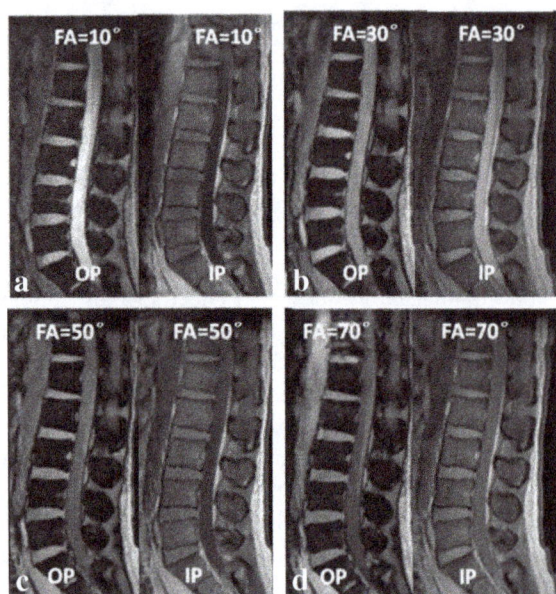

Fig. 5 Representative images of chemical shift MR imaging in different flip angles (FA, flip angle). (**a**) in-phase and opposed-phase images acquired when flip angle = 10°; (**b**) in-phase and opposed-phase images acquired when flip angle = 30°; (**c**) in-phase and opposed-phase images acquired when flip angle = 50°; (**d**) in-phase and opposed-phase images acquired when flip angle = 70°

study, we did find no significant difference between the group of flip angle 50° versus 70° while there were significant differences between other groups. Moreover, the mean SII values increased with the augment of flip angle. The reason may be that a low flip angle could decrease the SNR leading to a bias in measuring SII and smaller estimates, and/or that due to the shorter T1 of fat, a low flip angle would influence full T1 recovery and make the ratio TE/TR changed.

The result of our study indicated that chemical shit MR imaging might be applicable as a biomarker in the lumbar spine, even in multicenter studies combining different vendors and different field strengths. For instance, studies that focus on treatment-induced SII value differences can be performed with any combination of MR systems. Ongoing research could focus on providing correction factors for intervendor or interfiled strength comparisons or further optimizations of SNR to reduce overall test-retest variability.

Our study still have some limitations. Firstly, we included healthy volunteers instead of a phantom for measurements. But we aimed to simulate a clinical environment similar to clinical practice for our analysis. Secondly, we did not evaluate the reproducibility in subjects with pathology to make meaningful comparisons. A large number of patients with different diseases in various vertebrae or organs would be necessary. However, it may be difficult to acquire a large number of patients with the disease who would be willing to undergo three repeated measurements. Thirdly, subjected to the limited conditions, we did not strictly compare mean SII values between different filed strength at the same vendor. A next multicenter study will be performed to refine our research. Lastly, as SIIs measured in chemical shift MR imaging are not quantitative, quantitative MR measurement including T1 and T2 relaxation times, such as a proton density fat fraction (PDFF) should be intended in our further research.

Conclusion

In conclusion, the signal index (SII) using chemical shift MR imaging may be comparable between MR systems from different vendors and at different field strengths. In addition, high flip angles (50° or 70°) showed better stability for quantitative analysis of lumbar fat content, indicating that high flip angles should be chosen when other parameters are fixed.

Abbreviations
FA: Flip angle; ICC: Interclass correlation coefficients; IP: In phase; LOA: limits of agreement; MRI: Magnetic resonance imaging; OP: Out of phase; PDFF: Proton density fat fraction; SII: Signal intensity index; SNR: Signal-to-noise ratio; STIR: Short inversion time inversion-recovery; TR: Repetition time

Acknowledgements
None.

Funding
None.

Authors' contributions
ZX and JL participated in the design of the study, performed the experiments and the statistical analysis and drafted the manuscript. DC participated in the design of the study, performed the experiments and the statistical analysis. YZ participated in the design of the study and assisted with manuscript preparation. CL participated in the design of the study and assisted with manuscript preparation. DS assisted with manuscript preparation. All authors read and approved the final manuscript.

Competing interests
The authors declare that they have no competing interests.

Author details
[1]Department of Radiology, First Affiliated Hospital of Fujian Medical University, 20 Cha-Zhong Road, Fuzhou, Fujian 350005, China. [2]Department of Radiology, Sanming Hospital of Integrated Traditional and Western, Sanming, Fujian 365000, China.

References
1. Savci G, Yazici Z, Sahin N, Akgoz S, Tuncel E. Value of chemical shift subtraction MRI in characterization of adrenal masses. AJR Am J Roentgenol. 2006;186(1):130–5.
2. Chang JS, Taouli B, Salibi N, Hecht EM, Chin DG, Lee VS. Opposed-phase MRI for fat quantification in fat-water phantoms with 1H MR spectroscopy to resolve ambiguity of fat or water dominance. AJR Am J Roentgenol. 2006;187(1):W103–106.
3. Haider MA, Ghai S, Jhaveri K, Lockwood G. Chemical shift MR imaging of hyperattenuating (>10 HU) adrenal masses: does it still have a role? Radiology. 2004;231(3):711–6.
4. Kohl CA, Chivers FS, Lorans R, Roberts CC, Kransdorf MJ. Accuracy of chemical shift MR imaging in diagnosing indeterminate bone marrow lesions in the pelvis: review of a single institution's experience. Skeletal Radiol. 2014;43(8):1079–84.
5. Wang X, Hernando D, Reeder SB. Sensitivity of chemical shift-encoded fat quantification to calibration of fat MR spectrum. Magn Reson Med. 2016; 75(2):845–51.
6. Priola AM, Priola SM, Ciccone G, Evangelista A, Cataldi A, Gned D, Paze F, Ducco L, Moretti F, Brundu M, et al. Differentiation of rebound and lymphoid thymic hyperplasia from anterior mediastinal tumors with dual-echo chemical-shift MR imaging in adulthood: reliability of the chemical-shift ratio and signal intensity index. Radiology. 2015;274(1):238–49.
7. Tsushima Y, Ishizaka H, Matsumoto M. Adrenal masses: differentiation with chemical shift, fast low-angle shot MR imaging. Radiology. 1993;186(3):705–9.
8. Del Grande F, Santini F, Herzka DA, Aro MR, Dean CW, Gold GE, Carrino JA. Fat-suppression techniques for 3-T MR imaging of the musculoskeletal system. Radiographics. 2014;34(1):217–33.
9. Gokalp G, Mutlu FS, Yazici Z, Yildirim N. Evaluation of vertebral bone marrow fat content by chemical-shift MRI in osteoporosis. Skeletal Radiol. 2011;40(5):577–85.
10. Gokalp G, Yildirim N, Yazici Z, Ercan I. Using chemical-shift MR imaging to quantify fatty degeneration within supraspinatus muscle due to supraspinatus tendon injuries. Skeletal Radiol. 2010;39(12):1211–7.
11. Kransdorf MJ, Bridges MD. Current developments and recent advances in musculoskeletal tumor imaging. Semin Musculoskelet Radiol. 2013;17(2): 145–55.
12. Liney GP, Bernard CP, Manton DJ, Turnbull LW, Langton CM. Age, gender, and skeletal variation in bone marrow composition: a preliminary study at 3. 0 Tesla. J Magn Reson Imaging. 2007;26(3):787–93.
13. Ragab Y, Emad Y, Gheita T, Mansour M, Abou-Zeid A, Ferrari S, Rasker JJ. Differentiation of osteoporotic and neoplastic vertebral fractures by chemical shift {in-phase and out-of phase} MR imaging. Eur J Radiol. 2009; 72(1):125–33.
14. Regis-Arnaud A, Guiu B, Walker PM, Krause D, Ricolfi F, Ben Salem D. Bone marrow fat quantification of osteoporotic vertebral compression fractures: comparison of multi-voxel proton MR spectroscopy and chemical-shift gradient-echo MR imaging. Acta Radiol. 2011;52(9):1032–6.
15. Zajick Jr DC, Morrison WB, Schweitzer ME, Parellada JA, Carrino JA. Benign and malignant processes: normal values and differentiation with chemical shift MR imaging in vertebral marrow. Radiology. 2005;237(2):590–6.
16. Zampa V, Cosottini M, Michelassi C, Ortori S, Bruschini L, Bartolozzi C. Value of opposed-phase gradient-echo technique in distinguishing between benign and malignant vertebral lesions. Eur Radiol. 2002;12(7):1811–8.
17. Fujiyoshi F, Nakajo M, Fukukura Y, Tsuchimochi S. Characterization of adrenal tumors by chemical shift fast low-angle shot MR imaging: comparison of four methods of quantitative evaluation. AJR Am J Roentgenol. 2003;180(6):1649–57.
18. Bydder M, Yokoo T, Hamilton G, Middleton MS, Chavez AD, Schwimmer JB, Lavine JE, Sirlin CB. Relaxation effects in the quantification of fat using gradient echo imaging. Magn Reson Imaging. 2008;26(3):347–59.
19. Del Grande F, Subhawong T, Flammang A, Fayad LM. Chemical shift imaging at 3 Tesla: effect of echo time on assessing bone marrow abnormalities. Skeletal Radiol. 2014;43(8):1139–47.
20. Kuhn JP, Jahn C, Hernando D, Siegmund W, Hadlich S, Mayerle J, Pfannmoller J, Langner S, Reeder S. T1 bias in chemical shift-encoded liver fat-fraction: role of the flip angle. J Magn Reson Imaging. 2014;40(4):875–83.
21. Disler DG, McCauley TR, Ratner LM, Kesack CD, Cooper JA. In-phase and out-of-phase MR imaging of bone marrow: prediction of neoplasia based on the detection of coexistent fat and water. AJR Am J Roentgenol. 1997; 169(5):1439–47.

22. Schindera ST, Soher BJ, Delong DM, Dale BM, Merkle EM. Effect of echo time pair selection on quantitative analysis for adrenal tumor characterization with in-phase and opposed-phase MR imaging: initial experience. Radiology. 2008;248(1):140–7.

23. Busing KA, Kilian AK, Schaible T, Debus A, Weiss C, Neff KW. Reliability and validity of MR image lung volume measurement in fetuses with congenital diaphragmatic hernia and in vitro lung models. Radiology. 2008;246(2): 553–61.

24. Bland JM, Altman DG. Statistical methods for assessing agreement between two methods of clinical measurement. Lancet (London, England). 1986; 1(8476):307–10.

25. Bland JM, Altman DG. Measuring agreement in method comparison studies. Stat Methods Med Res. 1999;8(2):135–60.

26. Fishbein MH, Gardner KG, Potter CJ, Schmalbrock P, Smith MA. Introduction of fast MR imaging in the assessment of hepatic steatosis. Magn Reson Imaging. 1997;15(3):287–93.

27. Wismer GL, Rosen BR, Buxton R, Stark DD, Brady TJ. Chemical shift imaging of bone marrow: preliminary experience. AJR Am J Roentgenol. 1985;145(5): 1031–7.

28. Wu RH, Ducreux D, Crawley A, Lin R, Kong KM, Guo G, Luo XT, Lang ZJ, Terbrugge K, Mikulis DJ. Improving spatial signal homogeneity in MR 2D chemical shift imaging using outer volume saturation bands. Conf Proc IEEE Eng Med Biol Soc. 2004;2:1084–7.

5

T2 relaxation time for intervertebral disc degeneration in patients with upper back pain: initial results on the clinical use of 3.0 Tesla MRI

Raoying Xie[1,2†], linhui Ruan[3†], Lei chen[1†], Kai Zhou[1†], Jiandong Yuan[1†], Wei Ji[4†], Guangjian Jing[1], Xiaojing Huang[1], Qinglei Shi[5] and Chun Chen[1*]

Abstract

Background: Magnetic resonance imaging (MRI) is a useful non-invasive tool for evaluating abnormalities of intervertebral discs. However, there are few studies which applied functional MRI techniques to investigate degenerative changes in cervical and cervicothoracic junction (CTJ) spine among adults. The aim of this study was to compare T2 relaxation time measurement evaluation with morphological grading for assessing cervical and CTJ intervertebral discs (IVD) in the patients suffering neck, shoulder, and upper back pain.

Methods: Sixty-three patients (378 IVDs) and 60 asymptomatic volunteers (360 IVDs) of the cervical and CTJ discs were assessed using a 3.0 T magnetic resonance imaging (MRI) protocol, including an sagittal T2 relaxation time protocol. The relaxation time values of the nucleus pulposus (NP) were recorded and all discs were visually graded according to Pfirrman's grading system. The correlation between T2 relaxation time values and qualitative clinical grading of degeneration, patient age, sex and anatomic level were analyzed

Results: There is a clear trend of decreasing mean T2 values of the NP associate with increasing Pfirrmann grades (C2-T1) for both patients and asymptotic volunteers. Significant T2 differences were seen among grades I-V ($P < 0.05$). However, grade V was not observed in the CTJ. Linear correlation analysis revealed a strong negative association between T2 values of the NP and Pfirrmann grade ($r = -0.588$, $r = -0.808$) of C2-7 and C7T1. Age were also significantly correlated NP T2 values ($r = -0.525$, $r = -0.723$) for patients and volunteers. Moreover, the receiver operating characteristic analysis for average measures in a range from 0.70-0.79 (C2-7) to 0.84-0.89 (C7T1) for patients.

Conclusions: T2 quantitation provides a more sensitive and robust approach for detecting and characterizing the early stage of IVD degeneration and age-associated disc changes.

Keywords: Intervertebral Disc Degeneration, Cervical, T2 Relaxation Time, Magnetic Resonance Imaging, Cervicothoracic Junction

* Correspondence: chenchunkk@163.com
†Equal contributors
[1]Department of Orthopaedics, the First Affiliated Hospital, Wenzhou Medical University, Nan baixiang Road, Shangcai Village, Wenzhou 325000, Zhejiang, People's Republic of China
Full list of author information is available at the end of the article

Background

Cervical intervertebral disc (IVD) degeneration changes range from 5% to 10% in people between the ages of 20 and 30 years, to more than 50% by 45 years of age. Approximately, 90% of men over the age of 50 and 90% of women over the age of 60 have radiographic evidence of cervical spondylosis [1]. Although there are many factors that can cause chronic neck, shoulder, and upper back pain [2, 3], degeneration of the cervical spine is the most common condition contribution. Moreover, a degenerative IVD in the cervicothoracic junction (CTJ) can also result in above syndromes [4].

Magnetic resonance imaging (MRI) is a promising non-invasive examining tool for evaluating abnormalities of IVD. Age and degeneration can be reflected by signal variation of the discs on T2-weighted images (T2WIs), which allows for the determination of degree of disc degeneration [5]. Specifically, changes in MRI signal strength, which related to water and proteoglycan (PG) content in the nucleus pulposus (NP), can indicate disc degeneration according to Pfirrmann grading system [5, 6]. However, a reliable quantification characterized by loss of water or PG in an intact disc is not provided in such system to evaluate the degenerative degree in early intervertebral disc degeneration (IVDD) stages.

Recently, several quantitative MRI techniques for evaluation of IVD have been used for evaluating disc degeneration [7–9]. In particular, The T2 relaxation time is the decay constant for T2 signal intensity (SI) in MRI which is an intrinsic property of the tissue reflecting the molecular environment created in the disc by water, proteins, fat, collagen, and other solutes [8]. Increased T2 relaxation times is associated with increased disc water or glycosaminoglycan content, the primary component of PG [8, 9]. A good correlation of T2 values and water content in lumbar IVD tissue has been the subject of many previous studies [10–13] and has been widely validated. In cervical spine, our research firstly evaluated early cervical IVDD quantified by T2 values MRI in asymptomatic young adults [11]. The results in our study confirmed that T2 relaxation time can be potentially used as a clinical tool to identify early IVDD and to formalize a reliable quantitative scale. However, to our knowledge, there are few studies to investigate degenerative changes in cervical and CTJ spine of adults using this functional MRI technique.

Therefore, the purpose of this study was to use the quantitative T2 relaxation time measurement of 3.0 T MRI to evaluate the degree of cervical and CTJ degenerative IVDs, comparing with Pfirrmann grading in a larger cohort of young-to-middle-aged patients with neck, shoulder, and upper back pain.

Methods

Ethics statement and study sample

The study was approved by the institutional review board of the First Affiliated Hospital, Wenzhou Medical University and all participants provided written informed consent prior to enrollment. This study involved 63 patients (26 male, 37 female, average age, 39.88 ± 12.47 years; range: 20–76 Y/O., 378 discs in total) and 60 asymptomatic volunteers (32 male, 28 female; average age, 37.64 ± 10.65 years, range: 22–70 Y/O., 360 discs in total) in our initial study, who accepted MRI scan of their cervical spine from C2 to T1. They were consecutively recruited and evaluated from September 2014 to May 2015. The subjects were excluded if they had diabetes mellitus, major systemic disease, serious illness (e.g., tumor, infection), back surgery, spinal fractures, or osteoporosis. They consisted of patients with back pain and/or brachial plexus neuralgia. The following inclusion criteria was applied: the patients had significant neurological symptoms, which were defined as upper back pain for > 2 weeks and severe enough to require physician consultation or treatment, including neck or arm weakness, numbness, or tingling [14]. In parallel, inclusion criteria of asymptomatic volunteers referenced are reported by Pfirrmann et al. [5], which observed the process of normal aging in the lumbar discs, as follows: 1) no upper back pain within the last 5 years, 2) never absent from work due to upper back pain or numbness, and 3) no history of consulting a physician due to upper back pain, arm weakness, numbness or tingling [11].

MR image acquisition

A GE Signa HDx 3.0 T MRI machine (GE Healthcare, Milwaukee, WI, USA) with a spine coil was used for MRI scanning. All MR images in this study were obtained in the afternoon to minimize the diurnal variation of T2 values in the IVDs [15]. Sagittal T1-weighted fast spin echo (FSE), and sagittal, transversal, and axial T2-WIs-FSE sequences were used for morphological MRI. T2-WIs (Time repetition (TR) 2560 ms, Time echo (TE) 102 ms, received band width [RBW] ± 31.25 kHz, field of view [FOV] 24 × 24 cm, matrix 320 × 224, slice thickness/gap 3 mm/0.5 mm, number of excitations [NEX] 4, total scan time 2 min and 18 s) were obtained and a radiologist blindly ranked the severity of disc degeneration as grade I to V in the midsagittal section according to the Pfirrmann classification (see Additional file 1: Table S1). Thereafter, a T2 map was generated on the midsagittal section, which was chosen from sagittal sections of cervical midline, by using the optimal T2 values obtained at a sequence of 8 echo multi-spin echo (TR/first echo TE, last echo TE, 3000/8.5-67.9, RBW ±31.25 kHz, FOV 18 × 18 cm, matrix 256 × 160, slice thickness/gap 3 mm/0.5 mm, NEX 1, total scan time

4 min and 27 s). All T2 map images were generated on the Advantage Workstation (version 4.3, Functool; GE Healthcare, Milwaukee, WA, USA) [10]. However, the first echo from the multi-spin system was excluded to minimize the effect of the stimulated echo.

Image analysis

Evaluation of all morphological images were performed by two radiologists in consensus, one with more than 10 years of experience and a special interest in musculo-skeletal radiology, and the other one with more than 20 years of experience in orthopedic radiology. Though challenging to appraise cervical or lumbar MRI [13], no obvious transitional vertebrae were detected. For measurement, to evaluate regions of interest (ROIs) in a standardized and reproducible way, we decided to adopt a previous reported method [7, 16, 17]. By using T2-WI as reference, regions of interest (ROIs) were manually drawn over the T2 map of the discs by an orthopedic consultant (GJ) with 20 years' experience reading MRI images. The geometrical center of the ellipses were defined to the intervertebral area ROIs only included the NP area. All ROIs were selected on the morphological images and transferred via "copy and paste" into the T2 maps with areas of 9.25 ± 1.38 mm^2 to cover the NP using the software. All of data was measured by three times in order to reduce error. The exemplary Pfirrmann grades were shown in Fig. 1.

Inter- and intraobserver analysis

The intra- and interobserver variability of the ROI evaluation was assessed. Two central sagittal slices of T2 map were evaluated as already described. The evaluation was performed by two independent observers with different skill levels (musculoskeletal radiologist with 15 years of experience [observer 1], orthopedic surgeon with 20 years of experience [observer 2]). In addition, observer A and B performed the same analysis twice, with an interval of one month, to test intraobserver agreement.

Statistical analysis

Statistical analysis and graph drawing were performed using SPSS 19.0 (SPSS Inc., Chicago, IL, USA). Descriptive statistical data are given as mean ± standard deviation (Mean ± SD). To evaluate the reliability of Pfirrmann grading, intraobserver and interobserver agreements were graded through Kappa statistics. The degree of internal consistency was considered as: strong consistency, $k \geq 0.7$; moderate consistency, $0.7 \geq k > 0.4$; and weak consistency $k \leq 0.4$. One-way ANOVA and Student Newman-Keuls test were used to detect the statistical differences of T2 values between different Pfirrmann grades. Additionally, Receiver operating characteristic (ROC) curves were plotted to test the sensitivity and specificity of T2 measures in assessment of Pfirrmann grade. Areas under the ROC curves were calculated. The statistical difference of T2 measures used to evaluate Pfirrmann grade was determined by U-test. All tests above were considered significant with $P < 0.05$.

Results

Morphological MRI findings

Tables 1 and 2 show the characteristics of all analyzed discs sorted by the Pfirrmann degeneration grade of C2-T1 of patients and asymptomatic volunteers, respectively. According to the Pfirrmann grades, 13 and 48 discs (3.43%, 13.33%) were classified as grade I, 117 and 84 discs (30.95%, 23.33%) as grade II, 142 and 107 discs

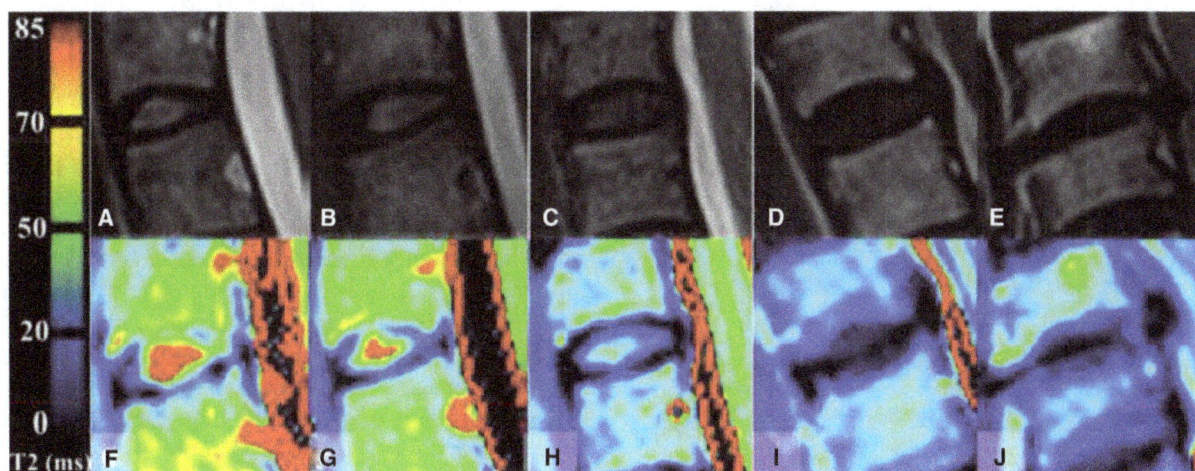

Fig. 1 Sagittal T2-weighted FSE images and corresponding T2 maps of discs with different Pfirrmann grades. **a** and **f** grade I; (**b** and **g**) grade II; P (**c** and **h**) grade III; (**d** and **i**) grade IV; (**e** and **j**) grade V

Table 1 Degeneration grade according to Pfirrmann scale, and disc level of the cervical intervertebral discs of patients analyzed in study

Degeneration Grade/N	Disc Levels						
	C2-3	C3-4	C4-5	C5-6	C6-7	C7T1	Total
I	3	1	2	0	0	7	13
II	19	23	23	11	15	26	117
III	25	24	26	22	25	20	142
IV	10	9	11	18	14	10	72
V	6	6	1	12	9	0	34
Total	63	63	63	63	63	63	378

(37.56%, 29.72%) as grade III, 72 and 69 disc (19.04%, 19.16%) as grade IV, and 34 and 52 discs as grade V (8.99%, 14.44%).

Inter- and intraobserver agreement
Regarding the Pfirrmann grading reproducibility by the 2 readers, the intraobserver test yielded k values ranging from 0.826 ($p = 0.000$) to 0.793 ($P = 0.000$), whereas the interobserver test produced k values of 0.757 ($P = 0.000$).

Results regarding pfirrmann classification
The mean value of T2 relaxation time at different regions of each Pfirrmann grade are presented in table 2 and table 3. As to patients, in the NP of C2-T1, T2 values tended to decrease with increasing Pfirrmann grades, and T2 values were significantly different when comparing grades I to V ($P < 0.01$, Table 3). However, Pfirrmann grade V was not observed among C7T1 discs. Regarding the T2 values of NP, significance was detected between T2 values of asymptomatic volunteers in the different Pfirrmann grades (Table 2). The Spearman

Table 2 T2 values in different level groups of asymptomatic volunteers

Pfirrmann Grade	No.	T2 values (mean, ms) C2-7	No.	T2 values (mean, ms) C7T1
I	35	71.98 ± 12.34	13	85.45 ± 19.53
II	68	64.25 ± 11.28@	16	73.49 ± 15.44$
III	87	62.76 ± 9.37@	20	67.72 ± 9.71$%
IV	58	50.39 ± 10.75@#^	11	54.60 ± 8.11$%~
V	52	41.23 ± 7.73@#^&	—	—
Total/average	300	59.65 ± 9.55	60	68.71 ± 13.14

Mean values (±standard deviation) of T2 relaxation times in milliseconds in different compartments of the cervical intervertebral disc for different Pfirrmann groups are shown. NP, nucleus pulposus. @ Compared with T2 values of NP of grade I for C2-7, $P < 0.000$; #Compared with T2 values of NP of grade II for C2-7, $P < 0.000$; ^Compared with T2 values of NP of grade III for C2-7, $P < 0.002$; &Compared with T2 values of NP of grade V for C2-7, $P < 0.05$; $ Compared with T2 values of NP of grade I for C7T1, $P < 0.004$; %Compared with T2 values of NP of grade II for C7T1, $P < 0.000$; ~Compared with T2 values of NP of grade III for C7T1, $P < 0.05$

Table 3 T2 values for discs with different Pfirrmann grades

Grade	T2 (mean ± SD, ms, C2-7)		T2 (mean ± SD, ms, C7T1)	
	No.	NP	No.	NP
I	6	62.99 ± 13.47	7	83.20 ± 17.59
II	91	50.75 ± 7.75@	26	58.46 ± 8.42$
III	122	44.83 ± 6.95@#	20	46.91 ± 4.98$%
IV	62	40.20 ± 5.62@#^	10	39.13 ± 5.13$~
V	34	34.93 ± 9.53@#^&	—	
Total	315	46.19 ± 9.37	63	57.02 ± 16.01

Mean values (±standard deviation) of T2 relaxation times in milliseconds in different compartments of the cervical intervertebral disc for different Pfirrmann groups are shown. NP, nucleus pulposus. @ Compared with T2 values of NP of grade I for C2-7, $P < 0.000$; #Compared with T2 values of NP of grade II for C2-7, $P < 0.000$; ^Compared with T2 values of NP of grade III for C2-7, $P < 0.002$; &Compared with T2 values of NP of grade V for C2-7, $P < 0.05$; $ Compared with T2 values of NP of grade I for C7T1, $P < 0.004$; %Compared with T2 values of NP of grade II for C7T1, $P < 0.000$; ~Compared with T2 values of NP of grade III for C7T1, $P < 0.05$

correlation analysis indicated a strong negative correlation between the Pfirrmann grade and the T2 values of NP ($r = -0.588$; $P = 0.000$; $r = -0.808$, $P = 0.000$) of C2-7 and C7T1. Furthermore, significant correlation between age and T2 value of NP was demonstrated both in patient group ($r = -0.525$, $P = 0.000$) and volunteer group ($r = -0.723$, $P = 0.000$). The overall mean value of T2 relaxation time of volunteer group was 59.65 ± 9.55 ms, which was significantly larger than its counterpart of patient group (46.19 ± 9.37 ms, 23.57% reduction, $P < 0.01$). Similarly, the mean value of T2 value of the 315 discs from patient group was significantly lower than that from volunteer group (57.02 ± 16.01 ms versus 68.71 ± 13.14 ms, 8.29% reduction, $P < 0.05$). At the same degeneration grade, the T2 values of patients were relatively smaller comparing to the T2 values of volunteers. As shown in table 4, the significant differences of sensitivity, specificity, area under the ROC curve (AUC) and T2 cut-off value between different Pfirrmann grades of C2-7 and C7T1, were demonstrated respectively ($P < 0.05$) by conducting U-test.

Discussion
In this prospective study, we developed and investigated an MRI method, applicable for conventional 3.0 Tesla units, for sagittal T2 mapping of cervical and CTJ IVDs in symptomatic patients and asymptomatic volunteers and then compared against the Pfirrmann grades which can be used in a clinical set-up. The results of this study suggest that negative correlations between T2 values and disc degeneration grades. More important, the results indicate that the IVDD of CTJ exist, range from grade I to IV. To the best of our knowledge, the present study is the first who use asymptomatic volunteers and symptomatic population to investigate the correlation between T2

values and Pfirrmann changes in the inner portion of cervical IVDs. This study suggests that T2 relaxation time can be sensitive to early degenerative changes in cervical IVDD.

MRI is commonly used in the clinical setting for examination of the degeneration of bone, cartilage and other tissues [6, 8, 13, 14]. Additionally, T2 mapping MRI has greater advantages over other methods of detecting matrix content [18]. The T2 relaxation time is able to provide superior information of early molecular and physiological alterations in IVDs as follows: 1) improving identification of IVDD in its early stages; 2) evaluating outcomes of biological treatments and 3) implementing continuous quantitative assessments of IVDD [8, 9, 12]. With the development of IVD tissue engineering, the T2 values can be used to follow regenerative progress of the NP, non-invasively.

Most previous studies emphasized T2 changes in the lumbar IVDD without consideration of cervical and CTJ [4]. Only our previous study reported a decrease of NP T2 values in asymptomatic healthy young adults [10]. Comparing with healthy young adults, the different grades of T2 values were smaller (grade I: 62.99 vs. 72.25 ms; II: 50.75 vs.59.36 ms; III: 44.83 vs. 51.73 ms) [10]. However, the T2 values of asymptomatic volunteers were relatively lager comparing with results in current study. The 3.0 T field used in the study and the different composition of subjects might contribute to the difference. The increase of regional T2 values will occur due to the magic angle effect when collagen fibers are oriented 54.7° relative to the orientation of the static magnetic field (B0) [19]. This effect can be shown inevitably in the annulus fibrosus, especially near its surface [20]. In view of this situation, the ROI in the present study only encompassed NP and inner annulus fibrosus. In our study, the T2 values of the discs with Pfirrmann grade IV-V (40.20 ms; 34.93 ms) were substantially lower than the discs with Pfirrmann grade I-III. There was a significant difference between the T2 values of the NPs with Pfirrmann grade IV and V. Previous studies have demonstrated that T2 values in the NP and AF decrease in accordance with lumbar IVDD, and, ultimately, difference in T2 SI between this two anatomical structures close to zero [21], which is consistent with results of the former study. Thus, comparison of T2 values of NP may also be valuable in the evaluation of disc degeneration. Moreover, the T2 values in cervical discs were lower than those previously results in healthy lumbar discs [12, 13, 22].

A degeneration IVD can also occur in CTJ. Strictly speaking, CTJ should contain the C7 vertebra, the disc between C7 and T1, and attachment of ligaments [4]. C7T1 disc herniation is responsible for less than 5% of all the cervical disc herniations [23]. In most of these patients, the common presenting symptom involving hand weakness and pain radiating to the lateral aspect of the hand were the same symptom as C2-7 IVD herniation [23]. Moreover, previous study reported that the incidence of the disc degeneration at C7T1 is 42% [24]. Another study reported cases that C7T1 IVDD occurred after C5-7 fusion [25]. Therefore, the clinical importance of the CTJ region may be related to the claimed concerning of region with neck and shoulder pain [26] and should be emphasized. In our study, T2 values of NP of C7T1 were higher than C2-7 with regard to Pfirrmann I and II, however, we found that most observations of C7T1 show no difference with the results of C2-7, The same as C2-7, the decreasing T2 values among different grades might attribute to decreasing water content and structural disorganization with severity increasing of disc degeneration.

Some previous studies showed no significant difference in T2 values between grade IV and V [12, 13] of lumbar which was in disagree with our present study. This difference may attribute to the various biochemical properties between cervical and lumbar IVDs, and measurement method. In accordance with our previous study, the T2 values were lower than former reported in lumbar discs [9, 13] which was a result of different biochemical changes among cervical, thoracic and lumbar [21].

It is important to realize that the correlation coefficients of T2 values of NP referring to grades and T2 values obtained in this study range between moderate and strong. This might be attributed to the relative large sample size. Moreover, the results also explained that the T2 value in the IVD is known to be sensitive to the composition of the collagen network structure and water content. Previous study reported that the T2 values are influenced by both rotational and translational motion which result in dipole-dipole interaction of water molecules in the collagen matrix [6].

Sekhon et al. confirmed a good to excellent correlation of T2 values, water content and PG content in IVD tissue [27]. Moreover, the inverse correlation has been observed between age and T2 values in the current study and several former studies [28]. As we known, it is difficult to distinguish a painful degenerative disc from one with age-related physiologic changes, therefore, we recruited a well-defined asymptomatic population for the current study for inspecting the effect of aging on T2 values. Given that previous studies recruited and analyzed IVDs of asymptomatic volunteers [11, 28], we had a much wider range of age resemble those researches and were a discrepancy compared to that in a previous study [29], which confirmed the inverse correlation between age and T2 values only for grade II discs in 20 patients with lumbar back pain or radiculopathy. However, it is important to point out that we did not consider the equivalence of age range and the balanced age distribution, that could introduce influence when analyze difference of disc degeneration for both the asymptomatic and symptomatic groups. Nevertheless, some authors also confirmed that T2 value is useful to evaluate IVDD after either distinguishing age groups or not [12].

The T2 maps can be generated and measured immediately after MRI scan, and the ROI analysis takes about 3 min for each patient. Moreover, an automated segmentation of the IVDs may facilitate acquiring promising initial data attribute to ongoing efforts in the future. Therefore, quantitative information reflecting the biochemical composition of IVDs can be provided without extensive increase in time.

ROC between each grade of the NP generated cut-off values obtaining from area under the curve (AUC) values for disc degeneration quantification via T2 SI. In this study, it was in consistent with previous study [12, 13] that all AUC values were within the moderate accuracy range, indicating a moderate level of reliability. These data demonstrated that this T2 value-based grade scale for the NP is a useful distinguishing system. Furthermore, the high correlation in the inter- and intraobserver analysis suggest that our standardized ROI positioning is adequately reproducible.

Naturally, this study has some limitations. Firstly, the major limitation of our study is no histological or biochemical analysis of IVDs performing. Secondly, partial volume effects still existed attributing to subjectivity and bias of ROIs selection. Thirdly, we did not compare some other imaging techniques such as T1p, T2*(star) or ADC and so on to results of T2 relaxation time [22, 30, 31], however, many studies had verified the practicability of this technique alone to diagnose lumbar IVDD [15, 32]. Additionally, the CTJ structure is not strictly defined. Some investigators involve thoracic 2 and sometimes thoracic 3 vertebrae and thoracic 2–3 disc and associated ligaments when discussing the CTJ, however, lesions involving the thoracic 2 and thoracic 3 vertebrae often face similar difficulties in reaching them through an anterior approach [4]. What's more, a selection bias surely exists in the subject enrollment of all clinical prospective studies and cannot be fully removed. Exclusion criteria used in our study included diseases such as diabetes mellitus, major systemic disease, tumor, infection, back surgery, and so on, of which back pain is the main complain, and the IVDs of the patients who suffering those diseases are prone to degeneration [33, 34]. We established the same exclusion criteria for all participants in order to minimize the influence of selection bias. Furthermore, thoracic 2–3 IVDs should be studied in the future for better understanding of CTJ.

Conclusions

In summary, our results proved a negative correlation between T2 values of cervical and CTJ IVDs and the Pfirrmann grades regarding IVDD. What should be highlighted is that we proposed the distinct cut-off values of the classification based on quantitative evaluation. Thus, the T2 value-based measurements of IVD water content and PG may be useful for estimating cervical and CTJ degenerative disc diseases.

Abbreviations

AF: Annulus fibrosus; AUC: Area under the curve; C: Cervical; CTJ: Cervicothoracic junction; FOV: Field of view; FSE: Fast spin echo; IVD: Intervertebral disc; IVDD: Intervertebral disc degeneration; MRI: Magnetic resonance imaging; NEX: Number of excitations; NP: Nucleus pulposus; PG: Proteoglycan; RBW: Received band width; ROC: Receiver operating characteristic; ROI: Regions of interest; SD: Standard deviation.; SI: Signal intensity; T2WIs: T2-weighted images; TE: Echo time; TR: Repetition time

Acknowledgements

Not applicable.

Funding

This work was supported by the Wenzhou Public Welfare Science and Technology Research Project (Y20160130) the Projects of Medical and Health Technology program in Zhejiang province (2017175018) .

Authors' contributions

JD, GJ, QL and XJ analyzed the data. CC, LH, and LC participated in the design of the study and performed the statistical analysis. CC RY WJ, QL and KZ conceived of the study, and participated in its design and coordination and helped to draft the manuscript. All authors read and approved the final manuscript.

Authors' information

Not applicable.

Competing interests

The authors declare that they have no competing interests.

Author details

[1]Department of Orthopaedics, the First Affiliated Hospital, Wenzhou Medical University, Nan baixiang Road, Shangcai Village, Wenzhou 325000, Zhejiang, People's Republic of China. [2]Department of Radiation and chemotherapy division, the First Affiliated Hospital, Wenzhou Medical University, Wenzhou, Zhejiang, People's Republic of China. [3]Department of Neurosurgery, the First Affiliated Hospital of Wenzhou Medical University, Wenzhou, Zhejiang, People's Republic of China. [4]Department of Orthopaedics, Navy General Hospital, Beijing, People's Republic of China. [5]Siemens Ltd, China Healthcare Sector MR Business Group, Beijing, People's Republic of China.

References

1. Grob D. Surgery in the degenerative cervical spine. Spine. 1998;23:2674–83.
2. Trinh K, Cui X, Wang YJ. Chinese herbal medicine for chronic neck pain due to cervical degenerative disc disease. Spine (Phila Pa 1976). 2010;35:2121–7.
3. Ehrmann Feldman D, Shrier I, Rossignol M, Abenhaim L. Risk factors for the development of neck and upper limb pain in adolescents. Spine (Phila Pa 1976). 2002;27:523–8.
4. Williams FM, Sambrook PN. Neck and back pain and intervertebral disc degeneration: role of occupational factors. Best Pract Res Clin Rheumatol. 2011;25:69–79.
5. Wang VY, Chou D. The cervicothoracic junction. Neurosurg Clin N Am. 2007; 18:365–71.
6. Pfirrmann CW, Metzdorf A, Zanetti M, Hodler J, Boos N. Magnetic resonance classification of lumbar intervertebral disc degeneration. Spine (Phila Pa 1976). 2001;26:1873–78.
7. Zou J, Yang H, Miyazaki M, Morishita Y, Wei F, McGovern S, et al. Dynamic bulging of intervertebral discs in the degenerative lumbar spine. Spine (Phila Pa 1976). 2009;34:2545–50.
8. Chen C, Jia Z, Han Z, Gu T, Li W, Li H, et al. Quantitative T2 relaxation time and magnetic transfer ratio predict endplate biochemical content of intervertebral disc degeneration in a canine model. BMC Musculoskelet Disord. 2015;16:157.
9. Fields AJ, Han M, Krug R, Lotz JC. Cartilaginous end plates: quantitative MR imaging with very short echo times-orientation dependence and correlation with biochemical composition. Radiology. 2015;274:482–9.
10. Ogon I, Takebayashi T, Takashima H, Tanimoto K, Ida K, Yoshimoto M, et al. Analysis of chronic low back pain with magnetic resonance imaging T2 mapping of lumbar intervertebral disc. J Orthop Sci. 2015;20:295–301.
11. Chen C, Huang M, Han Z, Shao L, Xie Y, Wu J, et al. Quantitative T2 magnetic resonance imaging compared to morphological grading of the early cervical intervertebral disc degeneration: an evaluation approach in asymptomatic young adults. PLoS One. 2014;9:e87856.
12. Niu G, Yu X, Yang J, Wang R, Zhang S, Guo Y. Apparent diffusion coefficient in normal and abnormal pattern of intervertebral lumbar discs: initial experience. J Biomed Res. 2011;25:197–203.
13. Stelzeneder D, Welsch GH, Kovacs BK, Goed S, Paternostro-Sluga T, Vlychou M, et al. Quantitative T2 evaluation at 3.0T compared to morphological grading of the lumbar intervertebral disc: a standardized evaluation approach in patients with low back pain. Eur J Radiol. 2012;81:324–30.
14. Takashima H, Takebayashi T, Yoshimoto M, Terashima Y, Tsuda H, Ida K, et al. Correlation between T2 relaxation time and intervertebral disk degeneration. Skeletal Radiol. 2012;41:163–7.
15. Hanvold TN, Veiersted KB, Waersted M. A prospective study of neck, shoulder, and upper back pain among technical school students entering working life. J Adolesc Health. 2010;46:488–94.
16. Souza RB, Baum T, Wu S, Feeley BT, Kadel N, Li X, et al. Effects of unloading on knee articular cartilage T1rho and T2 magnetic resonance imaging relaxation times: a case series. J Orthop Sports Phys Ther. 2012;42:511–20.
17. Nagashima M, Abe H, Amaya K, Matsumoto H, Yanaihara H, Nishiwaki Y, et al. A method for quantifying intervertebral disc signal intensity on T2-weighted imaging. Acta Radiol. 2012;53:1059–65.
18. Cai F, Wu XT, Xie XH, Wang F, Hong X, Zhuang SY, et al. Evaluation of intervertebral disc regeneration with implantation of bone marrow mesenchymal stem cells (BMSCs) using quantitative T2 mapping: a study in rabbits. Int Orthop. 2015;39:149–59.
19. Wang YX, Zhao F, Griffith JF, Mok GS, Leung JC, Ahuja AT, et al. T1rho and T2 relaxation times for lumbar disc degeneration: an in vivo comparative study at 3.0-tesla MRI. Eur Radiol. 2013;23:228–34.
20. Xia Y. Magic-angle effect in magnetic resonance imaging of articular cartilage: a review. Invest Radiol. 2000;35:602–21.
21. Van Breuseghem I, Bosmans HT, Elst LV, Maes F, Pans SD, Brys PP, et al. T2 mapping of human femorotibial cartilage with turbo mixed MR imaging at 1.5 T: feasibility. Radiology. 2004;233:609–14.
22. Blumenkrantz G, Zuo J, Li X, Kornak J, Link TM, Majumdar S. In vivo 3.0-tesla magnetic resonance T1rho and T2 relaxation mapping in subjects with intervertebral disc degeneration and clinical symptoms. Magn Reson Med. 2010;63:1193–200.
23. Chiu EJ, Newitt DC, Segal MR, Hu SS, Lotz JC, Majumdar S. Magnetic resonance imaging measurement of relaxation and water diffusion in the human lumbar intervertebral disc under compression in vitro. Spine (Phila Pa 1976). 2001;26:E437-44.
24. An HS, Anderson PA, Haughton VM, Iatridis JC, Kang JD, Lotz JC, et al. Introduction: disc degeneration: summary. Spine (Phila Pa 1976). 2004;29:2677–8.
25. Maquer G, Laurent M, Brandejsky V, Pretterklieber ML, Zysset PK. Finite element-based Non-linear normalization of human lumbar intervertebral disc stiffness to account for its morphology. J Biomech Eng. 2014;136:061003.
26. Post NH, Cooper PR, Frempong-Boadu AK, Costa ME. Unique features of herniated discs at the cervicothoracic junction: clinical presentation, imaging, operative management, and outcome after anterior decompressive operation in 10 patients. Neurosurgery. 2006;58:497–501.
27. Sekhon L. Cervicothoracic junction arthroplasty after previous fusion surgery for adjacent segment degeneration: case report. Neurosurgery. 2005;56: E205.
28. Norlander S, Gustavsson BA, Lindell J, Nordgren B. Reduced mobility in the cervico-thoracic motion segment–a risk factor for musculoskeletal neck-shoulder pain: a two-year prospective follow-up study. Scand J Rehabil Med. 1997;29:167–74.
29. Wang YX, Griffith JF, Leung JC, Yuan J. Age related reduction of T1rho and T2 magnetic resonance relaxation times of lumbar intervertebral disc. Quant Imaging Med Surg. 2014;4:259–64.
30. Noriega DC, Marcia S, Ardura F, Lite IS, Marras M, Saba L. Diffusion-weighted MRI assessment of adjacent disc degeneration after thoracolumbar vertebral fractures. Cardiovasc Intervent Radiol. 2016;39:1306–14.
31. Huang M, Guo Y, Ye Q, Chen L, Zhou K, Wang Q, et al. Correlation between T2* (T2 star) relaxation time and cervical intervertebral disc degeneration: an observational study. Medicine (Baltimore). 2016;95:e4502.
32. Zobel BB, Vadala G, Del Vescovo R, Battisti S, Martina FM, Stellato L, et al. T1rho magnetic resonance imaging quantification of early lumbar intervertebral disc degeneration in healthy young adults. Spine (Phila Pa 1976). 2012;37:1224–30.
33. Lotan R, Oron A, Anekstein Y, Shalmon E, Mirovsky Y. Lumbar stenosis and systemic diseases: is there any relevance? J Spinal Disord Tech. 2008;21:247–51.
34. Sierra-Jimenez G, Sanchez-Ortiz A, Aceves-Avila FJ, Hernandez-Rios G, Durán-Barragán S, Ramos-Remus C. Tendinous and ligamentous derangements in systemic lupus erythematosus. J Rheumatol. 2008;35:2187–91.

6

Preoperative axillary lymph node staging by ultrasound-guided cytology using a four-level sonographic score

Caroline De Coninck[*], Jean-Christophe Noël, Rachel Boutemy and Philippe Simon

Abstract

Background: The staging of axillary lymph nodes is critical to the management and prognosis of breast cancer, the most frequent cancer in females. Neoadjuvant therapy and lymph node dissection are recommended when malignant cells invade the lymph nodes. Therefore the pre-operative examination of these lymph nodes is crucial to treatment.

Methods: In this study, we examined the effectiveness of cytology through ultrasound-guided fine needle aspiration (USG-FNA) and ultrasound (US) imaging using an established classification system in correctly identifying lymph node status compared to the final histological results after surgery.

Results: Cytology by USG-FNA and US classification were found to be promising methods of axillary lymph node staging.

Conclusions: US and CB offer minimally invasive techniques to pre-operatively examine these lymph nodes in patients with primary breast cancer.

Keywords: Axillary lymph nodes, Breast cancer, Ultrasound, Cytology, Metastasis

Background

Breast cancer is the most frequent female cancer [1] and the second leading cause of female cancer death in Belgium [2]. Therefore, breast cancer management is critically important. When an axillary lymph node is invaded, neoadjuvant chemotherapy and axillary lymph node dissection are indicated [3, 4]. In terms of survival, it is now widely accepted that there are advantages of neoadjuvant chemotherapy in patients with node-positive breast cancer [3, 4]. Axillary lymph node status is an important factor in the prognosis and management of breast cancer. Several methods to detect positive axillary lymph nodes during the pre-operative diagnosis have been evaluated, including ultrasound-guided fine needle aspiration (USG-FNA) cytology, ultrasound-guided biopsy and, as an imaging method, axillary ultrasound [5]. If a positive lymph node is not found during the pre-operative evaluation, a less invasive sentinel node biopsy will be utilized instead of axillary lymph

node dissection [6]. The goal of this study was to compare the results of axillary lymph node status by cell-block obtained through fine-needle aspiration [7] and by axillary ultrasound, according to a classification system derived from Stavros [8].

Methods

Patient dataset

The Hôpital Erasme ethics committee approved this study. All the results were analyzed retrospectively and anonymously.

This study included a series of 208 cell or cyto-blocks (CB) of axillary or para-axillary (chest wall, subclavicular and intra-mammary) lymph nodes from 184 patients (141 patients with one, 18 patients with two, one patient with three, and one patient with four evaluated lymph nodes) with primary breast cancer from a university center collected between October 2008 and August 2012.

Fine-needle aspirations were performed on all patients by a radiologist using a 21-gauge, ultrasonographic (US)-

* Correspondence: caroline.de.coninck@ulb.ac.be
Erasme Hospital, 808 route de Lennik, 1070 Anderlecht, Belgium

guided needle prior to any operative procedure on the breast or axilla, regardless of whether the nodes appeared normal or abnormal.

Lymph node classification

Lymph nodes were classified into four categories according to criteria derived from Stavros' classification: normal "N", minimally suspect "+", mildly suspect "++" and highly suspect "+++". The details of these classifications are as follows:

- "+": lymph node with a maximum size of cortical thickness of 3 mm with regular capsular thickening
- "++": lymph node with irregular capsular thickening (with notches) or with regular capsular thickening and cortical thickness greater than 3 mm in size
- "+++": complete loss of lymph node structure; irregular cortex or absence of lymph node hilum.

Normal or "+" lymph nodes were considered non-suspicious, and "++" and "+++" lymph nodes were considered suspicious (Fig. 1).

Cytoblock and cytospin techniques

The sample obtained by US-guided fine-needle aspiration (USG-FNA) was placed in Saccomanno fluid and sent to the laboratory where it was separated into two samples: one for the CB technique and one for the cytospin technique. Both samples were centrifuged at 1400 rpm for 10 min. The cytospin sample was placed in a Shandon EZ Cytofunnel® with a few drops of concentration solution, then placed in the Shandon Cytospin®4 centrifuge for 10 min at 500 rpm. It was then placed on a microscope slide for cytologic analysis. For CB, 2–4 drops of Reagent 2 from the cytoblock kit were added to the pellet, and it was resuspended and incubated for one minute. Two to four drops of Reagent 1 from the kit were added, causing polymerization. After one minute, the resulting polymerized material was placed between two sponges in a standard cassette and routinely processed with other biopsies and paraffin-embedded blocks. Four-micron sections were cut and stained with hematoxylin and eosin. Immunohistochemistry (IHC) was performed on each cytoblock using broad-spectrum cytokeratin primary antibodies (clone AE1-AE3, dilution: 1/100, Dakocytomation, Glostrup, Denmark).

The CB results were classified into one of three categories: "C1" inadequate, "C2" negative and "C5" malignant.

Histological assessment

From the 208 CBs, only 93 had final histological confirmation of axillary lymph nodes after axillary lymph node dissection or sentinel node biopsy. These were categorized as either negative, when all of the examined lymph nodes were negative for metastasis, or positive, when there was evidence of metastasis in one or more lymph nodes. The same histopathologist performed histological assessments. Of the 93 results, only 54 had no neoadjuvant chemotherapy and were thus interpretable (Fig. 2).

The results were analyzed according to the type of breast cancer, the size of the evaluated lymph nodes, type of surgery (sentinel node biopsy or axillary lymph node dissection), surgeon, radiologist, patient's age, patient's BMI, and the presence or absence of neoadjuvant chemotherapy.

Results

Ninety-three CBs from 80 patients who underwent surgery had histological confirmation of axillary lymph nodes after sentinel node biopsy or axillary lymph node dissection. The 80 patients were between 28 and 84 years old. Tumor size was between 4 and 85 mm, and the axillary lymph node size was between 5 and 42 mm. In 73 cases, an axillary lymph node dissection was performed, and in 20 cases a sentinel node biopsy was performed.

Because 39 patients received neoadjuvant chemotherapy, the histological results from their surgeries were not interpretable. In effect, only the 54 patients who did not receive neoadjuvant chemotherapy were analyzed. Among these, 15 had non-suspicious lymph nodes (N), 23 were minimally suspect, nine were mildly suspect, and seven were highly suspect (Table 1). Five CBs were inadequate, 39 were negative, and 10 were positive (Table 2).

Of the 54 cases without neoadjuvant chemotherapy, 34 had a negative histological result and 20 had a positive histological result. Of the 34 negative results, 14 had an echo of N, 18 echo of + (also considered non-suspicious) and only two had an echo of ++. Of the 20 positive results, one had an echo N, five had + echoes, seven had ++ echoes, and seven had +++ echoes.

Of the 54 cases without neoadjuvant chemotherapy, 34 had a negative histological result and 20 had a positive histological result. Of the 34 negative results, only 2 had non-contributory CB (C1), 32 had negative CB (C2) and there were no positive CB (C5). Of the 20 positive results, 3 had non-contributory CB (C1), 7 had negative CB (C2) and 10 had positive CB (C5).

The final histological result was negative for 34 cases and positive for 20 cases.

Of the 38 non-suspicious lymph nodes based on US (N or "+") in patients who did not have neoadjuvant therapy, lymph node metastasis was found in six cases (15.8 %), whereas there were no malignant cells in 32 cases (84.2 %) (Table 1).

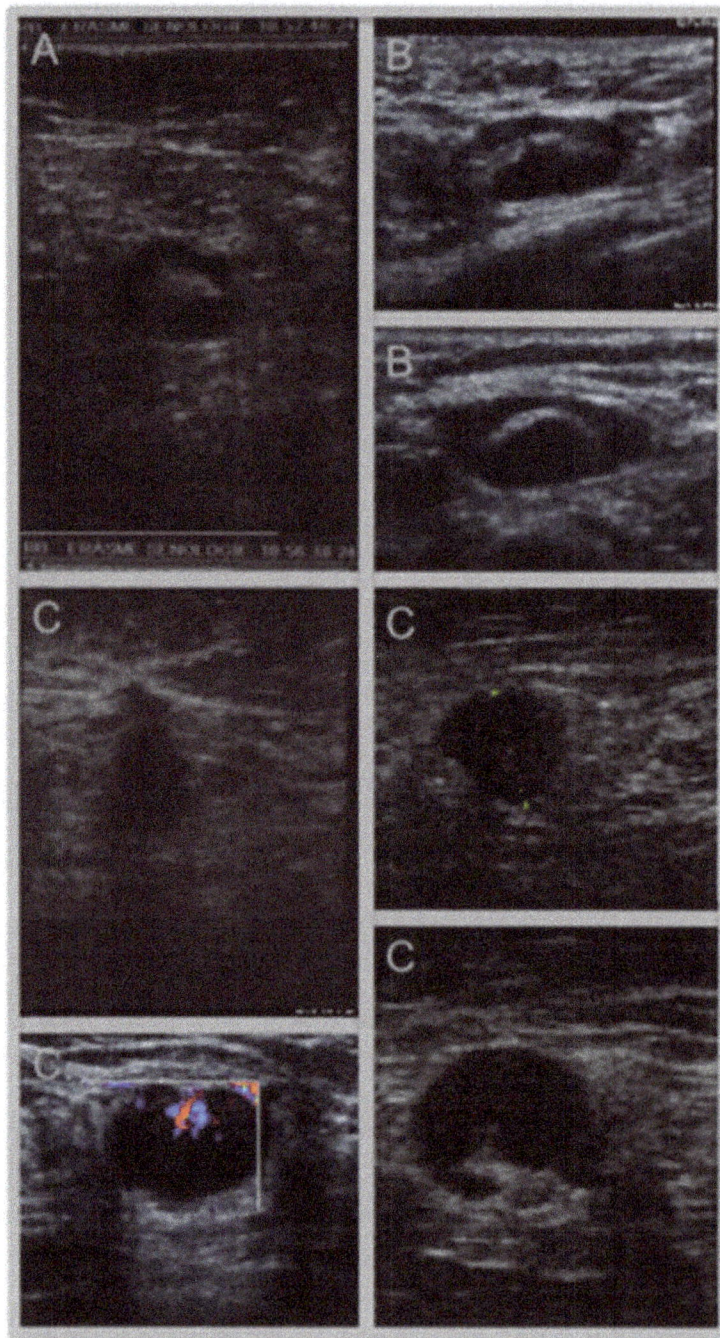

Fig. 1 Sonographic images of a minimally suspect axillary lymph node "+" (**A**), a mildly suspect axillary lymph node "++" (**B**) and highly suspect axillary lymph node "+++" (**C**)

Of the 16 suspicious lymph nodes based on US ("++" or "+++") in patients who did not receive neoadjuvant therapy, lymph node metastasis was found in 14 cases (87.5 %), and no malignant cells were detected in two cases (12.5 %) (Table 1).

All metastatic axillary lymph nodes identified by CB preparation in the absence of neoadjuvant chemotherapy (C5) had positive final histological results (100 %) (Table 2).

Of the 39 axillary lymph nodes in which metastasis was not found by CB preparation (C2), 32 had negative final histological results in the absence of neoadjuvant chemotherapy (82 %), and seven had positive final histological results (18 %) (Table 2).

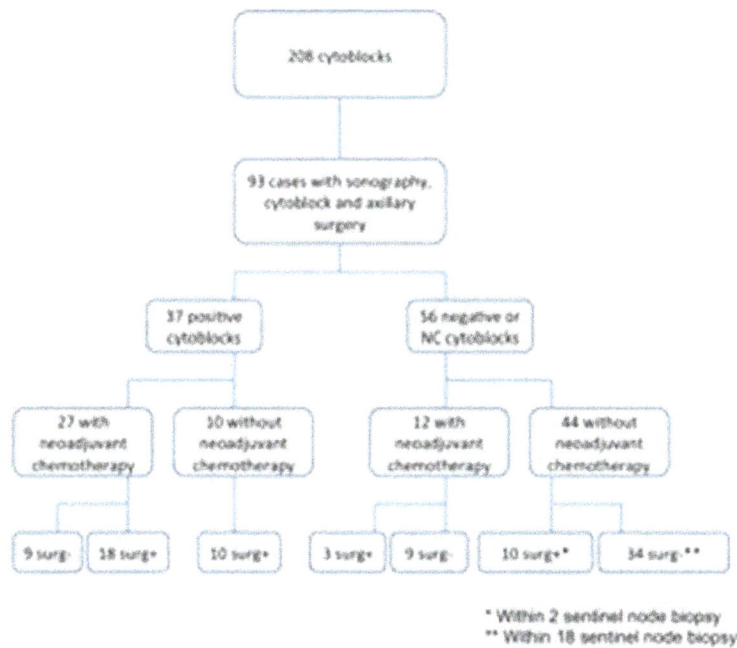

Fig. 2 Two hundred and eight cytoblocks (CB) were performed at Erasme Hospital between October 2008 and August 2012. Of these, 93 cases had sonography, cytoblock and axillary surgery. Of the CBs performed, 37 were positive and 56 were negative or non-contributory (NC). Of the 37 positive CB, 10 did not receive neoadjuvant therapy. Of the 56 negative or NC cytoblocks, 44 did not receive neoadjuvant chemotherapy

The results of the pre-operative lymph node staging by US and by CB preparation with the final histological result were compared using a χ^2 statistical test. A statistically significant correlation was found between the results in the two cases (Table 2). The results obtained were statistically significant (χ^2 23.691 ($p = 0.00000717$) for CB and χ^2 25.381 ($p = 0.00000046$) for US.

Of the C5 lymph nodes (10 cases) or those found by US to be suspicious (9 "++" and 7 "+++") in the pre-operative evaluations (26 cases), only two cases of "++" were ultimately negative in the absence of neoadjuvant therapy in the final histological results.

To determine whether some of the variables could explain a discordance in the results, or whether the rate of contribution changed depending on these variables, the impact of the variables on the results were analyzed using a χ^2 statistical test. None of the variables were found to be statistically significant.

In comparing the results of the CB preparation to those of the cytospins (57 cases), only three cases were discordant: three cases of inadequate CB had cytospin results of C3, C4 or C5.

A comparison of axillary lymph node status between CB preparation or US, and the final histological results of lymph nodes after surgery in the absence of neoadjuvant chemotherapy, indicated that false-negative results for metastasis were identified by CB in seven cases (7/39, 18 %) compared to one "N" (1/15, 6.67 %) and five "+++" (5/23, 21.7 %) cases obtained by US alone (6/38, 15.8 %). Moreover, the CB technique showed 0 % false-positive cases compared to 12.5 % (two "++", 16 "++", and "+++") false-positive cases obtained by US alone. The results summarized in Table 3 show the sensitivities, specificities, positive predictive values (PPV) and negative predictive values (NPV) for US alone compared to CB, excluding CB cases with inadequate results, and patients who received neoadjuvant chemotherapy.

Table 1 Lymph nodes histological results according to pre-operative sonographic results

Echography		Negative (%)	Positive (%)	Total
		Histological results from surgery		
	Echo N	14 (93)	1 (7)	15 (100)
	Echo +	18 (78)	5 (22)	23 (100)
	Echo ++	2 (22)	7 (78)	9 (100)
	Echo +++	0	7 (100)	7 (100)
	Total	34 (63)	20 (27)	54 (100)

Table 2 Lymph nodes histological results according to pre-operative cytoblock results

Cytoblock		Negative (%)	Positive (%)	Total
		Histological results from surgery		
	C 1	2 (40)	3 (60)	5 (100)
	C 2	32 (82)	7 (18)	39 (100)
	C 5	0	10 (100)	10 (100)
	Total	34 (63)	20 (37)	54 (100)

Table 3 Statistical peformance

	Sensibility (%)	Specificity (%)	PPV (%)	NPV (%)
Echography*	68.4	94.1	86.7	84
Cytoblock	58.8	100	100	82.1
Echography* + Cytoblock	75.0	94.1	88.2	86.5

* Echography N and + considered as non suspicious; echography ++ and +++ considered as suspicious

Based on the values displayed in Tables 1 and 2, we calculated the sensitivity, specificity, positive predictive value (PPV) and negative predictive value (NPV) of echography* and cytoblock both alone and together. *Echoes of N and + were considered non-suspicious; echoes of ++ and +++ considered suspicious.

For the "++" and "+++" lymph nodes classified as suspicious in the absence of neoadjuvant therapy, the sensitivity of CB in the 54 cases was 58.8 % compared to 68.4 % for US. The specificity (100 % versus 94.1 %), PPV (100 % versus 86.7 %) and NPV (82.1 % versus 84 %) values were high for both diagnostic methods (Table 3).

In cases where only the "+++" lymph nodes were considered suspicious, the sensitivity of CB in the 54 cases was 58.8 % compared to 85.7 % for US. Specificity was 100 % versus 100 %, PPV was 100 % versus 100 %, and NPV was 82.1 % versus 93.3 % (Table 3).

For non-suspicious lymph nodes with N or "+" results from US and C2 (a combination of the CB and US techniques) without neoadjuvant therapy, the sensitivity was 75 %, specificity was 94.1 %, PPV was 88.2 % and NPV was 86 % (Table 3).

These results support the hypothesis that pre-operative CB from USG-FNA biopsy of axillary lymph nodes, and axillary US using a modified version of Stavros' classification, are two promising methods of pre-operative axillary staging, with axillary US being the preferred means of staging.

Discussion

This study is based on a series of CBs from USG-FNA and sonography of axillary lymph nodes in patients with primary invasive breast cancer. Among non-invasive approaches, US and USG-FNA cytology have been reported to have high accuracy for staging axillary lymph nodes. Published estimates of USG-FNA cytology show a sensitivity varying from 25 to 87 %, a specificity ranging from 14 to 100 %, an NPV between 54 and 78 % and a PPV ranging from 37 to 100 % [6, 7, 9–13]. The results obtained in our study are similar to and even exceed these published findings. The only study to have previously described results from the CB technique, Engohan et al., has results very similar to those described here, with a

better sensitivity (73 % versus 58 %), a lower NPV (78 % versus 82 %) and same specificity and PPV (100 %). Analysis of our results showed that for patients with positive nodes by CB (C5) or positive nodes by US ("+++"), the probability of having axillary nodal metastasis upon surgery in the absence of neoadjuvant therapy is 100 % (PPV). Similarly, for patients with negative nodes by the CB technique and by US (N or "+"), the probability of having no axillary nodal metastasis upon surgery is 86.5 % (NPV) in the absence of neoadjuvant chemotherapy.

We found seven false-negative cases by the CB technique and by US, including one that had an inadequate CB result. Another false-negative lymph node was evaluated simultaneously with an ipsilateral lymph node that was positive at pre-operative staging; surgery showed two positive lymph nodes out of 12 analyzed. In effect, the second node was confirmed as positive without insurance, because the pathologist could not prove which one was the one diagnosed before surgery. We also found two false-positive cases by US when the CB result was negative, and the size of the pre-operative lymph node, as determined by US, was not the same as that measured by the pathologist after surgery.

This analysis reveals some limitations to our study. First, it is possible that the lymph node analyzed by the pathologist after surgery (sentinel node biopsy or axillary lymph node dissection) was not the same one as that evaluated by US and USG-FNA during pre-operative staging.

Additionally, there were 39 cases of lymph nodes from patients who had received neodajuvant chemotherapy. For those cases, it is not possible to compare the pre-operative and final histological results.

Conclusion

Axillary lymph node status is an important component of staging and treatment planning in breast cancer. Our study confirms that the use of a combination of US and CB may improve the evaluation of axillary lymph nodes in patients with primary breast cancer. These techniques are simple, inexpensive, minimally invasive, and allow for immunostaining. They also permit the referral of patients with primary breast cancer to neoadjuvant chemotherapy if the CB result is C5 or if the US result is "+++". In the same way, for patients with a CB result of C2 and US result N or "+", these techniques may preclude the use of neoadjuvant chemotherapy. Given the limited number of cases in our study, additional, new studies will be necessary.

Abbreviations

CB: cytoblock; IHC: immunohistochemistry; NPV: negative predictive value; PPV: positive predictive value; US: ultrasound; USG-FNA: ultrasound-guided fine needle aspiration.

Competing interests

The authors declare that they have no competing interests.

Authors' contributions

CDC participated in the conception and design of the study, management of samples and acquisition of data, drafting of the manuscript, and final approval of the version to be published. RB participated in the acquisition of echographic data, and critical revision of the version to be published. JCN and PHS were involved in the conception and design of the study, or acquisition of data, or analysis and interpretation of data, and critical revision of the version to be published. All authors have read and approved the final manuscript.

Acknowledgements

None to report.

References

1. Belgian Cancer Registry. Incidence Fact Sheet. Female Breast Cancer. ICD10: C50. Belgium 2012. 2015. Accessed 1 January 2014.
2. SPF Economie, PME, Classes moyennes et Energie. Décès par groupe de causes initiales de décès, (Liste spéciale 1 de l'OMS). 2015. Accessed 1 January 2014.
3. Aigner J, Schneeweiss A, Sohn C, Marmé F. The role of neoadjuvant chemotherapy in the management of primary breast cancer. Minerva Ginecol. 2011;63(3):261–74.
4. National Comprehensive Cancer Network Guidelines, version 2.2013. Accessed 1 January 2014.
5. Holwitt D, Swatske ME, Gillanders WE, Monsees BS, Gao F, Aft RL, et al. Scientific Presentation Award: The combination of axillary ultrasound and ultrasound-guided biopsy is an accurate predictor of axillary stage in clinically node-negative breast cancer patients. Am J Surg. 2008;196(4):477–82.
6. Fraile M, Rull M, Julian FJ, Fuste F, Barnadas A, Llatjos M, et al. Sentinel node biopsy as a practical alternative to axillary lymph node dissection in breast cancer patients: an approach to its validity. Ann Oncol. 2000;11(6):701–5.
7. Engohan-Aloghe C, Hottat N, Noël JC. Accuracy of lymph node cell block preparation according to ultrasound features in preoperative staging of breast cancer. Diagn Cytopathol. 2010;38(1):5–8.
8. Stavros AT. Evaluation of regional lymph nodes in breast cancer patients. In: Stavros AT, editor. Breast Ultrasound. Philadelphia: Lippincott; 2004. p. 834–76.
9. Cools-Lartigue J, Sinclair A, Trabulsi N, Meguerditchian A, Mesurolle B, Fuhrer R, et al. Preoperative axillary ultrasound and fine-needle aspiration biopsy in the diagnosis of axillary metastases in patients with breast cancer: predictors of accuracy and future implications. Ann Surg Oncol. 2013;20(3):819–27.
10. Leenders MWH, Broeders M, Croese C, Richir MC, Go HLS, Langenhorst BLAM, et al. Ultrasound and fine needle aspiration cytology of axillary lymph nodes in breast cancer. To do or not to do? Breast. 2012;21(4):578–83.
11. García Fernandez A, Fraile M, Giménez N, Reñe A, Torras M, Canales L, et al. Use of axillary ultrasound, ultrasound-fine needle aspiration biopsy and magnetic resonance imaging in the preoperative triage of breast cancer patients considered for sentinel node biopsy. Ultrasound Med Biol. 2011;37(1):16–22.
12. Mills P, Sever A, Weeks J, Fish D, Jones S, Jones P. Axillary ultrasound assessment in primary breast cancer: an audit of 653 cases. Breast J. 2010;16(5):460–3.
13. Mainiero MB, Cinelli CM, Koelliker SL, Graves TA, Chung MA. Axillary ultrasound and fine-needle aspiration in the preoperative evaluation of the breast cancer patient: an algorithm based on tumor size and lymph node appearance. AJR Am J Roentgenol. 2010;195(5):1261–7.

7

Time-resolved tracking of the atrioventricular plane displacement in Cardiovascular Magnetic Resonance (CMR) images

Felicia Seemann[1,2,3] (iD), Ulrika Pahlm[1], Katarina Steding-Ehrenborg[1,4], Ellen Ostenfeld[1], David Erlinge[5], Jean-Luc Dubois-Rande[6], Svend Eggert Jensen[7], Dan Atar[8], Håkan Arheden[1], Marcus Carlsson[1] and Einar Heiberg[1,3*]

Abstract

Background: Atrioventricular plane displacement (AVPD) is an indicator for systolic and diastolic function and accounts for 60% of the left ventricular, and 80% of the right ventricular stroke volume. AVPD is commonly measured clinically in echocardiography as mitral and tricuspid annular plane systolic excursion (MAPSE and TAPSE), but has not been applied widely in cardiovascular magnetic resonance (CMR). To date, there is no robust automatic algorithm available that allows the AVPD to be measured clinically in CMR with input in a single timeframe. This study aimed to develop, validate and provide a method that automatically tracks the left and right ventricular AVPD in CMR images, which can be used in the clinical setting or in applied cardiovascular research in multi-center studies.

Methods: The proposed algorithm is based on template tracking by normalized cross-correlation combined with a priori information by principal component analysis. The AVPD in each timeframe is calculated for the left and right ventricle separately using CMR long-axis cine images of the 2, 3, and 4-chamber views.
The algorithm was developed using a training set ($n = 40$), and validated in a test set ($n = 113$) of healthy subjects, athletes, and patients after ST-elevation myocardial infarction from 10 centers. Validation was done using manual measurements in end diastole and end systole as reference standard. Additionally, AVPD, peak emptying velocity, peak filling velocity, and atrial contraction was validated in 20 subjects, where time-resolved manual measurements were used as reference standard. Inter-observer variability was analyzed in 20 subjects.

Results: In end systole, the difference between the algorithm and the reference standard in the left ventricle was (mean $\pm$ SD) -0.6 $\pm$ 1.9 mm (R = 0.79), and −0.8 $\pm$ 2.1 mm (R = 0.88) in the right ventricle. Inter-observer variability in end systole was −0.6 $\pm$ 0.7 mm (R = 0.95), and −0.5 $\pm$ 1.4 mm (R = 0.95) for the left and right ventricle, respectively. Validation of peak emptying velocity, peak filling velocity, and atrial contraction yielded lower accuracy than the displacement measures.

Conclusions: The proposed algorithm show good agreement and low bias with the reference standard, and with an agreement in parity with inter-observer variability. Thus, it can be used as an automatic method of tracking and measuring AVPD in CMR.

Keywords: Atrioventricular plane displacement, Automated tracking, Normalized cross-correlation, Principal component analysis, Cardiac valve displacement

* Correspondence: einar.heiberg@med.lu.se
[1]Department of Clinical Physiology, Lund University, Skane University Hospital, Lund, Sweden
[3]Department of Biomedical Engineering, Faculty of Engineering, Lund University, Lund, Sweden
Full list of author information is available at the end of the article

Background

The atrioventricular (AV) plane is a fibrous region containing the cardiac valves, separating the atria from the ventricles. During a heartbeat the AV-plane moves as a piston pump, towards apex during systole and back to the initial position during diastole [1, 2]. The atrioventricular plane displacement (AVPD) has been shown to account for 60% of the left ventricular (LV) stroke volume, and 80% of the right ventricular (RV) stroke volume [3, 4] and is an indicator of both systolic and diastolic function [5, 6]. A reduced AVPD is associated with disease and aging [7–10], while regular exercise has been shown to increase AVPD in young male athletes [11] and maintain AVPD at a level similar to young subjects in male master athletes [10].

In echocardiography, it is clinical standard to measure AVPD [9, 12] and a reduced long-axis function has been shown to have prognostic significance for future clinical events [13–17]. Mitral annular plane systolic excursion (MAPSE) is easily used as a good marker for left ventricular function [14], and current guidelines suggest the quantification of tricuspid annular plane systolic excursion (TAPSE) for determining RV function [12, 18]. A number of algorithms has been proposed in order to automatically measure valve displacement with echocardiography [19–21].

In cardiovascular magnetic resonance (CMR) imaging, long-axis cine images, acquired in clinical routine, can be used for measuring AVPD. However, currently AVPD is rarely evaluated in a clinical setting and is not implemented in the consensus document for CMR assessment [22]. When AVPD is assessed in CMR, the required method is often manual measurements in the end diastolic and end systolic timeframe [3, 4, 10, 11, 17, 23–26]. These measurements are applicable for quantification of the maximum displacement over a cardiac cycle. However, it does not carry any information about the temporal distribution of the displacement throughout a heartbeat. Time-resolved measurements allow computation of the AVPD over the whole cardiac cycle, thus creating an AVPD curve. However, manual time-resolved measurements are time consuming and observer dependent. Derived from the AVPD curve, velocity at peak emptying and peak filling can be calculated. These velocities can be considered in parity to the peak systolic and diastolic annular velocity known from echocardiography. Furthermore, atrial contraction can also be derived from the AVPD curve. Automatic tracking of the AVPD reduces the subjectivity of different observers, as well as the time spent on manual image analysis.

A few semi-automatic methods for tracking valves in CMR images have been presented [27–32]. However, no previous method has presented an algorithm using standard clinical CMR images, and that only require manual input in a single timeframe to track the AV-plane in both the left and the right side of heart.

Therefore, the aim of this study was to develop and validate a method that use manually placed input points in a single timeframe and thereafter automatically track the left and right ventricular AV-plane motion in CMR images. This will be useful in the clinical setting as well as in applied cardiovascular research in multi-center studies.

Methods

Study population

A total of 153 subjects, who underwent CMR imaging in three previous studies, were included in this study. Subjects consisted of 32 elite athletes [33], 14 elderly normal subjects [10], 81 patients with first time ST-elevation myocardial infarction from the multi-center clinical cardioprotection trial MITOCARE [34], and 26 normal controls [33]. Ten centers participated in data inclusion. Each subject underwent CMR scanning in a 1.5 T scanner using a steady-state-free precession (SSFP) sequence with retrospective ECG gating under end-expiratory breath hold. Scanners were from Philips (Philips Healthcare, Best, The Netherlands), Siemens (Siemens Healthcare, Erlangen, Germany) or GE (GE Healthcare, Waukesha, WI, USA). Long-axis cine images of the 2-chamber, 3-chamber, and 4-chamber views were acquired. In all vendors, typical pixel resolution was 1.5×1.5 mm, 8 mm slice thickness, 30 timeframes per cardiac cycle. For Philips, MR sequence parameters ranges were: repetition time 2.6–4.0 ms; echo time 1.3–2.0 ms; flip angle 60°; field of view 151–430 mm; matrix size $(92–336) \times (92–336)$. For Siemens ranges were: repetition time 2.6–3.4 ms; echo time 1.1–1.4 ms; flip angle 47–80°; field of view 129–430 mm; matrix size $(73–256) \times (79–256)$. For GE: repetition time 3.1–4.0 ms; echo time 1.3–1.7 ms; flip angle 45–70°; field of view 143–400 mm; matrix size $(166–512) \times (166–512)$.

Subjects were divided into a training set for algorithm development and optimization ($n = 40$), and a test set for validation ($n = 113$). A subset of the test set ($n = 20$) was used for time-resolved validation while the whole test set was used for validation of the maximum AVPD. The training set consisted of 16 patients, 9 athletes, and 15 healthy controls and was selected manually prior to looking at the images of the included subjects. The time-resolved test set consisted of 7 patients, 6 athletes, 2 elderly normal subjects, and 5 normal controls. Additionally, a subset of $n = 20$ patients from the training set was used for inter-observer variability analysis in end diastole and end systole.

All studies were approved by the local ethical committees, and written informed consent was obtained from each individual.

Automatic tracking algorithm

The algorithm yield time-resolved curves of the AVPD throughout the cardiac cycle. It was implemented in the medical image analysis software Segment v2.0 R5024 [35] (http://segment.heiberg.se), and is freely available for research purposes. A total of 8 input points that mark the AV-plane are manually placed in the end diastolic timeframe as user input; 2 input points in the 2-chamber view, 3 input points in the 3-chamber, and 3 input points in the 4-chamber. The input points are placed in the most basal part of the compact myocardium in the left and right ventricle, as illustrated in Fig. 1, according to the methodology in the papers by Carlsson et al. [3, 4]. In short, left ventricular AVPD (LVAVPD) is calculated from two input points in each of the three long-axis views for the LV, which equals 6 input points. For the right ventricle, the mean of the two LV septal input points together with the input points of the RV lateral in the 4-chamber view and the RV outflow tract in the 3-chamber view are used for calculating the right ventricular AVPD (RVAVPD). The total LVAVPD and RVAVPD are calculated separately, as described by Carlsson et al. [3, 4]. The algorithm tracks each of the 8 input points separately, using template tracking by normalized cross-correlation [36] combined with a priori information by principal component analysis (PCA) [37].

Training of statistical model

The algorithm was developed and optimized using the time-resolved manual measurements in the training set ($n = 40$). The amount of timeframes in CMR images differs between the subjects. Hence, all measurements were interpolated to 30 timeframes and normalized by the curve amplitude. For each of the 8 input points, the data was stored as a matrix representation of size 40x30. Rows consisted of the input point displacement perpendicular to the AV-plane in mm for 40 subjects, columns represented the 30 timeframes. Principal component analysis is a method that find underlying structures of the data it is applied to, using statistics and eigenvalue decomposition. Each eigenvector represents a component of the underlying structures, a principal component, and have a corresponding eigenvalue that represent the variance of the structure. In PCA, the largest eigenvalue corresponds to the most dominant principal component of the data. By performing PCA decomposition on the constructed matrix with AVPD data, a statistical model describing the shape of an AVPD curve was constructed. This transforms the matrix into linearly uncorrelated principal components, enabling the information about AVPD from the training set to be represented in 30 dimensions. When analyzing the 30 eigenvalues yielded by the PCA, the sum of the 5 largest eigenvalues accounted for 99% of the sum of all eigenvalues. Hence, the AVPD curve shape and behavior could be reconstructed from 5 coefficient dimensions, using the eigenvectors corresponding to the 5 most significant eigenvalues of the data covariance matrix.

The mean displacement for each point was reconstructed using this model, in order to define a position prediction curve. The prediction points are used by the algorithm as an initial guess of where the input point tracked is located in each timeframe. Reconstruction is also applied on the algorithm tracking result, as a physiological filtering method that smooth the displacement of each tracked point.

The space spanned by the shape reconstruction for one input point, the septum point in the 4-chamber view, is illustrated in Fig. 2. The space was created by 10.000 randomly generated AVPD curves, using the five

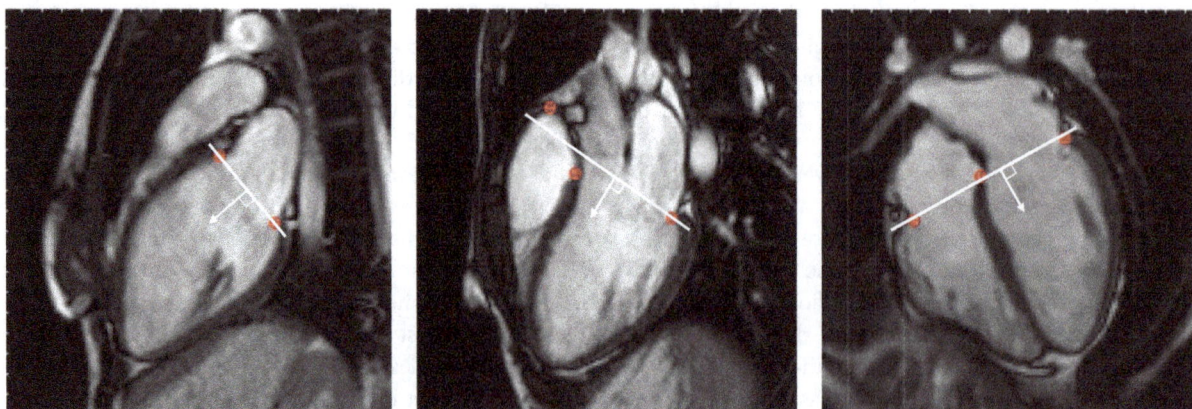

Fig. 1 Algorithm initialization and atrioventricular plane definition. The user marks the atrioventricular (AV) plane by placing 8 input points to be tracked, here seen in *red*, in the end diastolic timeframe in the 2-, 3-, and 4-chamber long-axis views. In step 1 of the algorithm, the AV-plane is defined in the end diastolic timeframe of each long-axis view (*white line*), and the direction perpendicular to the AV-plane towards the apex (*white arrow*) marks the direction of the AV-plane displacement (AVPD). In step 2, the a priori position prediction is placed according to the defined plane and direction

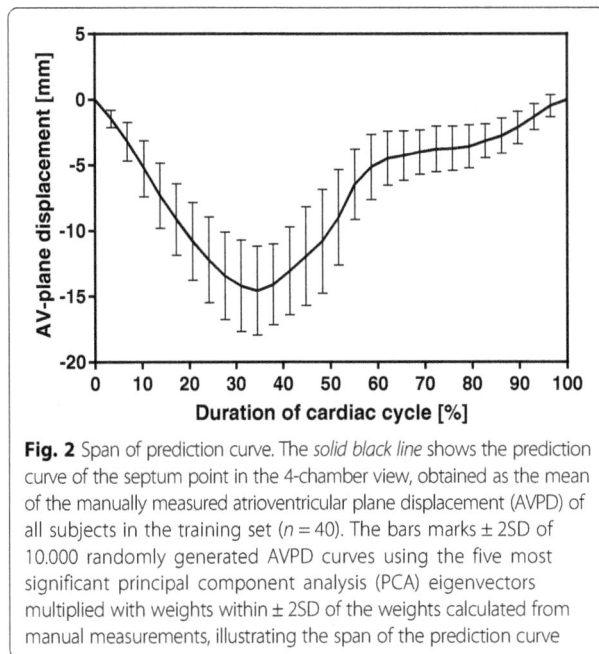

Fig. 2 Span of prediction curve. The *solid black line* shows the prediction curve of the septum point in the 4-chamber view, obtained as the mean of the manually measured atrioventricular plane displacement (AVPD) of all subjects in the training set ($n = 40$). The bars marks ± 2SD of 10.000 randomly generated AVPD curves using the five most significant principal component analysis (PCA) eigenvectors multiplied with weights within ± 2SD of the weights calculated from manual measurements, illustrating the span of the prediction curve

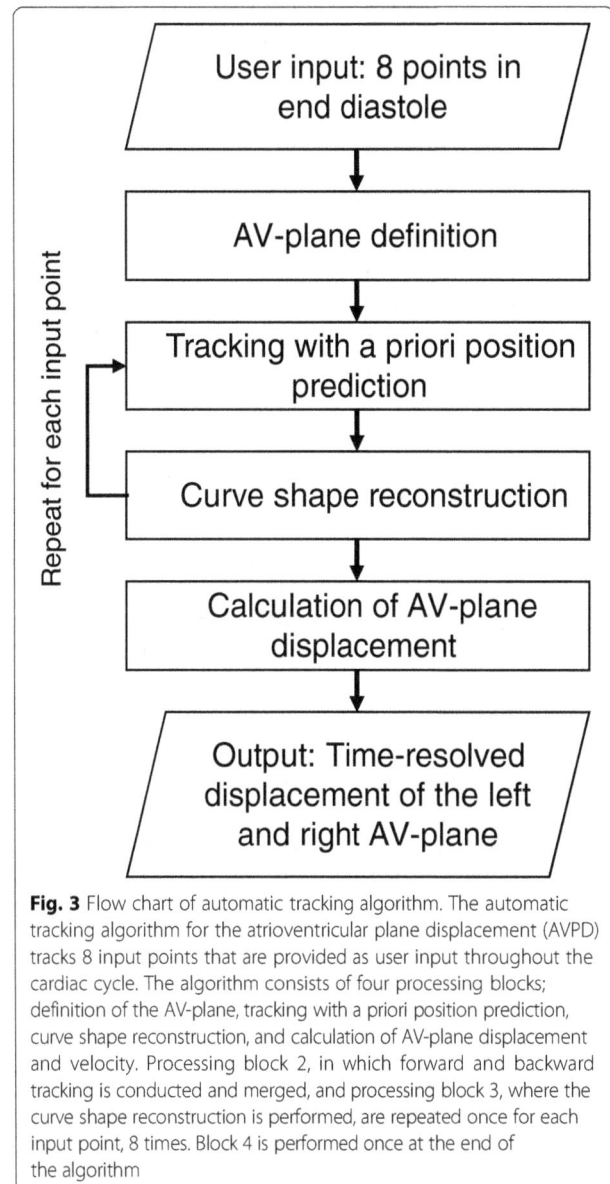

Fig. 3 Flow chart of automatic tracking algorithm. The automatic tracking algorithm for the atrioventricular plane displacement (AVPD) tracks 8 input points that are provided as user input throughout the cardiac cycle. The algorithm consists of four processing blocks; definition of the AV-plane, tracking with a priori position prediction, curve shape reconstruction, and calculation of AV-plane displacement and velocity. Processing block 2, in which forward and backward tracking is conducted and merged, and processing block 3, where the curve shape reconstruction is performed, are repeated once for each input point, 8 times. Block 4 is performed once at the end of the algorithm

first principal component eigenvectors multiplied by PCA weights within ± 2SD of the weights of the prediction curve. The spread of the space is shown as bars of ± 2SD over the mean AVPD curve from manual measurements in the training set. The ± 2SD in Fig. 2 has large spread, since the training set include AVPD measures ranging from a reduced AVPD in patients to an increased AVPD in male athletes.

Tracking and reconstruction process

Figure 3 show a flow chart of the automatic tracking algorithm. The process consists of 4 processing blocks; 1) definition of the AV-plane, 2) template tracking with position prediction, 3) curve shape reconstruction using PCA, and 4) calculation of the AVPD, peak emptying velocity, peak filling velocity, and atrial contraction.

Step 1: AV-plane definition

Only the perpendicular movement in relation to the AV-plane in end diastole is accounted for. The AV-plane is defined in each long-axis view. In the 2-chamber and 4-chamber view, the AV-plane is defined as the line where the residuals between the input points and plane are minimized. In the 3-chamber, the plane intersects the lateral input point of the LV and pass between the input points in septum and RV. This is illustrated in Fig. 1.

Step 2: tracking with a priori position prediction

The position of the input point throughout the cardiac cycle is predicted by placing prediction points in each timeframe, according to the prediction

curves obtained in the training process. Prediction points are positioned perpendicular to the AV-plane, and interpolated according to the duration of the cardiac cycle.

Tracking is performed by extracting the pixels in a region of interest (ROI), a square around the input point in the end diastolic timeframe. In the following timeframe a region of search (ROS) is extracted as a square centered on the prediction point. Normalized cross-correlation is performed for the ROI $\mathbf{I}$, indexed as $(\mathbf{x},\mathbf{y})$, and ROS $\mathbf{S}$, indexed $(\mathbf{u},\mathbf{v})$. The maximum correlation coefficient between the ROI and ROS, $\mathbf{\gamma}(\mathbf{u},\mathbf{v})$, indicate the best corresponding position of the input point in the second timeframe [36].

$$\gamma(u,v) = \frac{\sum_{x,y}\left[S(x,y)-\overline{S}_{u,v}\right]\left[I(x-u,\ y-v)-\overline{I}\right]}{\sqrt{\sum_{x,y}\left[S(x,y)-\overline{S}_{u,v}\right]^2 \sum_{x,y}\left[I(x-u,\ y-v)-\overline{I}\right]^2}}$$

Around this tracked point, a new ROI is extracted and a ROS is extracted around the prediction point in the next timeframe, and normalized cross-correlation is applied again. The procedure is repeated twice for each input point. First, the tracking is initiated in end diastole, proceeding forward to the next timeframe until reaching the last timeframe. The tracking is then repeated according to the same principle, but instead of forward tracking, the input points in end diastole are tracked backwards.

Step 3: curve shape reconstruction
Displacement curves from the forward and backward tracking are calculated and merged as a weighted sum of the curves. The forward tracking displacement is weighted linearly from 1 to 0, assigning the displacement in the first timeframe the weight 1 and the last timeframe the weight 0. Accordingly, the displacement in the first timeframe from backward tracking has the weight 1, and the last timeframe the weight 0. To ensure a smooth and physiologically behaving curve, the merged displacement curve for each point is projected using PCA weights and the 5 most significant eigenvectors.

Each of the 8 input points are tracked separately, hence step 2–3 are repeated 8 times before the fourth processing block is executed. The corresponding position of each input point is visualized in every timeframe in Segment.

Step 4: calculation of AV-plane displacement
After tracking, the total LVAVPD and RVAVPD curves are calculated according to Carlsson et al. [3, 4]. The total LVAVPD is the mean displacement curve of the 6 tracked points located in the left side of heart. The sum of the displacement curves of the 2 tracked points in the right side of heart, plus the mean of the displacement curves of the 2 points in septum, divided by 3 gives the total RVAVPD. End systole is defined as the timeframe where the AVPD curve is at its minimum, that is, where the AV-plane is the farthest away from the starting point in end diastole.

In order to calculate the velocity at peak emptying and peak filling, the moving average of 3 data samples of the AVPD curve of each side of the heart are calculated, then the first order derivative by forward differentiation is calculated. Peak emptying velocity is calculated as the slope of the line drawn from 2 timeframes before and 2 timeframes after the timeframe where the first order derivative is at its maximum. Peak filling velocity is calculated as the slope of the line from 1 timeframe before and 2 timeframes after the minimum of the first order derivative, see Fig. 4. Atrial contraction is calculated as the distance between the AVPD in end diastole and the AVPD at the timeframe where absolute value of the second derivative of the moving average displacement curve is at its minimum, divided by the AVPD at end systole.

A 3 dimensional (3D) AV-plane was defined for comparison to the 2 dimensional (2D) planes defined in step 1. The 3D plane was defined by the best fit in the least square sense between the input points in all long axis views, using the 3D coordinate system from the MR scanner.

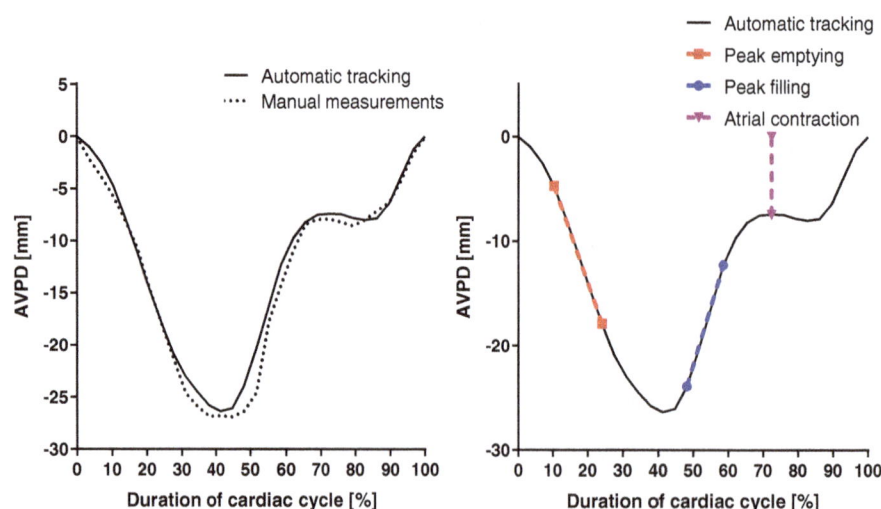

Fig. 4 Example of automatic tracking result. A typical result of the atrioventricular plane displacement (AVPD) in the left ventricle (LV) by automatic tracking is shown as a *solid black line* in the left and right panel. A more negative AVPD correspond to a larger displacement. In the *left panel*, the corresponding manually measured AVPD in the LV is shown as a *dotted line*. The *right panel* illustrate how the peak emptying velocity, peak filling velocity, and atrial contraction are obtained. The slope of the *dashed red line* corresponds to the peak emptying velocity, and the slope of the *dashed blue line* corresponds to the peak filling velocity. The length of the *purple dashed line* divided by the AVPD at end systole gives the atrial contraction in %

Parameter optimization

The sizes of the region of interest, ROI, and region of search, ROS, for all 8 input points were optimized by using the time-resolved measurements in the training set as reference. The training set ($n = 40$) consisted of 16 patients, 9 athletes, and 15 healthy controls. The size of each ROI and ROS in mm was optimized over a range of combinations using 10-fold cross-validation. Correlation R value, bias, and standard deviation, SD, was calculated between manual and tracked AVPD in the end systolic timeframe for each parameter combination in an exhaustive search. Also, the 2-norm of the difference between the manual and tracked AVPD curves was calculated for each subject, as a measure of similarity between the manual and automatic AVPD curves, where the value 0 would indicate that the two curves are identical. The ROI and ROS size for each input point was chosen by optimizing the combination of the mean of R value, bias, SD, and 2-norm difference for each fold. The parameter combination yielding the minimum SD was sought out, combined with the requirement that constraints defined for R, bias, and 2-norm were fulfilled. The constraint for R was all parameter combinations yielding an R value above the 75th percentile of all calculated R. For bias, the constraint was parameter combinations yielding a bias below the 25th percentile. The 2-norm constraint was parameter combinations yielding a 2-norm value below the 75th percentile. For 2 out of 8 parameter combinations, the constraints were fulfilled for the global minimum of all calculated standard deviations. The same ROI and ROS sizes are used for the forward and the backward tracking and are presented in Additional file 1.

Validation

The AV-plane displacement was measured manually by expert readers in all subjects. The automatic tracking algorithm was validated against manual measurements of the total displacement in mm from end diastole to end systole in the whole test set ($n = 113$), as well as separately in the patient ($n = 65$), healthy control ($n = 24$), and athlete ($n = 24$) populations. For the time-resolved subset of the test set ($n = 20$), the AVPD resulting from the automatic tracking algorithm in each timeframe was compared to manual measurements. In the time-resolved test set, the minimum velocity at peak emptying (cm/s), the maximum velocity at peak filling (cm/s), and the atrial contraction (%) was compared for the automatic tracking algorithm and manual measurements. The distance between the manual and automatic AVPD curves was assessed by taking the 2-norm of the difference of the manual and automatic curves in each timeframe. Inter-observer variability of the AVPD in end

systole was performed in a subset of 20 patients with first time myocardial infarction.

Since the starting point for the algorithm is the 8 input points provided by the user in the end diastolic timeframe, different input points will result in different tracking results, even if placed only slightly differently. In order to ensure that the same points were compared, the automatic tracking was provided the exact same input points in end diastole as in the manual measurements. To measure how the algorithm results may differ due to different positions of the input points, inter-observer analysis of the algorithm was analyzed. For the inter-observer analysis, both of the algorithm and for manual measurements, the input points in end diastole were placed separately for each observer. All manual measurements were verified by a second observer.

Statistical analysis

Comparisons were performed using modified Bland-Altman plots with manual measurements as reference standard (mean with limits of agreement (± 2SD)) [38], and linear regression analysis (correlation coefficient).

Automatic tracking of the LVAVPD and RVAVPD was compared to manual measurements in end systole for the test set ($n = 113$). In the time-resolved test set ($n = 20$), the displacement in the automatic tracking was compared to time-resolved manual measurements of the displacement in each timeframe. Also, the peak emptying velocity, peak filling velocity, and atrial contraction was compared in the time-resolved test set. Inter-observer variability in end systole was assessed.

Results

An example of a tracked AVPD curve together with the corresponding manual curve is shown in Fig. 4, showing high similarity of the curves in amplitude and phase. Three movies are available as additional files illustrating typical tracking results in a 2-chamber (Additional file 2), 3-chamber (Additional file 3), and 4-chamber long-axis view (Additional file 4).

Manual measurements compared to automatic tracking results at end systole ($n = 113$) are shown in Fig. 5, and the displacement difference of the time-resolved manual measurements ($n = 20$) compared to automatic tracking in each timeframe are shown in Fig. 6. For both displacement measures, strong correlation and low bias was found between manual and automatic AVPD measurements. The results for the velocity at peak emptying ($n = 20$) for manual compared to automatic measurements are shown in Fig. 7, and the results for the velocity at peak filling ($n = 20$) in Fig. 8. The algorithm tends to overestimate the left peak emptying velocity, and underestimate the left and right peak filling velocity. Figure 9 shows the results for the atrial contraction ($n = 20$).

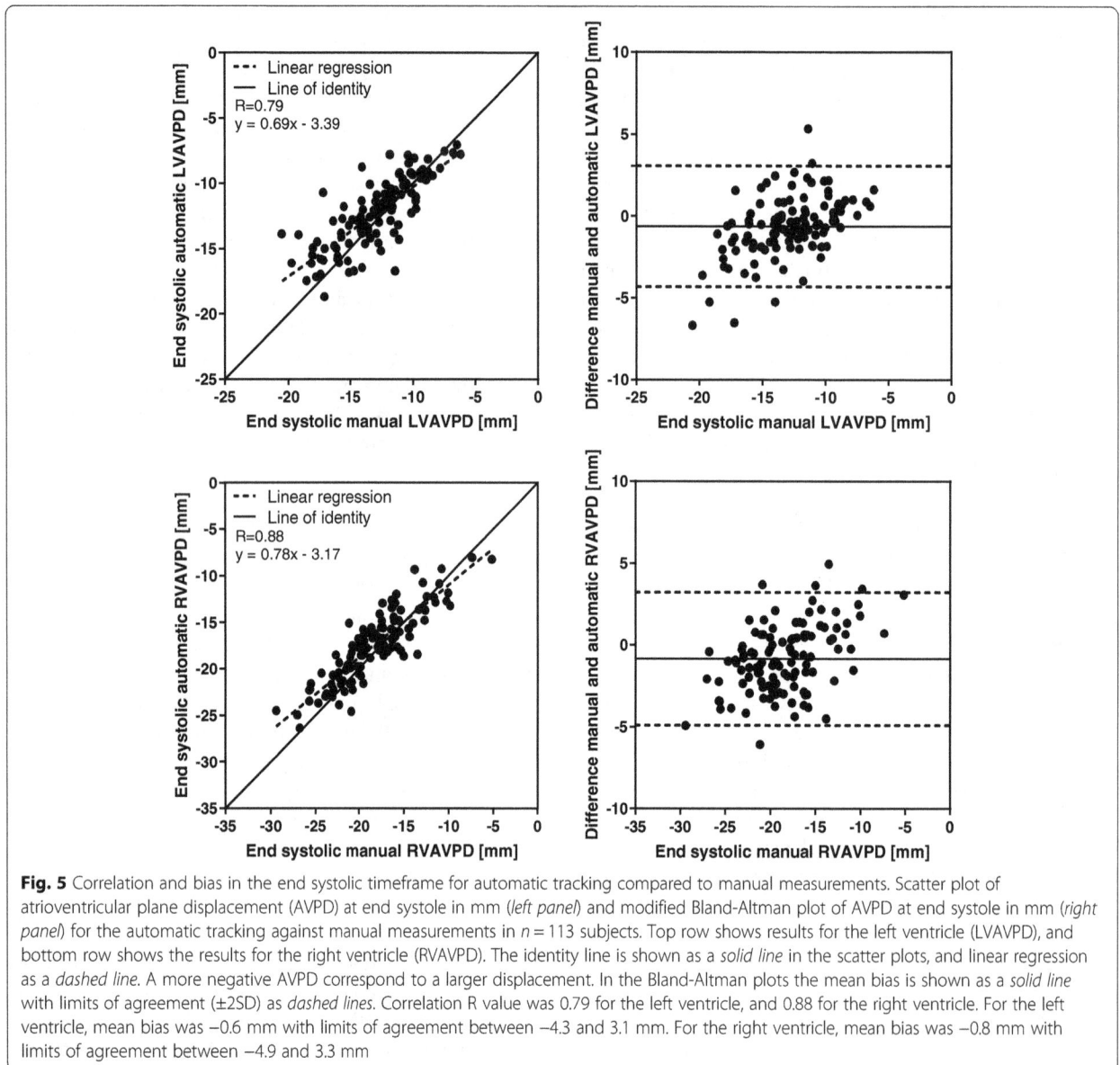

Fig. 5 Correlation and bias in the end systolic timeframe for automatic tracking compared to manual measurements. Scatter plot of atrioventricular plane displacement (AVPD) at end systole in mm (*left panel*) and modified Bland-Altman plot of AVPD at end systole in mm (*right panel*) for the automatic tracking against manual measurements in $n = 113$ subjects. Top row shows results for the left ventricle (LVAVPD), and bottom row shows the results for the right ventricle (RVAVPD). The identity line is shown as a *solid line* in the scatter plots, and linear regression as a *dashed line*. A more negative AVPD correspond to a larger displacement. In the Bland-Altman plots the mean bias is shown as a *solid line* with limits of agreement (±2SD) as *dashed lines*. Correlation R value was 0.79 for the left ventricle, and 0.88 for the right ventricle. For the left ventricle, mean bias was −0.6 mm with limits of agreement between −4.3 and 3.1 mm. For the right ventricle, mean bias was −0.8 mm with limits of agreement between −4.9 and 3.3 mm

Manual and automatic measurements of the AV-plane displacement in all subjects ($n = 113$) are presented in Table 1 as correlation R value and bias ± SD, while Table 2 present the population based AVPD results for patients ($n = 65$), healthy controls ($n = 24$), and athletes ($n = 24$). LVAVPD correlation R value was lower in athletes than for healthy subjects and patients. Otherwise, displacement results in the different populations are in parity to those in all subjects. Results for automatically calculated peak emptying velocity, peak filling velocity, and atrial contraction are presented in Table 3. The 2-norm of the difference between the time-resolved manual and tracked AVPD curves was 10 ± 5 for the left side of the heart, and 11 ± 6 for the right side of the heart. The tracking yielded displacement results agreeing with

manual measurements, with a low bias and high correlation R value. For the peak emptying velocity, peak filling velocity, and atrial contraction, the results presented a higher bias and SD than for the displacement results.

Inter-observer variability for manual measurements in end systole ($n = 20$) was -0.6 ± 0.7 mm, R = 0.95, for the LVAVPD and -0.5 ± 1.4 mm, R = 0.95, for the RVAVPD. Thus, inter-observer variability was similar to the difference between manual and automatic algorithm measurement of AVPD. Inter-observer variability of the algorithm in end systole ($n = 20$) was 0.2 ± 1.4 mm, R = 0.69, for the LVAVPD and 0.0 ± 0.7 mm, R = 0.98, for the RVAVPD. The average time for tracking and calculation of the AVPD for both the left and the right heart was 0.6 s per subject, using a standard laptop computer.

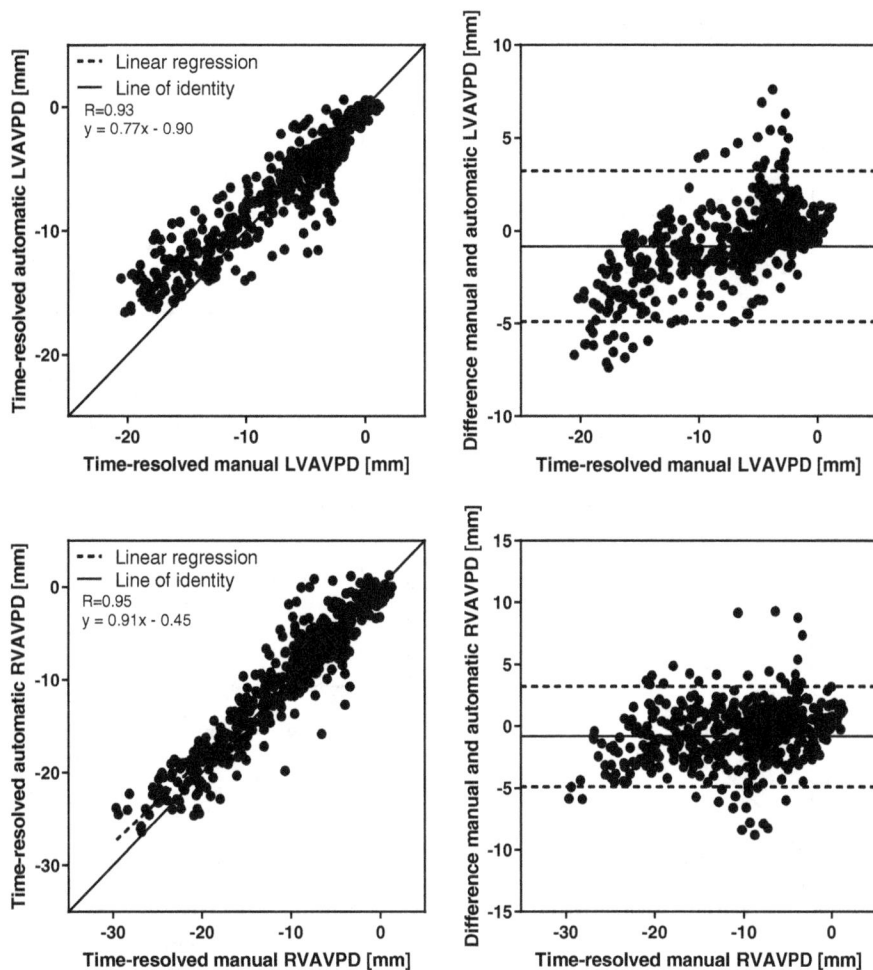

Fig. 6 Correlation and bias in all timeframes for automatic tracking compared to manual measurements. Scatter plot (*left panel*) and modified Bland-Altman plot (*right panel*) for automatic tracking against manual measurements of the atrioventricular plane displacement (AVPD) in *n* = 20 subjects in all timeframes. Top row shows results for the left ventricle (LVAVPD), and the bottom row shows the results for the right ventricle (RVAVPD). The identity line is shown as a *solid line* in the scatter plots, and linear regression as a *dashed line*. A more negative AVPD correspond to a larger displacement. In the modified Bland-Altman plots the mean bias is shown as a solid line with limits of agreement (±2SD) as *dashed lines*. Correlation R value was 0.93 for the left ventricle, and 0.95 for the right ventricle. For the left ventricle, mean bias was −0.6 mm with limits of agreement between −4.5 and 3.3 mm. For the right ventricle, mean bias was −0.5 mm with limits of agreement between −4.8 and 3.8 mm

Figure 10 illustrates the added value, in terms of the 2-norm of the difference between the time-resolved manual and tracked AVPD curves, for four steps in the algorithm; only tracking forward without position prediction, merging the tracking forward and backwards, merging curves using point prediction, and finally when also adding the curve shape reconstruction. Each processing block yielded results with lower variability.

Comparison of tracking results using 2D and 3D AV-planes in the time-resolved test set (*n* = 20) showed a low variability and strong correlation. LVAVPD results was −0.1 ± 0.5 mm, R = 0.99. RVAVPD results was −0.1 ± 0.6 mm, R = 1.00.

Discussion

In this study, an automatic algorithm for time-resolved tracking of the AVPD from standard long-axis CMR cine images has been developed and validated. The algorithm is based on template tracking by normalized cross-correlation and a priori information by principal component analysis, and yield the position of the AV-plane in all timeframes. The input needed by the user is the marking of the AV-plane in end diastole at eight points. The validation of the algorithm in 113 subjects from multi-center and multi-vendor studies showed low bias and high correlation to expert manual measurements.

Forward template tracking can be quite unstable. If the tracking fails in one timeframe, the error will

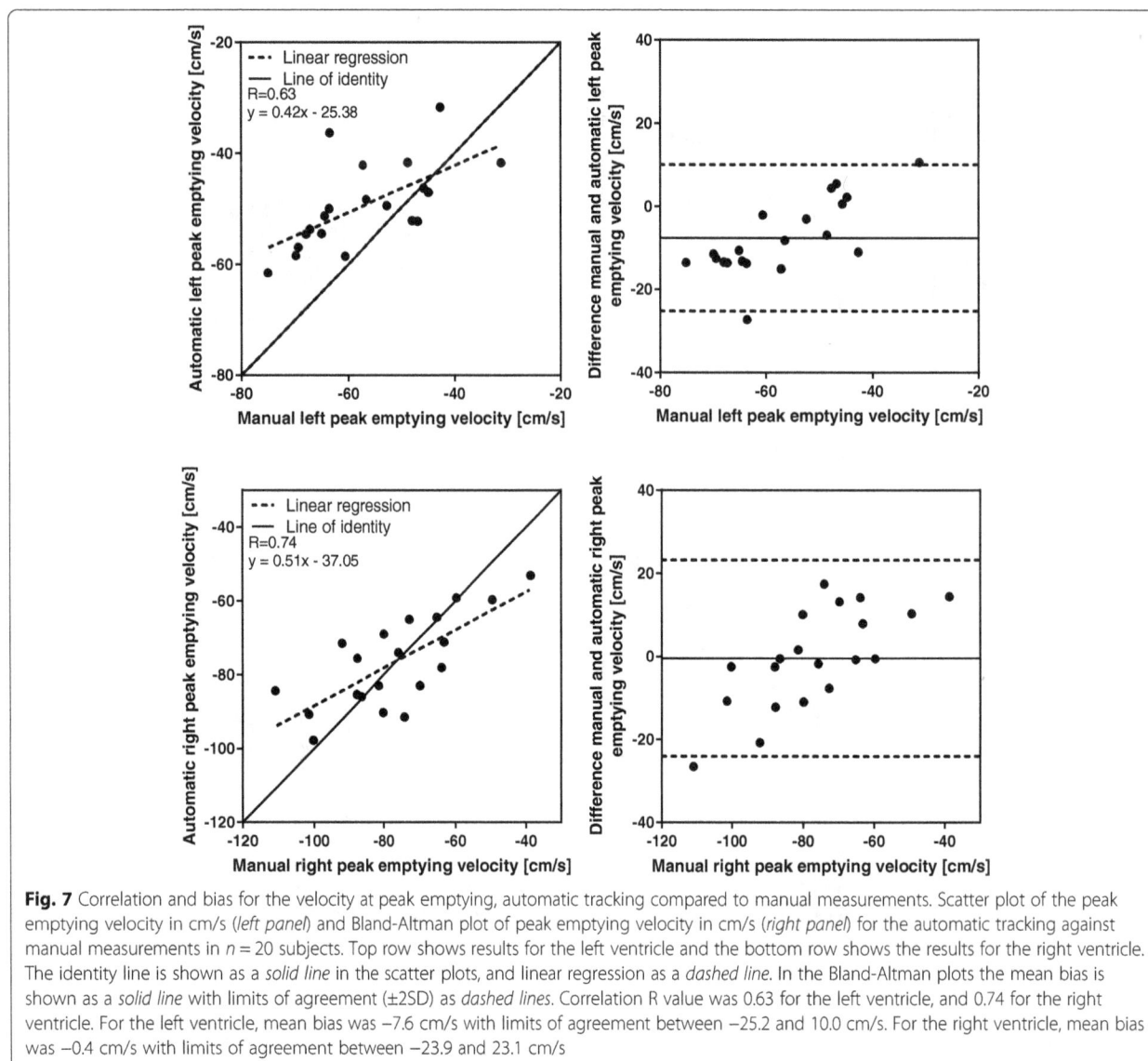

Fig. 7 Correlation and bias for the velocity at peak emptying, automatic tracking compared to manual measurements. Scatter plot of the peak emptying velocity in cm/s (*left panel*) and Bland-Altman plot of peak emptying velocity in cm/s (*right panel*) for the automatic tracking against manual measurements in $n = 20$ subjects. Top row shows results for the left ventricle and the bottom row shows the results for the right ventricle. The identity line is shown as a *solid line* in the scatter plots, and linear regression as a *dashed line*. In the Bland-Altman plots the mean bias is shown as a *solid line* with limits of agreement (±2SD) as *dashed lines*. Correlation R value was 0.63 for the left ventricle, and 0.74 for the right ventricle. For the left ventricle, mean bias was −7.6 cm/s with limits of agreement between −25.2 and 10.0 cm/s. For the right ventricle, mean bias was −0.4 cm/s with limits of agreement between −23.9 and 23.1 cm/s

propagate since another point than the intended will be tracked in the coming timeframes. This might occur at any timeframe for various reasons such as poor image quality, or a region of search (ROS) that does not cover the intended match. This problem has previously been approached in different ways. In the method presented by Wu et al. [29], the user was encouraged to interactively adjust unsatisfactory tracking results, and then run the algorithm again based on the corrections. In the work by Leng et al. [28], stability is obtained by placing input points in several timeframes, and tracking is performed in the timeframes between these input points. In the method presented by Maffessanti et al. [27], manual input is required in the end diastolic and end systolic timeframes. A novelty in the presented algorithm compared to previous approaches is that input points are only required in the end diastolic timeframe and merges

the tracking results from both forward and backward tracking in order to approach the stability issues with forward tracking. In case the template tracking drifts off at some point, the weighted sum of the two displacement curves aids in improving the final AVPD curve. Also, the use of a priori information specific to each input point tracked is used as a prediction for the tracking, thus always placing the ROS in a region where the match is expected, which stabilizes the forward tracking. The prediction adapts according to the number of timeframes in the data set, varying heart rates, and the parameter optimization of ROI and ROS sizes in mm allow the algorithm to adapt to different spatial resolutions. The incremental value of merging two tracking results, using position prediction and curve shape reconstruction can be seen in Fig. 10, suggesting that these steps improves the tracking results comparing

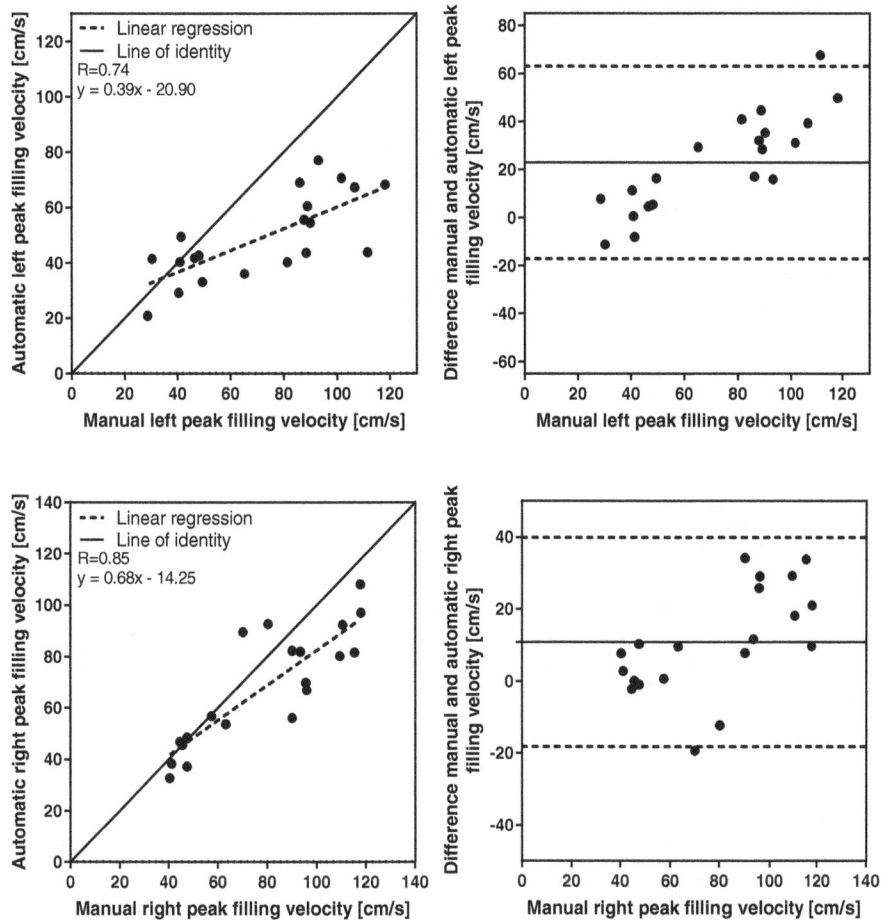

Fig. 8 Correlation and bias for the velocity at peak filling, automatic tracking compared to manual measurements. Scatter plot of the peak filling velocity in cm/s (*left panel*) and Bland-Altman plot of peak filling velocity in cm/s (*right panel*) for the automatic tracking against manual measurements in *n* = 20 subjects. Top row shows results for the left ventricle and the bottom row shows the results for the right ventricle. The identity line is shown as a *solid line* in the scatter plots, and linear regression as a *dashed line*. In the Bland-Altman plots the mean bias is shown as a *solid line* with limits of agreement (±2SD) as *dashed lines*. Correlation R value was 0.74 for the left ventricle, and 0.85 for the right ventricle. For the left ventricle, mean bias was 23.0 cm/s with limits of agreement between −17.0 and 63.0 cm/s. For the right ventricle, mean bias was 10.8 cm/s with limits of agreement between −18.2 and 39.8 cm/s

to only performing forward tracking without any position prediction.

Other researchers have implemented valve tracking for different purposes than to quantify AV-plane displacement per se. Quantification of mitral valve displacement and velocity in 4-chamber view cine images was presented by Saba et al. [30], and a similar method quantifying the tricuspid valve displacement and velocity has been described by Ito et al. [31]. The method by Saba et al. [30] was later on expanded to a three-dimensional volume tracking method, based on semi-automated tracking of the mitral valve in the 2, 3, and 4-chamber views [29]. Also, Westenberg et al. implemented retrospective valve tracking in order to measure three-dimensional blood flow in CMR [32]. The presented algorithm in this study aimed to quantify the AV-plane displacement in both the left and the right side of the

heart, using cine images of the 2, 3, and 4-chamber view that are acquired as clinical standard. To the best of our knowledge, this approach of using images acquired as clinical standard to quantify both the left and right ventricular AVPD has not be published before.

Manual inter-observer variability in end systole was performed on 20 subjects and showed a low bias and variability, and manual measurements were used as reference standard. The inter-observer variability of the algorithm in end systole had a similar agreement as for the manual inter-observer variability in the right side of the heart. In the left side of the heart, the algorithm inter-observer had a lower correlation R value than for the manual inter-observer, but low bias and SD. Hence, the overall algorithm performance varies about as much as manual measurements vary for different observers. Also, the displacement results of the algorithm had an

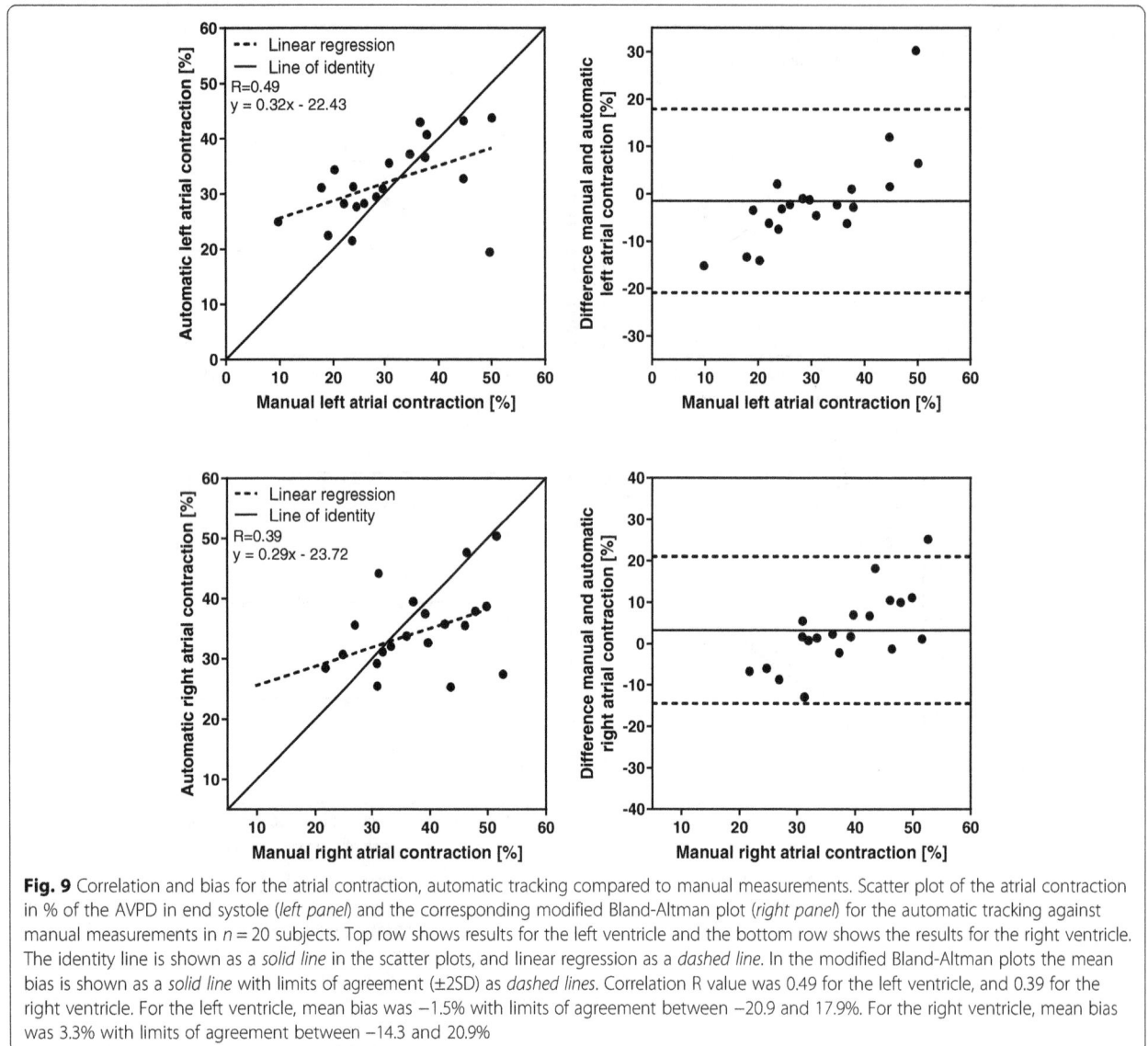

Fig. 9 Correlation and bias for the atrial contraction, automatic tracking compared to manual measurements. Scatter plot of the atrial contraction in % of the AVPD in end systole (*left panel*) and the corresponding modified Bland-Altman plot (*right panel*) for the automatic tracking against manual measurements in $n = 20$ subjects. Top row shows results for the left ventricle and the bottom row shows the results for the right ventricle. The identity line is shown as a *solid line* in the scatter plots, and linear regression as a *dashed line*. In the modified Bland-Altman plots the mean bias is shown as a *solid line* with limits of agreement ($\pm 2SD$) as *dashed lines*. Correlation R value was 0.49 for the left ventricle, and 0.39 for the right ventricle. For the left ventricle, mean bias was -1.5% with limits of agreement between -20.9 and 17.9%. For the right ventricle, mean bias was 3.3% with limits of agreement between -14.3 and 20.9%

agreement in parity with the manual inter-observer variability, and bias was below pixel resolution for both automatic and manual displacement measurements. The end systolic results for both the LVAVPD and the RVAVPD were interchangeable with the inter-observer variability. In the three population groups (consisting of patients, healthy controls, and athletes), similar displacement results were obtained, although the correlation R value was stronger in the LVAVPD for patients compared to healthy controls and athletes.

The AV-plane determined in 2D, by defining a line in each long axis view, was compared to an approach where

Table 1 Displacement results. Manual and automatic measurement results of atrioventricular plane displacement (AVPD) as mean $\pm$ SD in the left (LVAVPD) and right ventricle (RVAVPD). Comparison of automatic tracking vs manual measurements as correlation R value and bias $\pm$ SD of the AVPD. In the time-resolved measure, the AVPD in each timeframe is compared for $n = 20$ subjects. The validation in end systole was performed on $n = 113$ subjects

Measure	Manual	Automatic	R	Bias $\pm$ SD
LVAVPD in end systole [mm]	-13 ± 3	-12 ± 3	0.79	-0.6 ± 1.9
RVAVPD in end systole [mm]	-18 ± 4	-18 ± 4	0.88	-0.8 ± 2.1
Time-resolved LVAVPD [mm]	-	-	0.93	-0.6 ± 2.0
Time-resolved RVAVPD [mm]	-	-	0.95	-0.5 ± 2.2

Table 2 Population based end systolic displacement results. Manual and automatic measurement results of atrioventricular plane displacement (AVPD) in end systole as mean ± SD in the left (LVAVPD) and right ventricle (RVAVPD) for patients (n = 65), healthy controls (n = 24), and athletes (n = 24). Comparison of automatic tracking vs manual measurements as correlation R value and bias ± SD of the AVPD

Measure	Manual	Automatic	R	Bias ± SD
LVAVPD in patients [mm]	−11 ± 2	−11 ± 2	0.81	−0.6 ± 1.3
RVAVPD in patients [mm]	−17 ± 4	−15 ± 3	0.83	−1.0 ± 2.2
LVAVPD in healthy controls [mm]	−14 ± 3	−14 ± 2	0.49	0.0 ± 2.5
RVAVPD in healthy controls [mm]	−20 ± 4	−20 ± 3	0.88	−0.4 ± 1.7
LVAVPD in athletes [mm]	−16 ± 2	−15 ± 2	0.44	−1.3 ± 2.3
RVAVPD in athletes [mm]	−22 ± 3	−21 ± 2	0.77	−0.7 ± 2.2

the AV-plane was defined in 3D, by a best fit all input points in a least square sense. The comparison showed a strong correlation, low bias and variability between both methods. Images were acquired during end-expiratory breath hold and the apex is essentially stationary during the heart beat [39], hence the global heart movement was minimized during the data collection. However, in case the subject move during the MR scan, the 3D coordinate system from the MR scanner might not correspond well to the obtained long axis image positions. Therefore, the 2D implementation was used in this study.

Peak emptying and peak filling are usually calculated from ventricular volume curves and reported as a volumetric flow rate in ml/s. In this study the velocity of the AV-plane at peak emptying and peak filling are quantified in cm/s. Since the AVPD accounts for 60% of the stroke volume in the left side of the heart and 80% in the right side [4], the AV-plane velocity could be an indirect measure of the emptying and filling of the ventricles. A study by Leng et al. showed a good correlation between early diastolic filling from tissue Doppler echocardiography and CMR measures of the AV-plane velocity which would support this [28]. The derivative of a distance curve must be calculated in order to determine velocity estimations. The tracking yields a time-resolved AVPD curve, and even though the curve shape is reconstructed and smoothed using PCA eigenvectors, this curve can appear noisy in between the timeframes. Also,

difficulties are to be expected since CMR cine images can be rather noisy in the timeframes where the peak emptying velocity and peak filling velocity occur. Therefore, taking the numerical first order derivative of the AVPD curve results in an even noisier velocity curve, where it is hard to extract an accurate maximum and minimum velocity. Hence, taking the moving average of the displacement curves prior to differentiating them, and calculating the slope of the straight line over the timeframes where the maximum and minimum velocity occur was considered a more stable approach in this study. The results for the peak emptying velocity have an agreement for manual and automatic measurements in the left and the right side of the heart. When comparing the results of the peak filling velocity, the automatic measurements tends to underestimate the velocities and both bias and SD are quite large.

In general, it is difficult to automatically determine the atrial contraction in the AVPD curve, since the duration of the diastasis can vary from about 20% of the cardiac cycle for low heart rates, to non-existing for high heart rates [40]. The proposed algorithm is programmed to calculate atrial contraction to be the difference in AVPD between end diastole and where the absolute value of the second derivative of the AVPD curve is at its minimum, but the user might change the interval by observing the tracked curve. By design, the algorithm forces the AVPD curve to return to its original position at the

Table 3 Results for automatically calculated peak velocities and atrial contraction. Manual and automatic measurement results of automatically calculated peak emptying velocity, peak filling velocity, and atrial contraction as mean ± SD in the left and right side of the heart. Comparison of automatic tracking vs manual measurements as correlation R value and bias ± SD. The validation was performed on n = 20 subjects. The atrial contraction is given in % of the atrioventricular plane displacement (AVPD) in end systole

Measure	Manual	Automatic	R	Bias ± SD
Left peak emptying velocity [cm/s]	−57 ± 12	−49 ± 8	0.63	−7.6 ± 9.0
Right peak emptying velocity [cm/s]	−77 ± 18	−77 ± 12	0.74	−0.4 ± 12.0
Left peak filling velocity [cm/s]	72 ± 29	49 ± 15	0.74	23.0 ± 20.4
Right peak filling velocity [cm/s]	79 ± 28	68 ± 23	0.85	10.8 ± 14.8
Left atrial contraction [%]	31 ± 11	32 ± 7	0.49	−1.5 ± 9.9
Right atrial contraction [%]	38 ± 9	35 ± 7	0.39	3.3 ± 9.0

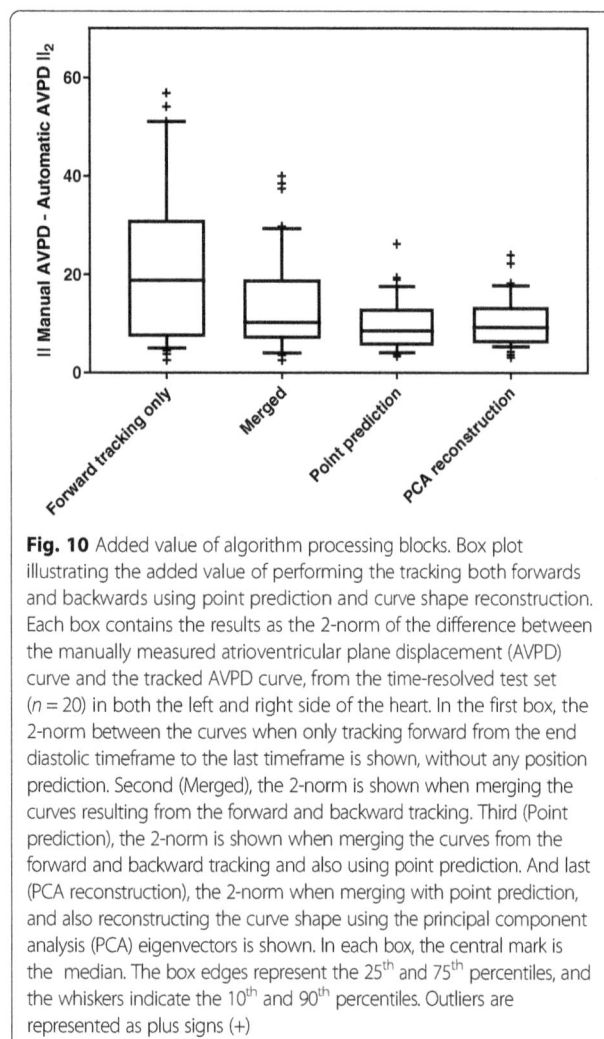

Fig. 10 Added value of algorithm processing blocks. Box plot illustrating the added value of performing the tracking both forwards and backwards using point prediction and curve shape reconstruction. Each box contains the results as the 2-norm of the difference between the manually measured atrioventricular plane displacement (AVPD) curve and the tracked AVPD curve, from the time-resolved test set (*n* = 20) in both the left and right side of the heart. In the first box, the 2-norm between the curves when only tracking forward from the end diastolic timeframe to the last timeframe is shown, without any position prediction. Second (Merged), the 2-norm is shown when merging the curves resulting from the forward and backward tracking. Third (Point prediction), the 2-norm is shown when merging the curves from the forward and backward tracking and also using point prediction. And last (PCA reconstruction), the 2-norm when merging with point prediction, and also reconstructing the curve shape using the principal component analysis (PCA) eigenvectors is shown. In each box, the central mark is the median. The box edges represent the 25th and 75th percentiles, and the whiskers indicate the 10th and 90th percentiles. Outliers are represented as plus signs (+)

end of the cardiac cycle. Hence, if the AVPD tracking is far away from the original position at diastasis, the atrial contraction will be represented as a very steep segment in the AVPD curve. This might explain why the SDs of the atrial contraction was large. Also, the diastasis can be hard to detect for high heart rates.

An underestimation can be seen for large displacements in both the end systolic and time-resolved AVPD measurements (Figs. 5 and 6), as well as in the results of high peak velocities and large atrial contractions (Figs. 7, 8 and 9). The cause of this underestimation is unknown. However, one source for the underestimation could be an effect of overtraining of the algorithm. In order to evaluate if overtraining could be a cause, the proportion of subjects in the training and test sets were compared. The proportion of healthy controls in the training set was 38% whereas in the test set it was 21%, thus the training set included more subjects with a higher AVPD compared to the test set. The proportion of athletes in both the training and test set were the same (23%

and 21%, respectively). This should rather be a source for overestimation than underestimation. Another potential source of error might be that the algorithm has difficulties in tracking the AV-plane when it is moving at high velocities. On the other hand, the overall tracked displacement curve has a good agreement to manual measurements, according to the time-resolved displacement validation and the low distance between the automatic and manual AVPD curves, measured by the 2-norm.

Limitations

Limitations of this study comprises that patients included in the training and test set were only patients with first time ST-elevation myocardial infarction. The algorithm is based on a priori information extracted from manual measurements in the training set. Hence other patient categories and anatomic variations may have been missed when constructing the AVPD prediction model, such as patients with very low AVPD. Including such patients might be necessary for the algorithm to track very low AV-plane motions, but it might also reduce the accuracy of the tracking results in healthy subjects if the prediction curve is reduced in amplitude. On the other hand, the lower limit of agreement of LVAVPD was 7 mm, why this limitation might be of less significance.

The algorithm is not expected to work on prospective ECG gated CMR data, since the backward tracking, PCA prediction, and curve shape reconstruction are designed on data comprising the whole cardiac cycle. All images in this study were acquired during end-expiratory breath hold. In images acquired during breathing, the calculation of the AVPD might be obfuscated by the chest movement.

The input points to be tracked are chosen by the user, and variations in placements of these input points may result in some points being hard to track for the algorithm. Heart sizes impacts the amplitude of the AVPD curve, where for example athletes have larger hearts and therefore are expected to have a larger AVPD, while elderly and different patient groups often have a reduced AVPD. The amplitude of the tracking predictor is not scaled according to the specific subject, and even though the size of the ROS's for each input point has been optimized for a large range of AVPD amplitudes, the true match may not be present in the ROS for varying heart sizes. The curve shape reconstruction ensures that the AV-plane trajectory is transformed to a smooth and physiological movement. If the chosen input point does not move as physiologically expected, for example due to anatomical variations, severe disease, or an incorrect input by the user, the calculated displacement may not represent the true AVPD. Therefore, manual monitoring and manual corrections are important for research and clinical use, as for any automatic image analysis algorithm. The same applies to the estimated peak emptying velocity, peak filling velocity, and atrial contraction, where the user should check that the interval of the lines defining the measures are placed in agreement with the appearance of the AVPD curve. The use of the proposed automatic tracking algorithm will reduce time input and user variability, which are important aspects for clinical use. Also, this allow the researcher or clinician to observe not only the total AVPD in end systole, which is the commonly used reference standard today, but also the whole AVPD trajectory throughout the whole cardiac cycle.

Future work

Atrial contraction results were not satisfactory, comprising many outliers (Fig. 9). Further studies of the algorithm can verify if this is a recurring issue.

In order to implement a fully automatized algorithm for AVPD tracking, the 8 manually placed input points in the end diastolic timeframe may possibly be replaced by automatic input point detection. The tracking algorithm predict the position of each input point in the next timeframe, using a priori information gathered from normal controls, athletes and patients with first time myocardial infarction. Gathering information from other physiological variations and patient groups might improve the prediction model. An automatic adaptive approach to scale the prediction curve based on the physiology of each individual data set could also increase the robustness of the algorithm and yield more accurate results for displacement, peak velocities, and atrial contraction.

Conclusion

The developed automatic algorithm performs time-resolved tracking of the AVDP in CMR images using normalized cross-correlation and a priori information based on principal component analysis. The algorithm performs well with regards to displacement against manual measurements in healthy controls of a wide age spread, athletes, and first time myocardial infarction patients from multi-center and multi-vendor data. Further, the algorithm yields displacement results in parity with inter-observer variability.

Therefore, an algorithm based on normalized cross-correlation and principal component analysis may be introduced as a method for measuring the atrioventricular plane displacement in CMR imaging.

Abbreviations

AV: Atrioventricular; AVPD: Atrioventricular plane displacement; CMR: Cardiovascular magnetic resonance; LV: Left ventricle; LVAVPD: Left ventricular atrioventricular plane displacement; MAPSE: Mitral annular plane systolic excursion; PCA: Principal component analysis; ROI: Region of interest; ROS: Region of search; RV: Right ventricle; RVAVPD: Right ventricular atrioventricular plane displacement; SD: Standard deviations; TAPSE: Tricuspid annular plane systolic excursion

Acknowledgements

Not applicable.

Funding

This study was founded by the Swedish Research Council (2012–4944), The Swedish Heart Lung Foundation (20140624) and the Region of Scania, Sweden. Funding for the MITOCARE trial was received from the European Commission within the 7th Framework Program for RTD – Project MITOCARE – Grant Agreement HEALTH-2010-261034. The inclusion of elderly normal subjects was funded by Novo Nordisk and the Swedish Heart Association.

Authors' contributions

FS developed and implemented the algorithm, analyzed the results, performed time-resolved manual measurements in the training and test set, the inter-observer analysis, drafted the manuscript, and helped conceive the study. UP contributed by performing manual measurements of the patient data, and second observer analysis on the time-resolved measurements in the training and test set, and in the inter-observer analysis. KE included healthy subjects and athletes, and performed manual measurements in them. EO performed the inter-observer analysis. DE, SJ, and JR collected patient data. DA was responsible for the collection of patient data. HA helped in conceiving the study. MC contributed to the design of the algorithm and conceived the study. EH contributed to the design of the study, the algorithm design, and conceived the study. Further, FS, EH, UP, EO, KE, MC contributed with intellectual discussion and consensus definition of the AV-plane. All authors have revised the manuscript and approved the final version.

Competing interests

EH is the founder of Medviso AB, Lund, Sweden, which sells a commercial version of the software Segment. HA is a shareholder of Imacor AB, Lund, Sweden, which performs core lab analysis of CMR images. HA and MC have been part-time consultants to Imacor AB. The other authors declare that they do not have any competing interests.

Author details

[1]Department of Clinical Physiology, Lund University, Skane University Hospital, Lund, Sweden. [2]Department of Numerical Analysis, Faculty of Engineering, Lund University, Lund, Sweden. [3]Department of Biomedical Engineering, Faculty of Engineering, Lund University, Lund, Sweden. [4]Department of Health Sciences, Physiotherapy, Lund University, Lund, Sweden. [5]Department of Cardiology, Clinical Sciences, Lund University, Lund, Sweden. [6]Assistance Publique Hôpitaux de Paris, Hôpital Henri Mondor, Créteil, France. [7]Department of Cardiology, Aalborg University Hospital, Aalborg, Denmark. [8]Department of Cardiology B, Oslo University Hospital Ullevål and Faculty of Medicine, University of Oslo, Oslo, Norway.

References

1. Henein MY, Gibson DG. Normal long axis function. Heart. 1999;81:111–3.
2. Henein MY, Gibson DG. Long axis function in disease. Heart. 1999;81:229–31.
3. Carlsson M, Ugander M, Mosen H, Buhre T, Arheden H. Atrioventricular plane displacement is the major contributor to left ventricular pumping in healthy adults, athletes, and patients with dilated cardiomyopathy. AJP Heart Circ Physiol. 2006;292:H1452–9.
4. Carlsson M, Ugander M, Heiberg E, Arheden H. The quantitative relationship between longitudinal and radial function in left, right, and total heart pumping in humans. AJP Heart Circ Physiol. 2007;293:H636–44.
5. Willenheimer R, Israelsson B, Cline C, Rydberg E, Broms K, Erhardt L. Left atrioventricular plane displacement is related to both systolic and diastolic left ventricular performance in patients with chronic heart failure. Eur Heart J. 1999;20:612–8.
6. Carlhäll CJ, Lindström L, Wranne B, Nylander E. Atrioventricular plane displacement correlates closely to circulatory dimensions but not to ejection fraction in normal young subjects. Clin Physiol. 2001;21:621–8.
7. Willenheimer R, Cline C, Erhardt L, Israelsson B. Left ventricular atrioventricular plane displacement: an echocardiographic technique for rapid assessment of prognosis in heart failure. Heart. 1997;78:230–6.
8. Wandt B, Bojö L, Wranne B. Influence of body size and age on mitral ring motion. Clin Physiol. 1997;17:635–46.
9. Caballero L, Kou S, Dulgheru R, Gonjilashvili N, Athanassopoulos GD, Barone D, Baroni M, Cardim N, Gomez de Diego JJ, Oliva MJ, Hagendorff A, Hristova K, Lopez T, Magne J, Martinez C, de la Morena G, Popescu BA, Penicka M, Ozyigit T, Rodrigo Carbonero JD, Salustri A, Van De Veire N, Von Bardeleben RS, Vinereanu D, Voigt J-U, Zamorano JL, Bernard A, Donal E, Lang RM, Badano LP, et al. Echocardiographic reference ranges for normal cardiac Doppler data: results from the NORRE Study. Eur Hear J Cardiovasc Imaging. 2015;16(9):1031–41.
10. Steding-Ehrenborg K, Boushel RC, Calbet JA, Åkeson P, Mortensen SP. Left ventricular atrioventricular plane displacement is preserved with lifelong endurance training and is the main determinant of maximal cardiac output. J Physiol. 2015;593:5157–66.
11. Steding-Ehrenborg K, Carlsson M, Stephensen S, Arheden H. Atrial aspiration from pulmonary and caval veins is caused by ventricular contraction and secures 70% of the total stroke volume independent of resting heart rate and heart size. Clin Physiol Funct Imaging. 2013;33:233–40.
12. Lang RM, Badano LP, Mor-Avi V, Afilalo J, Armstrong A, Ernande L, Flachskampf FA, Foster E, Goldstein SA, Kuznetsova T, Lancellotti P, Muraru D, Picard MH, Rietzschel ER, Rudski L, Spencer KT, Tsang W, Voigt J-U. Recommendations for cardiac chamber quantification by echocardiography in adults: an update from the american society of echocardiography and the european association of cardiovascular imaging. J Am Soc Echocardiogr. 2015;28:1–39. e14.
13. Sanderson JE. Left and right ventricular long-axis function and prognosis. Heart. 2008;94:262–3.
14. Hu K, Liu D, Herrmann S, Niemann M, Gaudron PD, Voelker W, Ertl G, Bijnens B, Weidemann F. Clinical implication of mitral annular plane systolic excursion for patients with cardiovascular disease. Eur Heart J Cardiovasc Imaging. 2013;14:205–12.
15. Kalam K, Otahal P, Marwick TH. Prognostic implications of global LV dysfunction: a systematic review and meta-analysis of global longitudinal strain and ejection fraction. Heart. 2014;100:1673–80.
16. Galiè N, Humbert M, Vachiery J-L, Gibbs S, Lang I, Torbicki A, Simonneau G, Peacock A, Vonk Noordegraaf A, Beghetti M, Ghofrani A, Gomez Sanchez MA, Hansmann G, Klepetko W, Lancellotti P, Matucci M, McDonagh T, Pierard LA, Trindade PT, Zompatori M, Hoeper M. 2015 ESC/ERS Guidelines for the diagnosis and treatment of pulmonary hypertension. Eur Respir J. 2015;46:903–75.
17. Rangarajan V, Chacko SJ, Romano S, Jue J, Jariwala N, Chung J, Farzaneh-Far A. Left ventricular long axis function assessed during cine-cardiovascular magnetic resonance is an independent predictor of adverse cardiac events. J Cardiovasc Magn Reson. 2016;18:35.
18. Rudski LG, Lai WW, Afilalo J, Hua L, Handschumacher MD, Chandrasekaran K, Solomon SD, Louie EK, Schiller NB. Guidelines for the echocardiographic assessment of the right heart in adults: a report from the american society of echocardiography. J Am Soc Echocardiogr. 2010;23:685–713.
19. Nevo ST, van Stralen M, Vossepoel AM, Reiber JHC, de Jong N, van der Steen AFW, Bosch JG. Automated tracking of the mitral valve annulus motion in apical echocardiographic images using multidimensional dynamic programming. Ultrasound Med Biol. 2007;33:1389–99.
20. Behar V, Adam D, Lysyansky P, Friedman Z. The combined effect of nonlinear filtration and window size on the accuracy of tissue displacement estimation using detected echo signals. Ultrasonics. 2004;41:743–53.
21. Eto Y, Yamada H, Shin J-H, Agler DA, Tsujino H, Qin J-X, Saracino G, Greenberg NL, Thomas JD, Shiota T. Automated mitral annular tracking: a novel method for evaluating mitral annular motion using two-dimensional echocardiography. J Am Soc Echocardiogr. 2005;18:306–12.
22. Schulz-Menger J, Bluemke DA, Bremerich J, Flamm SD, Fogel MA, Friedrich MG, Kim RJ, von Knobelsdorff-Brenkenhoff F, Kramer CM, Pennell DJ, Plein S, Nagel E. Standardized image interpretation and post processing in cardiovascular magnetic resonance: Society for Cardiovascular Magnetic Resonance (SCMR) board of trustees task force on standardized post processing. J Cardiovasc Magn Reson. 2013;15:35.
23. Arvidsson PM, Toger J, Heiberg E, Carlsson M, Arheden H. Quantification of left and right atrial kinetic energy using four-dimensional intracardiac magnetic resonance imaging flow measurements. J Appl Physiol. 2013;114:1472–81.
24. Stephensen S, Steding-Ehrenborg K, Munkhammar P, Heiberg E, Arheden H, Carlsson M. The relationship between longitudinal, lateral, and septal contribution to stroke volume in patients with pulmonary regurgitation and healthy volunteers. AJP Heart Circ Physiol. 2014;306:H895–903.
25. Jorstig S, Emilsson K, Lidén M, Thunberg P. A study to determine the contribution to right ventricle stroke volume from pulmonary and tricuspid valve displacement volumes. Clin Physiol Funct Imaging. 2015; 35:283–90.
26. Ostenfeld E, Stephensen SS, Steding-Ehrenborg K, Heiberg E, Arheden H, Rådegran G, Holm J, Carlsson M. Regional contribution to ventricular stroke volume is affected on the left side, but not on the right in patients with pulmonary hypertension. Int J Cardiovasc Imaging. 2016; 32(8):1243–53.
27. Maffessanti F, Gripari P, Pontone G, Andreini D, Bertella E, Mushtaq S, Tamborini G, Fusini L, Pepi M, Caiani EG. Three-dimensional dynamic assessment of tricuspid and mitral annuli using cardiovascular magnetic resonance. Eur Heart J Cardiovasc Imaging. 2013;14:986–95.
28. Leng S, Zhao X-D, Huang F-Q, Wong J-I, Su B-Y, Allen JC, Kassab GS, Tan R-S, Zhong L. Automated quantitative assessment of cardiovascular magnetic resonance-derived atrioventricular junction velocities. Am J Physiol Heart Circ Physiol. 2015;309:H1923–35.
29. Wu V, Chyou JY, Chung S, Bhagavatula S, Axel L. Evaluation of diastolic function by three-dimensional volume tracking of the mitral annulus with cardiovascular magnetic resonance: comparison with tissue Doppler imaging. J Cardiovasc Magn Reson. 2014;16:71.
30. Saba SG, Chung S, Bhagavatula S, Donnino R, Srichai MB, Saric M, Katz SD, Axel L. A novel and practical cardiovascular magnetic resonance method to quantify mitral annular excursion and recoil applied to hypertrophic cardiomyopathy. J Cardiovasc Magn Reson. 2014;16:35.
31. Ito S, McElhinney DB, Adams R, Bhatla P, Chung S, Axel L. Preliminary assessment of tricuspid valve annular velocity parameters by cardiac magnetic resonance imaging in adults with a volume-overloaded right ventricle: comparison of unrepaired atrial septal defect and repaired tetralogy of fallot. Pediatr Cardiol. 2015;36:1294–300.
32. Westenberg JJM, Roes SD, Ajmone Marsan N, Binnendijk NMJ, Doornbos J, Bax JJ, Reiber JHC, de Roos A, van der Geest RJ. Mitral valve and tricuspid valve blood flow: accurate quantification with 3D velocity-encoded MR imaging with retrospective valve tracking. Radiology. 2008;249:792–800.
33. Steding K, Engblom H, Buhre T, Carlsson M, Mosén H, Wohlfart B, Arheden H. Relation between cardiac dimensions and peak oxygen uptake. J Cardiovasc Magn Reson. 2010;12:8.
34. Atar D, Arheden H, Berdeaux A, Bonnet J-L, Carlsson M, Clemmensen P, Cuvier V, Danchin N, Dubois-Rande J-L, Engblom H, Erlinge D, Firat H, Halvorsen S, Hansen HS, Hauke W, Heiberg E, Koul S, Larsen A-I, Le Corvoisier P, Nordrehaug JE, Paganelli F, Pruss RM, Rousseau H, Schaller S, Sonou G, Tuseth V, Veys J, Vicaut E, Jensen SE. Effect of intravenous TRO40303 as an adjunct to primary percutaneous coronary intervention for acute ST-elevation myocardial infarction: MITOCARE study results. Eur Heart J. 2015;36:112–9.
35. Heiberg E, Sjögren J, Ugander M, Carlsson M, Engblom H, Arheden H. Design and validation of Segment–freely available software for cardiovascular image analysis. BMC Med Imaging. 2010;10:1.
36. Lewis JP. Fast normalized cross-correlation. Vis interface. 1995;10(1):120–23.
37. Pearson K. LIII. On lines and planes of closest fit to systems of points in space. Philos Mag Ser 6. 1901;2:559–72.

8

Image quality improvement using model-based iterative reconstruction in low dose chest CT for children with necrotizing pneumonia

Jihang Sun[1], Tong Yu[1], Jinrong Liu[2], Xiaomin Duan[1], Di Hu[1], Yong liu[1] and Yun Peng[1*]

Abstract

Background: Model-based iterative reconstruction (MBIR) is a promising reconstruction method which could improve CT image quality with low radiation dose. The purpose of this study was to demonstrate the advantage of using MBIR for noise reduction and image quality improvement in low dose chest CT for children with necrotizing pneumonia, over the adaptive statistical iterative reconstruction (ASIR) and conventional filtered back-projection (FBP) technique.

Methods: Twenty-six children with necrotizing pneumonia (aged 2 months to 11 years) who underwent standard of care low dose CT scans were included. Thinner-slice (0.625 mm) images were retrospectively reconstructed using MBIR, ASIR and conventional FBP techniques. Image noise and signal-to-noise ratio (SNR) for these thin-slice images were measured and statistically analyzed using ANOVA. Two radiologists independently analyzed the image quality for detecting necrotic lesions, and results were compared using a Friedman's test.

Results: Radiation dose for the overall patient population was 0.59 mSv. There was a significant improvement in the high-density and low-contrast resolution of the MBIR reconstruction resulting in more detection and better identification of necrotic lesions (38 lesions in 0.625 mm MBIR images vs. 29 lesions in 0.625 mm FBP images). The subjective display scores (mean ± standard deviation) for the detection of necrotic lesions were 5.0 ± 0.0, 2.8 ± 0.4 and 2.5 ± 0.5 with MBIR, ASIR and FBP reconstruction, respectively, and the respective objective image noise was 13.9 ± 4.0HU, 24.9 ± 6.6HU and 33.8 ± 8.7HU. The image noise decreased by 58.9 and 26.3% in MBIR images as compared to FBP and ASIR images. Additionally, the SNR of MBIR images was significantly higher than FBP images and ASIR images.

Conclusions: The quality of chest CT images obtained by MBIR in children with necrotizing pneumonia was significantly improved by the MBIR technique as compared to the ASIR and FBP reconstruction, to provide a more confident and accurate diagnosis for necrotizing pneumonia.

Keywords: Computed tomography (CT), Model-based iterative reconstruction, Filtered back-projection, Necrotizing pneumonia, Child

* Correspondence: ppengyun@yahoo.com
[1]Imaging Center, Beijing Children's Hospital, Capital Medical University, No.56, Nanlishi Road, Xicheng District, Beijing 100045, People's Republic of China
Full list of author information is available at the end of the article

Background

With the increased demand for CT, the desire to reduce radiation dose also increases. This is especially true in pediatric CT imaging. However, the conventional filtered back-projection (FBP) reconstruction limits the possibility of further reducing the radiation dosage, especially when higher spatial resolution and thinner image slice thickness are desirable. Hence, the intention of reducing the radiation dosage in CT has in recent years shifted focus from hardware upgrades and tube current decrease only to the development of advanced reconstruction algorithms. Noise model-based iterative reconstruction, such as adaptive statistical iterative reconstruction (ASIR), iDose and Sinogram affirmed iterative reconstruction (SAFIRE) [1–5], is a new type of CT reconstruction algorithm using statistical models to reduce image noise and produce better image quality [6, 7]. These new iterative reconstruction techniques have been applied in clinical practice and have demonstrated the ability to provide clinically acceptable images for diagnosis with significantly reduced radiation dosage by 32–65% [7].

Recently, a full model-based iterative reconstruction (MBIR) algorithm that incorporates both the noise mode and the optical model of the whole detection system for significantly decreasing image noise and improving spatial resolution at the same time has been introduced. MBIR algorithm has been used in adults for reducing image noise and radiation dose in chest and lung field [8–12], but few studies have been done in children [13, 14], and there is no research about the effect of iterative algorithm on image quality and dose in children with necrotic lesions. The purpose of this study was to evaluate the improvements in chest CT image quality and diagnostic performance with MBIR over FBP and ASIR in children with necrotizing pneumonia (NP) in simulated extremely low signal (radiation dose) CT scans.

Methods

Patient population

This retrospective study was approved by the Ethics Committees of Beijing Children's Hospital for using the data, and parent consent was waived. One hundred and forty-one children with suspected NP, congenital lung diseases, trachea malformation or vessel malformation underwent low dose enhanced chest CT scans in our hospital between March 11, 2012 and August 31, 2013. Of these, 26 children (aged 2 months to 11 years with a median age of 4.0 years) were clinically diagnosed for NP. There were 3 patients in the 0–12 month age group, 5 in the 1–2 years and 18 in the 3–17 years age groups. Among these, 15 children had *Mycoplasma pneumoniae* (combined with *Klebsiella pneumonia* infection in one patient), two children had group A beta-hemolytic *Streptococci*, two children had *Streptococcus pneumonia*

infections, and seven children had no clear etiological diagnosis. The time interval between the enhanced CT examination and the onset of the symptoms (fever, cough, or other symptoms) was 30.2 ± 11.1 days. In total, 33 necrotic lesions were observed in 28 pulmonary lobes in the standard CT images (5 mm thickness FBP image). Twenty of the lesions involved 17 lobes in the right lung (1 lesion in 1 upper lobe; 3 lesions in 3 middle lobes; 16 lesions in 13 lower lobes) and 13 lesions involved 11 lobes in the left lung (2 lesions in 2 upper lobes; 4 lesions in 3 middle lobes; 7 lesions in 6 lower lobes).

Data acquisition

All patients underwent a contrast-enhanced low dose CT scan on a 64 rows high definition CT (HDCT) scanner (Discovery CT 750 HD, GE Healthcare, Waukesha, WI USA) with a tube voltage of 120 kVp, pitch of 1.375, detector collimation was 64x0.625 mm for a 40 mm total coverage in a single rotation, and rotation speed of 0.8 s. The tube current was set between 10 and 350 mA, and modulated with the automatic tube current modulation (ATCM) system. Age-dependent noise index (NI) settings for a 5 mm thick image were used for the acquisition: $NI = 11$ for 0–12month old, $NI = 13$ for 1–2 years old and $NI = 15$ for 3–17years old. Most children were too young to cooperate and were sedated with oral chloral hydrate (10%, 0.5 mL/kg) before scanning. The CT scan covered the area between the entrance to the chest and the base of the lungs. Iodinated contrast (Iodixanol 320, 320 mg I/mL, visipaque™; GE Healthcare, Ireland, IDA Business Park Carrigtohill Co. Cork) was intravenously administered; contrast dose was based on body weight with 1.8, 1.6, 1.4, 1.2, and 1.0 mL/kg, for children weighing 3–5 kg, 5–10 kg, 10–15 kg, 15–35 kg, and >35 kg, respectively. Contrast was administered using a single-head power injector at injection rates of 0.4–3.0 mL/s adjusted to a fixed injection time of 15 s. Enhanced scans started at 45 s after the start of contrast injection.

Subjective assessment of the image quality

The original image sets were reconstructed at 5 mm slice thickness with a filtered back-projection (FBP) algorithm according to the standard protocol for image review and diagnosis. The scan data were further retrospectively reconstructed into three groups with thinner slice thickness of 0.625 mm based on the reconstruction algorithm: series A with MBIR technique, series B with 30%ASIR (blending of 30% of ASIR and 70% of FBP reconstruction), which was recommended by vendor to have balanced image noise and spatial resolution, series C with FBP technique. The division of image slice thickness from 5 to 0.625 mm was used to simulate an extremely low signal but higher resolution study. All images were transferred to a GE

AW4.5 CT workstation for analysis. The reviewers were blinded to background information about the children, scanning parameters and reconstruction algorithms. Two experienced radiologists (one with 13 years of experience in adult radiography, and 6 years' experience in pediatric radiography, and the other one with 3 years of experience in adult radiography and 4 years of experience in pediatric radiography) evaluated the images independently. The objective image quality evaluation was performed on the three 0.625 mm slice thickness image sets (with MBIR, ASIR and FBP). The images were displayed initially in the mediastinal window, but the reviewers could adjust the window width and window level as per their preference. Multi-planar reconstruction (MPR) and Volume rendering (VR) images were also available for viewing. The thickness of MPR was also 0.625 mm.

Subjective display ability for necrotic lesions and confidence in diagnosis were used to rate image quality, with a 5-point scale. The ability for the necrotic lesions display was scored as follows: 5 = lesion(s) border displayed clearly with excellent contrast to surrounding tissue; 4 = lesion(s) margin displayed clearly with good contrast; 3 = lesion(s) displayed with marginal contrast, but a little blurry; 2 = lesion(s) margin displayed with poor contrast and incompletely; and 1 = cannot distinguish necrosis lesions from surrounding tissue. Diagnosis confidence was scored as, 5 = the whole image displayed perfectly with excellent confidence; 4 = the whole image has small amount of noise but with good confidence; 3 = there are some noise but image quality is good enough for diagnosis; 2 = whole image is not clear enough for confident diagnosis; and 1 = very hard to distinguish structures and cannot make any diagnosis.

Evaluation of the objective noise

Quantitative image noise measurement was performed on all 4 image sets: both 5 and 0.625 mm slice thickness images with FBP reconstruction, 0.625 mm slice thickness with ASIR algorithm and 0.625 mm slice thickness with MBIR algorithm. After the qualitative evaluation, the two radiologists selected the largest cross-section area of the consolidated lesion (Le) and necrotic area (Nec) in the lesion and drew regions of interest (ROI) together in consensus. The CT density was measured in an area of ROI of 8–39 mm^2, and the standard deviation (SD) was calculated. CT densities and SD of the back muscles (Mus) and background air (Air) in the same cross section were also measured. The objective image noise was represented using the average SD for these areas. Signal-to-noise ratio (SNR) for all tissues was calculated using the following formula: $SNR = CT\ density_{(ROI)}/SD_{(ROI)}$. Contrast noise ratio (CNR) for the consolidated lesion to necrotic area ($CNR_{(L-C)}$) and consolidated lesion to air ($CNR_{(L-A)}$) were calculated using

the following formula: $CNR_{(L-C)} = (CT\ density_{(Le)} - CT\ density_{(Nec)})/SD_{(muscle)}$, $CNR_{(L-A)} = (CT\ density_{(Le)} - CT\ density_{(Air)})/SD_{(Air)}$. The ROI was generally about 1 quarter of the cross-section area of the descending aorta at the same image layer, and the shape of the region was variable in the evaluation.

Statistical analysis

The objective noise, SNR and CNR measurements and subjective image quality evaluation were recorded in detail and were presented as Mean ± SD. Objective measurements between MBIR, ASIR and FBP (0.625 and 5 mm) were compared statistically using one way ANOVA, To account for multiple statistical, a 'Tukey' post-hoc analysis was applied. And subjective image quality evaluation was compared using the Friedman's test. Kappa statistics were used to evaluate the consistency between the two radiologists' diagnoses. All statistical analyses were performed using SPSS17.0 (SPSS Inc., Chicago, IL, USA). A 2-tailed P value < 0.05 was deemed significant.

Radiation dosage

Parameters of the X-ray radiation dosages including the volumetric CT dose index (CTDIvol) and dose length product (DLP) were recorded. Effective dose (ED) was calculated using the following formula: $ED = DLP \times W$, where W is the patient age-dependent conversion factor for the chest area of pediatric patients. For our study, we used W values of 0.039, 0.026, and 0.018 for the patient age groups of 0–12 months, 1–2 years, and 3–6 years, respectively, based on the European guidelines on quality criteria for computed tomography to calculate an age-weighted conversion factor.

Results

The CTDIvol, DLP, and overall radiation dose for the present study was 1.14 ± 0.56 mGy, 26.96 ± 9.86 mGy.cm, and 0.59 ± 0.19 mSv (using the age-weighted conversion factor of 0.022 $mSv.mGy^{-1}.cm^{-1}$ based on the age distribution of patient population in this study), respectively.

There were 33 necrotic lesions in 28 lobes detected in the standard 5 mm FBP images. In the 0.625 mm MBIR images, 38 necrotic lesions were found in the same 28 lobes; 3 necrotic lesions were missed in the 0.625 mm ASIR images, and only 29 necrotic lesions could be certain in the 0.625 mm FBP images due to high image noise.

Subjective assessment of the image quality

The subjective image quality evaluation for the 3 thin image slice series are displayed in Table 1. MBIR images showed significantly better subjective image quality with significantly lower granular noise artifacts. There were significant differences between the 3 groups ($P < 0.05$).

Table 1 Subjective image quality evaluation among different reconstructions

Algorithm	Doctor A				Doctor B			
	Overall diagnosis confidence	P	Display ability for necrotic lesions	P	Overall diagnosis confidence	P	Display ability for necrotic lesions	P
MBIR	4.6 ± 0.5	-	5.0 ± 0.0	-	5.0 ± 0.0	-	5.0 ± 0.0	-
ASIR	2.9 ± 0.3	<0.01	2.6 ± 0.5	<0.01	3.0 ± 0.2	<0.01	3.0 ± 0.2	<0.01
FBP	2.7 ± 0.5	<0.01	2.3 ± 0.5	<0.01	2.9 ± 0.3	<0.01	2.6 ± 0.5	<0.01

Objective image quality measurement

Figure 1 displays the objective image noise measurements; Fig. 2 displays the SNR and CNR results for all 4 image series. There were significant differences in the objective noise value among the 0.625 mm MBIR, ASIR and FBP images ($F = 61.5$, $P < 0.05$). There was significantly less objective noise for the consolidated lesions with the 0.625 mm thickness MBIR images than the thin slice ASIR and FBP images, and even the conventional 5 mm slice FBP images. The objective noise of consolidated lesions in the MBIR images was reduced by 44.2, 18.7 and 58.9%, compared with the 0.625 mm ASIR, 5 mm FBP and 0.625 mm FBP images, respectively (Fig. 3). Similarly, for the noise measurement in air, MBIR images reduced noise by a respective 67.9, 30.8 and 76.0%. The objective noise for the muscle in the 0.625 mm MBIR images was reduced by 46.7 and 60.6% compared to the 0.625 mm ASIR and FBP images, respectively, but image noise was statistically the same between the 0.625 mm MBIR and the 5 mm FBP images. The noise measurements in the necrotic area were similar to those in muscle, MBIR image reduced noise by 57.8 and 68.9% compared to the 0.625 mm ASIR and FBP images, and was not significant different from the 5 mm FBP images. SNR values for the consolidated lesion of 0.625 mm MBIR image increased by 89.7, 150.0 and 34.1%, compared with the 0.625 mm ASIR, 0.625 mm FBP and 5 mm FBP, respectively ($F = 43.5$, $P < 0.05$), (Table 2). The $CNR_{(L-C)}$ of 0.625 mm MBIR image was increased by 100.0, 23.1 and 166.7%, compared with the 0.625 mm ASIR, 5 mm FBP and 0.625 mm FBP images, ($F = 27.0$, $P < 0.05$), and $CNR_{(L-A)}$ was increased by 343.2, 101.3 and 491.6%, respectively ($F = 22.9$, $P < 0.05$), (Table 3).

Inter-observer consistency

The inter-observer *Kappa* value for the subjective quality scores was 0.66, showing a good consistency between the two observers.

Discussion

Necrotizing pneumonia (NP) has no clear definition today. According to Hacimustafaoglu, NP is necrosis in pulmonary consolidation [15], and patchy areas without contrast in a CT scan [16]. Hyewon Seo et al pointed out that NP is distinct form lung abscess, with a characteristic performance of poorly defined foci of low density, and unassociated with enhancing margins in

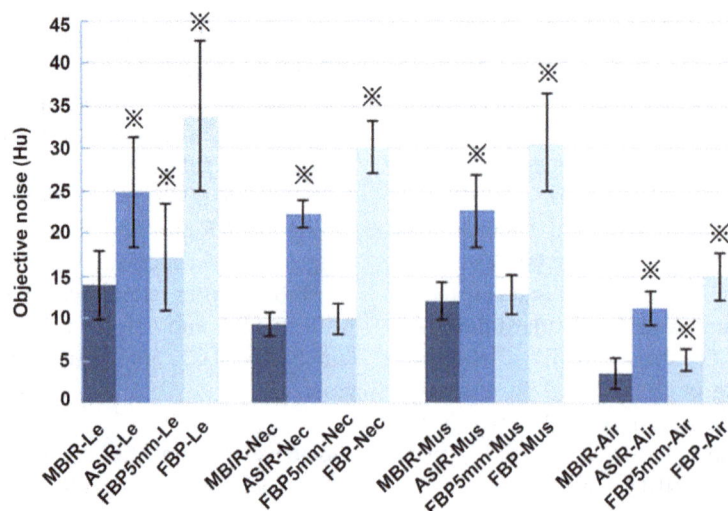

Fig. 1 Average number and standard deviation of objective image noise of 4 algorithms on different tissues. Images were 0.625 mm in thickness unless stated otherwise. Le: consolidated lesion; Nec: necrotic area; Mus: muscle; Air: background air around body. ※ Significant difference of image noise compared with the 0.625 mm MBIR image

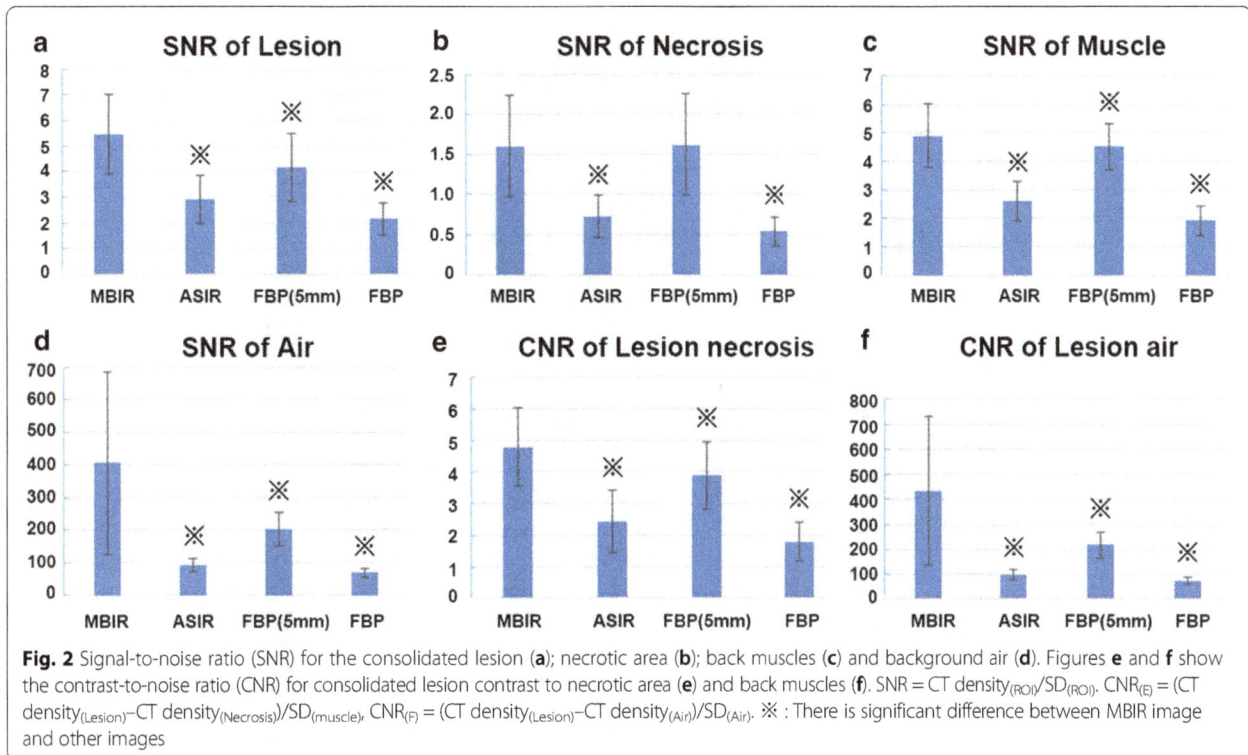

Fig. 2 Signal-to-noise ratio (SNR) for the consolidated lesion (**a**); necrotic area (**b**); back muscles (**c**) and background air (**d**). Figures **e** and **f** show the contrast-to-noise ratio (CNR) for consolidated lesion contrast to necrotic area (**e**) and back muscles (**f**). SNR = CT density$_{(ROI)}$/SD$_{(ROI)}$. CNR$_{(E)}$ = (CT density$_{(Lesion)}$−CT density$_{(Necrosis)}$)/SD$_{(muscle)}$, CNR$_{(F)}$ = (CT density$_{(Lesion)}$−CT density$_{(Air)}$)/SD$_{(Air)}$. ※ : There is significant difference between MBIR image and other images

enhanced chest CT [17]. Our own experience indicated that it is very difficult to find necrotic lesions in unenhanced CT, so the standard protocol for NP in our hospital was to perform low dose enhanced CT. NP is currently diagnosed clinically and necrotic lesions are determined in CT images according to experience. Since necrotic lesions have an important significance in the diagnosis of NP, timely and accurate diagnosis is important for guiding future treatment, increasing awareness of complications, follow-up and in providing appropriate recommendations to parents of patients recovering from NP [16]. Previous research on children chest imaging has indicated that MBIR can increase both image quality and image contrast-noise-ratio due to its ability to dramatically decrease image noise and increase spatial resolution [13, 14]. In this study we used the existing standard of care (SOC) low dose CT data. Since SOC low dose CT images meet the clinical diagnostic image quality requirements at 5 mm slice thickness in terms of image noise, by reconstructing the images into 0.625 mm slice thickness, we substantially reduce the signal strength in the thinner slice images to simulate extremely low dose scan conditions while improving the image spatial resolution. The thin-slice (0.625 mm) images were then reconstructed with MBIR, ASIR and conventional FBP algorithms, and the results demonstrated that MBIR algorithm increased image spatial resolution and improved image quality to better delineate necrotic lesions to aid the earlier detection and more confident diagnosis of NP.

Low-dose CT is widely used and necessary, but traditional FBP reconstruction technique provides limited image quality to balance spatial resolution and image noise when using low radiation dose CT scanning, because of the limitation of its mathematical model. More recent noise model-based iterative reconstruction techniques, such as ASIR, use complex statistical models to reduce noise and to produce acceptable image quality even with low-radiation dose [1–5]. The full mode-based iterative reconstruction (MBIR) algorithm further extends the noise reduction capability and at the same time improves the image spatial resolution [8–13] which is not standard on a Discovery CT 750 HD scanner and requires an additional software and hardware. We hypothesized that MBIR can help us to detect even tiny and low contrast necrotic lesions better at their early stage, especially for displaying small necrotic foci of necrosis pneumonia in pediatric patients, even with extremely low radiation doses. But due to paucity of such data, we simulated the extremely low signal situations by using clinically confirmed cases acquired at the standard of care low dosage to validate its capabilities. Since X-ray (signal) detected by the detector is proportional to the thickness of the detection cell, by reconstructing images into the 0.625 mm slice thickness from the standard 5 mm slice thickness, we effectively reduced the X-ray flux in each of the smaller detection cell (0.625 mm vs. 5 mm) by more than 85%, simulating an extremely low signal (low dose) situation. Therefore, the present

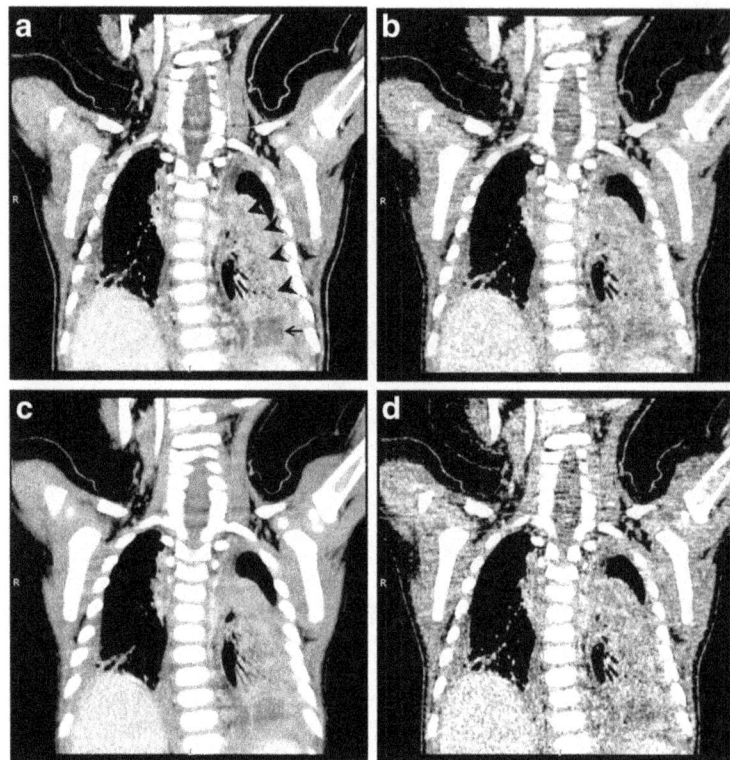

Fig. 3 A child with group A beta-hemolytic streptococcus infection. CT scan was acquired at 120 kV with automatic tube current modulation technique (19–22 mA). Multi-planar reconstruction (MPR) was used for image review. (**a**, **b**, **c**, **d**) were MPR images with mediastinal window. **a** MBIR image with 0.625 mm; **b** ASIR image with 0.625 mm; **c** FBP image with 5 mm; **d** FBP image with 0.625 mm. Image noise of in MBIR image (**a**) was reduced significantly compared with that of 0.625 mm ASIR image (**b**) and 0.625 mm FBP image (**d**), and was similar to that of 5 mm FBP image (**c**). Necrotic lesions (*arrowheads*) and encapsulated pleural effusion (*arrow*) in the MBIR image (**a**) were displayed much clearly and confidently than in the 0.625 mm ASIR (**b**) and FBP (**d**) images. 5 mm FBP image (**c**) was too thick to display boundaries and scope of necrotic lesions

research was based on the standard-of-care data acquired for clinical purpose. The data acquisition was completed with the conventional scanning procedures for clinical use with no additional operation on patients.

MBIR drastically reduced image noise in such a low signal condition in both lesion and muscle. Our results indicated that the image noise of the 0.625 mm MBIR images was statistically the same as the conventional 5 mm FBP images, and was about 60% lower than that of the 0.625 mm FBP images. In terms of subjective quality, MBIR images were significantly better than FBP and even ASIR images in the overall image quality and visibility of necrotic lesions (Fig. 1). In our study group, there were 33 necrotic lesions observed in 28 pulmonary lobes in the standard 5 mm FBP CT images. The conventional 5 mm images were often too thick to clearly show the boundaries of necrotic lesions, so, not all 33 lesions were confidently determined. The 0.625 mm MBIR images, with higher spatial resolution and much lower image noise, were able to provide clear boundaries for tiny necrotic lesions (Fig. 3). So the 0.625 mm MBIR images not only identified the 33 lesions confidently, but also detected 5 extra lesions (38 vs. 33) in the same 28

lobes. On the other hand, the 0.625 mm FBP images only identified 29 lesions, missing 4 small necrotic lesions from the standard 5 mm FBP images due to the much higher image noise caused by the extremely low signal in the thin slice imaging mode.

In the present study, all included patients were children, wherein the distribution of body fat and length are different from those of adults. Therefore, the association between the radiation dose and BMI was not clear in this population. Consequently, we divided the children into different groups based on their age instead of their body weight or BMI [13]. On the other hand, the body type of children display greater variations with age than adults. In order to obtain a similar proportion of region of interest area in children with different body type, a region with the area about one quarter of the cross-section of the aorta was chosen as the region of interest. Thus, the proportion of the area of the region of interest was the same in different individuals. In addition, the size of the region of interest could be modulated to facilitate the evaluation. Because the necrotic lesions are usually small, it limits the inclusion of a larger area, and a very small range affects the noise result, and hence, we

Table 2 Objective image noise measurements

Tissue	Image[a]	CT value Mean ± SD	P	Noise Mean ± SD	P	SNR Mean ± SD	P
Consolidated lesion	MBIR	71.1 ± 9.3	-	13.9 ± 4.0	-	5.5 ± 1.6	-
	ASIR	67.9 ± 12.7	0.13	24.9 ± 6.6	<0.01	2.9 ± 0.9	<0.01
	5 mm FBP	63.9 ± 7.9	<0.01	17.2 ± 6.4	0.02	4.1 ± 1.3	<0.01
	FBP	68.9 ± 12.1	0.10	33.8 ± 8.7	<0.01	2.2 ± 0.6	<0.01
Necrotic area	MBIR	14.8 ± 5.7	-	9.4 ± 1.4	-	1.6 ± 0.6	-
	ASIR	16.2 ± 5.5	0.02	22.3 ± 1.6	<0.01	0.7 ± 0.3	<0.01
	5 mm FBP	15.6 ± 5.0	0.19	9.9 ± 1.8	0.25	1.6 ± 0.6	0.92
	FBP	16.2 ± 5.0	0.05	30.2 ± 3.0	<0.01	0.5 ± 0.2	<0.01
Muscle	MBIR	57.4 ± 7.2	-	12.1 ± 2.2	-	4.9 ± 1.1	-
	ASIR	56.3 ± 6.6	0.48	22.7 ± 4.3	<0.01	2.6 ± 0.7	<0.01
	5 mm FBP	56.6 ± 6.6	0.49	12.9 ± 2.3	0.07	4.5 ± 0.8	0.04
	FBP	56.2 ± 8.9	0.21	30.7 ± 5.8	<0.01	1.9 ± 0.5	<0.01
Air	MBIR	−994.8 ± 4.3	-	3.6 ± 1.9	-	−407.9 ± 280.0	-
	ASIR	−996.7 ± 3.2	0.08	11.2 ± 2.1	<0.01	−92.3 ± 18.8	0.01
	5 mm FBP	−996.8 ± 2.6	0.09	5.2 ± 1.2	<0.01	−203.9 ± 51.4	0.02
	FBP	−996.5 ± 4.0	0.16	15.0 ± 2.7	<0.01	−69.0 ± 14.5	0.01

[a]Images were 0.625 mm in thickness unless stated otherwise

used the well-proportioned back muscle for noise measurement to correct this variation.

This study does have limitations. First, all examinations were performed using 120 kV scan according to the then (before December 2013) standard protocol in our institution. The scan protocols have since been optimized based on patient sizes and clinical tasks. However, we do not expect the tube voltage selection should affect the results of this study significantly, since same data were used with different reconstruction algorithms. Second, because NP is rare in children, the present study was limited by a small sample size. In addition, different noise index used in children with different age could also introduce bias. Further studies with larger sample sizes are necessary to confirm these findings. Third, since the MBIR image quality is much more superior to FBP image, true blinded study was impossible, and there could have been some bias in the subjective quality score. Doctor B provided maximum scores for all evaluation, and this could have possibly affected the fairness

of the image quality results to some extent. Third, MBIR is a complex algorithm, it needs quite a long reconstruction time (about 30 min per scan series at the current software version) which also limited the number of cases included in this study and further large-scale research is needed to confirm the conclusion. Finally, we demonstrated the ability of MBIR to dramatically reduce image noise and increase both the high and low contrast resolution compared with the other algorithms in a simulated extreme low signal scanning condition, further research on the performance of MBIR with actual reduced scanning conditions is needed to fully demonstrate it clinical ability.

Conclusions

The quality of chest CT images in children with necrotizing pneumonia significantly improved by the MBIR technique, especially in the extremely low signal condition, as compared to the FBP reconstruction and noise model-based iterative reconstruction (ASIR), to provide a more confident and accurate diagnosis for necrotizing pneumonia and to help clinicians to develop treatment programs earlier.

Table 3 CNR between model-based iterative reconstruction (MBIR) image and other reconstructions

Algorithm	Consolidated lesion-necrotic area CNR	P	Consolidated lesion -air CNR	P
MBIR (0.625 mm)	4.8 ± 1.3	-	436.6 ± 298.5	-
ASIR (0.625 mm)	2.4 ± 1.0	<0.01	98.5 ± 19.8	<0.01
FBP (5 mm)	3.9 ± 1.1	<0.01	216.9 ± 54.7	<0.01
FBP (0.625 mm)	1.8 ± 0.6	<0.01	73.8 ± 15.4	<0.01

Abbreviations
Air: Background air; ASIR: Adaptive statistical iterative reconstruction; ATCM: Automatic tube current modulation; CNR: Contrast noise ratio; CT: Computed tomography; CTDIvol: CT dose index; DLP: Dose length product; ED: Effective dose; FBP: Filtered back-projection; Le: Consolidated lesion; MBIR: Model-based iterative reconstruction; MPR: Multi-planar reconstruction; Mus: Back muscles; Nec: Necrotic area; NI: Noise index; NP: Necrotizing pneumonia; ROI: Regions of interest; SAFIRE: Sinogram affirmed iterative reconstruction; SD: Standard deviation; SNR: Signal-to-noise ratio; SOC: Standard of care; VR: Volume rendering

Acknowledgements

I would like to express my sincere thanks to Dr. Jianying Li for his technical support in understanding the model-based iterative reconstruction algorithm.

Funding

The authors gratefully acknowledge the financial supports by the National Science and Technology Major Project of the Ministry of Science and Technology of China and The Application Research of Clinical Characteristics of Beijing under Grant numbers Z141107002514005, and Beijing Children's Hospital Young Investigator Program under Grant numbers BCH-YIPB-2016-06.

Authors' contributions

JS and TY carried out the studies, participated in collecting data, and drafted the manuscript. JL and XD performed the statistical analysis and participated in its design. DH, YL and YP helped to draft the manuscript. All authors read and approved the final manuscript.

Competing interests

The authors declare that they have no competing interests.

Author details

[1]Imaging Center, Beijing Children's Hospital, Capital Medical University, No.56, Nanlishi Road, Xicheng District, Beijing 100045, People's Republic of China. [2]Department of respiratory, Beijing Children's Hospital, Capital Medical University, Beijing 100045, People's Republic of China.

References

1. Cornfeld D, Israel G, Detroy E, Bokhari J, Mojibian H. Impact of Adaptive Statistical Iterative Reconstruction (ASIR) on radiation dose and image quality in aortic dissection studies: a qualitative and quantitative analysis. Am J Roentgenol. 2011;196:W336–40.
2. Singh S, Kalra MK, Gilman MD, Hsieh J, Pien HH, Digumarthy SR, Shepard JA. Adaptive statistical iterative reconstruction technique for radiation dose reduction in chest CT: a pilot study. Radiology. 2011;259:565–73.
3. Singh S, Kalra MK, Hsieh J, Licato PE, Do S, Pien HH, Blake MA. Abdominal CT: Comparison of Adaptive Statistical Iterative and Filtered Back Projection Reconstruction Techniques 1. Radiology. 2010;257:373–83.
4. Sagara Y, Hara AK, Pavlicek W, Silva AC, Paden RG, Wu Q. Abdominal CT: comparison of low-dose CT with adaptive statistical iterative reconstruction and routine-dose CT with filtered back projection in 53 patients. AJR Am J Roentgenol. 2010;195:713–9.
5. Prakash P, Kalra MK, Kambadakone AK, Pien H, Hsieh J, Blake MA, Sahani DV. Reducing abdominal CT radiation dose with adaptive statistical iterative reconstruction technique. Investig Radiol. 2010;45:202–10.
6. Lee SH, Kim MJ, Yoon CS, Lee MJ. Radiation dose reduction with the adaptive statistical iterative reconstruction (ASIR) technique for chest CT in children: an intra-individual comparison. Eur J Radiol. 2012;81:e938–43.
7. Hara AK, Paden RG, Silva AC, Kujak JL, Lawder HJ, Pavlicek W. Iterative reconstruction technique for reducing body radiation dose at CT: feasibility study. AJR Am J Roentgenol. 2009;193:764–71.
8. Katsura M, Matsuda I, Akahane M, Yasaka K, Hanaoka S, Akai H, Sato J, Kunimatsu A, Ohtomo K. Model-based iterative reconstruction technique for ultralow-dose chest CT: comparison of pulmonary nodule detectability with the adaptive statistical iterative reconstruction technique. Investig Radiol. 2013;48:206–12.
9. Neroladaki A, Botsikas D, Boudabbous S, Becker CD, Montet X. Computed tomography of the chest with model-based iterative reconstruction using a radiation exposure similar to chest X-ray examination: preliminary observations. Eur Radiol. 2013;23:360–6.
10. Ichikawa Y, Kitagawa K, Nagasawa N, Murashima S, Sakuma H. CT of the chest with model-based, fully iterative reconstruction: comparison with adaptive statistical iterative reconstruction. BMC Med Imaging. 2013;13:27.
11. Chen B, Barnhart H, Richard S, Robins M, Colsher J, Samei E. Volumetric quantification of lung nodules in CT with iterative reconstruction (ASiR and MBIR). Med Phys. 2013;40:111902.
12. Yanagawa M, Gyobu T, Leung AN, Kawai M, Kawata Y, Sumikawa H, Honda O, Tomiyama N. Ultra-low-dose CT of the lung: effect of iterative reconstruction techniques on image quality. Acad Radiol. 2014;21:695–703.
13. Sun J, Peng Y, Duan X, Yu T, Zhang Q, Liu Y, Hu D. Image quality in children with low-radiation chest CT using adaptive statistical iterative reconstruction and model-based iterative reconstruction. PLoS One. 2014;9:e96045.
14. Sun J, Zhang Q, Hu D, Duan X, Peng Y. Improving pulmonary vessel image quality with a full model-based iterative reconstruction algorithm in 80kVp low-dose chest CT for pediatric patients aged 0–6 years. Acta Radiol. 2014. doi:10.1177/0284185114540884.
15. Hacimustafaoglu M, Celebi S, Sarimehmet H, Gurpinar A, Ercan I. Necrotizing pneumonia in children. Acta Paediatr. 2004;93:1172–7.
16. Reimel BA, Krishnadasen B, Cuschieri J, Klein MB, Gross J, Karmy-Jones R. Surgical management of acute necrotizing lung infections. Can Respir J. 2006;13:369–73.
17. Seo H, Cha SI, Shin KM, Lim J, Yoo SS, Lee J, Lee SY, Kim CH, Park JY. Focal necrotizing pneumonia is a distinct entity from lung abscess. Respirology. 2013;18:1095–100.

9

Analysis of the three-dimensional anatomical variance of the distal radius using 3D shape models

Sebastian F. Baumbach[1*], Jakob Binder[1], Alexander Synek[2], Fabian G. Mück[3], Yan Chevalier[4], Ekkehard Euler[1], Georg Langs[5] and Lukas Fischer[5,6]

Abstract

Background: Various medical fields rely on detailed anatomical knowledge of the distal radius. Current studies are limited to two-dimensional analysis and biased by varying measurement locations. The aims were to 1) generate 3D shape models of the distal radius and investigate variations in the 3D shape, 2) generate and assess morphometrics in standardized cut planes, and 3) test the model's classification accuracy.

Methods: The local radiographic database was screened for CT-scans of intact radii. 1) The data sets were segmented and 3D surface models generated. Statistical 3D shape models were computed (overall, gender and side separate) and the 3D shape variation assessed by evaluating the number of modes. 2) Anatomical landmarks were assigned and used to define three standardized cross-sectional cut planes perpendicular to the main axis. Cut planes were generated for the mean shape models and each individual radius. For each cut plane, the following morphometric parameters were calculated and compared: maximum width and depth, perimeter and area. 3) The overall shape model was utilized to evaluate the predictive value (leave one out cross validation) for gender and side identification within the study population.

Results: Eighty-six radii (45 left, 44% female, 40 ± 18 years) were included. 1) Overall, side and gender specific statistical 3D models were successfully generated. The first mode explained 37% of the overall variance. Left radii had a higher shape variance (number of modes: 20 female / 23 male) compared to right radii (number of modes: 6 female / 6 male). 2) Standardized cut planes could be defined using anatomical landmarks. All morphometric parameters decreased from distal to proximal. Male radii were larger than female radii with no significant side difference. 3) The overall shape model had a combined median classification probability for side and gender of 80%.

Conclusions: Statistical 3D shape models of the distal radius can be generated using clinical CT-data sets. These models can be used to assess overall bone variance, define and analyze standardized cut-planes, and identify the gender of an unknown sample. These data highlight the potential of shape models to assess the 3D anatomy and anatomical variance of human bones.

Keywords: Image processing, Anatomical model, Distal radius, Statistical model, Computed tomography

* Correspondence: sebastian.baumbach@med.uni-muenchen.de
[1]Department of General, Trauma and Reconstructive Surgery, University Hospital LMU Munich, Nussbaumstr. 20, Munich 80336, Germany
Full list of author information is available at the end of the article

Background

Various medical fields rely on detailed anatomical knowledge of the distal radius. This is required to understand joint kinematics, improve fracture pattern analysis, plan surgical procedures [1, 2], design novel osteosynthetic devices [3–5], and identify human remains [6, 7]. Up to now, literature on the anatomy of the distal radius is limited to morphologic (shape) and morphometric (size) studies based on radiographs [8] or single computed tomography (CT) slices [9–11]. Limiting the analysis to two-dimensional (2-D) results has two predominant limitations: first, it does not allow the display of three-dimensional (3D) shape variation of the distal radius; second, the use of single CT slices may impair inter-subject comparability due to inconsistent slice position and orientation.

A well-established methodology in assessment of 3D anatomy and anatomical variances of bones are statistical shape models. These can be generated from a database of CT scans. Following 3D surface segmentation, a dense set of corresponding surface landmarks is generated for each bone. Based on this information, 3D shape models can be calculated and the variation of each surface point within the population illustrated. These variations are referred to as modes. A further application of these 3D shape models is the generation of two-dimensional (2D) slices of each bone within the database with identical matching location and orientation. Finally, the 3D shape models can be used to classify anatomical geometries into groups, for instance to determine gender of unidentified bones.

Statistical shape models have been applied for segmentation of vertebra [12], femora [13, 14], or brain structures [15]. Van Giessen and colleges [16] used this methodology to analyze wrist bone motion patterns. No study has yet applied this methodology to assess the general 3D anatomy and population based variation of the distal radius, or generated inter-specimen consistent (position and orientation) cut planes. Therefore, the primary aim of this study was to generate and analyze a statistical 3D shape model of the intact distal radius. Specifically, 3D shape models were generated to 1) investigate the 3D shape variation, 2) generate standardized cut planes and evaluate morphometric parameters, and 3) test the model's classification accuracy for radius side and gender.

Methods

Study design

A retrospective, CT-based image processing study was designed to investigate anatomical variance of the distal radius. It was organized in three steps: First, 3D shape models were generationed; Second, corresponding, uniform cut-planes were computed and morphometric

parameters analized; Third, the model's classification accuracy for side and gender was assessed. The local ethics committee approved the study (Ref. Nr. 126-13).

Patient identification

Consecutive CT-scans of intact radii were identified using the local radiographic database (University Hospital LMU Munich). The search period was 2 years, the search terms used were: CT-scan AND wrist OR scaphoid; Eligibility criteria were 18 year of age, sufficiently large region of interest, identical scan and reconstruction parameters (i.e. identical scan protocol, bone kernel reconstructions, 1.25 mm axial slice thickness; Discovery HD 750, GE Healthcare, Waukesha IL/USA), no signs of current/previous fractures or morphologic changes such as osteoarthritis, bone cysts or tumors. If both radii of one person were eligible, only the right radius was included. No sample size calculation could be conducted due to missing preliminary data. Previous studies investigating the volar cortical angle of the distal radius included 74 ± 23 patients on average [9–11, 17–19]. Therefore, we aimed at a study population of 90 radii (mean + 1SD) and a gender ratio of 50% female.

3D shape model generation and analysis

The DICOM datasets of all distal radii were anonymized. The general workflow is outlined in Fig. 1. The CT-images (Fig. 1 3D Volumes) were segmented manually (Slicer 3D, [20]). Triangulated surfaces (0.1 mm side length, according to [21]) were generated using custom Python codes and CGAL libraries [22]. These were then registered to one radius to achieve a uniform alignment of the surface models (Fig. 1 Alignment). A Point Distribution Model (PDM) [23] was used to construct the shape model by computing the significant eigenmodes and thereby the shape variation of the data set. These shapes consisted of a set of n 3-dimensional landmarks. Correspondences between the shape landmarks were derived utilizing minimum description length (MDL) [24]. The shape information was then used to build models (Fig. 1 Statistical 3-D Shape Models), which allowed representation of the original shapes and generalization of new shapes within the distribution of shapes in the data set. The detailed process is outlined in Additional file 1. Three shape models were generated for all radii, as well as separately for gender and side. The gender and side specific models were used to analyze the general morphology of the distal radius. The 3D shape variation was assessed by evaluating the number of modes of the side and gender specific shape models. The number of modes was determined based on a 95% explained variance threshold. The first 5 modes were plotted. All calculations were performed in Matlab

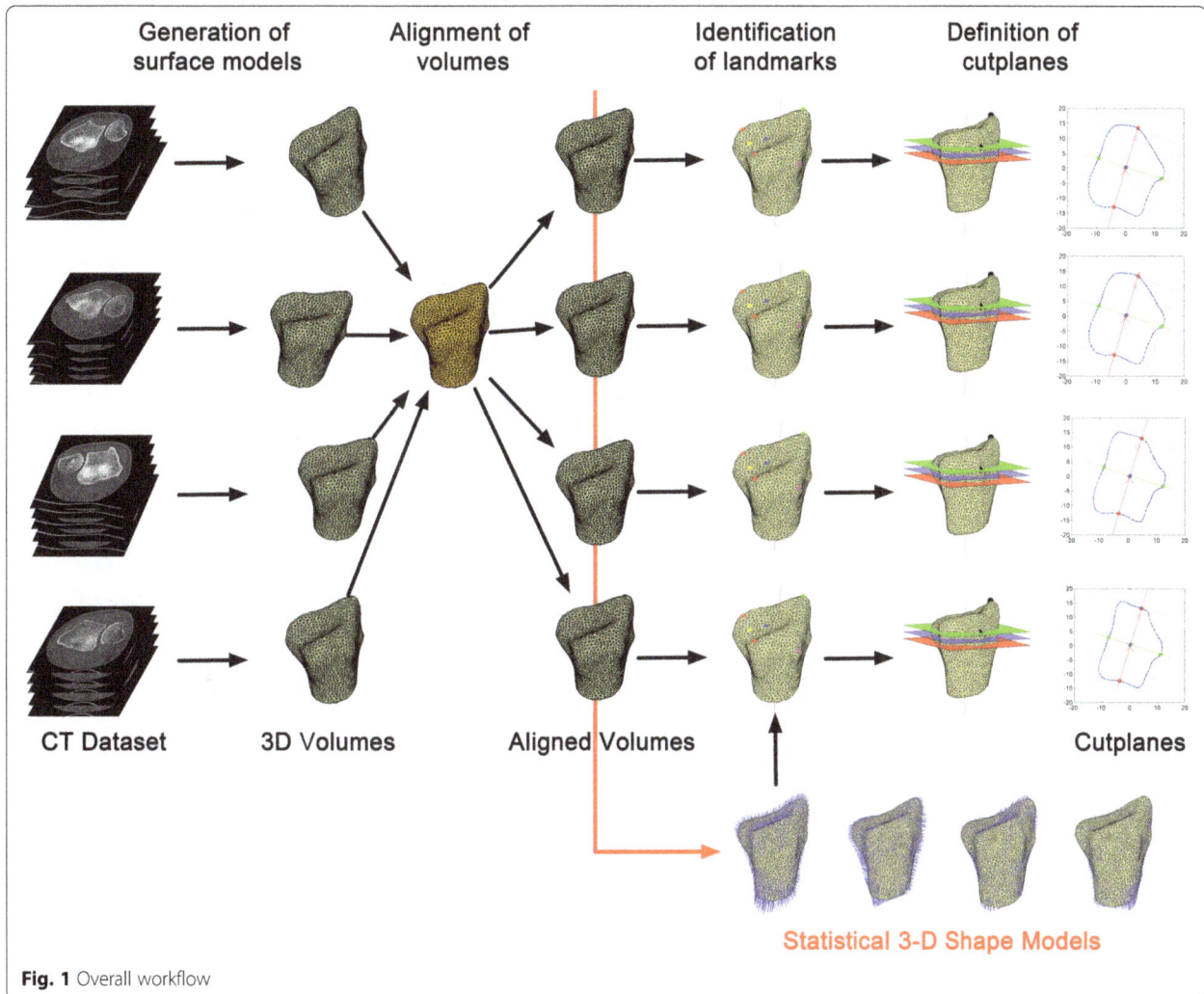

Fig. 1 Overall workflow

R2015a (The MathWorks, Inc., Natick, Massachusetts, United States).

Standardized cross-sectional cut planes and morphometric parameters

Three cross-sectional cut planes were defined for further morphometric analysis based on size-independent landmarks. These were the styloid process and the most dorsal point of the tuberculum listerii (Fig. 1 identification of landmarks and cut planes). Standardized three-dimensional sample orientation allowed the definition of cross-sectional cut planes perpendicular to the main axis. The following cross-sectional cut planes (Fig. 2) were chosen: *Distal*: The most dorsal point of the tuberculum listerii (Fig. 2B.1); *Proximal*: 50% of the distance between the tip of the styloid process and the most dorsal point of the tuberculum listerii (Fig. 2B.3); *Middle*: Half way between the distal and proximal sectional plane (Fig. 2B.2). Cross-sectional cut planes were calculated for the mean shape models as well as for

each individual radius. An animated illustration of the cross-sectional cut planes is presented in Additional file 2. For each sectional plane the maximum width and depth, perimeter and area were calculated (Fig. 2 Legend).

Classification accuracy for side and gender

The overall shape model was utilized to evaluate the predictive value for gender and side identification within our population. To do so leave-one-out cross validation (LOOCV) by repeatedly (100 iterations) removing one test shape and training a classifier (random forest with 50 decision trees) on the remaining shape model coefficients was conducted. The resulting classification accuracy was calculated. All computations were performed in Matlab R2015a.

Statistics

Statistical differences in morphometric parameters (maximum width and depth, perimeter and area) between side and gender were calculated using SPSS 22.0

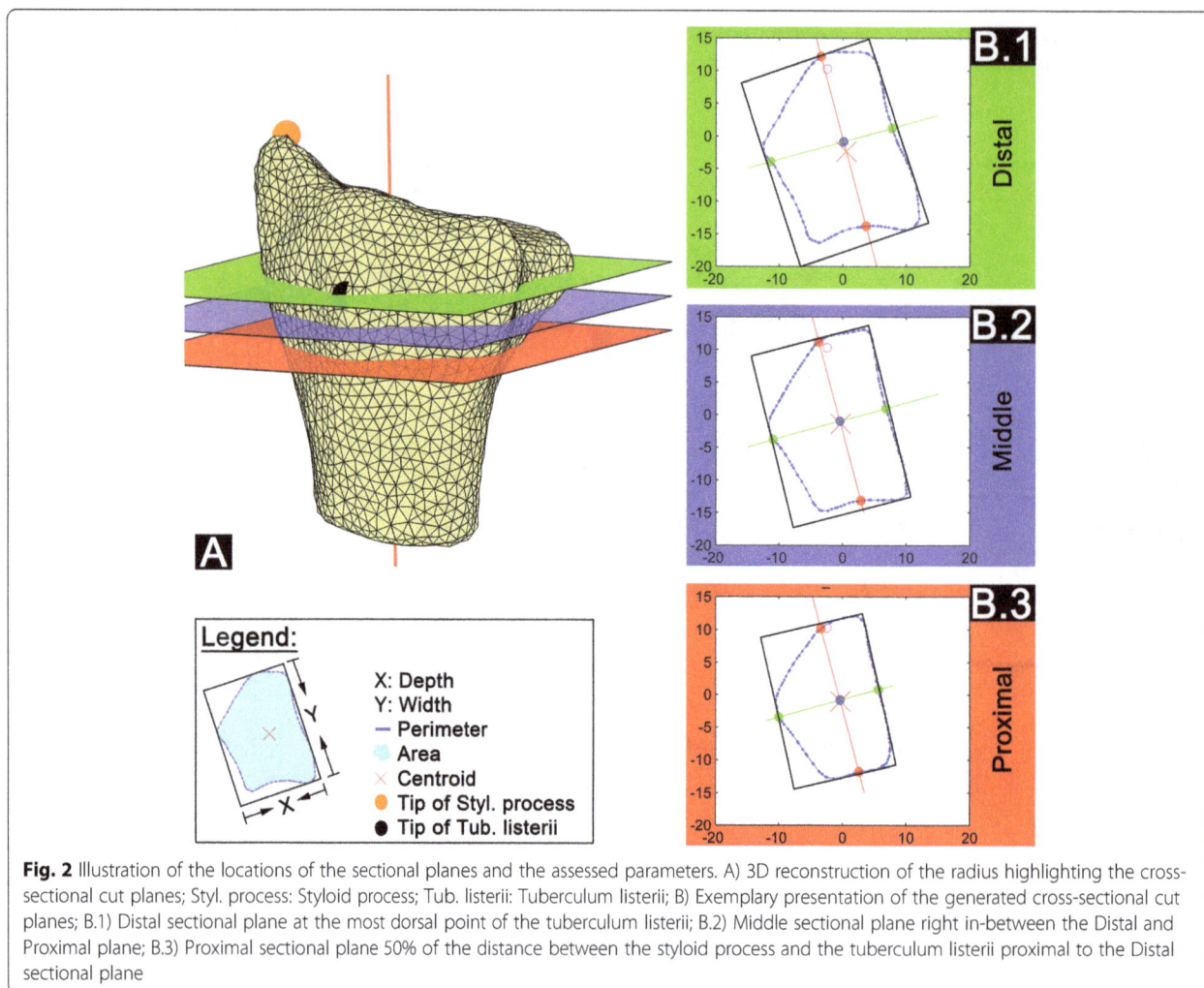

Fig. 2 Illustration of the locations of the sectional planes and the assessed parameters. A) 3D reconstruction of the radius highlighting the cross-sectional cut planes; Styl. process: Styloid process; Tub. listerii: Tuberculum listerii; B) Exemplary presentation of the generated cross-sectional cut planes; B.1) Distal sectional plane at the most dorsal point of the tuberculum listerii; B.2) Middle sectional plane right in-between the Distal and Proximal plane; B.3) Proximal sectional plane 50% of the distance between the styloid process and the tuberculum listerii proximal to the Distal sectional plane

(IBM, Chicago, IL, USA). The Kolmogorov-Smirnov test was used to verify that data was normally distributed. General morphology statistics comprised of descriptive analysis, an independent sample t-Test and an ANOVA (post hoc test: Bonferroni). Due to multiple testing, a Bonferroni correction was conducted ($p < 0.013$). The ratio between correctly and incorrectly classified radii was used to calculate the classification accuracy of the overall shape model.

Results

Patient sample

One thousand two hundred nine radii were screened, 96 radii met the inclusion criteria. 1113 radii were excluded for the following reasons: fracture ($n = 585$), region of interest too small ($n = 388$), duplicates ($n = 77$), morphometric changes ($n = 53$), and age ($n = 10$). Ten more radii were excluded as they were used for pretests. The remaining 86 radii (45 left radii, 44% female, no pairs, mean age 40 ± 18 years (18–88 years)) were used to

compute the models. The CT-indications for those radii were suspected distal radius- (25%) or suspected carpal fractures (75%).

3D shape model analysis

All shape models were computed successfully. Figure 3 illustrates the gender and side specific models including their first mode. The first mode explained 37% of the overall variance and 41% / 34% / 25% / 50% of the variance of female / male / left / right radii respectively. Animated illustrations of the first five modes of all models are presented in Additional file 3A-D. Left radii had a higher shape variance (number of modes: 20 female / 23 male) compared to right radii (number of modes: 6 female / 6 male) (Additional file 4). Predominant shape variation directions (1. mode) for female radii were disto-proximal, while in the axial plane for the male left radii. The shape variation in male radii was curved, from lateral to medio-distal.

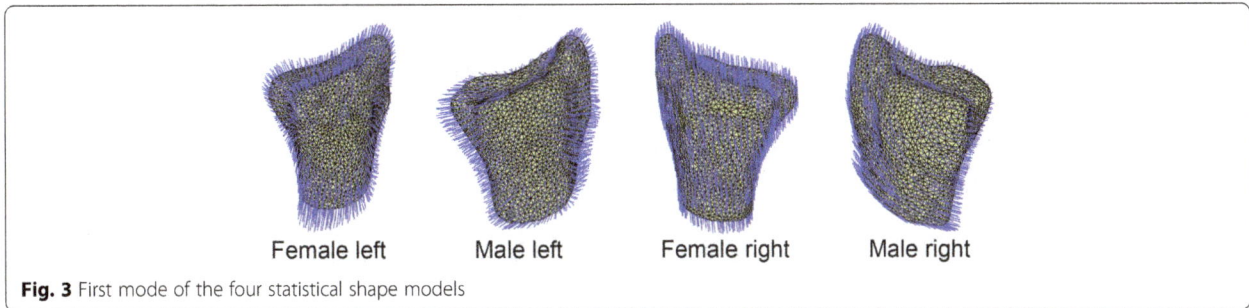

Fig. 3 First mode of the four statistical shape models

Standardized cross-sectional cut planes and morphometric parameters

Uniform cut planes were generated for the first mode of each mean shape model and every radius separately. Morphometric parameters, i.e. maximum width and depth, perimeter, and area (Fig. 2 Legend) were calculated. Figure 4 illustrates side and gender specific cross-sectional cut planes and their morphometric values for the mean shape model. The cross-sectional cut planes for ±1SD of the mean shape models are presented in Additional file 5, the subsequent morphometric values in Additional file 6. Overall, male radii were larger than female radii with no

significant side difference. All morphometric parameters decreased from distal to proximal.

Furthermore, the three standardized cut planes were calculated for all 86 radii separately. The cross-sectional cut planes were on average 3.5 ± 0.6 mm apart from each other. Table 1 summarizes their descriptive morphometric parameters. All assessed plane parameters were significantly greater in male than in female patients ($p \leq 0.001$). No significant side differences could be found. Comparing the morphometric parameters between the cross-sectional cut planes (ANOVA) gender separately revealed overall significant differences. The

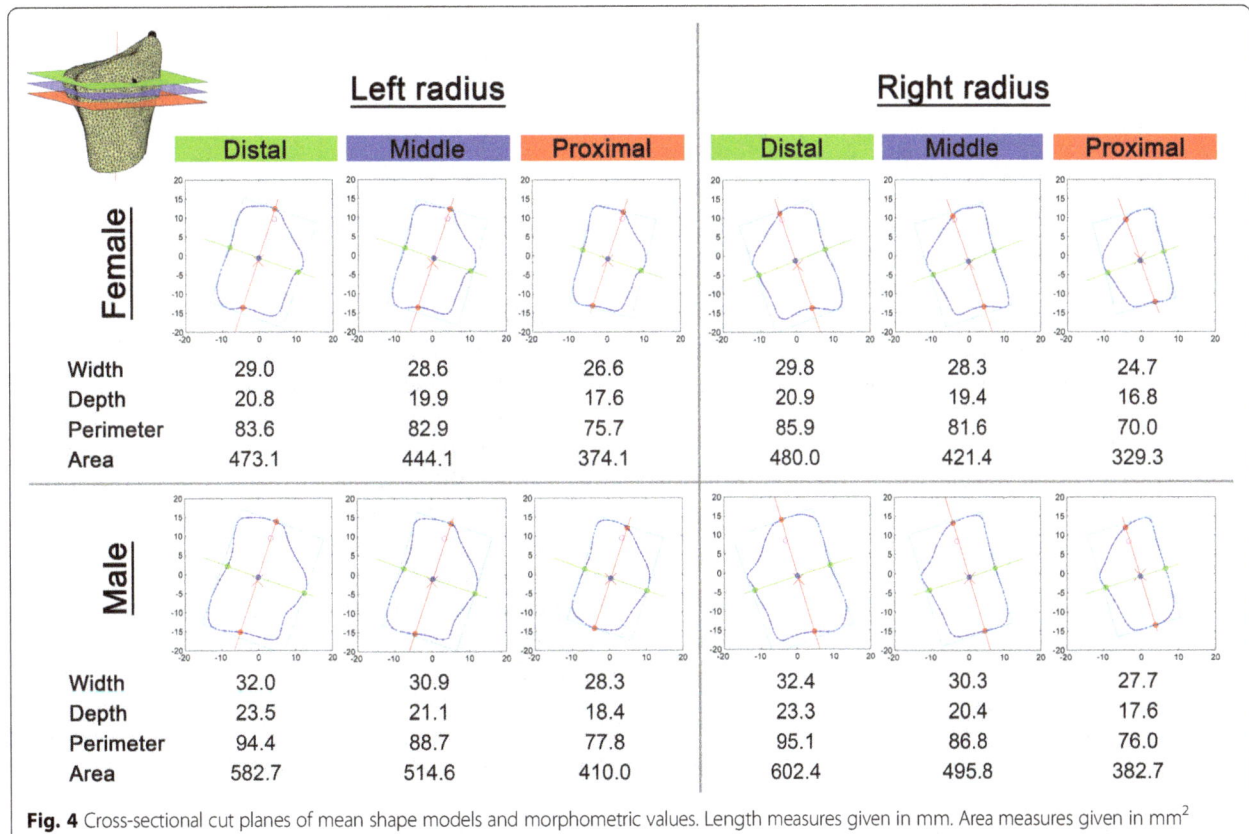

Fig. 4 Cross-sectional cut planes of mean shape models and morphometric values. Length measures given in mm. Area measures given in mm²

Table 1 Summary (mean +/- SD) of morphometric parameters of three different cross-sectional cut planes calculated directly from the CT slices (n = 86)

			Female	Female left	Female right	Male	Male left	Male right
Distal	Width	Mean ± SD	29.0 ± 2.1	28.7 ± 1.9	29.4 ± 2.4	33.0 ± 2.1	32.5 ± 2.1	33.5 ± 2.1
		Range	24.0–35.0	24.0–32.7	26.1–35.0	28.5–37.6	28.5–37.6	29.0–37.5
	Depth	Mean ± SD	21.0 ± 1.7	20.8 ± 1.7	21.2 ± 1.6	23.8 ± 1.4	23.5 ± 1.3	24.0 ± 1.5
		Range	17.3–24.7	17.3–24.7	18.9–24.6	21.0–26.3	21.8–26.3	21.0–26.2
	Perimeter	Mean ± SD	86.1 ± 6.1	84.9 ± 4.6	87.5 ± 7.4	96.5 ± 6.0	94.9 ± 5.8	98.2 ± 5.9
		Range	76.9–102.7	77.4–94.5	76.8–102.7	85.7–110.0	86.8–106.1	85.7–110.0
	Area	Mean ± SD	472.6 ± 70.2	464.0 ± 67.1	483.2 ± 74.5	593.1 ± 62.1	573.3 ± 57.4	612.9 ± 61.4
		Range	302.3–663.4	302.3–591.9	384.1–663.4	477.9–717.0	477.9–685.0	478.3–717.0
Middle	Width	Mean ± SD	28.2 ± 2.3	27.9 ± 1.9	28.6 ± 2.8	31.2 ± 2.2	30.9 ± 1.8	31.4 ± 2.6
		Range	24.3–34.2	24.6–31.9	24.3–34.2	25.9–37.5	27.4–34.8	25.9–37.5
	Depth	Mean ± SD	19.5 ± 1.8	19.4 ± 1.6	19.6 ± 2.0	21.6 ± 1.7	21.5 ± 1.4	21.7 ± 2.0
		Range	16.3–23.2	16.3–22.3	16.3–23.2	18.5–26.6	19.4–24.8	18.5–26.6
	Perimeter	Mean ± SD	81.5 ± 7.0	80.4 ± 5.4	82.9 ± 8.5	90.4 ± 6.7	89.3 ± 5.6	91.5 ± 7.6
		Range	68.5–99.5	72.7–91.2	68.5–99.5	75.1–107.5	79.5–100.8	75.1–107.5
	Area	Mean ± SD	427.5 ± 69.3	421.0 ± 60.8	435.6 ± 79.7	516.9 ± 67.7	507.2 ± 57.4	526.6 ± 76.6
		Range	315.5–586.9	337.6–556.9	315.5–586.9	372.3–706.9	427.3–669.1	372.3–706.9
Proximal	Width	Mean ± SD	26.3 ± 2.4	26.0 ± 2.1	26.5 ± 2.7	28.6 ± 2.4	28.5 ± 2.0	28.7 ± 2.7
		Range	21.4–31.8	21.4–30.2	22.0–31.8	23.4–35.8	24.9–33.3	23.4–35.8
	Depth	Mean ± SD	17.2 ± 1.7	17.2 ± 1.6	17.2 ± 1.9	18.6 ± 1.9	18.6 ± 1.6	18.7 ± 2.3
		Range	13.7–20.6	14.8–20.1	13.7–20.6	15.4–25.7	16.7–23.3	15.4–25.7
	Perimeter	Mean ± SD	73.4 ± 7.4	72.8 ± 6.3	74.1 ± 8.7	79.7 ± 7.7	79.1 ± 6.6	80.3 ± 8.8
		Range	59.9–92.1	63.1–85.3	59.9–92.1	64.1–106.0	70.1–97.7	64.1–106.0
	Area	Mean ± SD	353.2 ± 66.0	352.3 ± 63.9	354.3 ± 70.4	416.0 ± 71.4	410.7 ± 62.4	421.4 ± 80.4
		Range	242.7–486.8	254.2–486.8	242.7–479.2	280.7–640.8	328.1–612.0	280.7–640.8

Distal: Tuberculum dorsale; Proximal: ½ distance of proc. styl. rad. and the most dorsal point of the tub. dorsale; Middle: Plane in-between the disal and proximal plane

post-hoc analysis (Bonferroni) showed significant sectional plane differences for all parameters except female width, perimeter and area between the distal and middle sectional plane.

Finally, the morphometric parameters generated from the cut planes of the mean shape models were well within one standard deviation range of those of the individual radii values. The overall mean differences were distal: -0.8 ± 1.7 mm; middle: -1.0 ± 3.4 mm; proximal: -2.1 ± 4.4 mm.

Classification accuracy of the overall shape model

The overall shape model allowed accurate discrimination between left and right radii with a median classification probability of 98%. Testing for gender differences, 70% of the tested radii were classified correctly. Conducting the same analysis step-wise predictive, i.e. by firstly identifing the side, then the gender, yielded a median classification probability of 80% independent of the radii side.

The predictive quality of the overall shape model is illustrated in Fig. 5.

Discussion

A large dataset of clinical CT images was used to generate the first 3D mean shape model of the distal radius, define and analyze uniformly oriented cross-sectional cut planes, and finally provide good classification accuracy regarding side and gender.

Previous studies have predominantly been limited to the 2D anatomy of the distal radius. These assessed gross measurements (distal sagittal and axial width) [8–10, 25] or the cross-sectional anatomy of the distal radius [11, 26, 27]. Some studies indicated to assess the 3D anatomy of the distal radius. Hamilton et al. [27] analyzed various morphometric parameters at different locations of the distal radius. Oppermann et al. [11] analyzed longitudinal and transverse slices of 49 cadaver distal radii. Recent studies have attempted to analyze specific landmarks, such as the dorsal tubercle (Lister's tubercle) [1, 28, 29], the

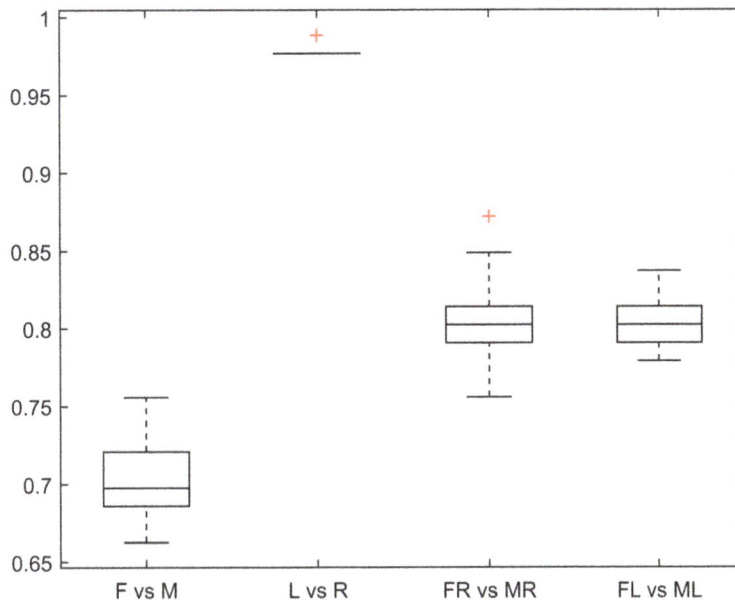

Fig. 5 Predictive quality of the overall shape model. F: Female; M: Male; L: Left; R: Right

volar surface [11, 18, 19], the promatory of the radius [5] or the radiocarpal surface [30]. However, these studies based their analysis on single slices.

This study is the first to approach the three-dimensional anatomy of the distal radius and examine its variability within a population. The morphometric parameters calculated from the mean shape model, correlated well with those from the individual cut planes. Moreover, these morphometric values mirror data from previous studies in similar populations [2, 8]. However, published morphometric distal radius values have shown a broad range, even within a population. This may either be due to a natural wide variability, or variations in measurement location between these studies.

This study highlights the significant influence of the measurement location on morphometric parameters. Although the generated cut-planes were only 3.5 ± 0.6 mm apart from each other on average, almost all morphometric parameters varied significantly. Therefore, two-dimensional analysis of cut-planes requires careful attention to the measurement location. Consistent measurement location may facilitate inter-study comparison. In future, however 3D anatomical models eliminate this confounder.

The retrospective dataset, generated from patients presenting with wrist/hand pain, is a limitation of this study. One may assume, that this patient cohort differs from a prospectively assessed, asymptomatic patient sample. However, patients who present at our level 1 trauma center are of an assumed random population. All CT-datasets were carefully reviewed by a fellow-trained orthopedic surgeon and radiologist to assure an intact bony architecture. Although trauma may have had an impact on the

intra-osseos architecture, i.e. trabecular microfractures, we belive this most likely did not alter the cortical architecture of the distal radius. Therefore, as the cortical surface was used to generate the 3D-surface models, the initial trauma should not compromise the results.

One further point that warrants discussion is sexual dimorphism and the identification of handedness. A forensic study by Ruiz Mediavilla et al. [7] avoided the bias of measurement location by assessing the volume of 127 distal radii (twentieth century) to analyze the potential of volume measurements in order to determine the gender of fragmentary remains. For the distal radius, they reported significant greater values for male and right radii compared to female and left radii respectively. The current study, as well as previous studies, also found significant gender differences, but no such differences for side [11]. Moreover, Ruiz Mediavilla et al. [7] reported a gender classification function accuracy of their volumetric measurements of 95.5% for right and 88.5% for left radii. These values are higher than reported herein. This may either be due to our limited sample size or a greater gender difference in the volume rather than the shape.

Interestingly, a greater shape variance (number of modes) was determined in left compared to right radii. As no further quantitative analyses could be conducted on the total 3D shape models, we computed their cross-sectional cut planes (mean, ±1SD). The greater shape variance of left radii may be explained by the functional adaptation of bone to stress [31]. Previous studies showed a difference in metacarpal bone size depending on hand dominance [32]. With most of the population being right-handed, this could explain the herein observed shape variance between left and right radii.

3D surface models bear various advantages. Firstly, they are well established for the application in a medical context, such as assessing bone morphology [33–35], temporal-lobe morphology [36], or anthropometric shape evaluations of the human scalp [37]. Secondly, the methodology can quickly and efficiently process large data and generate 3D shape models based on clinical CT datasets. Therefore it may easily be adapted to various anatomical locations. Finally, although the overall shape variance could not be further analyzed quantitatively, this may be possible for specific anatomical landmarks. Future studies should, for example, assess the surface area and the 3D curve of the distal volar surface. This is of particular interest to the design of pre-shaped plates used in osteosynthesis in distal radius factures [3, 38].

Conclusions

A novel 3D shape model of the distal radius was constructed allowing descriptive analysis of shape variance. Based on the shape model, uniform cut-planes were defined and analyzed. Assessment of the the model's side and gender classification accuracy was 80%. Future studies may apply these models to other anatomical locations and assess specific anatomical landmarks.

Additional files

Additional file 1: Detailed description of the process of shape model generation. (DOCX 92 kb)

Additional file 2: Animated illustration of the cross-sectional cut planes. Green plane: Proximal plane (50% of the distance between the tip of the styloid process and the most dorsal point of the tuberculum listerii); Blue plane: Middle plane (Half way between the distal and proximal sectional plane); Red plane: Distal plane (The most dorsal point of the tuberculum listerii). (PDF 140 kb)

Additional file 3: Animated illustrations of the first five modes of all radius models. A: Female left radii model; B: Female right radii model; C: Male left radii model; D: Male right radii model. (ZIP 9547 kb)

Additional file 4: Illustration of the shape variance (number of modes) for each radius model. (TIF 57327 kb)

Additional file 5: Illustration of the cross-sectional cut planes for ±1SD of the mean shape models. SD: Standard deviation; Distal: Distal plane; Middle: Middle plane; Proximal: Proximal plane. (TIF 9568 kb)

Additional file 6: Summary of morphometric parameters (Mean, ±1SD) of the mean shape model for all three sectional planes. SD: Standard deviation; Distal: Distal plane; Middle: Middle plane; Proximal: Proximal plane. (DOCX 113 kb)

Abbreviations
2D: Two-dimensional; 3D: Three-dimensional; CPD: Coherent point drift; CT: Computed tomography; DICOM: Digital imaging and communications in medicine; e: eigenvectors; Fig: Figure; I: Mean shape; LOOCV: Leave one out cross validation; n: number; PCA: Principle component analysis; SD: Standard deviation; Supp: Supplement; λ: Eigenvalues

Acknowledgements
The authors would like to Bela Turk for proof-reading.

Funding
The study was funded by a research grant of the Medical University of Munich (LMU, FöFoLe #828). Georg Langs was supported by FWF (I 2714-B31) and OeNB (15356, 15929).

Authors' contributions
SFB had the study idea, wrote the proposal for the ethics committee, conducted the statistics and wrote the paper. JB was responsible for data generation, rendering of the radii and participated in writing the paper. FGM conducted CT scans, helped prepare and analyze the data and proof-read the paper. AS was involved in study planning and conducted parts of the data analysis. YC conducted rendering of the radii and participated in manuscript preparation. EE was one of the study initiators, helped with the ethics proposal, data interpretation and proof-read the paper. GL supervised data generation and analysis and proof-read the paper. LF conducted the data analysis, model generation and prepared parts of the paper. All authors read and approved the final manuscript.

Authors' information
Not applicable.

Competing interests
The authors declare that they have no competing interests.

Author details
[1]Department of General, Trauma and Reconstructive Surgery, University Hospital LMU Munich, Nussbaumstr. 20, Munich 80336, Germany. [2]Institute of Lightweight Design and Structural Biomechanics, Vienna University of Technology, Getreidemarkt 9, Vienna 1060, Austria. [3]Department of Clinical Radiology, University Hospital LMU Munich, Nussbaumstr. 20, Munich 80336, Germany. [4]Department of Orthopaedic Surgery, Physical Medicine and Rehabilitation, University Hospital LMU Munich, Campus Grosshadern, Marchioninistraße 15, Munich 81377, Germany. [5]Computational Imaging Research Laboratory, Department of Biomedical Imaging and Image-guided Therapy, Medical University of Vienna, Waehringer Guertel 18-20, Vienna 1090, Austria. [6]Software Competence Center Hagenberg GmbH, Softwarepark 21, Hagenberg 4232, Austria.

References
1. Ağır I, Aytekin MN, Küçükdurmaz F, Gökhan S, Cavuş UY. Anatomical Localization of Lister's Tubercle and its Clinical and Surgical Importance. Open Orthop J. 2014;8:74–7. doi:10.2174/1874325001408010074.
2. Barrier ILO, L'Abbé EN. Sex determination from the radius and ulna in a modern South African sample. Forensic Sci Int. 2008;179(1):85.e1–7. doi:10.1016/j.forsciint.2008.04.012.
3. Oppermann J, Bredow J, Beyer F, Neiss WF, Spies CK, Eysel P et al. Distal radius: anatomical morphometric gender characteristics. Do anatomical pre-shaped plates pay attention on it? Arch Orthop Trauma Surg. 2014. doi:10.1007/s00402-014-2112-7.
4. Vroemen JC, Dobbe JGG, Sierevelt IN, Strackee SD, Streekstra GJ. Accuracy of distal radius positioning using an anatomical plate. Orthopedics. 2013;36(4):e457–62. doi:10.3928/01477447-20130327-22.
5. Windisch G, Clement H, Tanzer K, Feigl G, Grechenig W, Anderhuber F, et al. Promontory of radius: a new anatomical description on the distal radius. Surg Radiol Anat. 2007;29(8):629–33. doi:10.1007/s00276-007-0264-7.
6. Akhlaghi M, Sheikhazadi A, Ebrahimnia A, Hedayati M, Nazparvar B, Saberi Anary SH. The value of radius bone in prediction of sex and height in the

Iranian population. J Forensic Legal Med. 2012;19(4):219–22. doi:10.1016/j.jflm.2011.12.030.

7. Ruiz Mediavilla E, Perea Pérez B, Labajo González E, Sánchez Sánchez JA, Santiago Sáez A, Dorado FE. Determining sex by bone volume from 3D images: discriminating analysis of the tali and radii in a contemporary Spanish reference collection. Int J Legal Med. 2012;126(4):623–31. doi:10.1007/s00414-012-0715-5.

8. Baumbach SF, Krusche-Mandl I, Huf W, Mall G, Fialka C. Linear intra-bone geometry dependencies of the radius: Radius length determination by maximum distal width. Eur J Radiol. 2012;81(5):947–50. doi:10.1016/j.ejrad.2011.02.030.

9. Gasse N, Lepage D, Pem R, Bernard C, Lerais JM, Garbuio P, et al. Anatomical and radiological study applied to distal radius surgery. Surg Radiol Anat. 2011;33(6):485–90. doi:10.1007/s00276-010-0754-x.

10. Pichler W, Clement H, Hausleitner L, Tanzer K, Tesch NP, Grechenig W. Various circular arc radii of the distal volar radius and the implications on volar plate osteosynthesis. Orthopedics. 2008;31(12). https://www.ncbi.nlm.nih.gov/pubmed/?term=Pichler+W%2C+Clement+H%2C+Hausleitner+L%2C+Tanzer+K%2C+Tesch+NP%2C+Grechenig+W.+Various+circular+arc+radii+of+the+distal+volar+radius+and+the+implications+on+volar+plate+osteosynthesis.

11. Oppermann J, Wacker M, Stein G, Springorum H-P, Neiss WF, Burkhart KJ, et al. Anatomical fit of seven different palmar distal radius plates. Arch Orthop Trauma Surg. 2014;134(10):1483–9. doi:10.1007/s00402-014-2072-y.

12. Pekar V, Kaus MR, Lorenz C, Lobregt S, Truyen R, Weese J. Shape-modelbased adaptation of 3D deformable meshes for segmentation of medical images. In: Sonka M, Hanson KM, Editors. Proc SPIE Medical Imaging: Image Processing. vol 4322, San Diego; 2001. http://proceedings.spiedigitallibrary.org/solr/searchresults.aspx#q=%2C%20Weese%20J.%20Shape-modelbased%20adaptation%20of%203D%20deformable%20meshes%20for%20segmentation%20of%20medical%20images&SearchSourceType=1.

13. Josephson K, Ericsson A, Karlsson J. Segmentation of medical images using three-dimensional active shape models. In: Proc Scandinavian Conference on Image Analysis LNCS, vol 3540 Springer. 2005.

14. Tang TSY, Ellis RE. 2D/3D deformable registration using a hybrid atlas. In: Proc MICCAI LNCS, vol 3750 Springer. 2005.

15. Zhao Z, Aylward SR, Teoh EK. A novel 3D partitioned active shape model for segmentation of brain MR images. In: Proc MICCAI LNCS, vol 3749 Springer.

16. van de Giessen M, Foumani M, Vos FM, Strackee SD, Maas M, Van Vliet LJ, et al. A 4D statistical model of wrist bone motion patterns. IEEE Trans Med Imaging. 2012;31(3):613–25. doi:10.1109/TMI.2011.2174159.

17. Bassi RS, Krishnan KM, Dhillon SS, Deshmukh SC. Palmar cortical angle of the distal radius: a radiological study. J Hand Surg Eur Vol. 2003;28(2):163–4.

18. Evans S, Ramasamy A, Deshmukh SC. Distal volar radial plates: how anatomical are they? Orthop Traumatol Surg Res. 2014;100(3):293–5. doi:10.1016/j.otsr.2013.11.014.

19. Oura K, Oka K, Kawanishi Y, Sugamoto K, Yoshikawa H, Murase T. Volar morphology of the distal radius in axial planes: A quantitative analysis. J Orthop Res. 2014. doi:10.1002/jor.22780.

20. Slicer 3D. http://www.slicer.org/. Accessed 5 June 2016.

21. Chevalier Y. Numerical Methodology to Evaluate the Effects of Bone Density and Cement Augmentation on Fixation Stiffness of Bone-Anchoring Devices. J Biomech Eng. 2015;137(9). doi:10.1115/1.4030943.

22. CGAL Project. http://www.cgal.org/. Accessed 5 June 2016.

23. Cootes TF, Taylor CJ, Cooper DH, Graham J. Training Models of Shape from Sets of Examples. In: Proceedings of the British Machine Vision Conference. 1992. p. 9–18. doi:10.1007/978-1-4471-3201-1_2.

24. Thodberg HH. Minimum Description Length shape and appearance models. Inf Process Med Imaging. 2003;18:51–62.

25. Celbis O, Agritmis H. Estimation of stature and determination of sex from radial and ulnar bone lengths in a Turkish corpse sample. Surg Radiol Anat. 2006;158(2-3):135–9. doi:10.1016/j.forsciint.2005.05.016.

26. Bouxsein ML, Myburgh KH, van der Meulen MC, Lindenberger E, Marcus R. Age-related differences in cross-sectional geometry of the forearm bones in healthy women. Calcif Tissue Int. 1994;54(2):113–8.

27. Hamilton CJ, Thomas SG, Jamal SA. Associations between leisure physical activity participation and cortical bone mass and geometry at the radius and tibia in a Canadian cohort of postmenopausal women. Bone. 2010;46(3):774–9. doi:10.1016/j.bone.2009.10.041.

28. Clement H, Pichler W, Nelson D, Hausleitner L, Tesch NP, Grechenig W. Morphometric analysis of lister's tubercle and its consequences on volar plate fixation of distal radius fractures. J Hand Surg Am. 2008;33(10):1716–9. doi:10.1016/j.jhsa.2008.08.012.

29. Pichler W, Windisch G, Schaffler G, Rienmüller R, Grechenig W. Computer tomography aided 3D analysis of the distal dorsal radius surface and the effects on volar plate osteosynthesis. J Hand Surg Eur Vol. 2009;34(5):598–602. doi:10.1177/1753193409101471.

30. Andermahr J, Lozano-Calderon S, Trafton T, Crisco JJ, Ring D. The volar extension of the lunate facet of the distal radius: a quantitative anatomic study. J Hand Surg Am. 2006;31(6):892–5. doi:10.1016/j.jhsa.2006.03.010.

31. Goodship AE, Lanyon LE, McFie H. Functional adaptation of bone to increased stress. An experimental study. J Bone Joint Surg Am. 1979;61(4):539–46.

32. Plato CC, Wood JL, Norris AH. Bilateral asymmetry in bone measurements of the hand and lateral hand dominance. Am J Phys Anthropol. 1980;52(1):27–31. doi:10.1002/ajpa.1330520105.

33. Varzi D, Coupaud SAF, Purcell M, Allan DB, Gregory JS, Barr RJ. Bone morphology of the femur and tibia captured by statistical shape modelling predicts rapid bone loss in acute spinal cord injury patients. Bone. 2015;81:495–501. doi:10.1016/j.bone.2015.08.026.

34. Schneider MTY, Zhang J, Crisco JJ, Weiss APC, Ladd AL, Nielsen P, et al. Men and women have similarly shaped carpometacarpal joint bones. J Biomech. 2015;48(12):3420–6. doi:10.1016/j.jbiomech.2015.05.031.

35. Lindner C, Thiagarajah S, Wilkinson JM, Panoutsopoulou K, Day-Williams AG, Consortium A, et al. Investigation of association between hip osteoarthritis susceptibility loci and radiographic proximal femur shape. Arthritis Rheumatol (Hoboken, NJ). 2015;67(8):2076–84. doi:10.1002/art.39186.

36. Ramezani M, Johnsrude I, Rasoulian A, Bosma R, Tong R, Hollenstein T, et al. Temporal-lobe morphology differs between healthy adolescents and those with early-onset of depression. Neuroimage Clin. 2014;6:145–55. doi:10.1016/j.nicl.2014.08.007.

37. Lacko D, Huysmans T, Parizel PM, De Bruyne G, Verwulgen S, Van Hulle MM, et al. Evaluation of an anthropometric shape model of the human scalp. Appl Ergon. 2015;48:70–85. doi:10.1016/j.apergo.2014.11.008.

38. Schneppendahl J, Windolf J, Kaufmann RA. Distal radius fractures: current concepts. J Hand Surg Am. 2012;37(8):1718–25. doi:10.1016/j.jhsa.2012.06.001.

10

Evaluation of dynamic infrared thermography as an alternative to CT angiography for perforator mapping in breast reconstruction

Sven Weum[1,2*], James B. Mercer[1,2] and Louis de Weerd[1,3]

Abstract

Background: The current gold standard for preoperative perforator mapping in breast reconstruction with a DIEP flap is CT angiography (CTA). Dynamic infrared thermography (DIRT) is an imaging method that does not require ionizing radiation or contrast injection. We evaluated if DIRT could be an alternative to CTA in perforator mapping.

Methods: Twenty-five patients scheduled for secondary breast reconstruction with a DIEP flap were included. Preoperatively, the lower abdomen was examined with hand-held Doppler, DIRT and CTA. Arterial Doppler sound locations were marked on the skin. DIRT examination involved rewarming of the abdominal skin after a mild cold challenge. The locations of hot spots on DIRT were compared with the arterial Doppler sound locations. The rate and pattern of rewarming of the hot spots were analyzed. Multiplanar CT reconstructions were used to see if hot spots were related to perforators on CTA. All flaps were based on the perforator selected with DIRT and the surgical outcome was analyzed.

Results: First appearing hot spots were always associated with arterial Doppler sounds and clearly visible perforators on CTA. The hot spots on DIRT images were always slightly laterally located in relation to the exit points of the associated perforators through the rectus abdominis fascia on CTA. Some periumbilical perforators were not associated with hot spots and showed communication with the superficial inferior epigastric vein on CTA. The selected perforators adequately perfused all flaps.

Conclusion: This study confirms that perforators selected with DIRT have arterial Doppler sound, are clearly visible on CTA and provide adequate perfusion for DIEP breast reconstruction.

Trial registration: Retrospectively registered at ClinicalTrials.gov with identifier NCT02806518.

Keywords: Deep Inferior Epigastric Perforator (DIEP), Medical thermography, Perforator flap surgery, Perforator imaging, CT angiography, Radiology, Plastic surgery, Reconstructive surgery, Breast reconstruction

* Correspondence: sven.weum@unn.no
[1]Medical Imaging Research Group, Department of Clinical Medicine, UiT The Arctic University of Norway, 9037 Tromsø, Norway
[2]Department of Radiology, University Hospital of North Norway, Sykehusveien 38, P.O. Box 103, 9038 Tromsø, Norway
Full list of author information is available at the end of the article

Background

Breast reconstruction with a deep inferior epigastric perforator (DIEP) flap utilizing skin and subcutaneous tissue from the patient's lower abdomen has become a popular option for women treated for breast cancer. The DIEP flap receives its blood supply from a perforator consisting of an artery and one or two comitant veins arising from the deep inferior epigastric artery (DIEA) and vein [1, 2]. In DIEP breast reconstruction the blood supply to the DIEP flap is reestablished by anastomosing the perforator to the internal mammary vessels.

The selected perforator is crucial for flap survival as it is the only source of blood supply to the flap. Although intraoperative perforator selection without preoperative perforator mapping is possible, the large variability in the numbers, locations and diameters of perforators makes this rather difficult [3–5]. A multicenter consensus study considered CTA the preferred method for preoperative perforator mapping [6]. CTA allows for precise anatomical description of the origin of perforators, their intramuscular course and point of fascia penetration. The main disadvantages of CTA are exposure to ionizing radiation and the use of intravenous contrast medium. The use of CTA is also associated with high costs. CTA can be time consuming due to delays in obtaining CTA preoperatively leading to delay in surgery, time the patient has to expend to obtain the CTA, and time of the surgeon and radiologist to review the imaging.

In 1993 Itoh and Arai described for the first time in English literature the use of dynamic infrared thermography (DIRT) for perforator mapping in DIEP flaps [7, 8]. Perforators that transport blood to the subdermal plexus cause a local heating at the skin surface that can be visualized as hot spots on infrared images. In DIRT a cold challenge is applied to the skin surface and temperature changes at the hot spots during the rewarming period are registered with an infrared camera. It might be beneficial for patients if DIRT could replace CTA in preoperative perforating mapping as DIRT, unlike CTA, does not involve the exposure to ionizing radiation or the use of intravenous contrast medium. DIRT has been used in the preoperative planning as well as intraoperative and postoperative monitoring of flap perfusion [9–14]. To our knowledge there are no studies that systematically have compared DIRT with other techniques for preoperative perforator mapping.

In this study the results of preoperative perforator mapping in DIEP breast reconstruction with DIRT were compared with those obtained with the most frequently used techniques hand-held Doppler and CTA. As flap survival is dependent on the selected perforator, all breast reconstructions were based on the perforator selected with DIRT and the surgical outcome was evaluated.

Methods

This prospective clinical study was approved by the Regional Committee for Research Ethics. After giving informed consent to participation and publication of data, 25 women with mean age 57 years (range 38–69) and mean body mass index 27.2 kg/m^2 (range 21.6–32.4) scheduled for DIEP breast reconstruction were included. Perforator mapping on the lower abdomen was performed with hand-held Doppler, DIRT and CTA in the same supine position. In all cases the DIEP breast reconstruction was based on the perforator selected with DIRT. The DIRT results were compared to the results obtained with the hand-held Doppler and CTA. Evaluation of the surgical outcome related to flap survival was made.

The flap was marked on the lower abdomen. The lateral border of each rectus abdominis muscle was marked following palpation before and during muscle contraction. To describe the locations of perforators, a quadrant system was used. The flap surface overlying each rectus fascia was divided into 4 quadrants (Fig. 1). The vertical line at the midline between the upper and lower border of the flap is bisected in two equal lengths and defines the horizontal line between upper and lower quadrants. The area between the lateral border of each rectus abdominis muscle and the linea alba is bisected in equal parts by a vertical line.

Hand-held Doppler (8 MHz, Multi Dopplex II, Huntleigh Healthcare, Cardiff, UK) was used to locate arterial Doppler sounds within the quadrants and these were marked as black dots on the skin. DIRT included a 5-min acclimatization of the exposed abdomen at room temperature (22–24 °C).

An infrared camera (FLIR ThermaCAM S65 HS, FLIR Systems, Boston, MA) was used to capture video sequences of thermal images before, during and after exposure of the lower abdomen to a cold challenge. This cold challenge was provided by blowing air at room temperature for 2 min over the abdomen using a desktop fan (Fig. 2). The temperature changes were well within the physiological range. After a recovery period of 3 min, the presence of arterial Doppler sounds at the first appearing hot spots was evaluated with hand-held Doppler. If present at a hot spot, its location was marked with a cross on the skin. A digital photo of the abdomen was taken at the end of the DIRT examination using the same angle as the infrared camera (Fig. 3). Thermal images and photos were stored on the hospital's picture archiving and communication system (PACS).

The thermal images were qualitatively analyzed for the rate and pattern of rewarming of the hot spots. The first appearing hot spots and their associated quadrants were registered and named with increasing identification numbers based on their order of appearance. Hot spots showing the same rate of rewarming were ranked on basis of

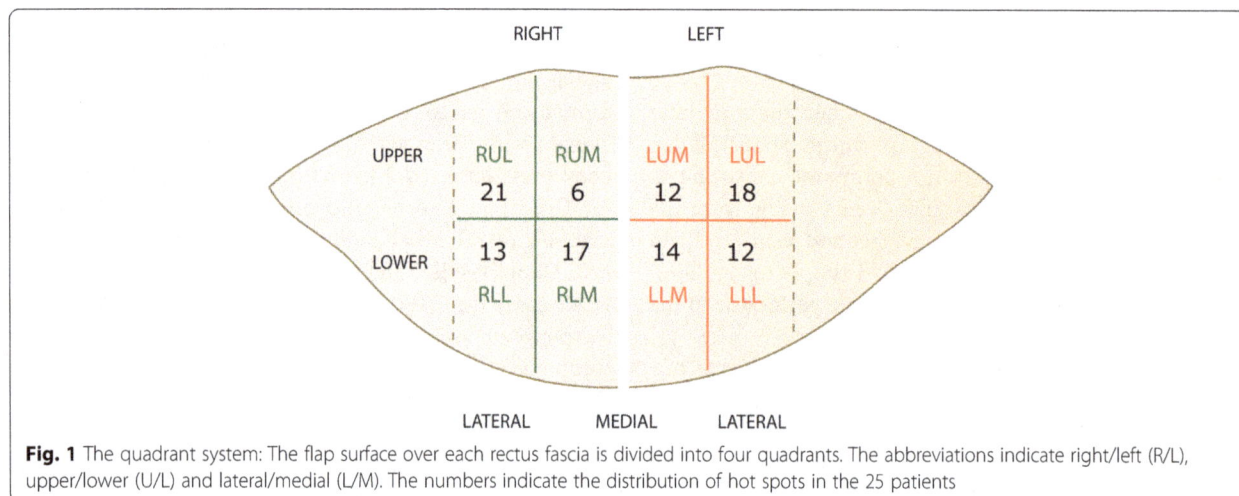

Fig. 1 The quadrant system: The flap surface over each rectus fascia is divided into four quadrants. The abbreviations indicate right/left (R/L), upper/lower (U/L) and lateral/medial (L/M). The numbers indicate the distribution of hot spots in the 25 patients

rewarming of the area around the hot spot. The hot spot with most progressive rewarming was given the lowest number.

CTA was performed (SOMATOM Sensation 16, Siemens Medical Solutions, Erlangen, Germany) after intravenous

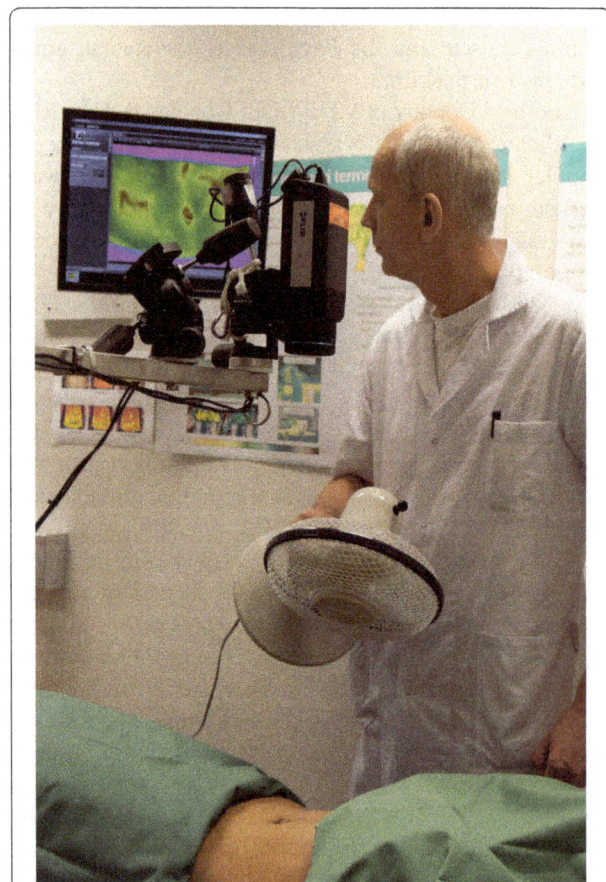

Fig. 2 An infrared camera captures video sequences of thermal images before, during and after a cold challenge delivered by a desktop fan

injection of contrast medium (Ultravist 370, Schering AG, Berlin, Germany or Iomeron 350, Bracco, Milan, Italy) with bolus triggering on the distal aorta. Scan parameters are summarized in Table 1. Three- dimensional (3D) and multiplanar reconstructions (MPR) were used to evaluate the DIEA and its perforators within the flap area (OsiriX version 4.0, OsiriX foundation, Geneva, Switzerland). On coronal thick maximum intensity projection (MIP) images the course and ramifications of the DIEA were evaluated on both sides. Axial thick MIP images were used to evaluate if there was a dominating DIEA system with perforators suitable for a DIEP reconstruction.

CTA images were analyzed by consensus between a radiologist (SW) and plastic surgeon (LdW). MPR images were used to see if the locations of the first appearing hot spots could be related to perforators from the DIEA. Axial images were used to decide if perforators were classified as lateral or medial. Sagittal images were used to decide if perforators were cranially or caudally located to the level midway between the umbilicus and the pubic symphysis.

Results
Preoperative results
DIRT revealed a large variability in location, size, and number of hot spots between patients. This variability was also seen between the left and right side. Hot spots were always associated with arterial Doppler sounds. First appearing hot spots during rewarming were brighter than those appearing later. The hand-held Doppler does not allow for quantitative volume registration but, subjectively, the brightness of hot spots was related to the volume of Doppler sounds. All first appearing hot spots were also associated with clearly visible perforators on CTA and located in the same quadrants (Fig. 4). Hot spots were always slightly laterally located to the exit points of the perforators through the rectus fascia as seen on CTA.

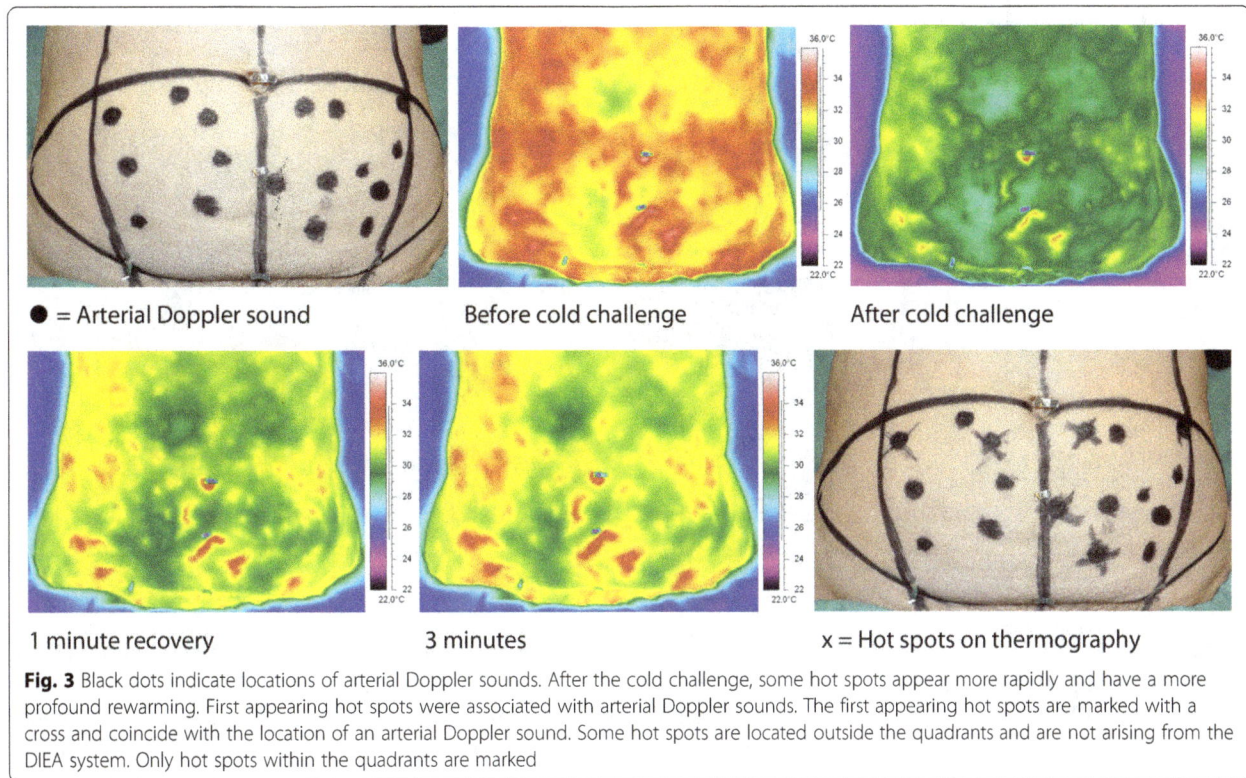

● = Arterial Doppler sound   Before cold challenge   After cold challenge

1 minute recovery   3 minutes   x = Hot spots on thermography

Fig. 3 Black dots indicate locations of arterial Doppler sounds. After the cold challenge, some hot spots appear more rapidly and have a more profound rewarming. First appearing hot spots were associated with arterial Doppler sounds. The first appearing hot spots are marked with a cross and coincide with the location of an arterial Doppler sound. Some hot spots are located outside the quadrants and are not arising from the DIEA system. Only hot spots within the quadrants are marked

In our 25 patients 113 hot spots were registered using DIRT and 108 (95.6 %) corresponded to a perforator in the same quadrant seen on CTA (Fig. 1). The remaining 5 hot spots (4.4 %) were all found in the lower part of the lower quadrants and corresponded to perforators coming from other arteries than the DIEA. The 113 hot spots were evenly distributed between the right and left side (57/56), as well as between the upper and lower quadrants (57/56). In the upper quadrants there were fewer medial than lateral hot spots (18/39).

Some large periumbilical perforators on CTA were associated with arterial Doppler sounds but not with hot spots. In these cases 3D reconstruction revealed a connection between the perforator and the superficial inferior epigastric vein in the periumbilical area. Not all arterial Doppler sounds locations could be associated with a hot spot on DIRT or a perforator on CTA.

Surgical results

In all cases, the selected hot spots could be related to perforators found intraoperatively. Large periumbilical perforators that were not associated with a hot spot consisted of a small artery with one or two large comitant veins. The marked hot spots were always slightly laterally located to the exit points of the perforator through the fascia. While all first appearing hot spots could be related to suitable perforators, not all arterial Doppler sound locations on the skin could be related to suitable perforators intraoperatively. All flaps were based on the selected perforator from DIRT and were adequately perfused. Of the 25 flaps, 24 survived. One flap was lost on the second postoperative day due to a bleeding beneath the flap that was diagnosed too late to save the flap. This complication could not be related to the selected perforator. The mean flap weight was 713 grams (range 302–1270). Twelve flaps were based on one perforator, nine flaps on two perforators, two flaps on three perforators and two flaps on four perforators. In all cases the selected perforator visualized with DIRT was the most suitable perforator, additional perforators were added in cases with large volume flaps to guarantee adequate flap perfusion.

Table 1 CT scan parameters

Patient position: Head first supine

Range: 3 cm cranial of umbilicus to symphysis

Bolus tracking: Abdominal aorta 2 cm cranial to bifurcation

Contrast medium: 120 mL Ultravist 370 or Iomeron 350, 4.0 mL/s

Voltage: 120 kV

Current: 150–200 mA

Slice collimation: 0.75 mm

Kernel: B20f medium

Slice width/increment: 1.0 mm/0.7 mm reconstruction

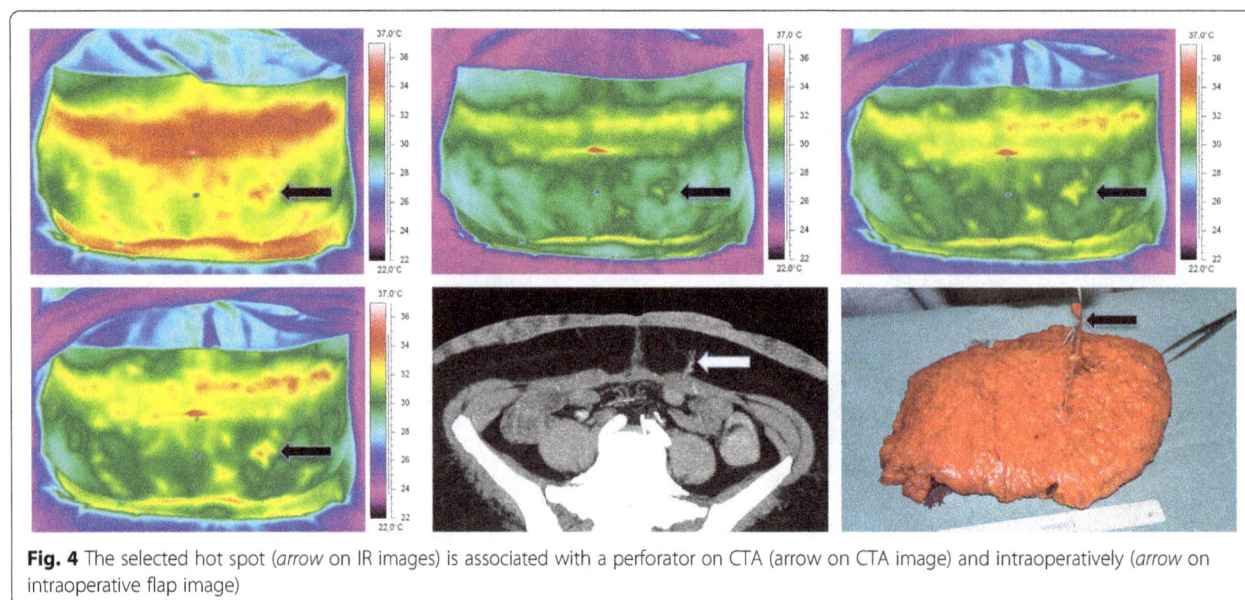

Fig. 4 The selected hot spot (*arrow* on IR images) is associated with a perforator on CTA (arrow on CTA image) and intraoperatively (*arrow* on intraoperative flap image)

Discussion

The main finding of this study is that the first appearing hot spots on DIRT were always associated with arterial Doppler sounds as well as clearly visible perforators on CTA and intraoperatively. The use of DIRT in preoperative perforator mapping provided a suitable perforator for DIEP breast reconstruction in all 25 cases.

Surgeons want information on the hemodynamic properties of a perforator as well as its location. Hand-held Doppler is frequently used for preoperative perforator mapping. Giunta et al. attributed the high number of false-positive results in their study to the relative high sensitivity of the hand-held Doppler [15]. Very small perforating vessels were also located, unsuitable for perforator flaps because of their narrow caliber. Others have abandoned hand-held Doppler because the results often proved to be aberrant from the intraoperative observations [16]. Similar to Giunta we found arterial Doppler sounds that could not be associated with hot spots, nor with suitable perforators intraoperatively.

CTA has become the current gold standard for perforator mapping and is based on the perfusion of the perforators with contrast medium during the arterial phase. It provides information on the caliber of each perforator, its intramuscular course and its exit point through the anterior rectus fascia [6]. However, a recent study by Cina et al. revealed that the sum of the diameter of the perforating artery and vein with color Doppler was in agreement with the diameter of the presumed artery on CTA [2]. However, there was a significant disagreement between the measured diameters of the arteries measured with color Doppler and CTA, as well as for CTA and intraoperative findings. Thus, measurement of the assumed perforating artery on CTA may in fact constitute the sum of

the diameters of the perforating artery and vein(s). Mathes et al. warned against sole reliance on CTA perforator mapping as they had to make a significant number of changes intraoperatively [17]. Important disadvantages of CTA are exposure to ionizing radiation and the use of intravenous contrast medium. A method without these disadvantages would be beneficial.

In our study, the rate and pattern of rewarming of the hot spots were analyzed. There was a large variability in the number of hot spots and in the rate and pattern of rewarming. As first appearing hot spots were associated with perforators on CTA and arterial Doppler sounds, the rewarming at the hot spot is a result of blood perfusion through the perforator to the skin surface.

During the rewarming period all perforators compete with each other in skin rewarming. A rapid rewarming indicates that the associated perforator transports more blood to the skin surface than a perforator that produces a slower rewarming. Progressive rewarming around the hot spot indicates a well-developed vascular network around this hot spot. A well-developed branching pattern is also considered an important criterion when selecting a perforator on CTA [18, 19]. By analyzing the rate and pattern of rewarming, the surgeon obtains information on the perforator's hemodynamic properties.

Information on the location where the suitable perforator can be found is of great value to the surgeon. Chubb et al. reported their preliminary results with DIRT and reported that this technique matched the accuracy of CTA for perforator location [20]. We found, however, that the hot spot on the skin was always slightly laterally located in relation to the perforator's exit point through the rectus abdominis fascia. Using CTA, Rozen et al. found in their perforator angiosome study that lateral row perforators have a long and laterally directed course, whereas the medial perforators show a straighter course from the rectus sheath towards the skin [21]. An explanation for this lateral orientation of vessels was given by the eminent anatomist John Hunter (1728–1793), who saw it as a product of growth that occurs from the stage of fetus to adulthood [22]. In contrast to CTA, DIRT does not provide information on the intramuscular course of the perforator. Although the main goal of perforator mapping is to find a perforator that can provide adequate blood perfusion of the flap, a perforator with a short intramuscular course is preferred to a perforator with the same caliber and a longer intramuscular course. Interestingly, de Weerd et al. found in a DIRT study that first appearing hot spots were often associated with perforators passing through the tendineous intersection [19]. These perforators have a very short intramuscular course. A further advantage of CTA over DIRT is that CTA can provide information on the continuity of the deep inferior epigastric system in patients that have been previously operated in that area. In cases with large flap volumes, additional perforators were added to the selected perforator to optimize flap perfusion, as also reported by Gill et al. in their retrospective study [23].

Our results showed cases in which large periumbilical perforators on CTA could not be associated with hot spots. This indicates that these perforators do not transport much blood the skin surface. We postulate that such perforators consist of a small caliber artery and one or two large caliber comitant veins and that these large veins communicate with the superficial inferior epigastric vein. This postulation is supported by our intraoperative findings and CTA. The existence of these communications was already described by Carramenha e Costa et al. in an anatomic study and nicely illustrated with the use of CTA by Rozen at al. in a study on the venous anatomy of the abdominal wall [24, 25].

One of the disadvantages of DIRT is that only perforators that transport blood to the skin surface are detected. It is possible that a perforator that ends in the subcutaneous tissue might be a suitable perforator for DIEP breast reconstruction. Such a perforator can be detected with CTA but not with DIRT. From earlier studies it is known that the subdermal plexus contributes to the perfusion of the underlying subcutaneous tissue. In their cross sectional radiographic study, Taylor et al. revealed blood supply to the subcutaneous layer caused by "raining down" from the subdermal plexus, a result confirmed by Schaverien et al. [26, 27]. Initially, the perfusion of the DIEP flap depends on this mechanism. During the first postoperative week, the interconnections between the vascular structures within the flap increase in size and, as a result, tissue perfusion improves [28]. The main limitation of this study is the small number of 25 patients. Because of the small study size our results are indicative and should be interpreted within the context of this limitation. One limitation in this study is that we were unable to objectively measure perfusion of subcutaneous tissue. Such is possible using indocyanine green angiography intraoperatively [29]. Inadequate perfusion of subcutaneous tissue fat may cause fat necrosis or wound-healing problems. None of our patients had a wound-healing problem at the reconstructed site or required a reoperation for fat necrosis. Another limitation is that DIRT was used in relatively healthy patients. The mean BMI was 27.2 kg/m^2 (range 21.6–32.4). Further studies are required to evaluate the usefulness of DIRT in preoperative perforator mapping in patients with co-morbidities and obesity.

Conclusions

We conclude that the locations of first appearing hot spots on DIRT are associated with arterial Doppler sounds and with perforators on CTA. In addition, the surgical results revealed that DIEP breast reconstruction could reliably be performed using DIRT for perforator selection. DIRT provides information on the location of the perforator and its hemodynamic properties. DIRT is easy to interpret and it does not involve exposure to ionizing radiation or the use of intravenous contrast medium. Based on our results we conclude that DIRT is a promising alternative to CTA for preoperative perforator mapping in DIEP breast reconstruction.

Abbreviations
3D, Three-dimensional; CT, Computed tomography; CTA, Computed tomographic angiography; DIEA, Deep inferior epigastric artery; DIEP, Deep inferior epigastric artery perforator; DIRT, Dynamic infrared thermography; MIP, Maximum intensity projection; MPR, Multiplanar reconstruction; PACS, Picture archiving and communication system

Acknowledgements
Not applicable.

Funding
The corresponding author has received research grants provided by the Norwegian Research School in Medical Imaging (MedIm) and Northern Norway Regional Health Authority (Helse Nord RHF). The other authors have not received any funding.

Authors' contributions
All three authors have participated in the planning of the study, the collection of data, interpretation of data and writing of the manuscript. All authors read and approved the final manuscript.

Authors' information
SW is a Consultant Radiologist and Associate Professor at the University Hospital of North Norway and Head of Medical Imaging Research Group at UiT the Arctic University of Norway. JM is a Professor at UiT the Arctic University of Norway and the University Hospital of North Norway where he is responsible for the thermography laboratory. JM was the President of European Association of Thermology from 2009 to 2015. LdW is a Plastic Surgeon and Professor at the University Hospital of North Norway. LdW specializes in reconstructive surgery and the development of new surgical techniques in plastic surgery.

Competing interests

The authors declare that they have no competing interests.

Author details

[1]Medical Imaging Research Group, Department of Clinical Medicine, UiT The Arctic University of Norway, 9037 Tromsø, Norway. [2]Department of Radiology, University Hospital of North Norway, Sykehusveien 38, P.O. Box 103, 9038 Tromsø, Norway. [3]Department of Plastic Surgery and Hand Surgery, University Hospital of North Norway, P.O. Box 66, 9038 Tromsø, Norway.

References

1. El-Mrakby HH, Milner RH. The vascular anatomy of the lower anterior abdominal wall: a microdissection study on the deep inferior epigastric vessels and the perforator branches. Plast Reconstr Surg. 2002;109(2):539–43. discussion 544–537.
2. Cina A, Salgarello M, Barone-Adesi L, Rinaldi P, Bonomo L. Planning breast reconstruction with deep inferior epigastric artery perforating vessels: multidetector CT angiography versus color Doppler US. Radiology. 2010; 255(3):979–87.
3. Blondeel PN. One hundred free DIEP flap breast reconstructions: a personal experience. Br J Plast Surg. 1999;52(2):104–11.
4. Mathes DW, Neligan PC. Current techniques in preoperative imaging for abdomen-based perforator flap microsurgical breast reconstruction. J Reconstr Microsurg. 2010;26(1):3–10.
5. Blondeel PN, Beyens G, Verhaeghe R, Van Landuyt K, Tonnard P, Monstrey SJ, Matton G. Doppler flowmetry in the planning of perforator flaps. Br J Plast Surg. 1998;51(3):202–9.
6. Rozen WM, Garcia-Tutor E, Alonso-Burgos A, Acosta R, Stillaert F, Zubieta JL, Hamdi M, Whitaker IS, Ashton MW. Planning and optimising DIEP flaps with virtual surgery: the Navarra experience. J Plast Reconstr Aesthet Surg. 2010; 63(2):289–97.
7. Itoh Y, Arai K. The deep inferior epigastric artery free skin flap: anatomic study and clinical application. Plast Reconstr Surg. 1993;91(5):853–63. discussion 864.
8. Itoh Y, Arai K. Use of recovery-enhanced thermography to localize cutaneous perforators. Ann Plast Surg. 1995;34(5):507–11.
9. Lohman RF, Ozturk CN, Ozturk C, Jayaprakash V, Djohan R. An analysis of current techniques used for intraoperative flap evaluation. Ann Plast Surg. 2014.
10. Tenorio X, Mahajan AL, Wettstein R, Harder Y, Pawlovski M, Pittet B. Early detection of flap failure using a new thermographic device. J Surg Res. 2009;151(1):15–21.
11. Salmi AM, Tukiainen E, Asko-Seljavaara S. Thermographic mapping of perforators and skin blood flow in the free transverse rectus abdominis musculocutaneous flap. Ann Plast Surg. 1995;35(2):159–64.
12. de Weerd L, Mercer JB, Weum S. Dynamic infrared thermography. Clin Plast Surg. 2011;38(2):277–92.
13. Whitaker IS, Lie KH, Rozen WM, Chubb D, Ashton MW. Dynamic infrared thermography for the preoperative planning of microsurgical breast reconstruction: a comparison with CTA. J Plast Reconstr Aesthet Surg. 2012;65(1):130–2.
14. Kalra S, Dancey A, Waters R. Intraoperative selection of dominant perforator vessel in DIEP free flaps based on perfusion strength using digital infrared thermography - a pilot study. J Plast Reconstr Aesthet Surg. 2007;60(12): 1365–8.
15. Giunta RE, Geisweid A, Feller AM. The value of preoperative Doppler sonography for planning free perforator flaps. Plast Reconstr Surg. 2000; 105(7):2381–6.
16. Vandevoort M, Vranckx JJ, Fabre G. Perforator topography of the deep inferior epigastric perforator flap in 100 cases of breast reconstruction. Plast Reconstr Surg. 2002;109(6):1912–8.
17. Mathes D, Keys S, Said H, Louie O, Neligan P. The clinical utility of CT angiography in deep inferior epigastric perforator (DIEP) flap microsurgical breast reconstruction. In: Proceedings world congress reconstructive surgery Helsinki. 2011.
18. Hijjawi JB, Blondeel PN. Advancing deep inferior epigastric artery perforator flap breast reconstruction through multidetector row computed tomography: an evolution in preoperative imaging. J Reconstr Microsurg. 2010;26(1):11–20.
19. de Weerd L, Weum S, Mercer JB. The value of dynamic infrared thermography (DIRT) in perforatorselection and planning of free DIEP flaps. Ann Plast Surg. 2009;63(3):274–9.
20. Chubb D, Rozen WM, Whitaker IS, Ashton MW. Images in plastic surgery: digital thermographic photography ("thermal imaging") for preoperative perforator mapping. Ann Plast Surg. 2011;66(4):324–5.
21. Rozen WM, Ashton MW, Le Roux CM, Pan WR, Corlett RJ. The perforator angiosome: a new concept in the design of deep inferior epigastric artery perforator flaps for breast reconstruction. Microsurgery. 2010;30(1):1–7.
22. Taylor GI, Palmer JH. The vascular territories (angiosomes) of the body: experimental study and clinical applications. Br J Plast Surg. 1987;40(2):113–41.
23. Gill PS, Hunt JP, Guerra AB, Dellacroce FJ, Sullivan SK, Boraski J, Metzinger SE, Dupin CL, Allen RJ. A 10-year retrospective review of 758 DIEP flaps for breast reconstruction. Plast Reconstr Surg. 2004;113(4):1153–60.
24. Carramenha e Costa MA, Carriquiry C, Vasconez LO, Grotting JC, Herrera RH, Windle BH. An anatomic study of the venous drainage of the transverse rectus abdominis musculocutaneous flap. Plast Reconstr Surg. 1987;79(2):208–17.
25. Rozen WM, Pan WR, Le Roux CM, Taylor GI, Ashton MW. The venous anatomy of the anterior abdominal wall: an anatomical and clinical study. Plast Reconstr Surg. 2009;124(3):848–53.
26. Taylor G, Ian AO. Vascular anatomy of the lower anterior abdominal wall: a microdissection study on the deep inferior epigastric vessels and the perforator branches by Hamdy H. El-Mrakby, M.D. Richard H. Milner, M.D. Plast Reconstr Surg. 2002;109(2):544–7.
27. Schaverien M, Saint-Cyr M, Arbique G, Brown SA. Arterial and venous anatomies of the deep inferior epigastric perforator and superficial inferior epigastric artery flaps. Plast Reconstr Surg. 2008;121(6):1909–19.
28. de Weerd L, Miland AO, Mercer JB. Perfusion dynamics of free DIEP and SIEA flaps during the first postoperative week monitored with dynamic infrared thermography. Ann Plast Surg. 2009;62(1):42–7.
29. Gurtner GC, Jones GE, Neligan PC, Newman MI, Phillips BT, Sacks JM, Zenn MR. Intraoperative laser angiography using the SPY system: review of the literature and recommendations for use. Ann Surg Innov Res. 2013;7(1):1.

11

Increased enhancement of the liver adjacent to the gallbladder seen with contrast ultrasound: comparison between acute cholecystitis and non-cholecystitis

Ryousuke Kawai[1*], Jiro Hata[1], Noriaki Manabe[1], Hiroshi Imamura[1], Ai Iida[1], Nobuko Koyama[2] and Hiroaki Kusunoki[3]

Abstract

Background: This study was performed to evaluate the ability of contrast-enhanced ultrasonography (CEUS) with time-intensity curve analysis to demonstrate an increased enhancement of the liver parenchyma adjacent to the inflamed gallbladder, as seen on contrast-enhanced computed tomography.

Methods: The Ethics Committee of our institution approved the study protocol (Kawasaki Medical School, registration number 1277). From April to November 2013, 11 consecutive patients with acute cholecystitis and 16 patients without cholecystitis consented to CEUS (Sonazoid™) and were enrolled in this study. The gallbladder and liver were scanned by one gastroenterologist using harmonic imaging with a low mechanical index. The raw imaging data were stored. Another physician, blinded to all clinical information, constructed the time-intensity curve. The major axis of the region of interest (ROI) was set in segment 5 (pericholecystic area), and the control ROI in segment 8 at the same depth. The intensity ratio (IR) was defined as the peak intensity of segment 5 divided by the simultaneous value of segment 8. The characteristics of the patient with and without acute cholecystitis were compared. The correlation between the IR and the presence of acute cholecystitis was analyzed using binomial logistic regression analysis. A receiver operating characteristic (ROC) curve analysis was performed as well.

Results: The IR was significantly higher in the group with than without acute cholecystitis ($p = 0.006$). The IR correlated significantly with the presence of acute gallbladder inflammation ($p = 0.043$). The area under the ROC curve was estimated as 0.852 (95 % confidence interval, 0.709–0.995). A cut-off value of 2.72 had a sensitivity of 81.8 % and a specificity of 81.3 %.

Conclusions: The IR obtained by CEUS with time-intensity curve analysis generally demonstrated increased enhancement of the liver parenchyma adjacent to the inflamed gallbladder.

Keywords: Acute cholecystitis, Contrast-enhanced ultrasound, Time-intensity curve analysis

Background

Transabdominal ultrasonography (US) is regarded as the first-line noninvasive bedside examination for the diagnosis of acute abdominal diseases [1], including acute cholecystitis [2, 3], because it is safe, widely available, and inexpensive. Only patients with negative or inconclusive US findings should undergo computed tomography (CT), according to the general diagnostic strategy for acute abdominal pain, which aims for the highest sensitivity for urgent conditions and for the lowest radiation exposure [1]. Magnetic resonance imaging and cholescintigraphy are also useful for the diagnosis of acute cholecystitis [2, 3], although they are less available.

Imaging findings of gallbladder inflammation are needed for the diagnosis of acute cholecystitis according to the Tokyo Guideline 2013 (TG13) criteria [4, 5]. The reported sensitivity and specificity of gray-scale US are 88 % and 80 %, respectively [6]. However, typical

* Correspondence: ryosuke@med.kawasaki-m.ac.jp
[1]Department of Clinical Pathology and Laboratory Medicine, Kawasaki Medical School, 577 Matsushima, Kurashiki, Okayama 701-0192, Japan
Full list of author information is available at the end of the article

imaging findings are not necessarily demonstrated in all cases. In our opinion, the diagnostic power of gray-scale US should be based on the patient's specific complaints and should especially include the presence of a sonographic Murphy sign. For example, in a surgical series of patients with gangrenous cholecystitis, 28 % of the 7patients had no US findings diagnostic for gallbladder inflammation, mainly because of the absence of both a sonographic Murphy sign and gallbladder wall thickening [7]. Furthermore, diagnosis of acute cholecystitis must often be made with limited clinical information in patients with difficulties in communicating for reasons such as septic shock, dementia, brain damage, or use of sedative agents. The presence of a sonographic Murphy sign in these patients is difficult to evaluate correctly.

Increased pericholecystic attenuation on contrast-enhanced CT (CECT) is an objective and useful finding in the identification of acute cholecystitis [8, 9]. Some reports have supported the utility of contrast-enhanced US (CEUS) in differentiating between acute and chronic cholecystitis [10–12], by evaluating the intensity of contrast agent in the gallbladder wall. However, there have been no reports describing the diagnosis of acute cholecystitis using the contrast agent perflubutane (Sonazoid™; Daiichi Sankyo, Tokyo, Japan) in CEUS with time-intensity curve analysis along with an evaluation of the intensity of the contrast agent in the liver parenchyma adjacent to the gallbladder.

We hypothesized that increased enhancement of the liver parenchyma adjacent to the inflamed gallbladder is seen on CEUS, just as on CECT, and that time-intensity curve analysis can be useful to quantitatively express the findings. Thus, the purpose of this study was to evaluate whether CEUS with time-intensity curve analysis of the liver parenchyma adjacent to the inflamed gallbladder can improve the diagnosis of acute cholecystitis.

Methods

Patient selection

The Ethics Committee of our institution approved the study protocol (Kawasaki Medical School, registration number 1277). Informed consent was obtained from all patients before the injection of contrast agent.

From April to November 2013, 11 consecutive patients with acute cholecystitis (acute cholecystitis group) and 16 patients without acute cholecystitis (control group) were enrolled in this study. Patients with a focal spared area in the liver parenchyma adjacent to the gallbladder, as seen on gray-scale US imaging, and with portal vein embolism detected by color Doppler imaging, which may alter the focal perfusion, were excluded. The four males and seven females in the acute cholecystitis group had a median age of 68.0 years (range, 55–89 years). The diagnosis of acute cholecystitis was based on the TG13

criteria and involved surgery in seven patients and follow-up without surgery in four patients. All 16 patients in the control group underwent CEUS to search for metastatic liver tumors that could not be detected by gray-scale US. They were enrolled in this study under the criterion that no metastatic tumor was detected on segment 5 or 8 according to Couinaud's classification. The 12 males and 4 females in the control group had a median age of 67.0 years (range, 40–86 years) and included patients with colon cancer ($n = 8$), gastric cancer ($n = 5$), lung cancer ($n = 2$), and duodenal cancer ($n = 1$).

US technique and interpretation

All US examinations were performed with a diagnostic ultrasound system (TUS-A500; Toshiba, Tokyo, Japan) equipped with a 3.75-MHz transducer. No special patient preparations were undertaken. Gray-scale US was performed within 10 min in all patients. Sonazoid™ was injected intravenously (bolus, 0.015 mL/kg) followed by 10 mL of saline within 10 s. The gallbladder and liver parenchyma adjacent to the gallbladder were then scanned through the intercostal view using harmonic imaging with a low mechanical index (0.2–0.3) by one gastroenterologist (J.H.) with 21 years of experience in US. The raw imaging data, from the injection of the contrast medium to the beginning of enhancement of the main portal vein, were stored. Another physician (R.K.), with 3 years of experience in US, who was blinded to all clinical information then analyzed the data and constructed the time-intensity curve (Fig. 1a, b). To construct the time-intensity curve, the major axis of the region of interest (ROI) was set in segment 5 (the liver parenchyma adjacent to the gallbladder), and the control ROI was set in segment 8 on the same image (Fig. 2). The two ROIs were placed at the same depth. Neither ROI included relatively large vessels detectable by CEUS. The intensity ratio (IR) was defined as the peak intensity of segment 5 divided by the simultaneous value of segment 8. We considered that the IR would be suitable to demonstrate increased enhancement of the adjacent liver parenchyma by comparison with another point at the same depth that could be investigated simultaneously under the same conditions.

Statistical analysis

The following patient characteristics were compared between the acute cholecystitis and control groups: sex, age, presence of liver cirrhosis, and clinical symptoms (fever or abdominal pain), white blood cell count, C-reactive protein level, liver enzyme concentrations (total bilirubin, aspartate aminotransferase, and alanine aminotransferase), gray-scale US findings (short-axis gallbladder diameter, presence of gallbladder stones, and presence of sonographic Murphy sign), and IR

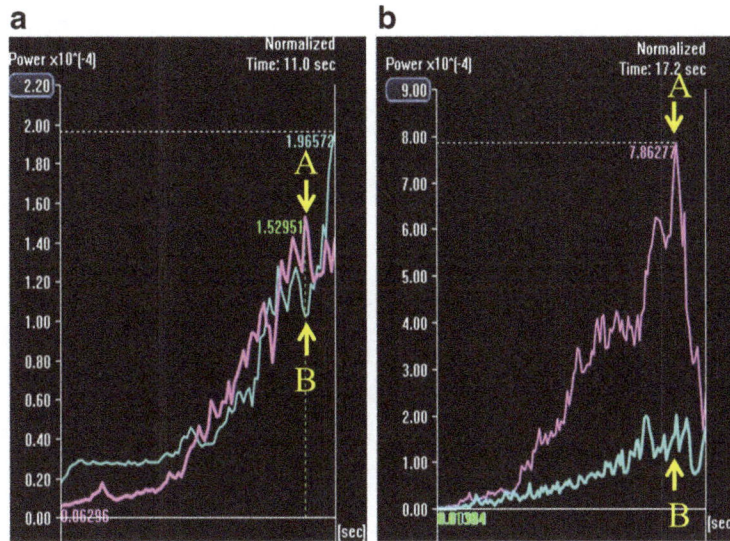

Fig. 1 Time-intensity curves. **a,** Time-intensity curve of the non-cholecystitis group. The intensity ratio was defined as follows: the peak intensity of segment 5 (*arrow A*) divided by the simultaneous value of segment 8 (*arrow B*). Red line, segment 5; blue line, segment 8. **b,** Time-intensity curve of the acute cholecystitis group. The intensity ratio was defined as follows: the peak intensity of segment 5 (*arrow A*) divided by the simultaneous value of segment 8 (*arrow B*). Red line, segment 5; blue line, segment 8

obtained by CEUS. All comparisons were performed using SPSS (version 19.0; IBM, Armonk, NY, USA). The Mann–Whitney U test for continuous values and Fisher's exact test for categorical values were used to evaluate the significance of the differences between the two groups. A p value of <0.05 was considered to indicate a statistically significant difference. The correlation between the IR and the existence of acute gallbladder inflammation was analyzed using binomial logistic regression. A receiver operating characteristic (ROC) analysis was performed. The sensitivity and specificity of the IR for diagnosing acute cholecystitis were determined for each cut-off value using the resulting curve.

Results

The characteristics of all 27 patients in the two groups are detailed in Table 1. Most patients in the acute cholecystitis group had acute illness with abdominal pain (81.8 %, 9/11) and a positive sonographic Murphy sign (90.9 %, 10/11) consistent with acute cholecystitis. No patients in either group had liver cirrhosis. There were no significant differences in the laboratory test results, the short-axis gallbladder diameter, or the presence of gallbladder stones between the two groups. The IR obtained by CEUS was significantly higher in the acute cholecystitis group than in the control group ($p = 0.006$) (Fig. 3).

Binomial logistic regression showed that the IR correlated significantly with the presence of acute gallbladder inflammation ($p = 0.043$). The odds ratio was 2.676 [95 % confidence interval (CI), 1.033–6.932].

Analysis of the ROC curve for the diagnosis of acute cholecystitis based on the IR (Fig. 4) showed that a cut-off value of 1.58 had a sensitivity of 100.0 % (11/11) with a 95 % CI of 67.9–100.0, and a specificity of 50.0 % (8/16) with a 95 % CI of 25.5–74.5. A cut-off of 2.72 had a sensitivity of 81.8 % (9/11) with a 95 % CI of 47.8–96.8, and specificity of 81.3 % (13/16) with a 95 % CI 53.7–95.0. A cut-off of 5.81 had a sensitivity of 36.4 % (4/11)

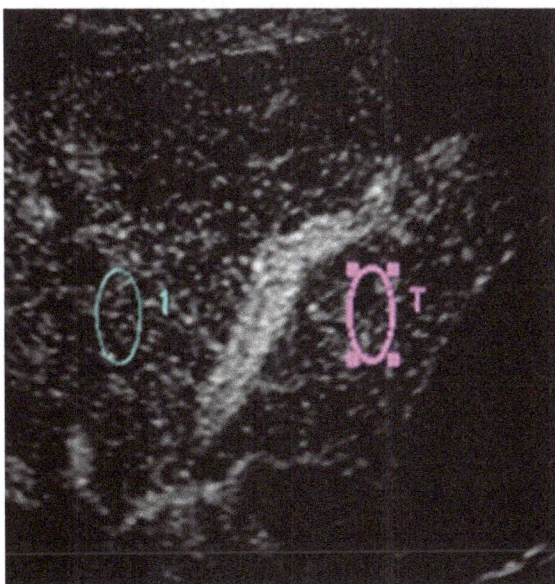

Fig. 2 Region of interest (ROI) for two points. A pericholecystic point (*red circle*, segment 5) and another point at the same depth (*blue circle*, segment 8), avoiding the large vessels

Table 1 Characteristics of the 27 patients in the acute cholecystitis and control groups

	Acute cholecystitis	Control	p value
Patients	11	16	
Male:female	4:7	12:4	0.061
Age, years	68.0 (64.0,81.0)	67.0 (56.5, 76.0)	1.000
Presence of liver cirrhosis, %	0 (0/11)	0 (0/16)	
Presence of fever (>37.5°), %	54.5 (6/11)	37.5 (6/16)	0.452
Presence of abdominal pain, %	81.8 (9/11)	31.3 (5/16)	0.018
White blood cell count, /μL	11010 (8615,13235)	6790 (5325, 8862.5)	0.054
C-reactive protein level, mg/dL	10.43 (3.77, 17.26)	0.56 (0.32, 4.89)	0.054
Total bilirubin level, mg/dL	0.90 (0.65, 1.20)	0.70 (0.50, 1.15)	0.452
AST level, IU/L	23.0 (17.0, 40.5)	40.5 (22.5, 63.3)	0.239
ALT level, IU/L	23.0 (14.5, 33.5)	34.0 (17.0, 53.5)	0.440
Short-axis gallbladder diameter, mm	30.0 (28.0, 35.5)	28.0 (22.0, 33.0)	0.198
Sonographic Murphy sign, positive, %	90.9 (10/11)	12.5 (2/16)	0.000
Gallbladder stones, positive, %	54.5 (6/11)	31.3 (5/16)	0.264
Intensity ratio	3.396 (2.90, 7.82)	1.595 (1.17, 2.50)	0.006

Data are presented as the median with the interquartile range (1st quartile, 3rd quartile)
AST aspartate aminotransferase; *ALT* alanine aminotransferase

with a 95 % CI of 12.4–68.4, and a specificity of 100.0 % (16/16) with a 95 % CI 75.9–100.0. The area under the curve was estimated as 0.852 (95 % CI, 0.709–0.995).

Five patients had an atypical IR: two in the acute cholecystitis group had a low IR (<2.72) and three in the control group had a high IR (>2.72).

Discussion

US is the first-line morphologic examination technique for the diagnosis of acute cholecystitis [2, 3]. However, US findings consistent with acute cholecystitis are often seen in patients with conditions other than acute cholecystitis. Thickening of the gallbladder wall and free fluid around the gallbladder are not specific for gallbladder inflammation in patients with cardiac failure, renal failure, hepatic cirrhosis, hepatitis, hypoalbuminemia, or blockage of the lymphatic or venous drainage of the gallbladder [13]. Furthermore, the diagnosis of acute cholecystitis is difficult in patients who cannot explain their symptoms correctly (e.g., patients who are in a coma, are critically ill, have dementia, or have myeloparalysis). The development of a reliable and quantitative sonographic technique for the diagnosis of acute cholecystitis is therefore very important, both in these patients and in others.

Acute gallbladder inflammation causes increased blood flow from the cystic artery to the gallbladder wall. Transient and focally increased attenuation of the liver parenchyma adjacent to the inflamed gallbladder is a common CECT finding of acute cholecystitis, with a reported sensitivity of 82.4 % [8]. This finding can perhaps be explained by cholecystitis-induced hepatic arterial hyperemia and early venous drainage from the gallbladder [14, 15]. However, it is often difficult to safely transport critically ill patients to the radiology unit for CECT, especially those in the intensive care unit. Furthermore, in patients with concomitant renal dysfunction, CT contrast agents should be avoided because of their nephrotoxicity. Therefore, for the diagnosis of acute cholecystitis, we emphasize the utility of CEUS with the contrast agent Sonazoid™ as a bedside procedure for the detection of

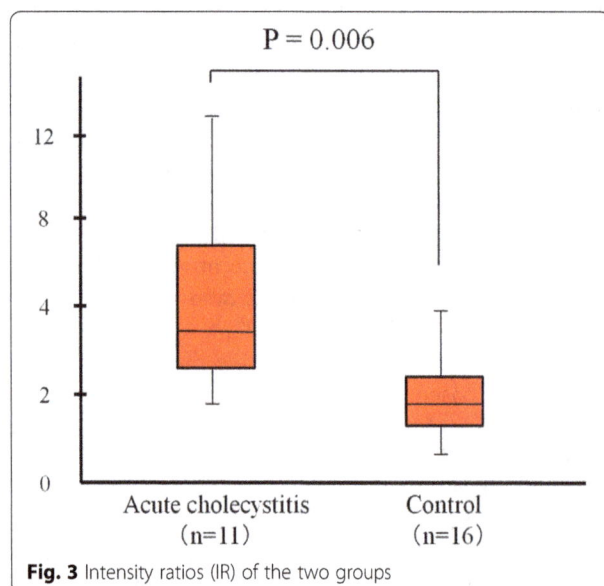

Fig. 3 Intensity ratios (IR) of the two groups

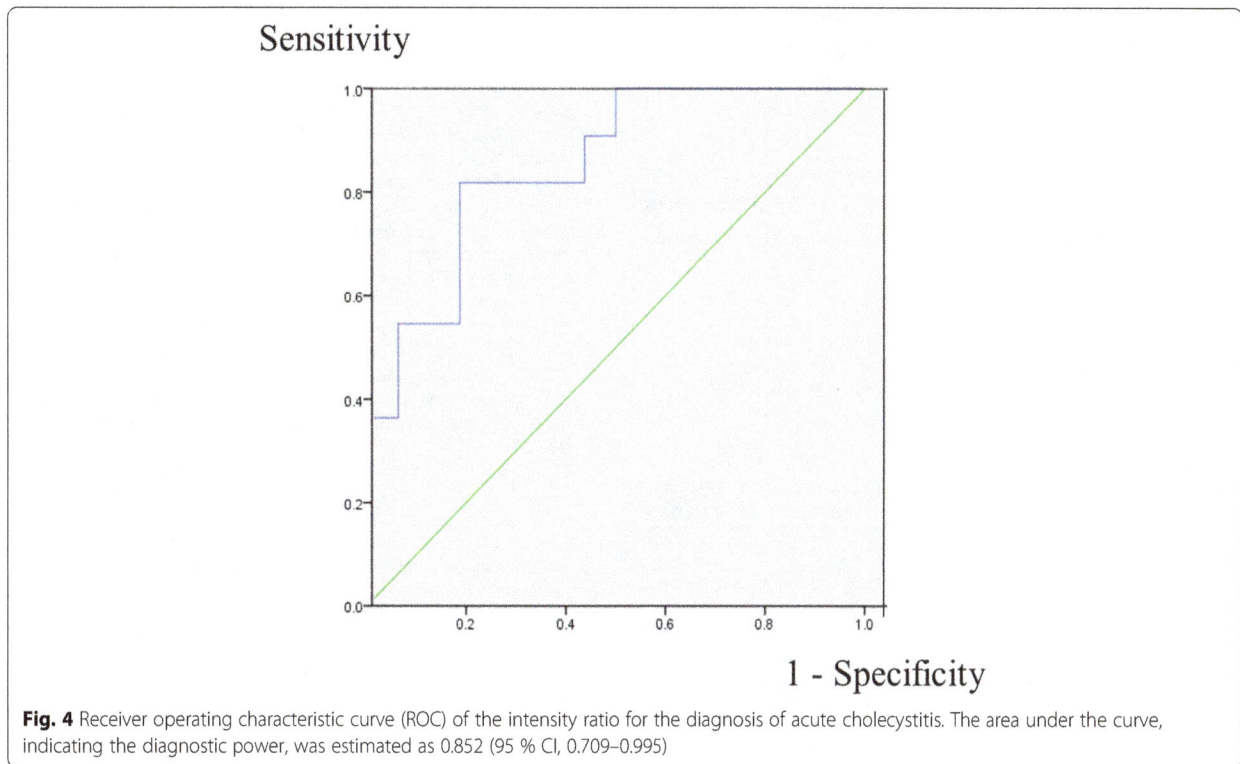

Fig. 4 Receiver operating characteristic curve (ROC) of the intensity ratio for the diagnosis of acute cholecystitis. The area under the curve, indicating the diagnostic power, was estimated as 0.852 (95 % CI, 0.709–0.995)

increased enhancement of the liver parenchyma adjacent to the inflamed gallbladder.

Adamietz et al. [10] used CEUS with SonoVue™ to examine 20 patients with acute cholecystitis and 8 with chronic cholecystitis. They reported that strong enhancement of the gallbladder wall was a very likely indicator of acute inflammation. However, our study is the first to demonstrate increased enhancement of the liver parenchyma adjacent to the inflamed gallbladder by CEUS together with time-intensity curve analysis. We used the IR, in which the peak intensity of the liver parenchyma adjacent to the gallbladder was divided by that of another point at the same depth, to avoid the interpatient variations caused by differences in the patients' health. Our results showed that the IR was higher in patients with acute cholecystitis, in agreement with the Adamietz et al. [10]. The area under the curve, which represents the diagnostic power of this method, was estimated as 0.852. In our opinion, this represents a clinically acceptable diagnostic ability; thus, the IR obtained by CEUS with time-intensity curve analysis can facilitate the diagnosis of acute cholecystitis.

In the present study, 2 of the 11 patients in the acute cholecystitis group had an atypically low IR (<2.72). One of these patients, with an IR of 1.71, had histopathologically confirmed gangrenous cholecystitis. Accordingly, our method may have certain limitations in diagnosing gangrenous cholecystitis, in

agreement with the results of a previous study [10]. The cause of the low IR (1.75) in the other patient remains unclear. In the control group, 3 of the 16 patients had a high IR (>2.72). The reason for this discrepancy is also unclear, but may have been due to the following: the mean IR among the other 13 patients in the control group was 1.52, indicating greater blood flow in segment 5 than in segment 8, even in patients without acute cholecystitis; this may be due to the normal venous return to segment 5 from the cystic artery. Additionally, anatomical variants of the cystic artery and the parabiliary venous system [16–19] may have contributed to these discrepancies. Furthermore, increased pericholecystic attenuation on contrast-enhanced CT is not pathognomonic for inflammation, as it is also observed in regions of focal fat deposition, cases of portal vein thrombosis, and similar conditions. Therefore, we excluded patients with a focal spared area in the liver parenchyma adjacent to the gallbladder by gray-scale US imaging and with portal vein embolism.

This study had several limitations. First, the number of patients was small. Second, we did not evaluate interobserver agreement. Finally, the patient selection of this study was based on the TG13. Therefore, the backgrounds of the two groups differed significantly in the clinical and gray-scale findings, which prevented an evaluation of the advantage of this method over the traditional diagnostic technique for acute cholecystitis using gray-scale imaging. This remains to be determined in further investigations.

Conclusion

The IR obtained by CEUS with time-intensity curve analysis can generally demonstrate an increased enhancement of the liver parenchyma adjacent to the inflamed gallbladder.

Abbreviations

US: Ultrasonography; *CEUS*: Contrast-enhanced ultrasonography; *CT*: Computed tomography; *CECT*: Contrast-enhanced computed tomography; *ROI*: Region of interest; *IR*: Intensity ratio; *ROC*: Receiver operating characteristic; *95% CI*: 95% confidence interval.

Competing interests

Ryousuke Kawai, Jiro Hata, Noriaki Manabe, Hiroshi Imamura, Ai Iida, Nobuko Koyama, and Hiroaki Kusunoki declare that they have no conflicts of interest.

Authors' contributions

RK: Study design, data collection, analysis and interpretation of data, drafting of the manuscript, critical revision of the manuscript, final approval of the submitted manuscript. JH: Study design, data collection, critical revision of the manuscript, final approval of the submitted manuscript. NM: Analysis and interpretation of data, final approval of the submitted manuscript. HI: Analysis and interpretation of data, final approval of the submitted manuscript. AI: Analysis and interpretation of data, final approval of the submitted manuscript. NK: Analysis and interpretation of data, final approval of the submitted manuscript. HK: Analysis and interpretation of data, final approval of the submitted manuscript.

Author details

[1]Department of Clinical Pathology and Laboratory Medicine, Kawasaki Medical School, 577 Matsushima, Kurashiki, Okayama 701-0192, Japan. [2]Department of Hepatology and Pancreatology, Kawasaki Medical School, 577 Matsushima, Kurashiki, Okayama 701-0192, Japan. [3]Department of General Medicine, Kawasaki Medical School, 577 Matsushima, Kurashiki, Okayama 701-0192, Japan.

References

1. Laméris W, van Randen A, van Es HW, van Heesewijk JP, van Ramshorst B, Bouma WH, et al. Imaging strategies for detection of urgent conditions in patients with acute abdominal pain diagnostic accuracy study. BMJ. 2009; 338:b2431.
2. Kiewiet JJ, Leeuwenburgh MM, Bipat S, Bossuyt PM, Stoker J, Boermeester MA. A systematic review and meta-analysis of diagnostic performance of imaging in acute cholecystitis. Radiology. 2012;264:708–20.
3. Van Santvoort HC. Imaging techniques in acute cholecystitis. Ned Tijdschr Geneeskd. 2013;157:A6028.
4. Miura F, Takada T, Strasberg SM, Solomkin JS, Pitt HA, Gouma DJ, et al. TG13 flowchart for the management of acute cholangitis and cholecystitis. J Hepatobiliary Pancreat Sci. 2013;20:47–54.
5. Okamoto K, Takada T, Strasberg SM, Solomkin JS, Pitt HA, Garden OJ, et al. TG13 management bundles for acute cholangitis and cholecystitis. J Hepatobiliary Pancreat Sci. 2013;20:55–9.
6. Trowbridge RL, Rutkowski NK, Shojania KG. Does this patient have acute cholecystitis? JAMA. 2003;289:80–6.
7. Hunt DR, Chu FC. Gangrenous cholecystitis in the laparoscopic era. Aust N Z J Surg. 2000;70:428–30.
8. Kim YK, Kwak HS, Kim CS, Han YM, Jeong TO, Kim IH, et al. CT findings of mild forms or early manifestations of acute cholecystitis. Clin Imaging. 2009; 33:274–80.
9. Yamashita K, Jin MJ, Hirose Y, Morikawa M, Sumioka H, Itoh K, et al. CT findings of transient focal increased attenuation of the liver adjacent to the gallbladder in acute cholecystitis. AJR Am J Roentgenol. 1995;164:343–6.
10. Adamietz B, Wenkel E, Uder M, Meyer T, Schneider I, Dimmler A, et al. Contrast enhanced sonography of the gallbladder: a tool in the diagnosis of cholecystitis? Eur J Radiol. 2007;61:262–6.
11. Kim KA, Park CM, Park SW, Cha SH, Seol HY, Cha IH, et al. Contrast-enhanced power Doppler US: is it useful in the differentiation of gallbladder disease? Clin Imaging. 2002;26:319–24.
12. Esteban JM, Maldonado L, Elia I, Ferrando F. Value of power Doppler ultrasonography with intravenous contrast medium (Levograf) in the diagnosis of acute cholecystitis. Gastroenterol Hepatol. 2002;25:79–83.
13. Teefey SA, Baron RL, Bigler SA. Sonography of the gallbladder: significance of striated (layered) thickening of the gallbladder wall. AJR Am J Roentgenol. 1991;156:945–7.
14. Ito K, Awaya H, Mitchell DG, Honjo K, Fujita T, Uchisako H, et al. Gallbladder disease: appearance of associated transient increased attenuation in the liver at biphasic, contrast-enhanced dynamic CT. Radiology. 1997;204:723–8.
15. Matsui O, Takashima T, Kadoya M, Konishi H, Kawamura I, Hirose J, et al. Staining in the liver surrounding gall bladder fossa on hepatic angiography caused by increased cystic venous drainage. Gastrointest Radiol. 1987;12: 307–12.
16. Michels NA. The hepatic, cystic and retroduodenal arteries and their relations to the biliary ducts with samples of the entire celiacal blood supply. Ann Surg. 1951;133:503–24.
17. Ramesh Babu CS, Sharma M. Biliary tract anatomy and its relationship with venous drainage. J Clin Exp Hepatol. 2014;4(S1):S18–26.
18. Couinaud C. The parabiliary venous system. Surg Radiol Anat. 1988;10:311–6.
19. Hasan MM, Reza E, Khan MR, Laila SZ, Rahman F, Mamun MH. Anatomical and congenital anomalies of extra hepatic biliary system encountered during cholecystectomy. Mymensingh Med J. 2013;22:20–6.

12

Usefulness of grayscale inverted images in addition to standard images in digital mammography

Ayşegül Altunkeser[1,3]* and M. Kazım Körez[2]

Abstract

Background: Mammography is essential for early diagnosis of breast cancer, which is the most common type of cancer in females that is associated with a high mortality rate. We investigated whether evaluation of the grayscale inverted images of mammograms would aid in increasing the diagnostic sensitivity of the mammographic imaging technique.

Methods: Our study included 636 mammograms of 159 women who had undergone digital mammography. Standard, grayscale inverted, and standard plus grayscale inverted images were sequentially examined three times, at 15-day intervals, for the presence or assessment of pathological changes in the skin, calcification, asymmetric density, mass lesions, structural distortions, and intramammary and axillary lymph nodes. To determine whether grayscale inverted image assessment improved detection rates, the results of the three assessment modes were compared using Cochran's Q test and the McNemar test ($p < 0.05$ was considered statistically significant).

Results: The average age of 159 patients was 50.4 years (range, 35–80 years). There were significant differences among the three assessment modes with respect to calcification and intramammary lymph nodes ($p < 0.05$); however, no significant differences were observed for the detection of other parameters.

Conclusions: Assessment of grayscale inverted images in addition to standard images facilitates the detection of microcalcification.

Keywords: Digital mammography, Macrocalcification, Microcalcification, Grayscale inverted images

Background

Breast cancer is the most frequent women's cancer, with high mortality rates in Turkey and other parts of the world. In Turkey, its incidence is 40.6 per 100,000 women (http://www.kanser.gov.tr/Dosya/ca_istatistik/2009kanseraporu). Early diagnosis can decrease the likelihood of mortality and requires scanning. It has been reported that scanning of women over 50 years of age reduces breast cancer-related mortality rates by 3–36% [1, 2].

Mammography is the most effective screening method for breast cancer [3]. However, mammographic assessment is difficult and requires experience owing to the complex structure of mammary tissue. The false negative

range in mammographic detection of breast cancer is 10–25%. Dense mammary structure, inferior mammogram quality, overlooked details of early breast cancers, and fatigue or carelessness of the radiologist may account for the high percentage of false negatives [4]. To lower this percentage, a double-reading system is recommended [5] but is costly and requires two professional readers and is thus impractical. Computer-aided detection (CAD) is an alternative method, especially in busy crowded centers that focus on mammography [6].

Unfortunately, not all mammography centers facilitate double reading or CAD system. In our center, one radiologist assesses the data obtained via digital mammography without CAD. In view of the fact that digital mammography is a digitalized system, digitalization allows different representations of the images. Therefore, in this paper we studied if the diagnostic assessment of grayscale inverted mammograms improved compared to a standard

---
* Correspondence: aaltunkeser@hotmail.com
[1]Department of Radiology, Konya Education and Research Hospital, Konya, Turkey
[3]Konya Eğitim ve Araştırma Hastanesi, Radyoloji Bölümü, Hacı Şaban Mah, Meram Yeni Yol Caddesi, No: 97, PK: 42090 Meram, Konya, Turkey
Full list of author information is available at the end of the article

representation of mammographic images when double-reading or CAD is impossible.

Methods

Our study included 636 mammograms of 159 women who had undergone mammography at Dr. Faruk Sükan Obstetrics and Pediatrics Hospital between January 5 and February 4, 2015. Scanning was performed for diagnostic purposes, in the mediolateral oblique and cranio-caudal views, and using a digital mammography device, which has ring shaped gantry, 24X30 cm Amorphous Selenium detector, Tungsten anode tube (Giotto Image 3D, IMS, Bologna, Italy). This study was approved by the ethics committee of Necmettin Erbakan University. Mammograms were evaluated by an experienced radiologist. Mammography was performed according to the Breast Imaging Reporting and Data System (BIRADS) as recommended by the American College of Radiology [7].

Initially, the parenchymal patterns on mammograms were evaluated. and categorized as follows: type A, the whole breast consists predominantly of fat tissue; type B, the whole breast contains fibroglandular densities as well as fat tissue; type C, the density of the breast parenchyma is heterogeneous; and type D, the breast parenchyma is highly dense [7]. Pathological changes in the skin (increased thickness, mass, or shrinkage), calcification, asymmetric density, mass lesion, structural distortion, and intramammary and axillary lymph nodes were then assessed and scored as present or absent. Calcifications were classified as macro or micro (<0.5 mm) regardless of their morphological properties and distribution patterns. Asymmetric density included both focal and regional asymmetric density detected in either or both views. Densities with a three-dimensional structure and observed in both views were defined as mass. Structural distortion was defined as shrinkage withdrawal without mass. Centrically radiolucent lymph nodes with regular margins and

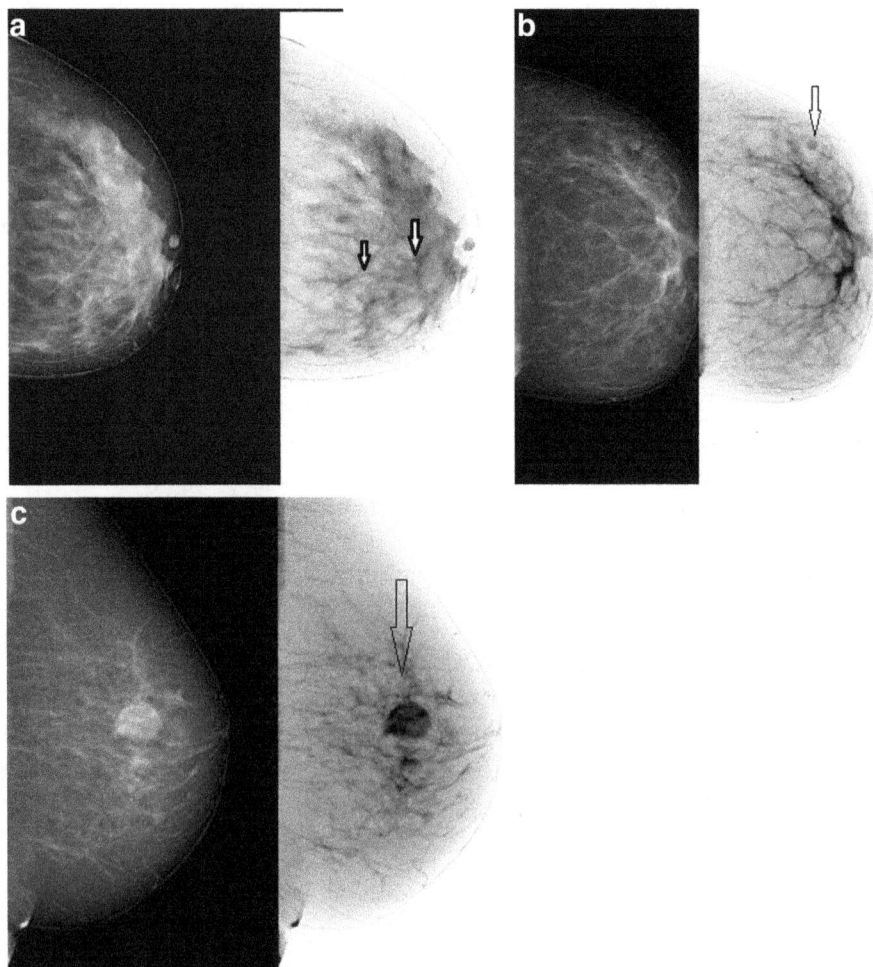

Fig. 1 a-c Standard and grayscale inverted image. *Arrows* indicate the early vascular macrocalcification, intramammary lymph node and nodular density with smooth contour respectively

oval-shaped nodular opacities were classified as intra-mammary (present in the breast parenchyma) or axillary (present in the axillary region).

Initial assessments were performed on standard images (the std method). Results were reported as present or absent or scored by using the BIRADS. In the final BIRADS assessment, BIRADS scores were defined as follows: 0, more examination needed; 1, normal; 2, benign; 3, probably benign; 4, suspicious; 5, highly suspicious; and 6, malignant [7]. At least 15 days after the first assessment, the same mammograms were evaluated as above using only the gray-scale inverted images (the gsi method). At least 15 days later, a third assessment was performed using both standard and grayscale inverted images (the std + gsi method) (Fig. 1a-c). Cochran's Q test was used to compare the results obtained with the three types of image evaluation. The McNemar multiple comparison test was used to compare the different methods ($p < 0.05$ was considered statistically significant). The intraobserver concordance among three assessment methods was measured by using the Fleiss' Kappa test.

Results

The average age of 159 patients in our study was 50.4 years (range, 35–80 years; standard deviation, 7.81 years). The parenchymal patterns on standard images were as follows: type A, 6 (3.8%) women; type B, 68 (42.8%) women; type C, 54 (34%) women; and type D, 31 (19.5%) women. According to the BIRADS, 45 (28.3%) mammograms were categorized as 0, 39 (24.5%) as 1, 74 (46.5%) as 2, and 1 (0.6%) as 3 (Table 1). There were no cases with BIRADS 4,5 and 6 score.

The intraobserver concordance for the results of the three assessment methods (standard, grayscale inverted, and std + gsi) is shown in Table 2. There were statistically significant differences in presence/absence of macrocalcifi-cation, microcalcification, and intramammary lymph nodes among the methods ($p < 0.05$) (Table 3), but not in the other parameters (Table 4).

Among the three assessment methods, a significant difference was observed in the detection of macrocalcifica-tion. In std + gsi images more macrocalcification (93 im-ages) were detected than in standard images (84 images) (Cochran's Q = 8.375, $p = 0.015$). There was also a signifi-cant difference in microcalcification detection among the methods. Multiple comparisons between the methods

Table 2 Intraobserver concordance assessment

Parameter	Fleiss Kappa	Concordance
Skin Pathology	0.908	Perfect Concordance
Macrocalcification	0.916	Perfect Concordance
Microcalcification	0.597	Moderate Concordance
Asymmetric Density	0.646	High Concordance
Structural Distortion	0.662	High Concordance
Mass	0.703	High Concordance
Intramammary Lymph Nodes	0.809	High Concordance
Axillary Lymph Nodes	0.905	Perfect Concordance

showed that microcalcification was more often observed in grayscale inverted (53 images) and std + gsi images (81 images) than in standard images (31 images). Moreover, microcalcification was the most often observed in std + gsi images (81 images) (Cochran's Q = 68.509, $p < 0.001$). Lastly, there was a significant difference in the detection of intramammary lymph nodes among the 3 assessment methods. In std + gsi images more intramammary lymph nodes (59 images) were detected than in standard images (49 images) (Cochran's Q =6.461, $p = 0.039$).

Discussion

In Turkey, yearly mammographic scanning beginning at 40 years of age is recommended [8]. The double-reading system is preferred as it decreases the false-negative rate in scanning mammograms. In previous studies, this system in-creased breast cancer detection rates by 4–15% [5, 9] and better detected small breast cancers owing to its relatively high sensitivity [10]. However, the double-reading system is impractical because it increases the cost of the mammo-gram and requires two readers. Moreover, it has been shown to decrease the positive estimation value and increase the recall rate and the patient's anxiety level [11].

The CAD system is an alternative to the double-reading system, especially in busy centers [6]. The CAD system directs the radiologist's attention to suspicious regions, thereby aiding detection of the lesion [12] Although the CAD system has existed for 10 years, its additive contribu-tion to routine scanning is controversial [13]. In the study by Fiona et al., the double-reading system and CAD system had similar detection rates [6]. However, another study suggested that the CAD system improved diagnostic performance and reduced assessment time [14]. An

Table 1 Parenchyma pattern of mammograms and BIRADS classification

Pattern	A	B	C	D				Total
Standard İmage	6 (3.8%)	68 (42.8%)	54 (34%)	31 (19.5%)				159 (100%)
BIRADS	0	1	2	3	4	5	6	Total
Standard İmage	45 (28.3%)	39 (24.5%)	74 (46.5%)	1 (0.6%)	0	0	0	159 (100%)

BIRADS Breast Imaging Reporting and Data System

Table 3 Significant differences between the image types

Parameter	Image type	No (%)	Yes (%)	Cochran's Q	p	Multiple comparison
Macro-calcification	(a) Standard	234 (73.58)	84 (26.42)	8.375	0.015*	(c)
	(b) Grayscale inverted	232 (72.96)	86 (27.04)			
	(c) Std + Gsi	225 (70.75)	93 (29.25)			(a)
Micro-calcification	(a) Standard	287 (90.25)	31 (9.75)	68.509	<0.001¶	(b) (c)
	(b) Grayscale inverted	265 (83.33)	53 (16.67)			(a) (c)
	(c) Std + Gsi	237 (74.53)	81 (25.47)			(a) (b)
Intramammary Lymph Nodes	(a) Standard	269 (84.59)	49 (15.41)	6.461	0.039†	(c)
	(b) Grayscale inverted	261 (82.08)	57 (17.92)			
	(c) Std + Gsi	259 (81.45)	59 (18.55)			(a)

Std + Gsi standard plus grayscale inverted image. *: a versus c. ¶: a versus b, a versus c, and b versus c. †: a versus c

additional benefit of the CAD system is its capacity to detect microcalcification even when used by radiologists with little experience [15, 16].

Mammographic sensitivity is lowest during the premenopausal period, at which time the fibroglandular tissue is especially dense. In this situation, digital mammography more efficiently detects lesions than does conventional mammography [17]. Digital mammography can also process the data in various formats because its image forming and display phases are different.

We assessed the usefulness of grayscale inverted images for detecting mammary abnormalities using digital mammography facilities when double reading or CAD system is not feasible. To our knowledge, there are previous studies in the medical literature that has performed such an assessment [18–20]. But we have not found a study on mammograms.

Including grayscale inverted images in mammogram assessments is not routine; however, it is not a difficult application (standard images can be converted to grayscale inverted images by the touch of a button in digital systems). However, evaluation of the negative image, as well as the standard image, somewhat prolongs the assessment time.

Our study did not examine the distribution pattern, number, or morphological properties of microcalcifications except for their size. Therefore, were unable to categorize them as benign, suspicious, or malignant. An advantage of grayscale inverted images for detection of microcalcification is that black spots indicative of microcalcification are easily seen and taken attention on white backgrounds and graphs. By altering the perception of the reader, even a single white spot not apparent on a standard image becomes

Table 4 Insignificant differences between the image types

Parameter	Image	No (%)	Yes (%)	Cochran's Q	p
Skin Pathology	Standard	314 (98.75)	4 (1.25)	2.000	0.367
	Grayscale inverted	315 (99.05)	3 (0.95)		
	Std + Gsi	314 (98.75)	4 (1.25)		
Asymmetric Density	Standard	288 (90.57)	30 (9.43)	0.266	0.875
	Grayscale inverted	286 (89.94)	32 (10.06)		
	Std + Gsi	286 (89.94)	32 (10.06)		
Structural Distortion	Standard	315 (99.06)	3 (0.94)	1.500	0.472
	Grayscale inverted	313 (98.43)	5 (1.57)		
	Std + Gsi	314 (98.74)	4 (1.26)		
Mass	Standard	293 (92.14)	25 (7.86)	3.111	0.211
	Grayscale inverted	299 (94.03)	19 (5.97)		
	Std + Gsi	297 (93.40)	21 (6.60)		
Axillary Lymph Node	Standard	248 (77.99)	70 (22.01)	2.375	0.305
	Grayscale inverted	246 (77.36)	72 (22.64)		
	Std + Gsi	243 (76.42)	75 (23.58)		

Std + Gsi standard plus grayscale inverted image

readily recognizable as a black spot on a negative image.

Additionally, intramammary lymph nodes were also easier to identify on grayscale inverted images than on standard images, which increases diagnostic and detection rates. We could readily detect the characteristic small fatty hilum of intramammary lymph nodes on negative images. However, grayscale inverted images provided no advantage in terms of detecting axillary lymph nodes, even though they also have a fatty hilum. In our opinion, this may be explained by the fact that the axillary lymph node hilum is large and therefore apparent on both negative and standard images. Evaluation of grayscale inverted images in addition to standard images aids diagnosis owing to the ease of detecting the small white fatty hila of intramammary lymph nodes, which appear as bean-shaped, darkly colored masses.

The limitations of our study are the small number of cases and the performance of the assessments by a single radiologist.

In our study, assessment of grayscale inverted images, compared with standard images, improved detection of microcalcifications and intramammary lymph nodes. We believe that this finding is important because microcalcification is a strong indicator of benign or malignant lesions. Hence, we recommend the use of grayscale inverted images for evaluating microcalcification.

Conclusions

Assessment of grayscale inverted images in addition to standard images improves mammographic evaluation and facilitates the detection of small but crucial signs of breast cancer such as microcalcification. Therefore, assessment of grayscale inverted images can be practicable especially in busy centers.

Abbreviations
ACR: American College of Radiology; BIRADS: Breast Imaging Reporting and Data System; CAD: Computer-aided detection; Gis: Grayscale inverted; Std + Gsi: Standard plus grayscale inverted image; Std: Standard

Acknowledgements
None

Funding
This study was not funded by any organization.

Authors' contributions
AA planned the study, and participated in its design and coordination and collected of data and drafted the manuscript. KK performed the statistical analysis and tables and interpreted the data. All the authors read and approved the final version of the manuscript.

Competing interests
The authors declare that they have no competing interests.

Author details
[1]Department of Radiology, Konya Education and Research Hospital, Konya, Turkey. [2]Department of Statistics, Faculty of Science, Selcuk University, Konya, Turkey. [3]Konya Eğitim ve Araştırma Hastanesi, Radyoloji Bölümü, Hacı Şaban Mah, Meram Yeni Yol Caddesi, No: 97, PK: 42090 Meram, Konya, Turkey.

References
1. Miller AB, et al. Canadian National Breast Screening Study: I and II. Can Med Assoc J. 1992;147:1459–88.
2. Frisell J, et al. Randomized study of mammography screening-preliminary report on mortality in the Stockholm trial. Breast Cancer Res Treat. 1991;18:49–56.
3. Fletcher SW, et al. Mammographic screening for breast cancer. N Engl J Med. 2003;348:1672–80.
4. Birdwell RL, et al. Computer-aided detection with screening mammography in a university hospital setting. Radiology. 2005;236:451–7.
5. Thurfjell EL, et al. Benefit of independent double reading in a population-based mammography screening program. Radiology. 1994;191:241–4.
6. Gilbert FJ, et al. Single reading with computer-aided detection for screening mammography. N Engl J Med. 2008;359(16):1675–84.
7. D'Orsi CJ, et al. ACR BI-RADS® Atlas, Breast Imaging Reporting and Data System. 5th ed. Reston: American College of Radiology; 2013.
8. Turkish Radiology Asssociation. Guide for Breast Cancer Scanning in Turkey. TRD Sufficiency Board; 2011.
9. Hofvind S, et al. Screening-detected breast cancers: discordant independent double reading in a population-based screening program. Radiology. 2009; 253:652–60.
10. Blanks RG, et al. Observer variability in cancer detection during routine repeat (incident) mammographic screening in a study of two versus one view mammography. J Med Screen. 1999;6:152–8.
11. Anderson ED, et al. The efficacy of double reading mammograms in breast screening. Clin Radiol. 1994;49(4):248–51.
12. Azavedo E, et al. Is single reading with computer-aided detection (CAD) as good as double reading in mammography screening? A systematic review. BMC Med Imaging. 2012;12:22. doi:10.1186/1471-2342-12-22.
13. Guerriero C, et al. Is computer aided detection (CAD) cost effective in screening mammography? A model based on the CADET II study. BMC Health Serv Res. 2011;11(1):11.
14. Jung NY, et al. Who could benefit the most from using a computer-aided detection system in full-field digital mammography? World J Surg Oncol. 2014;12:168. doi:10.1186/1477-7819-12-168.
15. Bolivar AV, et al. Computer-aided detection system applied to full-field digital mammograms. Acta Radiol. 2010;51:1086–92.
16. Dromain C, et al. Computed-aided diagnosis (CAD) in the detection of breast cancer. Eur J Radiol. 2013;82(3):417–23. doi:10.1016/j.ejrad.2012.03.005.
17. Pisano ED, et al. American College of Radiology Imaging Network digital mammographic imaging screening trial: objectives and methodology. Radiology. 2005;236:404–12.
18. Park JB, et al. Diagnostic accuracy of the inverted grayscale rib series for detection of rib fracture in minor chest trauma. Am J Emerg Med. 2015;33(4):548–52.
19. Thompson JD, et al. The impact of greyscale inversion for nodule detection in an anthropomorphic chest phantom: a free-response observer study. Br J Radiol. 2016;89:(1064):20160249.
20. Reese DJ, et al. Intra- and interobserver variability of board-certified veterinary radiologists and veterinary general practitioners for pulmonary nodule detection in standard and inverted display mode images of digital thoracic radiographs of dogs. J Am Vet Med Assoc. 2016;238(8):998–1003.

13

How to assess intra- and inter-observer agreement with quantitative PET using variance component analysis: a proposal for standardisation

Oke Gerke[1,2]*[iD], Mie Holm Vilstrup[1], Eivind Antonsen Segtnan[1], Ulrich Halekoh[3] and Poul Flemming Høilund-Carlsen[1,4]

Abstract

Background: Quantitative measurement procedures need to be accurate and precise to justify their clinical use. Precision reflects deviation of groups of measurement from another, often expressed as proportions of agreement, standard errors of measurement, coefficients of variation, or the Bland-Altman plot. We suggest variance component analysis (VCA) to estimate the influence of errors due to single elements of a PET scan (scanner, time point, observer, etc.) to express the composite uncertainty of repeated measurements and obtain relevant repeatability coefficients (RCs) which have a unique relation to Bland-Altman plots. Here, we present this approach for assessment of intra- and inter-observer variation with PET/CT exemplified with data from two clinical studies.

Methods: In study 1, 30 patients were scanned pre-operatively for the assessment of ovarian cancer, and their scans were assessed twice by the same observer to study intra-observer agreement. In study 2, 14 patients with glioma were scanned up to five times. Resulting 49 scans were assessed by three observers to examine inter-observer agreement. Outcome variables were SUVmax in study 1 and cerebral total hemispheric glycolysis (THG) in study 2.

Results: In study 1, we found a RC of 2.46 equalling half the width of the Bland-Altman limits of agreement. In study 2, the RC for identical conditions (same scanner, patient, time point, and observer) was 2392; allowing for different scanners increased the RC to 2543. Inter-observer differences were negligible compared to differences owing to other factors; between observer 1 and 2: −10 (95 % CI: −352 to 332) and between observer 1 vs 3: 28 (95 % CI: −313 to 370).

Conclusions: VCA is an appealing approach for weighing different sources of variation against each other, summarised as RCs. The involved linear mixed effects models require carefully considered sample sizes to account for the challenge of sufficiently accurately estimating variance components.

Keywords: Bland-Altman limits of agreement, Intra-observer, Inter-observer, Intraobserver, Interobserver, Intra-rater, Inter-rater, Repeatability coefficient, Sample size, Standardised uptake value

* Correspondence: oke.gerke@rsyd.dk
[1]Department of Nuclear Medicine, Odense University Hospital, Sdr. Boulevard 29, 5000 Odense C, Denmark
[2]Centre of Health Economics Research, University of Southern Denmark, Campusvej 55, 5230 Odense M, Denmark
Full list of author information is available at the end of the article

Background

Quantitative PET measurements

Molecular imaging is done by hybrid positron emission tomography/computed tomography (PET/CT) and PET/magnetic resonance imaging (MRI). The vast majority of PET scans worldwide is made with the glucose analogue ^{18}F-fluorodeoxyglucose (FDG) meaning that recorded tracer uptake corresponds to regional glucose metabolism. This makes FDG-PET imaging an extremely useful tool in cancer since (a) malignant cells have a higher energy turnover than non-malignant cells [1, 2] and (b) cancers vary geno- and phenotypically from primary tumour to regional and distant metastases which calls for generic rather than very specific tracers [3]. A popular measure of tumour uptake is the standardised uptake value (SUV) which is the ratio of recorded radioactivity in voxels of interest (numerator) and an assumed evenly distributed whole-body concentration of tracer (denominator). Several variants of SUV are in play, comprising SUVmax, i.e., the maximal uptake in a single voxel within a given region of interest (ROI), and SUVmean, i.e., the average tracer uptake across all pixels within a given 3-dimensional ROI [4, 5].

Nomenclature and concept

Terms used in agreement and reliability studies are applied ambiguously in practice (see Appendix for a glossary). Agreement measures the (absolute) closeness between readings and can be used to express accuracy and precision. Accuracy refers to deviation of a measurement from the true value of the quantity being measured (if available), while precision reflects deviation of groups of measurement from another. Since precision is a matter of closeness of two or more measurements to each other rather than to a standard value, it is possible for a group of values to be precise without being accurate, or to be accurate without being precise (see Fig. 1).

In biological research where nothing can be considered absolutely and exactly correct as in physical science, accuracy of a new measurement procedure is deemed present if the principle of measurement is sound and series of measurements do not deviate inappropriately much from a predefined standard or series of measurements made by an accepted reference method. What limit of deviation is acceptable must be arbitrarily defined *a priori*. Precision is usually calculated and discussed in terms of standard deviations and coefficients of variation (CV), proportions of agreement, standard errors of measurement, and Bland-Altman plots with respective limits of agreement [6]. Zaki and colleagues concluded in their systematic review on agreement studies published between 2007 and 2009 that the Bland-Altman approach was by far the most frequently used (178 studies (85 %)), followed by the Pearson correlation coefficient (27 %) and

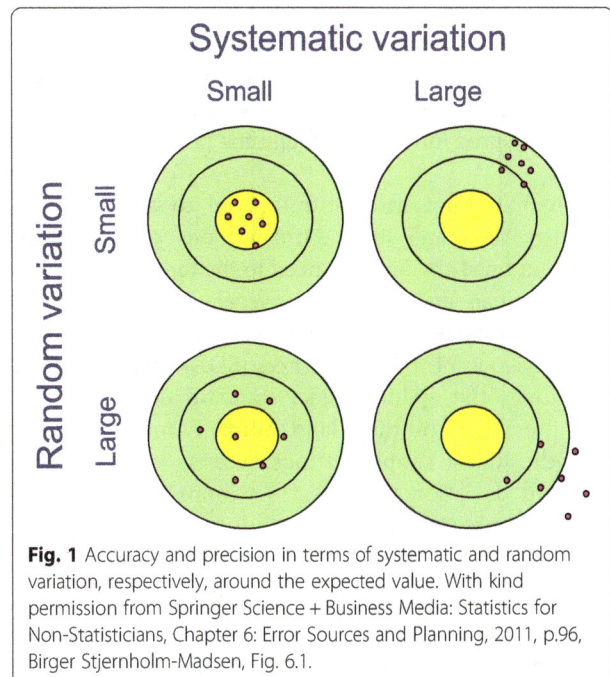

Fig. 1 Accuracy and precision in terms of systematic and random variation, respectively, around the expected value. With kind permission from Springer Science + Business Media: Statistics for Non-Statisticians, Chapter 6: Error Sources and Planning, 2011, p.96, Birger Stjernholm-Madsen, Fig. 6.1.

the comparison of means (18 %) [7]. Though Bland-Altman plots were proposed for the comparison of two methods of measurement [8–10], they were also valuable when comparing two observers (assessing inter-observer variability) or repeated measurements made by the same observer (assessing intra-observer variability). However, the Bland-Altman approach was not intended for assessment of inter-observer variability with more than two observers, nor was it designed to study single sources of variation in the data. Applying instead the concept of variance component analysis (VCA), we estimated the variances due to errors caused by separate elements of a PET scan (tracer, scanner, time point, patient, observer, etc.) to express the composite uncertainty of repeated measurements and obtain relevant repeatability coefficients (RCs), which have a unique relation to Bland-Altman plots in simple test-retest settings: the RC is the limit below which 95 % of differences will lie, holding different sources of variation fixed.

Reliability concerns the ability of a test to distinguish patients from each other, despite measurement error, while agreement focuses on the measurement error itself [11]. Reliability assessment is well established and usually done by means of intraclass correlation coefficients (ICC) [12, 13].

Purpose of this study

The aims of this paper are as follows:

- to apply VCA to the most simple setting of agreement assessment in PET studies – the study of intra-observer variability when differences between paired measurements are investigated;

- to apply VCA in settings, in which different sources of the observed variation in the data shall be accounted for, like observer, time point, or scanner.

The first point will naturally lead to a connection between VCA and Bland-Altman limits of agreement, which, in turn, are directly linked to the term RC: whereas Bland-Altman limits span the average of all differences between pairwise measurements +/− 1.96 times the standard deviation of these differences (SD_{diff}), the RC equals 2.77 times the within-subject standard deviation (S_w); half the width of the Bland-Altman limits coincides with the RC in simple settings because within-subject standard deviation is then synonymous with standard error of measurement (SEM):

$$2.77 \times S_w = 2.77 \times SEM = 1.96\sqrt{2} \times \frac{SD_{diff}}{\sqrt{2}} = 1.96 \times SD_{diff}.$$

The second point will demonstrate that the RC can be used more widely, as it is still estimable in more challenging settings and can serve as an evaluation tool when assessing the magnitude of various possible sources of variation observed in the data. In the following, we exemplify VCA by means of two studies conducted at our institution and discuss sample size considerations from a general point of view.

Methods

Study 1

At our institution, we are conducting a clinical study called *Dual Time PET/CT in the Preoperative Assessment of Ovarian Cancer* since summer 2013. Its primary hypothesis is that dual time FDG-PET/CT performed at 60 and 180 min. after injection of tracer will increase the diagnostic accuracy of FDG-PET/CT (routinely performed at 60 min.) in the preoperative assessment of resectability (provided optimal debulking is achievable). The target population consists of patients with suspicion of ovarian cancer in whom the clinical suspicion of malignancy is based on initial physical (including pelvic) examination, blood tests including CA-125, and transvaginal ultrasound. Patients are referred to the Department of Gynaecology and Obstetrics at our institution from other hospitals in the region of Southern Denmark or the region of Zealand and from private specialists and general practitioners. Inclusion is expected to go on until summer 2018 with a frequency of 1–2 patients per week. A total number of 180 patients in the study is aimed for, from which around 50 have been included by 1st September 2015. The assessment of the PET/CT scans performed at 60 min. in the first 30 patients was done twice and the second time in random sequence by author MHV in May and September 2015 in order to address the

intra-observer repeatability of the post imaging process. SUVmax (g/ml) was measured in the primary ovarian lesion when possible to identify; otherwise, the SUVmax in peritoneal carcinosis was used.

PET/CT scans were acquired on one of four available scanners: GE Discovery VCT, RX, 690, or 710 (GE Healthcare, Milwaukee, WI, USA). Patients were scanned according to guidelines [14], and the analysis of PET/CT including SUV measurements was done on a GE Advantage Workstation v. 4.4 by an experienced nuclear medicine physician with 10 years of experience with PET/CT. The scans were assessed in fused axial, coronal, and sagittal planes using the default color scale "hot iron". Due to often large, heterogeneous ovarian tumours, SUVmax was assessed to be more representative of malignant metabolism than SUVmean. When possible, the ovarian tumour was identified on the fused PET/CT images. A circular ROI was placed on the axial slices in the area with visually highest uptake making sure to exclude physiological uptake, for instance, nearby the bladder. If the highest uptake area was not clearly identified visually, multiple ROIs were drawn covering all areas with high uptake, and the maximum SUV lesion was used. When a primary ovarian lesion was not identified on PET/CT, a peritoneal lesion with high uptake was identified in a similar manner. The assessment and placement of ROIs are challenging because of the heterogeneity of primary tumour and multifocal peritoneal carcinosis, often accompanied by physiological uptake in adjacent organs such as colon and urine bladder/ureters and associated ascites.

Study 2

The second study focuses on diaschisis in gliomas, where diaschisis means a brain dysfunction remote from a focal brain lesion. A consecutive series of 14 glioma patients, referred from our Department of Neurosurgery with suspicion of cerebral malignancy (as assessed by histopathological findings of biopsy samples and MRI results from the clinical routine), underwent FDG-PET/CT examinations from 2012 to 2015. The patients were followed throughout the entire treatment course for 1 year or until death occurred, and FDG-PET/CT scans were done at up to five times: 1) at baseline (before treatment); 2) post operation; 3), 4) and 5) follow-up during chemotherapy or no treatment. Each patient was assigned to one of two scanners (GE Discovery 690 or 710, GE Healthcare, Milwaukee, WI, USA) at each time point, and a total of 49 FDG-PET/CT scans were collected. Using dedicated 3D-segmenatation software (ROVER version 2.1.26, ABX GmbH, Radeberg, Germany), total hemispheric glycolysis (THG) was assessed in the ipsilateral and contralateral hemisphere relative to the primary tumour. Two inexperienced medical students (observers 1 and 2) and one experienced neuro PET clinician (observer 3) drew

ROIs. THG is defined as the product of the segmented metabolic volume and the mean SUV in this volume ($cm^3 \times g/ml$), encompassing all voxels in one cerebral hemisphere; iterative thresholding with 40 % cutoff from SUVmax was applied. In the following, only THG measurements in the ipsilateral hemisphere are used.

Statistical analysis

The aim of VCA, which builds upon a linear mixed effects model, is to split the observed variance in the data and distribute its parts to factors of the statistical model [15]. The dependent variable was SUVmax in study 1 and THG in study 2. In study 1, we treated 'reading' (1st vs. 2nd) as fixed factor and 'patient' as random factor, i.e., we considered patients to be merely representatives of the target population, whereas the factor 'reading' referred to two concrete readings which we would like to make inferences about. In study 2, both 'observer' and 'time point' were considered fixed effects, whereas 'patient' and 'scanner' were treated as crossed random effects since the same images were evaluated by different observers. Using the estimated within-subject variance from these models, RCs were derived. The RC is the limit within which 95 % of differences between two measurements made at random on the same patient will lie in absolute terms, assuming differences to have an approximately normal distribution; the RC equals 2.77 times the estimated within-subject standard deviation [10, 16, 17]. In simple settings, such as our study 1, half the width of the Bland-Altman limits coincides with the RC. In study 2, we derived the RCs for repeated measurements for (a) the same patient at the same time point on the same scanner by the same observer and (b) the same patient at the same time point by the same observer, but studied by different scanners.

Data from study 1 were displayed graphically by Bland-Altman plots with respective limits of agreement which are defined by the mean estimated difference between readings +/− 1.96 times the standard deviation of the differences between readings. These plots were supplemented by lines stemming from linear regressions of the differences on the averages, also called the Bradley-Blackwood procedure [18], in order to support visual assessment of trends over the measurement scale. Data from study 2 were displayed by line plots over time by observer.

The level of significance was set to 5 %. Ninety-five percent confidence intervals (95 % CI) were supplemented where appropriate. All analyses were performed by using STATA/MP 14.1 (StataCorp LP, College Station, Texas 77845 USA). The package *concord* [19] was used for the generation of Bland-Altman plots. The STATA source code of VCA is accessible as Additional file 1.

Results
Study 1

The differences between the two readings of SUVmax in study 1 were all less than one in absolute terms, apart from those for patient no. 3, 5, 10, 23, and 26 (Additional file 2). The estimated mean difference between reading 1 and reading 2 was 0.43 (95 % CI: −0.02 to 0.88; Table 1), and Bland-Altman limits of agreement were −2.03 and 2.89. According to the respective Bland-Altman plot (Fig. 2, upper panel), the variance of the differences seemed to be quite homogenous across the whole range of measured values, but an increasing trend with increasing average of measurements was visible. However, this trend appeared to be triggered by one outlier, the removal of which would mean that the trend according to the Bradley-Blackwood regression line would disappear (Fig. 2, lower panel). Removal of this outlier would further nearly halve the estimated mean difference between readings (0.24) and lead to a smaller Bland-Altman band (−1.13 to 1.60).

According to VCA, patient and residual variance were estimated to 47.53 and 0.787, respectively, mirroring the between-patient variance to be the dominating source of variation in the data. The RC for a new reading of the same image by the same observer equalled 2.77 times $\sqrt{0.787} = 2.46$, which coincided with one half of the Bland-Altman band (here: 1.96 times 1.255 [not shown elsewhere]).

Study 2

THG measurements by all three observers had a median value of 2468.8 and ranged from 124.3 to 7509.4. The visual display of the data by patient and observer indicated good agreement between the three observers, except for patient no. 10 in whom one observer measured way below the other two observers at the second time point (Fig. 3). Note that only patients 1, 2, 4, and 5 had observations on all five time points, whereas no scan was available for patient 3 at time point 4 due to technical issues, and patients 6–14 were only scanned up to three times as they died during the study. The VCA revealed negligible mean differences in THG recorded by the three observers, but huge imprecision of estimates: observer 1 vs. 2: −10.03, 95 % CI: −351.91 to 331.85; observer 1 vs. 3: 28.39, 95 % CI: −313.49 to 370.27 (Table 2). Regarding

Table 1 Results from the linear mixed effects model (study 1)

Component	Factor level	Estimate	95 % CI	P-value
Reading	1st (reference)			
	2nd	0.43	−0.02 to 0.88	0.06
Constant		8.60	6.03 to 11.16	<0.0001
Patient variance		47.53	28.28 to 79.86	
Residual variance		0.787	0.470 to 1.317	

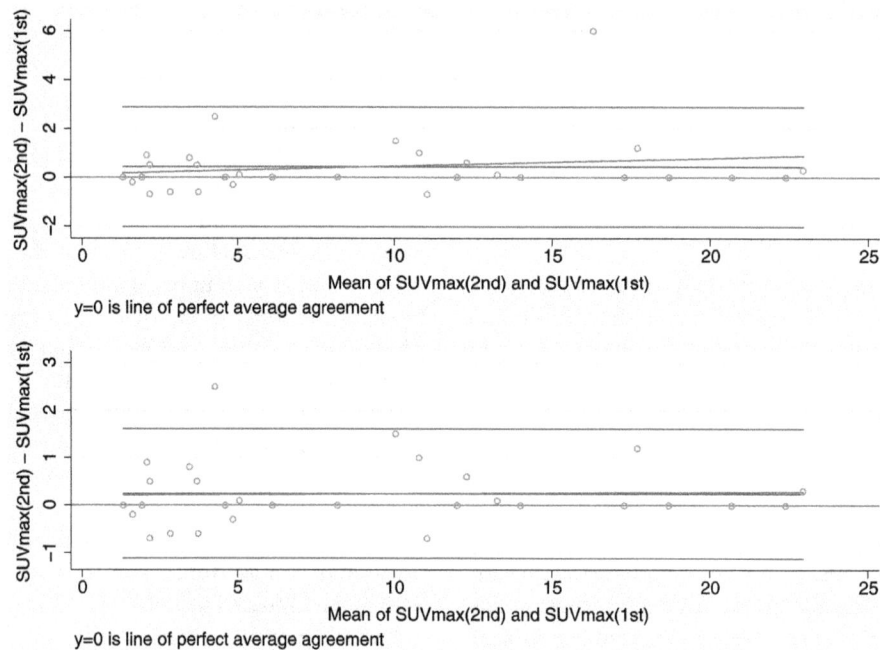

Fig. 2 Bland-Altman plots for study 1 (upper panel: N = 30; lower panel: N = 29). Graphical display of the means against their respective paired differences, the Bland-Altman limits of agreement (*red lines*), the estimated mean difference (*purple line*), the reference line of perfect average agreement (line at y = 0), and the regression line according to the Bradley-Blackwood procedure (*green line*). In the lower panel, one outlier was excluded.

changes from baseline, only measurements at the first time point after baseline (post operation) were statistically significantly decreased by −490.51 (95 % CI: −859.78 to −121.24; p = 0.009). Patient, scanner, and residual variance were estimated as 345668.5, 97156.9, and 745438.9, respectively. The RC for a new assessment of the same patient made at the same time point on the same scanner by the same observer equalled 2.77 times $\sqrt{745438.9} = 2391.6$; the RC for a new assessment of the same patient made at the same time point by the same observer, but using a different scanner increased to 2.77 times $\sqrt{(745438.9 + 97156.9)} = 2542.7$.

Discussion

In agreement studies with sole focus on the difference between paired measurements, as in our study 1, the data are ideally displayed by means of Bland-Altman plots, possibly optimised by using log transformation of the original data and accounting for heterogeneity and/or trends over the measurement scale [10, 20]. In study 1, we observed the duality between Bland-Altman limits of agreement on the one hand and the corresponding RC on the other hand. Actually, various authors of recently published agreement studies defined the repeatability coefficient (or coefficient of repeatability) as 1.96 times the standard deviation of the paired differences [21–25] which is algebraically the same as 2.77 times the within-subject standard deviation in simple settings as

our study 1. Lodge et al. referred to the RC as 2.77 times the within-subject standard deviation [26].

Modelling a more complex situation, in which both fixed and random effects shall be accounted for, leads naturally to a mixed effects model as in our study 2. Here, we applied VCA in order to provide relevant RCs. However, the estimation of both fixed effects and random components was prone to large uncertainty which was reflected by the widths of respective 95 % CIs. In general, the estimation of variance components requires larger sample sizes as the estimation of fixed effects, since the former relates to second moments and the latter to first moments of random variables [27]. How many observations suffice to demonstrate agreement?.

An ad hoc literature search in PubMed (using the search term *((reproducibility OR repeatability OR agreement)) AND SUV*) for the period 1st January 2013 to 30th June 2015 revealed 153 studies with sample sizes between eight [28] and 252 [29], where most studies included up to 40 patients. Despite the increased interest in the conduct of agreement and reliability studies over recent decades, investigations into sample size requirements remain scarce [30, 31]. Carstensen reckoned that little information is gained in a method comparison study beyond the inclusion of 50 study subjects, using three repetitions [20]. In the context of multivariable regression modelling, 10 to 20 observations should be available per continuous variable and level per categorical variable in order

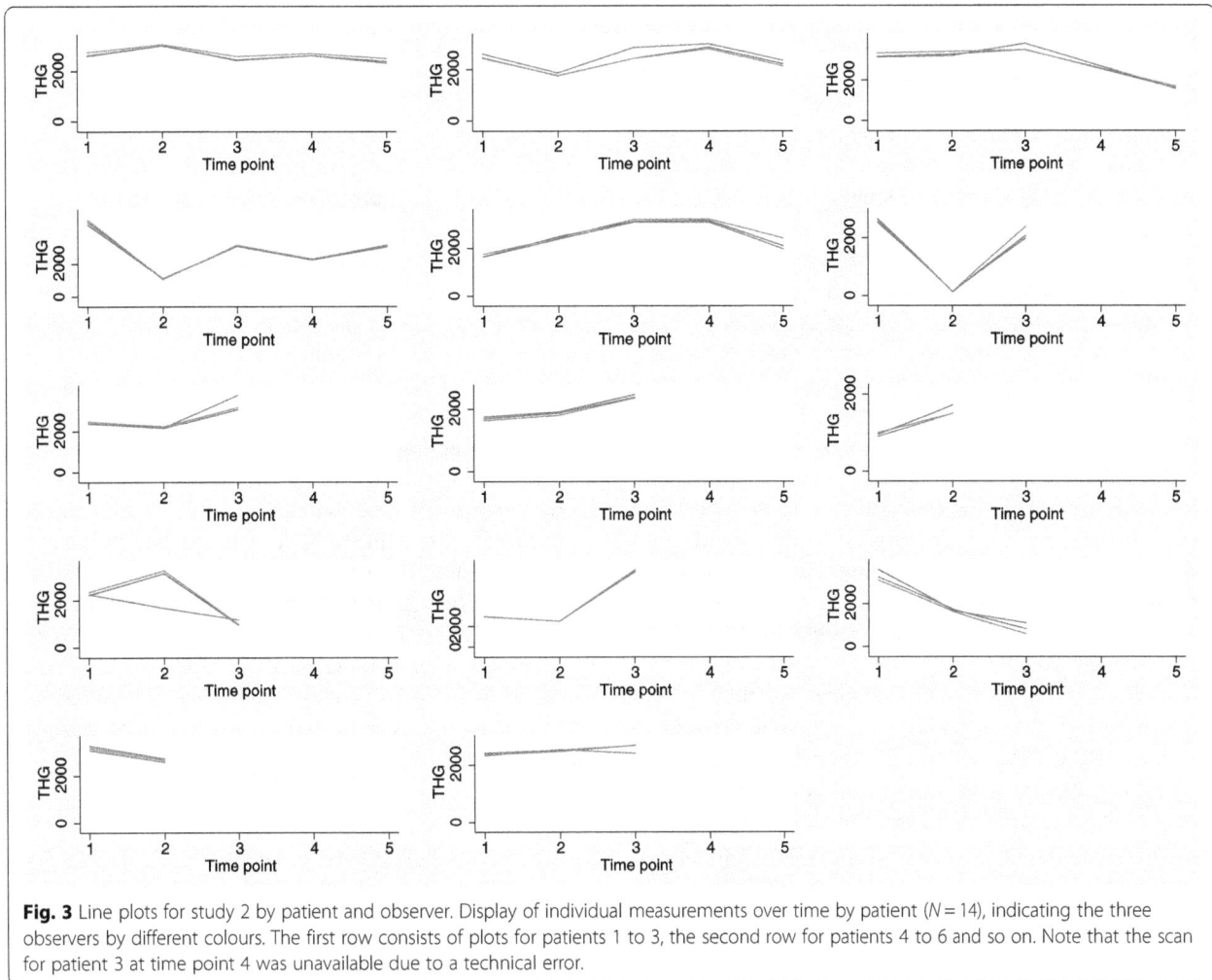

Fig. 3 Line plots for study 2 by patient and observer. Display of individual measurements over time by patient ($N = 14$), indicating the three observers by different colours. The first row consists of plots for patients 1 to 3, the second row for patients 4 to 6 and so on. Note that the scan for patient 3 at time point 4 was unavailable due to a technical error.

Table 2 Results from the linear mixed effects model (study 2)

Component	Factor level	Estimate	95 % CI	P-value
Observer	1st (reference)			
	2nd	−10.03	−351.91 to 331.85	0.95
	3rd	28.39	−313.49 to 370.27	0.87
Time point	Baseline (reference)			
	Post operation	−490.51	−859.78 to −121.24	0.009
	1. follow-up	185.90	−210.54 to 582.33	0.36
	2. follow-up	−89.89	−692.92 to 513.13	0.77
	3. follow-up	−389.29	−937.38 to 158.80	0.16
Constant		2675.03	2046.19 to 3303.86	<0.0001
Patient variance		345668.5	127739.2 to 935395.8	
Scanner variance		97156.9	2976.2 to 3171673	
Residual variance		745438.9	582229.8 to 954398.3	

to fit a statistical model, which results in sufficiently accurately estimated regression coefficients [32–37]. Level refers here to a category of a categorical variable; for instance the variable 'time point' in our study 2 had 5 levels, meaning five realised time points. The abovementioned rule-of-thumb can lead to large sample sizes in an agreement study, even though only few explanatory fixed and random variables are involved. In our study 2, we employed 10 levels all in all (five time points, three observers, and two scanners), leading to 10 times 20 = 200 observations. Unfortunately, we could only gather around 150 observations due to slow patient accrual, but we learned that at least 20 observations should be employed per continuous variable and level of a categorical variable in an agreement study in order to account for the challenge of sufficiently accurately estimating variance components. Note that subject-observer interaction, i.e., the extra variation in a subject due to a specific observer, can only be isolated when having repeated measurements per observer [16].

We understand repeatability as an agreement and not a reliability assessment (see Appendix), whereas the ICC happens to be used as repeatability assessment on occasions [38, 39]. Since the ICC is heavily dependent on between-subject variation and may produce high values for heterogeneous patient groups [30, 31], it should be used exclusively for the assessment of reliability. We hope to contribute to a more jointly agreed usage of terms in the future, being in line with the published guidelines for reporting reliability and agreement studies [6]. Further, we reckon that the biggest challenge most likely is a clear understanding of which exact question a researcher seeks answered, before undertaking an agreement or a reliability study. Guyatt, Walter, and Norman pointed out that reliability indices (like ICC) are used for discriminative purposes, whereas agreement parameters (like RC) are used for evaluative purposes [40].The former focuses on a test's ability to divide patients into groups of interest, despite measurement error, whereas the latter relies on the measurement error itself; with small measurement errors, it is possible to detect even small changes over time [11].

Moreover, the choice of independent variables of the linear mixed effects model (i.e., the potential sources of variation in the data) and the decision to treat a factor as fixed or random is far from trivial and requires thorough planning in order to reflect the clinical situation in the best possible, meaning most appropriate, way. Is the assessment of inter-observer variability limited to only few observers, as these are the only ones handling cases in daily routine (treating 'observer' as fixed effect), or is an observer merely a representative of the pool of several potential observers (treating 'observer' as random effect)? In the former case, every observer reads all scans; in the latter case, every observer assesses only a portion of all scans, to which he/she gets randomly assigned, which in turn distributes the assessment work on several observers (thereby easing data collection) and increases generalisability.

Apart from factors like observer, time point, and scanner, FDG PET quantification itself is affected by technical (e.g. relative calibration between PET scanner and dose calibrator, paravenous administration of FDG PET), biological (e.g. blood glucose level; patient motion or breathing), and physical factors (e.g. scan acquisition parameters, ROI, blood glucose level correction) [41]. In our studies, intra- and inter-observer agreement was assessed with respect to the post-imaging process; therefore, technical, biological, and most physical factors came not into play, whereas size and type of ROI used are observer-specific and, thus, cannot be modelled separately from the factor 'observer'. When investigating day-to-day variation of the scans and dealing with multi-centre trials, the PET procedure guideline [5] should be adhered to in order to maintain accuracy and precision of quantitative PET measurements best possible. The technical, biological, and physical factors which were discussed by Boellard [41], can, in principle, partly be included to a statistical model as explanatory variables; however, only those should be considered that justify a respective increase in sample size (see discussion on appropriate sample sizes above).

The guidelines for reporting reliability and agreement studies [6] include 15 issues to be addressed in order to improve the quality of reporting. Doing so can result in separate publications on agreement and/or reliability apart from the main study, as Kottner et al. put it [6]: "Studies may be conducted with the primary focus on reliability and agreement estimation itself or they may be a part of larger diagnostic accuracy studies, clinical trials, or epidemiological surveys. In the latter case, researchers report agreement and reliability as a quality control, either before the main study or by using data of the main study. Typically, results are reported in just a few sentences, and there is usually only limited space for reporting. Nevertheless, it seems desirable to address all issues listed in the following sections to allow data to be as useful as possible. Therefore, reliability and agreement estimates should be reported in another publication or reported as part of the main study."

Conclusions

Intra-observer agreement is excellently visualised with Bland-Altman limits of agreement, which in turn can be directly linked to RCs derived from VCA. Incorporating several sources of potential variation in the data (like using different observers) leads to extended models, from which appropriate RCs can be derived for the assessment of agreement. It is difficult to specify the required sample sizes for such linear mixed effects models, but as rule-of-thumb 20 observations should be included per continuous variable and factor level of categorical variable in the statistical model.

Appendix

The two most prominent authorities on how to define terms like accuracy or precision in biomedical research are the International Organization for Standardization (ISO) and the US Food and Drug Administration (FDA) [42, 43]. Barnhart, Haber, and Lin discussed thoroughly the differences in definitions and proposed a standardisation [12] which we adopted due to its focus on biomedical application and, hence, its appropriateness for molecular imaging studies.

- Accuracy vs. precision: Accuracy and precision have historically been used to measure systematic bias and random errors around the expected (true) value, respectively (see Fig. 1). Using accuracy as term for systematic bias, a 'true sense of accuracy' reflects a systematic shift from the truth if a reference is available, whereas a 'loose sense of accuracy' means a systematic shift between measurements if a reference is unavailable. In contrast, precision describes the closeness of agreement between independent test results under prescribed conditions. The term precision is intertwined with the terms repeatability and reproducibility (see below).

- Agreement: Measuring *closeness* between readings, agreement can be considered to be used in a broader sense which comprises both accuracy and precision.

- Repeatability vs. reproducibility: Repeatability ascertains the closeness of agreement between measures *under the same condition*, i.e., using the same laboratory, employing the same observer and the same equipment (PET scanner, image reconstruction software), within short intervals of time. Reproducibility targets the closeness of agreement between measures *under all possible conditions* on identical subjects, i.e., using different laboratories, observers, or PET scanners, or assessing day-to-day variation.

- Validity vs. reliability: An assessment of validity requires a reference standard and necessitates both accuracy and precision; for details on several types of validity (face, content, criterion, and construct validity), see for instance [44]. With respect to clinical trials, internal and external validity can be distinguished. The former assesses what can be accomplished with, for instance, a diagnostic test in a clinical trial setting under restricted conditions, whereas the latter reflects a diagnostic test's value in daily practice when applied to a broader and less selected patient population [45]. Reliability originated from test theory and was defined as the patient-specific score variance, divided by the observed total score variance [46, 47]. It is, therefore, interpreted as the proportion of the observed variance that is explained by the true score variance. In terms of the commonly used ICC, it represents the fraction of the variability between study subjects (patients) divided by the sum of between-subjects variability and a measurement error. Reliability addresses the question of how well patients can be distinguished from each other, despite measurement error [11].

Abbreviations
CT: Computed tomography; CV: Coefficient of variation; FDA: Food and Drug Administration; FDG: ^{18}F-fluorodeoxyglucose; ICC: Intraclass correlation coefficient; ISO: International Organization for Standardization; MRI: Magnetic resonance imaging; PET: Positron emission tomography; RC: Repeatability coefficient; ROI: Region of interest; SUV: Standardised uptake value; THG: Total hemispheric glycolysis; VCA: Variance component analysis

Acknowledgements
The authors thank their colleagues Sofie Christlieb and Peter Grupe for acting as observer 2 and 3 in study 2 and three reviewers for valuable comments on earlier versions of the manuscript.

Funding
None.

Author's contributions
OG designed the study, conducted the statistical analyses, and drafted the manuscript. MHV and EAS provided data from their respective clinical studies. UH participated in data interpretation and fine-tuning of the statistical analyses. PFHC contributed to the conceptual design and edited the manuscript. All authors revised former versions of the manuscript, and they read and approved the final manuscript.

Competing interests
The authors declare that they have no competing interests.

Author details
Department of Nuclear Medicine, Odense University Hospital, Sdr. Boulevard 29, 5000 Odense C, Denmark. [2]Centre of Health Economics Research, University of Southern Denmark, Campusvej 55, 5230 Odense M, Denmark. [1]Epidemiology, Biostatistics and Biodemography, University of Southern Denmark, J. B. Winsløws Vej 9b, 5000 Odense C, Denmark. [4]Department of Clinical Research, University of Southern Denmark, Winsløwparken 19, 5000 Odense C, Denmark.

References
1. Alavi A, Reivich M. The conception of FDG-PET imaging. Semin Nucl Med. 2002;32(1):2–5.
2. Hess S, Blomberg BA, Zhu HJ, Høilund-Carlsen PF, Alavi A. The pivotal role of FDG-PET/CT in modern medicine. Acad Radiol. 2014;21:232–49.
3. Kwee TC, Gholami S, Werner TJ, Rubello D, Alavi A, Høilund-Carlsen PF. 18 F-FDG, as a single imaging agent in assessing cancer, shows the ongoing biological phenomena in many domains: do we need additional tracers for clinical purposes? Nucl Med Commun. 2016;37(4):333–7.
4. Thie JA. Understanding the standardized uptake value, its methods, and implications for usage. J Nucl Med. 2004;45(9):1431–4.
5. Boellaard R, Delgado-Bolton R, Oyen WJ, Giammarile F, Tatsch K, Eschner W, et al. FDG PET/CT: EANM procedure guidelines for tumour imaging: version 2.0. Eur J Nucl Med Mol Imaging. 2015;42(2):328–54.
6. Kottner J, Audigé L, Brorson S, Donner A, Gajewski BJ, Hróbjartsson A, et al. Guidelines for reporting reliability and agreement studies (GRRAS) were proposed. J Clin Epidemiol. 2011;64(1):96–106.
7. Zaki R, Bulgiba A, Ismail R, Ismail NA. Statistical methods used to test for agreement of medical instruments measuring continuous variables in method comparison studies: a systematic review. PLoS ONE. 2012;7(5): e37908.
8. Bland JM, Altman DG. Statistical methods for assessing agreement between two methods of clinical measurement. Lancet. 1986;1(8476):307–10.
9. Bland JM, Altman DG. Difference versus mean plots. Ann Clin Biochem. 1997;34(5):570–1.

10. Bland JM, Altman DG. Measuring agreement in method comparison studies. Stat Methods Med Res. 1999;8(2):135–60.

11. de Vet HC, Terwee CB, Knol DL, Bouter LM. When to use agreement versus reliability measures. J Clin Epidemiol. 2006;59(10):1033–9.

12. Barnhart HX, Haber MJ, Lin LI. An overview on assessing agreement with continuous measurements. J Biopharm Stat. 2007;17(4):529–69.

13. Shrout PE, Fleiss JL. Intraclass correlations: uses in assessing rater reliability. Psychol Bull. 1979;86(2):420–8.

14. Boellaard R, O'Doherty MJ, Weber WA, Mottaghy FM, Lonsdale MN, Stroobants SG, et al. FDG PET and PET/CT: EANM procedure guidelines for tumour PET imaging: version 1.0. Eur J Nucl Med Mol Imaging. 2010;37(1):181–200.

15. Searle SR, Casella G, McCulloch CE. Variance Components. New York: Wiley; 1992.

16. Bland M. How do I analyse observer variation studies? 2004. https://www-users.york.ac.uk/~mb55/meas/observer.pdf. Accessed 2 Sept 2016.

17. Bland M. What is the origin of the formula for repeatability? 2005. https://www-users.york.ac.uk/~mb55/meas/repeat.htm. Accessed 2 Sept 2016.

18. Bradley EL, Blackwood LG. Comparing paired data: a simultaneous test for means and variances. American Statistician. 1989;43(4):234–5.

19. Steichen TJ, Cox NJ. Concordance correlation coefficient. Stata Technical Bulletin May 2008 (stb-43):35–39. http://www.stata.com/products/stb/journals/stb43.pdf. Accessed 2 Sept 2016.

20. Carstensen B. Comparing Clinical Measurement Methods: A Practical Guide. Chichester: Wiley; 2010.

21. Klaassen R, Bennink RJ, van Tienhoven G, Bijlsma MF, Besselink MG, van Berge Henegouwen MI, et al. Feasibility and repeatability of PET with the hypoxia tracer [(18)F]HX4 in oesophageal and pancreatic cancer. Radiother Oncol. 2015;116(1):94–9.

22. Rockall AG, Avril N, Lam R, Iannone R, Mozley PD, Parkinson C, et al. Repeatability of quantitative FDG-PET/CT and contrast-enhanced CT in recurrent ovarian carcinoma: test-retest measurements for tumor FDG uptake, diameter, and volume. Clin Cancer Res. 2014;20(10):2751–60.

23. Thorn SL, de Kemp RA, Dumouchel T, Klein R, Renaud JM, Wells RG, et al. Repeatable noninvasive measurement of mouse myocardial glucose uptake with 18 F-FDG: evaluation of tracer kinetics in a type 1 diabetes model. J Nucl Med. 2013;54(9):1637–44.

24. Heijmen L, de Geus-Oei LF, de Wilt JH, Visvikis D, Hatt M, Visser EP, et al. Reproducibility of functional volume and activity concentration in 18 F-FDG PET/CT of liver metastases in colorectal cancer. Eur J Nucl Med Mol Imaging. 2012;39(12):1858–67.

25. Lamoureux M, Thorn S, Dumouchel T, Renaud JM, Klein R, Mason S, et al. Uniformity and repeatability of normal resting myocardial blood flow in rats using [13 N]-ammonia and small animal PET. Nucl Med Commun. 2012;33(9):917–25.

26. Lodge MA, Jacene HA, Pili R, Wahl RL. Reproducibility of tumor blood flow quantification with 15O-water PET. J Nucl Med. 2008;49(10):1620–7.

27. Casella G, Berger RL. Statistical Inference. 2nd ed. Boston: Cengage Learning; 2008.

28. Beiderwellen KJ, Poeppel TD, Hartung-Knemeyer V, Buchbender C, Kuehl H, Bockisch A, et al. Simultaneous 68Ga-DOTATOC PET/MRI in patients with gastroenteropancreatic neuroendocrine tumors: initial results. Invest Radiol. 2013;48(5):273–9.

29. Hamill JJ, Sunderland JJ, LeBlanc AK, Kojima CJ, Wall J, Martin EB. Evaluation of CT-based lean-body SUV. Med Phys. 2013;40(9):092504.

30. Shoukri MM. Measures of Interobserver Agreement and Reliability. 2nd ed. Boca Raton: Chapman & Hall; 2010.

31. Dunn G. Statistical Evaluation of Measurement Errors. Design and Analysis of Reliability Studies. 2nd ed. Chichester: Wiley; 2004.

32. Altman DG. Practical Statistics for Medical Research. 1990. Chapman & Hall/CRC.

33. Peduzzi P, Concato J, Kemper E, Holford TR, Feinstein AR. A simulation study of the number of events per variable in logistic regression analysis. J Clin Epidemiol. 1996;49(12):1373–9.

34. Concato J, Peduzzi P, Holford TR, Feinstein AR. Importance of events per independent variable in proportional hazards analysis. I. Background, goals, and general strategy. J Clin Epidemiol. 1995;48(12):1495–501.

35. Peduzzi P, Concato J, Feinstein AR, Holford TR. Importance of events per independent variable in proportional hazards regression analysis. II. Accuracy and precision of regression estimates. J Clin Epidemiol. 1995;48(12):1503–10.

36. Harrell Jr FE, Lee KL, Matchar DB, Reichert TA. Regression models for prognostic prediction: advantages, problems, and suggested solutions. Cancer Treat Rep. 1985;69(10):1071–7.

37. Harrell Jr FE, Lee KL, Califf RM, Pryor DB, Rosati RA. Regression modelling strategies for improved prognostic prediction. Stat Med. 1984;3(2):143–52.

38. Tahari AK, Paidpally V, Chirindel A, Wahl RL, Subramaniam RM. Two-time-point FDG PET/CT: liver SULmean repeatability. Am J Roentgenol. 2015;204(2):402–7.

39. Menda Y, Ponto LL, Schultz MK, Zamba GK, Watkins GL, Bushnell DL, et al. Repeatability of gallium-68 DOTATOC positron emission tomographic imaging in neuroendocrine tumors. Pancreas. 2013;42(6):937–43.

40. Guyatt G, Walter S, Norman G. Measuring change over time: assessing the usefulness of evaluative instruments. J Chronic Dis. 1987;40(2):171–8.

41. Boellaard R. Standards for PET image acquisition and quantitative data analysis. J Nucl Med. 2009;50 Suppl 1:11S–20.

42. International Organization for Standardization (ISO). Accuracy (Trueness and Precision) of Measurement Methods and Results—Part 1: General Principles and Definitions (5725–1). Geneva: ISO; 1994. http://www.iso.org/iso/catalogue_detail.htm?csnumber=11833. Accessed 2 Sept 2016.

43. Food and Drug Administration (FDA). Guidance for Industry: Bioanalytical Method Validation. 2001. www.fda.gov/downloads/drugs/guidancecomplianceregulatoryinformation/guidances/ucm070107.pdf. Accessed 2 Sept 2016.

44. Litwin MS. How to Assess and Interpret Survey Psychometrics. 2nd ed. Thousands Oaks: Sage Publications; 2003.

45. Horton R. Common sense and figures: the rhetoric of validity in medicine (Bradford Hill Memorial Lecture 1999). Stat Med. 2000;19(23):3149–64.

46. Lord FM, Novick MR. Statistical Theories of Mental Test Scores. Reading: Addison-Wesley; 1968.

47. Cronbach LJ, Gleser GC, Nanda H, Rajaratnam N. The Dependability of Behavioral Measurements: Theory and Generalizability for Scores and Profiles. New York: Wiley; 1972.

14

Whole body cardiovascular magnetic resonance imaging to stratify symptomatic and asymptomatic atherosclerotic burden in patients with isolated cardiovascular disease

Jonathan R. Weir-McCall[1,2,5*], Suzanne L. Duce[1], Stephen J. Gandy[2,3], Shona Z. Matthew[1], Patricia Martin[2], Deirdre B. Cassidy[1], Lynne McCormick[1], Jill J. F. Belch[1], Allan D. Struthers[1], Helen M. Colhoun[4] and J. Graeme Houston[1,2]

Abstract

Background: The aim of this study was to use whole body cardiovascular magnetic resonance imaging (WB CVMR) to assess the heart and arterial network in a single examination, so as to describe the burden of atherosclerosis and subclinical disease in participants with symptomatic single site vascular disease.

Methods: 64 patients with a history of symptomatic single site vascular disease (38 coronary artery disease (CAD), 9 cerebrovascular disease, 17 peripheral arterial disease (PAD)) underwent whole body angiogram and cardiac MR in a 3 T scanner. The arterial tree was subdivided into 31 segments and each scored according to the degree of stenosis. From this a standardised atheroma score (SAS) was calculated. Cine and late gadolinium enhancement images of the left ventricle were obtained.

Results: Asymptomatic atherosclerotic disease with greater than 50 % stenosis in arteries other than that responsible for their presenting complain was detected in 37 % of CAD, 33 % of cerebrovascular and 47 % of PAD patients. Unrecognised myocardial infarcts were observed in 29 % of PAD patients. SAS was significantly higher in PAD patients 24 (17.5-30.5) compared to CAD 4 (2–11.25) or cerebrovascular disease patients 6 (2-10) (ANCOVA $p < 0.001$). Standardised atheroma score positively correlated with age (β 0.36 $p = 0.002$), smoking status (β 0.34 $p = 0.002$), and LV mass (β -0.61 $p = 0.001$) on multiple linear regression.

Conclusion: WB CVMR is an effective method for the stratification of cardiovascular disease. The high prevalence of asymptomatic arterial disease, and silent myocardial infarctions, particularly in the peripheral arterial disease group, demonstrates the importance of a systematic approach to the assessment of cardiovascular disease.

Keywords: Whole body magnetic resonance angiography, Atherosclerosis, Coronary artery disease, Peripheral arterial disease, Cerebrovascular disease, Atheroma burden

* Correspondence: j.weirmccall@dundee.ac.uk
Jonathan R. Weir-McCall and Suzanne L. Duce are joint first authors.
[1]Division of Cardiovascular and Diabetes Medicine, Medical Research Institute, University of Dundee, DD1 9SY, UK
[2]NHS Tayside Clinical Radiology, Ninewells Hospital, Dundee DD1 9SY, UK
Full list of author information is available at the end of the article

Background

Atherosclerosis with subsequent plaque formation is the underlying pathophysiological process in the leading causes of morbidity and mortality in the western world [1]. The widely distributed nature of atherosclerosis across the body has been appreciated for decades [2], however routine stratification or quantification of whole body disease burden is not routinely performed. Multimodal imaging studies of patients presenting with coronary artery disease [3, 4], cerebrovascular disease [5, 6] and peripheral arterial disease [7–9], have shown a high prevalence of atherosclerotic disease in other sites in addition to the presenting disease. Multimodal studies by their nature involved multiple examinations and typically require visits to different healthcare departments. An alternative option is whole body cardiovascular magnetic resonance imaging (WB CVMR), which can assess the heart and arterial network in a single examination, has the advantages of being non-invasive and avoids ionising radiation.

WB CVMR comprises of a suite of cardiac magnetic resonance (CMR) and whole body MR angiography (WB-MRA) sequences, allowing the systemic assessment of whole body atheroma burden, with cardiac structure, function and the detection of myocardial scarring, in a single imaging session. Global atheroma burden has been shown to correlate well with traditional cardiac risk factors, the prevalence of coronary artery disease and future major adverse cardiovascular events [10–13]. Previous studies have assessed the ability of WB-MRA to assess extra-site disease in coronary arterial disease, peripheral arterial disease and vasculitis [14–16]. However a direct comparison of extra-site disease and atheroma burden between cardiovascular disease groups has not been previously conducted. The aim of the study was therefore to determine the yield of WB CVMR in detecting asymptomatic cardiovascular disease, at sites other than at the clinically apparent location in different patient cohorts, and to compare atheroma burden between the groups.

Methods
Ethics

The protocols were reviewed and approved by the East of Scotland Research Ethics Committee and was conducted in accordance with the Declaration of Helsinki. All volunteers gave written informed consent to participate in this study.

Participants

Patients with isolated coronary, cerebrovascular or peripheral vascular disease were identified from existing clinical databases and from local cardiology, stroke, and vascular clinics. Sixty-four participants with a prior diagnosis of single territory vascular disease attended MRI appointments between March 2009 and December 2012. The subjects were categorised based on their history of cardiovascular disease; their demographics are summarised in Table 1. Group 1 contained those with clinical evidence of coronary artery disease (n = 38). Group 2 contained those who had had a cerebrovascular event (n = 9). Group 3 contained those with clinical evidence of peripheral arterial disease (n = 17).

Coronary arterial disease (Group 1) included non-fatal acute myocardial infarction, hospitalised acute coronary syndrome, resuscitated cardiac arrest (not attributed to a non CAD causes), coronary artery bypass graft (CABG) or any other coronary revascularisation procedure. Cerebrovascular disease (Group 2) inclusion criteria were non-fatal strokes or transient ischemic attacks (TIA) confirmed by a specialist stroke physician. Peripheral arterial disease (Group 3) inclusion criteria was ankle-brachial pressure index (ABPI) <0.9 with intermittent claudication, walking distance of not more than 200 yards, or abnormal toe systolic pressure. Volunteers were excluded if they had a clinical history of arterial disease at any site other than their primary diagnosis location. Other exclusion criteria included the possibility of metallic implants, history of claustrophobia, pregnancy, renal replacement therapy, end stage renal disease, therapy for any chronic inflammatory disease, atrial fibrillation or malignancy.

Table 1 Demographics and clinical characteristics in the study population

	Group 1 CAD	Group 2 CVD	Group 3 PAD
Number	38	9	17
Male [%]	31 (81.6)	4 (44.4)	13 (76.5)
Age [years]	66.0 ± 8	61.2 ± 8	68.7 ± 10
Weight [kg]	87.2 ± 13	77.4 ± 12	89.7 ± 28
Height [m]	1.69 ± 0.1	1.64 ± 0.1	1.7 ± 0.1
BMI [kg/m²]	30.6 ± 4	28.7 ± 2	28.8 ± 4
Systolic BP [mmHg]	135 ± 15	132 ± 12	137 ± 14
Diastolic BP [mmHg]	76 ± 9	74 ± 8	78 ± 8
Hypertension	32 (84.2)	6 (66.7)	13 (76.5)
Antiplatelet	34 (89)	9 (100)	15 (88)
Antihypertensive	37 (97)	8 (89)	14 (82)
Statin prescription	30 (79)	8 (89)	16 (94)
Type 2 Diabetes	19 (50)	5 (55.6)	6 (35.3)
Non-Smokers	16 (42)	1 (11)	1 (6)
Former-Smokers	20 (53)	8 (89)	11 (65)
Smokers	2 (5)	0 (0)	5 (29)

Values expressed as Mean ± SD, or N (%)
BMI body mass index, *BP* blood pressure, *CAD* coronary artery disease, *CVD* cerebrovascular disease, *PAD* peripheral arterial disease

Magnetic resonance imaging

Images were acquired on a 32 RF receiver channel, 3 Tesla MRI scanner (Magnetom Trio, Siemens, Erlangen, Germany) equipped with high-performance gradient system and electrocardiograph (ECG)-gating. For whole body coverage, a combination of six RF coils were used: head matrix (12 elements); neck matrix (4 elements); spine matrix (up to 24 elements); two body matrix (6 elements each); and peripheral angiography phased array RF surface coils (16 elements. Subjects were placed head first into the magnet bore and were examined in the supine position. Total scan time was of the order of 45 min.

Whole body magnetic resonance angiography protocol

For localisation, four low-resolution images were acquired from head to foot using gradient echo fast low angle shot (FLASH) sequences with 500 mm field of view (FOV). Whole body magnetic resonance angiography (WB-MRA) images involved the acquisition of 4 overlapping 3D data sets using a coronal spoiled FLASH (fast low angle shot) sequence (see Table 2 for acquisition parameters). Four anatomically distinct stations with field of view of 500 mm were: head and thorax (station 1), thorax and abdomen (station 2), abdomen and upper legs (stations 3) and lower legs (station 4). These were positioned with an overlap of at least 75 mm between each field of view. Anatomical paired images were acquired pre- and post-contrast. A standard dose of 25 ml gadoterate meglumine contrast agent (Dotarem, Guerbet, Villepinte, France) was administered by intravenous injection in the antecubital fossa in 2 separate boluses (10 ml and 15 ml respectively) using a Spectris Solaris power injector (MedRad, Pittsburgh, USA) at a rate of 1.5 ml/sec, each followed by a 20 ml bolus of saline. For station 1 and 4 imaging, post-contrast images were acquired after an injection of 10 ml of 0.5 mmol/ml gadoterate meglumine contrast agent. Station 1 image acquisition commenced when the bolus of contrast agent arrived at the top of the aortic arch in the '2D Care Bolus' images (Siemens, Erlangen, Germany). Station 4 image acquisition followed immediately after this, with three consecutive volumes of station 4 acquired

to ensure that peak arterial enhancement was caught. There was a delay before stations 2 and 3 image acquisition of at least 10 min to allow contrast washout and minimise venous contamination during the second injection and image acquisition [17]. Post-contrast images were acquired after an injection of 15 ml of 0.5 mmol/ml gadoterate meglumine contrast agent, again followed by a 20 ml saline bolus. Acquisition commenced once the contrast agent bolus was seen in the descending aorta in the coronal 2D Care Bolus image. Station 3 imaging commenced immediately after the completion of the acquisition of station 2.

Cardiac magnetic resonance (CMR) protocols

Cardiac magnetic resonance (CMR) imaging utilised a spine matrix and six-element body array matrix RF coils. Left ventricular assessment involved the acquisition of short axis, multi-slice 2D images from the atrio-ventricular ring to the apex using a CINE TrueFISP sequence with retrospective ECG-gating, with repeated end-expiratory breath-holds (Table 2). The slice thickness was 6 mm and inter-slice gap was 4 mm. Ten minutes after the injection of the first dose of contrast agent, the ECG-gated, breath-hold, end-diastole, short-axis, multi-slice late gadolinium enhanced (LGE) CMR images were acquired using a 2D phase sensitive inversion recovery (PSIR) sequence (Table 2).

WB-MRA image analysis

Researchers were blind to the participants' clinical history during image analysis. The 3D WB-MRA datasets were viewed offline as source images using both multi-planar reconstruction (MPR) and maximum intensity projections (MIP) (Carestream PACS Client Suite Version 10.1 sp1, Rochester, NY, USA) by a radiologist with experience of reporting over 400 whole body magnetic resonance angiograms. Based on previous pilot work, the arterial network was divided into 31 vessel segments extending from the internal and external carotid arteries to the trifurcation vessels of the lower limb (Fig. 1). Each arterial segment was scored according to maximal luminal stenosis within the vessel lumen. Categorical MRA scores from 0-4 were

Table 2 Imaging parameters for MRI sequences used for the combined CMR and WB-MRA protocol

	Location	Sequence	Plane	TR (ms)	TE (ms)	Flip Angle (°)	Pixel size (mm)	Slice thickness (mm)
WB-MRA	Station 1	FLASH	Coronal	2.68	1	19	1.1x1	1.1
WB-MRA	Station 2	FLASH	Coronal	2.6	0.96	16	1.3x1.1	1.3
WB-MRA	Station 3	FLASH	Coronal	3.47	1.21	37	1.5x1	1.4
WB MRA	Station 4	FLASH	Coronal	2.61	0.96	22	1.2x1.1	1
LVA	Heart LV	TrueFISP	Short axis	3.40	1.48	50-60	1.9x1.4	6
LGE-CMR	Heart LV	PSIR	Short axis	846.4/5.21	1.99	20	1.9x1.4	6

WB-MRA whole body magnetic resonance angiography, *LVA* left ventricular analysis, *LGE-CMR* Late gadolinium enhanced cardiac magnetic resonance images, *TR* repetition time, *TE* echo time

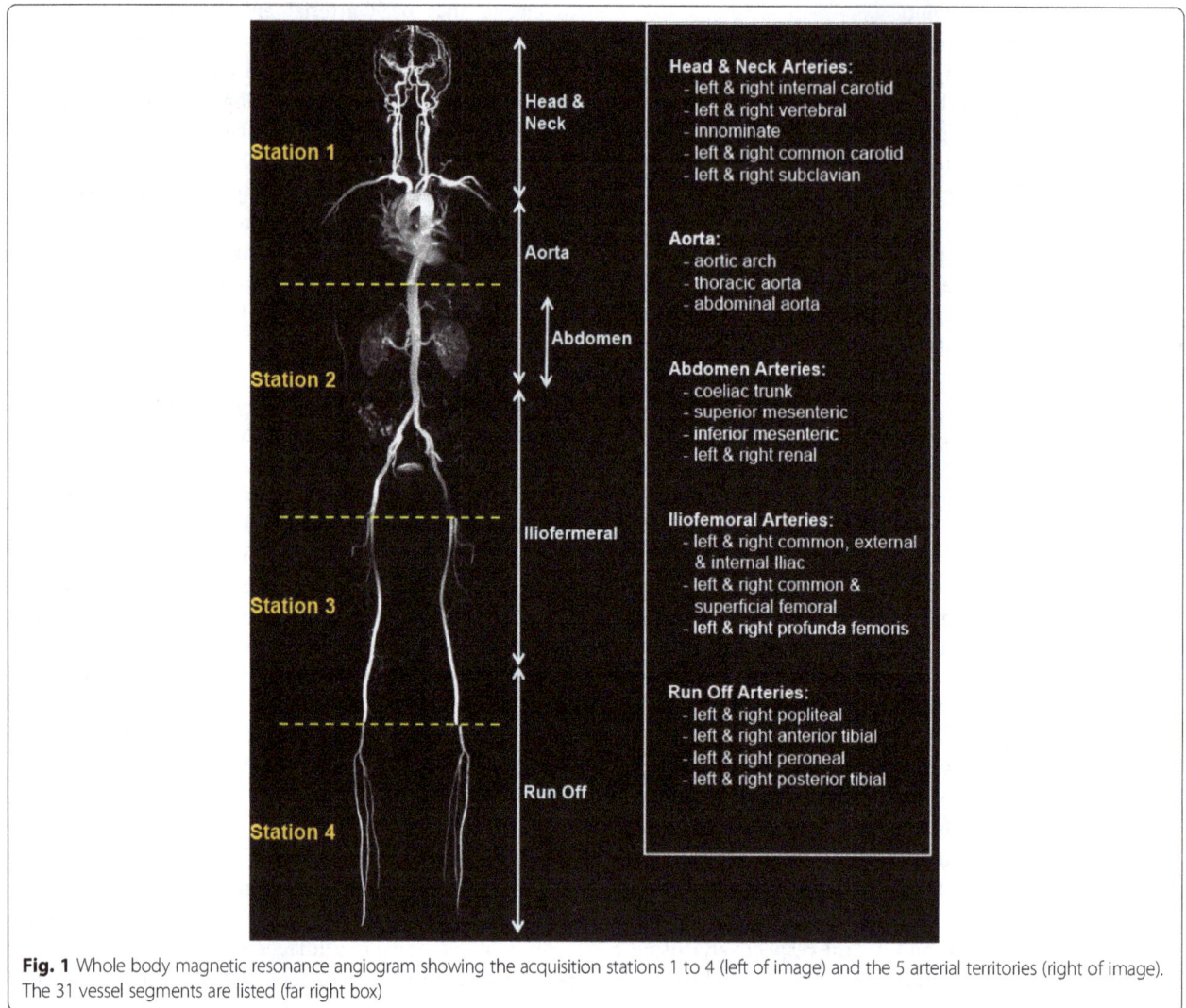

Fig. 1 Whole body magnetic resonance angiogram showing the acquisition stations 1 to 4 (left of image) and the 5 arterial territories (right of image). The 31 vessel segments are listed (far right box)

allocated to each vessel segment, where 0 = healthy segment with no stenosis, 1 = <50 % stenosis, 2 = 51-70 % stenosis, 3 = 71-99 % stenosis, 4 = vessel occlusion. For each participant, the 'standardised atheroma score' (SAS) was calculated using equation [1] where n is the number of diagnostic segments [18].

$$SAS = \left[\left(\frac{\Sigma \ MRA \ scores}{n} \right) \div 4 \right] \times 100 \quad (1)$$

The 31 vessel segments were subdivided into 5 anatomical territories: (i) the head and neck arteries, (ii) the aorta, (iii) the abdominal arteries, (iv) the ilio-femoral arteries and (v) the run off arteries in the lower limbs (Fig. 1). Regional standardised atheroma scores were calculated for each anatomical territory. For each patient the individual vessel segments that had MRA scores of 3 or 4 were noted, with the number of vessels with stenosis greater than 70 % being counted and their location

recorded, as luminal narrowing of greater than 70 % is considered clinically significant. In addition a moderate stenosis assessment recorded the number and location of vessel segments that had MRA scores equal to 2 (50-70 % stenosis), in a similar manner to that of the severe stenosis assessment.

(ii) CMR image analysis

Left ventricular analysis images were analysed offline using Argus software (Siemens, Erlangen, Germany) by two experienced CMR researchers. The manual 3D digital segmentation involved tracing endocardial and epicardial contours on the short-axis left ventricle images at end-diastolic and end-systolic phases of the cardiac cycle. Papillary muscles were treated as part of the blood pool volume unless they were indistinguishable from the myocardial wall, and then they were assigned as left ventricle muscle. The left ventricular mass (LVM), stroke volume (SV), ejection fraction (EF), end-diastolic

(EDV) and end-systolic volumes (ESV) were determined using an algorithm based on the Simpson rule [19]. Results were normalised to body surface area. Left ventricular hypertrophy was defined as an indexed LVM above the normal range for sex [19]. Late gadolinium enhanced images of the left ventricle were inspected for evidence of myocardial signal enhancement using a Carestream PACS workstation (Rochester, NY, USA). The location was recorded according to the AHA 17 segment model [20]. Delayed enhancement was defined as <50 % or >50 % wall thickness according to the maximum depth of delayed enhancement in any segment.

Statistical methods

Descriptive statistics were used for the analysis of the demographic and clinical features of the cohorts with data expressed as mean ± standard deviation (sd) for normally distributed data, and median (interquartile range) for non-normal distributed data. Normality tests were performed; if the test failed, where possible standard transformations such as square root, reciprocal or logarithmic transforms were used to generate a Gaussian distribution. To test the null hypothesis to determine if samples originated from the same distribution, one-way analysis of variance (ANOVA) with the Bonferroni post hoc adjustment was used for the parametric data, and Kruskal–Wallis ANOVA by ranks was used for the non-parametric data. ANCOVA was performed to confirm differences between the groups with the WB-SAS as the dependant variable. MANCOVA was used to determine the relations of the LV metrics to the demographic data with the LV metrics entered as the dependant variables. Pearson correlation coefficients between WB-SAS, LVA and population demographic metrics were reported. All variables with a p-value <0.3 on univariate analysis were entered into a multivariate regression analysis with the WB-SAS as the dependent variable and the remainder as independent variables. All data were analysed using SPSS statistical package (version 21.0, SPSS Inc. Chicago, Illinois). Significance was assumed when p < 0.05. A local statistician provided statistical support.

Results

CMR and whole body MRA images were acquired from 64 participants (75 % male, age 66.1 ± 8.5) with single site cardiovascular disease. There were no statistically significant differences in the demographic metrics between each of the diseased groups (Table 1), except for smoking status with significantly more people in the PAD group being current smokers than in either the CAD or cerebrovascular groups.

In the WB-MRA analysis, 1978 of the 1984 vessel segments (99.7 %) were interpretable. 6 segments in 4 of the 64 examinations were rated as 'non-diagnostic' due to movement artefact or incomplete vessel visualisation.

619 (31.3 %) of the 1978 arterial segments had evidence of luminal narrowing: 453 (22.9 %) had stenosis below 50 %, 61 (3.1 %) had stenosis between 50-70 %, 63 (3.2 %) had stenosis between 70-90 %, and 42 (2.1 %) had complete occlusion.

The PAD group had the highest whole body standardised atheroma score (WB-SAS) of 24.8 ± 9.9 and the CAD group had the lowest WB-SAS of 7.0 ± 6.2. The WB-SAS of the PAD patients was statistically significantly higher than those of either the CAD or cerebrovascular disease patients (ANOVA test: P ≤ 0.001). Differences between the groups persisted on ANCOVA (F = 15.18, p < 0.001), accounting for age, gender, smoking status, blood pressure, BMI and statin prescription. There was no significant difference in the WB-SAS between the CAD and cerebrovascular disease groups. Across all 5 anatomical territories, the PAD subjects' regional SAS were consistently higher compared to either the CAD or cerebrovascular groups' scores (Table 3). There were no statistically significant differences between any of the regional SAS of CAD and cerebrovascular group. On univariate analysis, there were positive correlations of SAS with age (r = 0.37 P = 0.002), smoking status (r = 0.397 P = 0.002), LV ejection fraction (r = -0.26 P = 0.034) and LV mass (r = -0.42 P = 0.001) and a trend towards an association with diastolic blood pressure (r = -0.23 P = 0.052) (Table 4). On multivariate analysis, age (β 0.36 p = 0.002), smoking status (β 0.34 p = 0.002), and LV mass (β -0.61 p = 0.001) continued to demonstrate a significant association with WB-SAS.

For each patient, the extent of stenosis was further investigated by counting the number of vessel segments that had either (a) severe stenosis with MRA score of 3 or 4 (associated with luminal narrowing of greater than 70 %) or (b) moderate stenosis with MRA score of 2 (associated with luminal narrowing of between 50 and 70 %). The results are summarised in Table 5. 100 % of PAD patients have severe stenosis detectable in at least one arterial vessel, with the ilio-femoral arteries being most affected. A third of the CAD patients had severe stenosis present in their MRA images, with the run off arteries most commonly affected (18.4 % of patients), while severe arterial stenosis was detected in only 22 % of the cerebrovascular patients. With luminal narrowing of greater than 70 % considered clinically significant, this analysis is useful for screening patients and highlighting those who require follow-up investigations.

The left ventricular assessment (Table 3) revealed that the PAD group have the largest mean left ventricular mass (LVM), end-diastolic (EDV), end-systolic volume (ESV), cardiac ejection fraction (EF) and stroke volume (SV), and these differences reached statistical significance for the LVM, EDV and SV values (ANOVA P ≤ 0.007). These differences persisted on MANCOVA (F = 8.87, p = 0.001 for

Table 3 Whole body cardiovascular magnetic resonance imaging (WB CVMR) data for each group including magnetic resonance angiography (MRA) scores, standardised stenosis scores (SAS), left ventricular analysis (LVA) and left ventricular late gadolinium enhancement (LGE) results

	Group 1	Group 2	Group 3
	CAD	CVD	PAD
WB-SAS	4 (2–11.25)	6 (2-10)	24 (17.5-30.5)
Head/Neck-SAS	2.8 (0–5.6)	8.3 (1.4–9.7)	19.4 (9.7-25)
Aorta-SAS	8.3 (0–16.7)	8.3 (8.3-12.5)	8.3 (8.3-16.7)
Abdomen-SAS	8.3 (0–10)	0 (0–5)	20 (5-27.5)
Ilio-Femoral-SAS	6.25 (0–20.8)	4.2 (2.1–14.6)	37.5 (27.1-52.1)
Run Off-SAS	0 (0–10.2)	0 (0–18.7)	31.3 (11-48.5)
LVM (g/m^2)	59.1 (54.1–64.5)	53.4 (47.4–71.1)	105.7 (67.8-124.5)
EDV (ml/m^2)	74.7 ± 18.8	72.4 ± 15.2	104.1 ± 34.9
ESV (ml/m^2)	25.3 (18.3–29.7)	22.4 (17.8–35.8)	33.8 (22.8-42.8)
EF (%)	64.5 ± 9.8	64.7 ± 13.4	66.4 ± 11.8
SV (ml/m^2)	46.8 (40.4–52)	46 (40.2–52.7)	73.7 (39.4-92.7)
LGE	16 (42.1 %)	0 (0 %)	5 (29.4 %)

Values expressed as Mean ± SD, Median (Interquartile range) or N (%)
CAD coronary artery disease, CVD cerebrovascular disease, PAD peripheral arterial disease, SAS standardised atheroma score, WB whole body, LVM indexed left ventricular mass, EDV indexed end diastolic volume, ESV indexed end systolic volume, EF ejection fraction, SV indexed stroke volume, LGE Late gadolinium enhancement

LVM, F = 3.27, p = 0.047 for EDV and F = 4.43, p = 0.018 for LVM). The differences between the CAD and cerebrovascular disease cohorts were relatively small and did not reach statistical significance. Left ventricular hypertrophy was detected in 16 % of the study population, while impaired left ventricular systolic function was present in 13 %.

Late gadolinium enhancement (LGE) was observed in 21 (32.8 %) of the 64 subjects. All subjects with LGE had

Table 4 Correlation of whole body standardised atheroma score with demographic and left ventricular parameters

	Pearson correlation	P-value
Age	0.461	<0.001
Gender	-0.19	0.091
Systolic BP	0.19	0.095
Diastolic BP	-0.23	0.052
BMI	-0.22	0.06
Hypertension	0.13	0.18
History of Smoking	0.4	0.002
T2DM	0.05	0.37
Statins	0.008	0.48
Left ventricular metrics		
LV End diastolic volume	0.11	0.22
LV End systolic volume	0.17	0.11
LV stroke volume	-0.18	0.11
Ejection fraction	-0.26	0.03
LV mass	-0.42	0.001

scarring in a subendocardial location with a territorial distribution typical of an ischaemic aetiology. The majority of the enhancement occurred in the CAD group, with 16 (42.1 %) CAD participants displaying evidence of myocardial scarring, affecting a total of 91 AHA segments. No myocardial LGE was observed in the cerebrovascular disease group images. Five (29.4 %) of the PAD group had evidence of unrecognised myocardial infarction (UMI), affecting a total of 21 AHA segments (See Figure 2). UMIs tended to occur in the inferior wall with 9/21 UMIs occurring in the inferior segments, with the second most common location being the inferoseptal segment with 4/21 UMIs occurring in this region. Recognised MIs demonstrated no territorial predominance. UMIs were smaller, involving an average of 4.2 AHA segments, compared with 6.1 AHA segments in the recognised MI group. 40 % of UMIs involved less than 50 % of the myocardial thickness in the affected segments while the remaining 60 % involved greater than 50 % of the myocardial thickness. In comparison, 73 % of recognised MIs involved >50 % of the myocardial thickness. No correlation was observed between WB-SAS and either the presence or the severity of the late gadolinium myocardial enhancement.

Discussion

We have shown that whole body cardiovascular MRI is a feasible solution to stratify the extent of atherosclerosis in arteries and the extent of cardiac dysfunction and myocardial scarring in a 45-min exam. This is also the first study to show a positive correlation between the

Table 5 The percentage of patients in each group that have at least one vessel segments with (a) severe stenosis (MRA score = 3 or 4) and (b) moderate stenosis (MRA score = 2) for the different anatomical territories. The bracketed number is the total number of vessel segments with the relevant degree of stenosis

Anatomical Territories	(a) Severe stenosis			(b) Moderate stenosis		
	Group 1	Group 2	Group 3	Group 1	Group 2	Group 3
	CAD	CVD	PAD	CAD	CVD	PAD
Whole body (%)	34.2 (26)	22.2 (6)	100 (73)	37 (21)	56 (6)	88 (34)
Head/Neck (%)	5.3 (4)	0 (0)	29.4 (8)	11 (4)	33 (3)	29 (7)
Aorta (%)	0 (0)	0 (0)	5.9 (1)	3 (1)	0 (0)	6 (1)
Abdomen (%)	7.9 (4)	11.1 (1)	52.9 (11)	18 (7)	0 (0)	12 (2)
Ilio-Femoral (%)	10.5 (6)	0 (0)	76 (28)	8 (5)	11 (1)	59 (15)
Run off (%)	18.4 (12)	22.2 (5)	58.8 (25)	8 (4)	22 (2)	41 (9)

CAD coronary artery disease, CVD cerebrovascular disease, PAD peripheral arterial disease

whole body atherosclerotic stenotic burden and left ventricular mass.

Stratified medicine has become a topic of increasing importance [21, 22]. This is as important in cardiovascular disease as it is in cancer, and requires accurate definition and quantification of disease. This is especially important given findings that polyvascular disease is associated with significantly higher rates for major adverse cardiovascular events than in single site vascular disease [23]. In our study we have demonstrated the ability of WB-MRA to stratify and quantify atherosclerotic burden throughout the body. Significant undetected arterial stenoses were found to be present in multiple sites in all disease groups. We found a 37 % prevalence

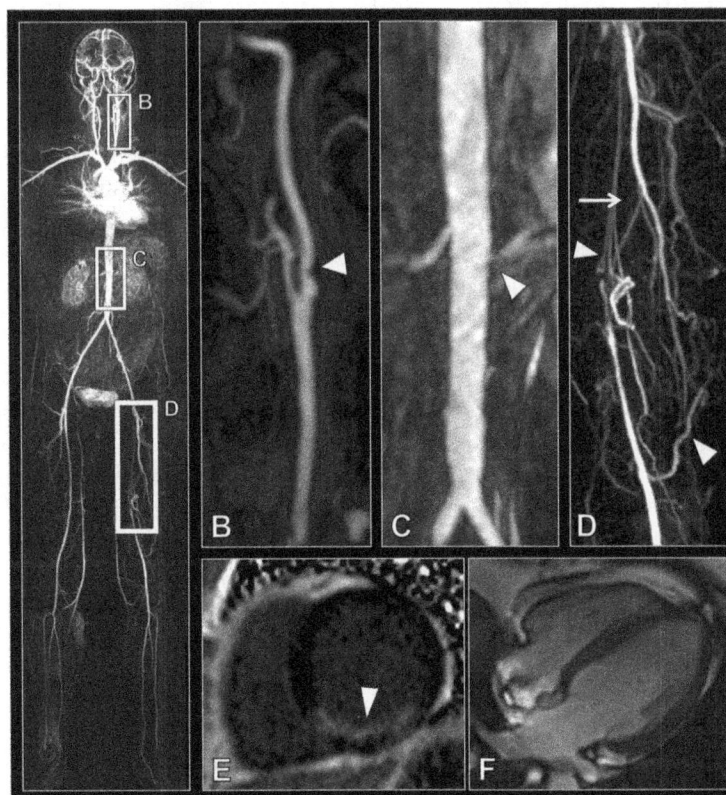

Fig. 2 a Whole body angiogram of a peripheral arterial disease patient. **b** Sagittal MIP (maximum intensity projection) of the bifurcation of the left carotid artery showing >50 % stenosis of the internal carotid artery (arrow head). **c** Coronal MIP of the renal arteries showing a normal right renal artery but a >70 % stenosis of the left renal artery (arrow head). **d** Coronal MIP showing a long segment occlusion of the left superficial femoral artery (arrow) with extensive collateral formation (arrow heads) with reformation distally. **e** Short axis late gadolinium enhancement showing a large unrecognised myocardial infarct (arrow head). **f** 4 chamber view of the heart showing normal dimensions of the ventricles

of extra-coronary arterial disease in CAD. This is lower than the 50 % reported in one study although this latter study did not exclude patients with known extra-coronary disease [16]. It is also lower than the 55 % reported in a more recent study [12], although this was performed at 1.5 T with a lower spatial resolution than obtained in the current study, thus the improved arterial definition may have led to a more accurate quantification of the degree of stenosis due to improved spatial resolution found at 3 T. We found that 33 % of cerebrovascular disease patients had significant disease outwith the head and neck. This is significantly lower than that reported by Paraskevas et al. [5], however their study only looked at patients with known unilateral internal carotid artery occlusion which is at the extreme end of the carotid disease spectrum, while our study used prior cerebrovascular events as inclusion criteria. Our PAD cohort demonstrated significant disease above the level of the abdominal aortic bifurcation in 47 % which is slightly higher than that previously reported on WB-MRA [15].

The standardised atheroma score was significantly higher in the peripheral arterial disease group than either the cerebrovascular or the coronary arterial disease group. Previous epidemiological studies have shown that patients with PAD have a 33 % higher composite risk of CV death, myocardial infarction, stroke, or hospitalisation for atherothrombotic event(s) than either cerebrovascular or coronary arterial disease groups [24]. As well as the intrinsic risk of arterial stenosis, part of the causative mechanism may be the effect the atherosclerotic burden has on the heart. We have shown for the first time the association between whole body arterial atheroma burden and left ventricular mass, which is known to be strongly associated with future cardiovascular events [25]. This may be due to the stiffening nature of the atherosclerosis on the arteries, as total atheroma burden has been shown to correlate with arterial stiffness, [26] which in turn is associated with left ventricular hypertrophy [27]. Given that both left ventricular mass and atheroma burden are associated with increased future risk of cardiac events, further work is required to extricate the interaction between these measures, to ascertain whether these need to be targeted individually, or whether there is a single linking aetiology which can be targeted.

Unrecognised myocardial infarctions are present in 29.4 % of patients with peripheral arterial disease. The rate in peripheral arterial disease patients is significantly higher than the 6 % reported in a previous PAD population using ECG and echocardiography during pre-operative work-up [28], or the 14 % reported in a series of patients undergoing pre-operative coronary angiography screening [29]. However ECG has been shown to only detect 6-29 % of unrecognised myocardial infarcts revealed on late gadolinium enhancement [30, 31]. Our observed incidence is closer to that expected from a previous study looking at whole body cardiovascular MR in a population cohort study which showed rates of unrecognised myocardial infarction in 19.7 % of 70 year olds and 30 % in 75 year olds [30, 32]. That the prevalence in the PAD population was on par with a 75 year old cohort despite having a mean age of 68 is in keeping with the higher prevalence of risks factors in our population, although a recent study has called into question the link between unrecognised myocardial infarctions and traditional risk factors [33]. None of the patients with cerebrovascular disease had evidence of unrecognised myocardial infarcts. This is surprising given the results of previous studies showing unrecognised myocardial infarcts in 32 %-52 % of patients but may be due to the small numbers of this group in the current study.

Recognition of unrecognised myocardial infarction is important as these have the same prognostic implications as recognised myocardial infarcts [34]. Furthermore these patients respond well to both conventional secondary prevention medication and percutaneous coronary intervention [35–37].

It could be argued that since patients with clinically apparent cardiovascular disease in one site will result in patients being treated for atherosclerotic risk factors that further information about disease elsewhere is superfluous. However this ignores several factors. Despite our study showing comparable rates of statin prescriptions between the different groups, a previous population study has shown that community prescription of risk modifying agents is markedly different between disease groups, with fewer patients with PAD being prescribed statins and antiplatelet agents compared with stroke or coronary artery disease groups [38]. This suggests poor appreciation of the extensive disease present elsewhere in the body, indeed, in our study the PAD population had the most extensive extra-primary site disease. The second is the additional prognostic information this provides. Multisite disease is associated with a significantly raised risk of future major adverse cardiac and cerebrovascular events (MACCE) compared with single site disease, and had a greater detrimental effect on future prognosis than the presence of diabetes [23, 38]. While these studies have focused on symptomatic disease, the significance of asymptomatic disease is supported by recent studies showing increased risk of MACCE in patients with higher global atherosclerotic burden on whole body MR angiography [10, 11]. Thus patients with polyvascular disease may warrant more intensive management and follow-up as well as being ideal candidates for future novel therapeutic agents [24]. For those being referred for a clinical MRA of a specific vascular territory, extension of this to a whole body cardiovascular MR would be a logical step, and indeed the added cost of extending a clinically indicated MRA to include the rest of the body is small when considered in relation to the high cost of the baseline exam, and in a peripheral arterial disease population has been shown to be cost effective due to its reductions in requirements for other imaging investigations (such as echocardiography and carotid Doppler) and alterations in patient management, although other cardiovascular disease cohorts have still to be assessed [39].

The limitations of the current study are: The study groups are unequal in size with a relatively small number of cerebrovascular patients and large number of coronary arterial disease. In addition the cerebrovascular group demonstrates a disproportionate number of females which could bias the results, however we demonstrated no significant correlation between SAS and sex, and accounting for sex using an analysis of covariance did not change the results. An intrinsic limitation of WB-MRA is its ability to only provide information on the prevalence of stenotic atherosclerosis, and will thus miss the earliest stages of the disease including vessel stiffening and remodelling. Additionally, while the prognostic effect of symptomatic multisite atherosclerosis is known, the effect of asymptomatic multisite disease still requires further work to elucidate.

Conclusion

WB CVMR is an effective method for the stratification of cardiovascular disease. The high prevalence of asymptomatic arterial disease, and silent myocardial infarctions, particularly in the peripheral arterial disease group, demonstrates the importance of a systematic approach to the assessment of cardiovascular disease.

Abbreviations
AHA: American Heart Association; CAD: coronary artery disease; CMR: cardiac magnetic resonance imaging; CVD: cerebrovascular disease; EDV: end diastolic volume; ESV: end systolic volume; LGE-CMR: late gadolinium enhanced cardiac magnetic resonance images; LVA: left ventricular analysis; LVH: left ventricular hypertrophy; LVM: left ventricular mass; MRA: magnetic resonance angiography; PAD: peripheral arterial disease; SAS: standardised atheroma score; SV: stroke volume; UMI: unrecognised myocardial infarct; WB-CVMR: whole body magnetic cardiovascular magnetic resonance; WB-MRA: whole body magnetic resonance angiography.

Competing interests
JWM has received monies from Guerbet for attending symposia, and for running educational meetings. HMC received monies from Pfizer for attending symposia, a speaker's bureau, as a member of staff and for consultancy. HMC has received research funds from Pfizer, Roche, Eli-Lilly, Boehringer Ingelheim (BI) and Astra Zeneca. HMC has shares in Roche. GH is director and Shareholder of Vascular Flow Technologies Ltd, and has received research funds from Guerbet.

Authors' contributions
JWM, SLD, HMC, JJF, ADS and GH conceived the study. JWM, SLD and SM analysed the MRI studies. JWM, SLD, DC analysed and interpreted the data. PM, SG and LM worked on the development of the MRI protocol. JWM and SLD drafted the manuscript. All authors revised the manuscript critically for important intellectual content, and read and approved the final manuscript.

Acknowledgements: Funding, disclosures
This is sub study of the multicentre SUMMIT study. SUMMIT receives support from the Innovative Medicines Initiative (IMI) Joint Undertaking under the grant agreement n° [115006], resources of which are composed of financial contribution from the European Union's Seventh Framework Programme (FP7/2007-2013) and EFPIA companies' in kind contribution. JRWM is supported by the Wellcome Trust through the Scottish Translational Medicine and Therapeutics Initiative (Grant no. WT 085664) in the form of a Clinical Research Fellowship. Neither groups had any role in: study design, the collection, analysis, and interpretation of data; in the writing of the manuscript; nor in the decision to submit the manuscript for publication.

Author details
[1]Division of Cardiovascular and Diabetes Medicine, Medical Research Institute, University of Dundee, DD1 9SY, UK. [2]NHS Tayside Clinical Radiology, Ninewells Hospital, Dundee DD1 9SY, UK. [3]NHS Tayside Medical Physics, Ninewells Hospital, Dundee DD1 9SY, UK. [4]Division of Population Health Sciences, Medical Research Institute, The Mackenzie Building, University of Dundee, DD2 4BF, UK. [5]Division of Cardiovascular and Diabetic Medicine, Level 7, Ninewells Hospital, Dundee DD1 9SY, UK.

References
1. Rosamond W, Flegal K, Furie K, Go A, Greenlund K, Haase N, Hailpern SM, Ho M, Howard V, Kissela B, Kissela B, Kittner S, Lloyd-Jones D, McDermott M, Meigs J, Moy C, Nichol G, O'Donnell C, Roger V, Sorlie P, Steinberger J, Thom T, Wilson M, Hong Y. Heart disease and stroke statistics–2008 update: a report from the American Heart Association Statistics Committee and Stroke Statistics Subcommittee. Circulation. 2008;117:e25–146.
2. Mitchell JR, Schwartz CJ. Relationship between arterial disease in different sites. A study of the aorta and coronary, carotid, and iliac arteries. Br Med J. 1962;1:1293–301.
3. Rigatelli G. Aortoiliac angiography during coronary artery angiography detects significant occult aortoiliac and renal artery atherosclerosis in patients with coronary atherosclerosis. Int J Cardiovasc Imaging. 2004;20:299–303.
4. Newman AB, Shemanski L, Manolio TA, Cushman M, Mittelmark M, Polak JF, Powe NR, Siscovick D. Ankle-arm index as a predictor of cardiovascular disease and mortality in the Cardiovascular Health Study. The Cardiovascular Health Study Group. Arterioscler Thromb Vasc Biol. 1999;19:538–45.
5. Paraskevas KI, Mikhailidis DP, Liapis CD. Internal carotid artery occlusion: association with atherosclerotic disease in other arterial beds and vascular risk factors. Angiology. 2007;58:329–35.
6. Kawarada O, Yokoi Y, Morioka N, Nakata S, Higashiue S, Mori T, Iwahashi M, Hatada A. Carotid stenosis and peripheral artery disease in Japanese patients with coronary artery disease undergoing coronary artery bypass grafting. Circ J. 2003;67:1003–6.
7. Wachtell K, Ibsen H, Olsen MH, Laybourn C, Christoffersen JK, Nørgaard H, Mantoni M, Lund JO. Prevalence of renal artery stenosis in patients with peripheral vascular disease and hypertension. J Hum Hypertens. 1996;10:83–5.
8. Alexandrova NA, Gibson WC, Norris JW, Maggisano R. Carotid artery stenosis in peripheral vascular disease. J Vasc Surg. 1996;23:645–9.
9. Von Kemp K, van den Brande P, Peterson T, Waegeneers S, Scheerlinck T, Danau W, van Tussenbroek F, Debing E, Staelens I. Screening for concomitant diseases in peripheral vascular patients. Results of a systematic approach. Int Angiol. 1997;16:114–22.
10. Bamberg F, Parhofer KG, Lochner E, Marcus RP, Theisen D, Findeisen HM, Hoffmann U, Schönberg SO, Schlett CL, Reiser MF, Weckbach S. Diabetes mellitus: long-term prognostic value of whole-body MR imaging for the occurrence of cardiac and cerebrovascular events. Radiology. 2013;269:730–7.
11. Lundberg C, Johansson L, Barbier CE, Lind L, Ahlström H, Hansen T. Total atherosclerotic burden by whole body magnetic resonance angiography predicts major adverse cardiovascular events. Atherosclerosis. 2013;228:148–52.
12. Lehrke S, Egenlauf B, Steen H, Lossnitzer D, Korosoglou G, Merten C, Ivandic BT, Giannitsis E, Katus H a. Prediction of coronary artery disease by a systemic atherosclerosis score index derived from whole-body MR angiography. J Cardiovasc Magn Reson. 2009;11:36.
13. Hansen T, Ahlström H, Wikström J, Lind L, Johansson L. A total atherosclerotic score for whole-body MRA and its relation to traditional cardiovascular risk factors. Eur Radiol. 2008;18:1174–80.

14. Lin J, Chen B, Wang J-H, Zeng M-S, Wang Y-X. Whole-body three-dimensional contrast-enhanced magnetic resonance (MR) angiography with parallel imaging techniques on a multichannel MR system for the detection of various systemic arterial diseases. Heart Vessels. 2006;21:395–8.

15. Goyen M, Herborn CU, Kröger K, Ruehm SG, Debatin JF. Total-body 3D magnetic resonance angiography influences the management of patients with peripheral arterial occlusive disease. Eur Radiol. 2006;16:685–91.

16. Ladd SC, Debatin JF, Stang A, Bromen K, Moebus S, Nuefer M, Gizewski E, Wanke I, Doerfler A, Ladd ME, Benemann J, Erbel R, Forsting M, Schmermund A, Jöckel K-H. Whole-body MR vascular screening detects unsuspected concomitant vascular disease in coronary heart disease patients. Eur Radiol. 2007;17:1035–45.

17. Waugh SA, Ramkumar PG, Gandy SJ, Nicholas RS, Martin P, Belch JJF, Struthers AD, Houston JG. Optimization of the contrast dose and injection rates in whole-body MR angiography at 3.0 T. J Magn Reson Imaging. 2009;30:1059–67.

18. Weir-McCall JR, Khan F, Lambert MA, Adamson CL, Gardner M, Gandy SJ, Ramkumar PG, Belch JJF, Struthers AD, Rauchhaus P, Morris AD, Houston JG. Common carotid intima media thickness and ankle-brachial pressure index correlate with local but not global atheroma burden: a cross sectional study using whole body magnetic resonance angiography. PLoS One. 2014;9:e99190.

19. Natori S, Lai S, Finn JP, Gomes AS, Hundley WG, Jerosch-Herold M, Pearson G, Sinha S, Arai A, Lima JAC, Bluemke DA. Cardiovascular function in multi-ethnic study of atherosclerosis: normal values by age, sex, and ethnicity. AJR Am J Roentgenol. 2006;186(6 Suppl 2):S357–65.

20. Cerqueira MD, Weissman NJ, Dilsizian V, Jacobs AK, Kaul S, Laskey WK, Pennell DJ, Rumberger JA, Ryan T, Verani MS. Standardized myocardial segmentation and nomenclature for tomographic imaging of the heart. A statement for healthcare professionals from the Cardiac Imaging Committee of the Council on Clinical Cardiology of the American Heart Association. Circulation. 2002;105:539–42.

21. The Academy of Medical Sciences. Realising the potential of stratified medicine. 2013.

22. Trusheim MR, Berndt ER, Douglas FL. Stratified medicine: strategic and economic implications of combining drugs and clinical biomarkers. Nat Rev Drug Discov. 2007;6:287–93.

23. Bhatt DL, Eagle K a, Ohman EM, Hirsch AT, Goto S, Mahoney EM, Wilson PWF, Alberts MJ, D'Agostino R, Liau C-S, Mas J-L, Röther J, Smith SC, Salette G, Contant CF, Massaro JM, Steg PG. Comparative determinants of 4-year cardiovascular event rates in stable outpatients at risk of or with atherothrombosis. JAMA. 2010;304:1350–7.

24. Steg PG, Bhatt DL, Wilson PWF, D'Agostino R, Ohman EM, Röther J, Liau C-S, Hirsch AT, Mas J-L, Ikeda Y, Pencina MJ, Goto S. One-year cardiovascular event rates in outpatients with atherothrombosis. JAMA. 2007;297:1197–206.

25. Bluemke D a, Kronmal R a, Lima J a C, Liu K, Olson J, Burke GL, Folsom AR. The relationship of left ventricular mass and geometry to incident cardiovascular events: the MESA (Multi-Ethnic Study of Atherosclerosis) study. J Am Coll Cardiol. 2008;52:2148–55.

26. Lind L, Andersson J, Hansen T, Johansson L, Ahlström H. Atherosclerosis measured by whole body magnetic resonance angiography and carotid artery ultrasound is related to arterial compliance, but not to endothelium-dependent vasodilation - the Prospective Investigation of the Vasculature in Uppsala Seniors (PIV. Clin Physiol Funct Imaging. 2009;29:321–9.

27. Laurent S, Cockcroft J, Van Bortel L, Boutouyrie P, Giannattasio C, Hayoz D, Pannier B, Vlachopoulos C, Wilkinson I, Struijker-Boudier H. Expert consensus document on arterial stiffness: methodological issues and clinical applications. Eur Heart J. 2006;27:2588–605.

28. Roghi A, Palmieri B, Crivellaro W, Faletra F, Puttini M. Relationship of unrecognised myocardial infarction, diabetes mellitus and type of surgery to postoperative cardiac outcomes in vascular surgery. Eur J Vasc Endovasc Surg. 2001;21:9–16.

29. Hertzer NR, Beven EG, Young JR, O'Hara PJ, Ruschhaupt WF, Graor RA, Dewolfe VG, Maljovec LC. Coronary artery disease in peripheral vascular patients. A classification of 1000 coronary angiograms and results of surgical management. Ann Surg. 1984;199:223–33.

30. Barbier CE, Bjerner T, Johansson L, Lind L, Ahlström H. Myocardial scars more frequent than expected: magnetic resonance imaging detects potential risk group. J Am Coll Cardiol. 2006;48:765–71.

31. Schelbert EB, Cao JJ, Sigurdsson S, Aspelund T, Kellman P, Aletras AH, Dyke CK, Thorgeirsson G, Eiriksdottir G, Launer LJ, Gudnason V, Harris TB, Arai AE. Prevalence and prognosis of unrecognized myocardial infarction determined by cardiac magnetic resonance in older adults. JAMA. 2012;308:890–6.

32. Barbier CE, Nylander R, Themudo R, Ahlström H, Lind L, Larsson E-M, Bjerner T, Johansson L. Prevalence of unrecognized myocardial infarction detected with magnetic resonance imaging and its relationship to cerebral ischemic lesions in both sexes. J Am Coll Cardiol. 2011;58:1372–7.

33. Ebeling Barbier C, Bjerner T, Hansen T, Andersson J, Lind L, Hulthe J, Johansson L, Ahlström H. Clinically unrecognized myocardial infarction detected at MR imaging may not be associated with atherosclerosis. Radiology. 2007;245:103–10.

34. Sheifer SE, Gersh BJ, Yanez ND, Ades PA, Burke GL, Manolio TA. Prevalence, predisposing factors, and prognosis of clinically unrecognized myocardial infarction in the elderly. J Am Coll Cardiol. 2000;35:119–26.

35. Erne P, Schoenenberger AW, Burckhardt D, Zuber M, Kiowski W, Buser PT, Dubach P, Resink TJ, Pfisterer M. Effects of percutaneous coronary interventions in silent ischemia after myocardial infarction: the SWISSI II randomized controlled trial. JAMA. 2007;297:1985–91.

36. Erne P, Schoenenberger AW, Zuber M, Burckhardt D, Kiowski W, Dubach P, Resink T, Pfisterer M. Effects of anti-ischaemic drug therapy in silent myocardial ischaemia type I: the Swiss Interventional Study on Silent Ischaemia type I (SWISSI I): a randomized, controlled pilot study. Eur Heart J. 2007;28:2110–7.

37. Faglia E, Manuela M, Antonella Q, Michela G, Vincenzo C, Maurizio C, Roberto M, Alberto M. Risk reduction of cardiac events by screening of unknown asymptomatic coronary artery disease in subjects with type 2 diabetes mellitus at high cardiovascular risk: an open-label randomized pilot study. Am Heart J. 2005;149:e1–6.

38. Hirsch AT, Criqui MH, Treat-Jacobson D, Regensteiner JG, Creager MA, Olin JW, Krook SH, Hunninghake DB, Comerota AJ, Walsh ME, McDermott MM, Hiatt WR. Peripheral arterial disease detection, awareness, and treatment in primary care. JAMA. 2001;286:1317–24.

39. Gassull D, Schulthess D, Suttie S, Houston G. Whole-Body Magnetic Resonance Angiography (WBMRA) as a tool for driving efficiency in the cost and treatment of Claudication Co-morbities. Heal Policy Technol. 2013;2:181–7.

15

Developing a nomogram based on multiparametric magnetic resonance imaging for forecasting high-grade prostate cancer to reduce unnecessary biopsies within the prostate-specific antigen gray zone

Xiang-ke Niu[1], Jun Li[2*], Susant Kumar Das[3], Yan Xiong[1], Chao-bing Yang[1] and Tao Peng[1]

Abstract

Background: Since 1980s the application of Prostate specific antigen (PSA) brought the revolution in prostate cancer diagnosis. However, it is important to underline that PSA is not the ideal screening tool due to its low specificity, which leads to the possible biopsy for the patient without High-grade prostate cancer (HGPCa). Therefore, the aim of this study was to establish a predictive nomogram for HGPCa in patients with PSA 4–10 ng/ml based on Prostate Imaging Reporting and Data System version 2 (PI-RADS v2), MRI-based prostate volume (PV), MRI-based PV-adjusted Prostate Specific Antigen Density (adjusted-PSAD) and other traditional classical parameters.

Methods: Between January 2014 and September 2015, Of 151 men who were eligible for analysis were formed the training cohort. A prediction model for HGPCa was built by using backward logistic regression and was presented on a nomogram. The prediction model was evaluated by a validation cohort between October 2015 and October 2016 ($n = 74$). The relationship between the nomogram-based risk-score as well as other parameters with Gleason score (GS) was evaluated. All patients underwent 12-core systematic biopsy and at least one core targeted biopsy with transrectal ultrasonographic guidance.

Results: The multivariate analysis revealed that patient age, PI-RADS v2 score and adjusted-PSAD were independent predictors for HGPCa. Logistic regression (LR) model had a larger AUC as compared with other parameters alone. The most discriminative cutoff value for LR model was 0.36, the sensitivity, specificity, positive predictive value and negative predictive value were 87.3, 78.4, 76.3, and 90.4%, respectively and the diagnostic performance measures retained similar values in the validation cohort (AUC 0.82 [95% CI, 0.76–0.89]). For all patients with HGPCa ($n = 50$), adjusted-PSAD and nomogram-based risk-score were positively correlated with the GS of HGPCa in PSA gray zone ($r = 0.455$, $P = 0.002$ and $r = 0.509$, $P = 0.001$, respectively).

Conclusion: The nomogram based on multiparametric magnetic resonance imaging (mp-MRI) for forecasting HGPCa is effective, which could reduce unnecessary prostate biopsies in patients with PSA 4–10 ng/ml and nomogram-based risk-score could provide a more robust parameter of assessing the aggressiveness of HGPCa in PSA gray zone.

Keywords: Prostate cancer, Prostate-specific antigen, Magnetic Resonance Imaging, PI-RADS, Nomogram

* Correspondence: niu051228@163.com
[2]Department of General Surgery, Affiliated Hospital of Chengdu University, No. 82 2nd North Section of Second Ring Road, Chengdu, Sichuan 610081, China
Full list of author information is available at the end of the article

Background

Prostate cancer (PCa) is the third leading cause of cancer death among men worldwide [1]. The introduction of prostate-specific antigen (PSA) in selecting men for prostate biopsy leads to earlier detection of prostate cancer (PCa) and, perhaps, a reduction in PCa-specific mortality [2]. However, there has been a steady rise in the detection of low-grade PCa (commonly referred to as over-diagnosis) and subsequent overtreatment [3]. This problem is attributable to the poor sensitivity and specificity profile of PSA. This is particularly the case in a PSA gray zone (4–10.0 ng/ml), at which 65–70% of men have a negative biopsy result [4]. Men with indolent disease who undergo treatment may experience complications without reducing their risk of dying from PCa [5].

Some PSA evolutional indexes are widely used clinically, such as free/total PSA ratio (PSA f/t ratio) and PSA density (PSAD). However, they are all provincial because of their dependence on PSA [6]. Furthermore, several other advanced attempts have been performed, such as 4 K score [7] and messenger RNA (mRNA) [8]. Though these models based on these new tests might be useful, the unavailable parameters limit the application. Nowadays, the growing availability of Multiparametric magnetic resonance imaging (mp-MRI) and increased standardisation has increased the role of prostate MRI in detecting of prostate cancer [9]. Prostate Imaging Reporting and Data System version 2 (PI-RADS v2), which was released online in the form of a 55-page document in December 2014, the overall five-point scale used in PI- RADS v2 is not designed for every cancer but for high-grade prostate cancer (HGPCa) that may require further work-up or target biopsy [10]. Therefore, the aim of this study was to develop a model combining prostate mp-MRI with traditional clinical risk factors that could be used to identify patients accurately with HGPCa (Gleason score $\geq$ 7) on reduction of unnecessary prostate biopsies in PSA gray zone.

Methods

Subjects

The retrospective study was approved by the regional ethical board of the Affiliated Hospital of Chengdu University. Informed written consent was obtained from all subjects prior to inclusion in the study. Inclusion criteria were suspicion of PCa owing to increased PSA levels combined with a suspicious abnormality at MR imaging eligible for target biopsy (TB) and available clinical data such as PSA level, DRE and TRUS results. Exclusion criteria were as follows: the patient had a history of prostate biopsy, the patient had benign prostatic hypertrophy treated with a 5a-reductase inhibitor, and the patient had a contraindication to transrectal US-guided biopsy (eg, anorectal stenosis). Two temporally separated patient cohorts were identified: January 2014 to September 2015 (training cohort) and October 2015 to October 2016 (validation cohort). In total, 225 consecutive patients with prebiopsy PSA between 4 ng/ml and 10 ng/ml were finally enrolled for evaluation.

MRI protocol

Subjects underwent mp-MRI using a 3.0 T MR imager (Tim Trio, Siemens Healthcare, Erlangen, Germany) with a six-channel phased-array body coil. To suppress bowel peristalsis all patients received 20 mg butylscopolamine (Buscopan; Boehringer, Ingelheim, Germany) intravenously. The main imaging protocols included high-resolution axial T2WI, DWI, and DCE-MRI. An axial fat saturation T2W turbo spin echo (TSE) sequence (TR/TE, 4000/100 ms; slice thickness, 3 mm; no interslice gap; echo train length, 23; averages, two; field of view [FOV], 200 × 200 mm) were acquired. Diffusion-weighted imaging (DWI) was acquired using a single-shot echoplanar imaging (EPI) sequence. The slice thickness was 3.0 mm with no intersection gap, matrix size 128 × 128, and the FOV 260 × 210 mm. The TR/TE 3700/80 ms, flip angle 90°, averages 6, with three b values of 0, 100, and 1000 s/mm^2 . ADC maps were then automatically generated on the basis of a voxelwise calculation. DCE was performed with a 3D spoiled gradient-echo sequence with TR/TE = 5/1.69 ms, flip-angle = 12°, FOV 260 × 260 mm, slice thickness was 3.0 mm with no interslice gap, temporal resolution = 5.7 s seconds, and 32 contrast-enhanced sets of images were acquired sequentially. The data acquisition of the dynamic contrast-enhanced images began simultaneously with the initiation of IV bolus administration of gadopentetate dimeglumine (Magnevist; Berlex, Wayne, NJ) at a flow rate of 4 ml/s, followed by a flush of 20 ml of saline solution.

Prostate volume estimation

The method for estimation of the total prostate volumes from T2-weighted MR images was reported previously [11] and the ITK-SNAP software (Penn Image Computing and Science Laboratory) was adapted for this manual correction task. Briefly, the entire prostate was semiautomatically segmented on T2-weighted MR images [12] and a radiologist (5 years experience in prostate MRI) reviewed and manually corrected the segmentation results, especially at the base and the apex of the prostate, to ensure accuracy. Finally, the adjusted-PSAD was calculated by dividing PSA concentration by the MR-based prostate volume.

MR image analysis

Two urogenital radiologists (3 and 5 years of experience, respectively, in prostate imaging) reviewed the images in consensus at a standard Picture Archive and Communication System (PACS) workstation ((Syngo, Siemens Healthcare, Erlangen, Germany). These two readers whom were blinded to initial mp-MR imaging reports and resultant clinical-pathologic outcomes, scored the examinations. The PI-RADS v2 scores were assessed on each of the sequences of T2WI, DWI, and DCE-MRI in turn to provide the overall PI-RADS v2 score [13]. If there were multiple lesions, the PI-RADS v2 score of the index lesion demonstrating the largest size or the most aggressive feature (i.e., extracapsular extension) was assigned to the patient.

Biopsy procedure and Histopathology

At time of biopsy, first, standardized 12-core transrectal US-guided systematic biopsy was performed by a urologist (who had 4 years of experience with prostate biopsy). Next, targeted biopsy was performed by same operator; these biopsies consisted of at least one additional core per target, the TB were using cognitive registration (cognitive TB [TB-COG]) on the basis of zonal anatomy or imaging landmarks (eg, cysts, remarkable nodules), which was described in a previously published studies [14, 15]. All biopsy cores were immediately fixed in formalin, stained with haematoxylin and eosin (H&E) and underwent routine histopathological evaluation. A Gleason score of ≥ 7 were defined as 'high-grade prostate cancer'.

Statistical analysis

As a primary analysis, we considered the statistical associations between the mp-MRI and clinical data with the binary outcome of HGPCa (present/absent). The data were presented as median (interquartile range) or mean (standard deviation), as appropriate. For comparison of continuous variables, the Welch t test was used or the Mann-Whitney-Wilcoxon test as a nonparametric alternative. A chi-square or Fisher exact test was applied to compare proportions.

Univariate and multivariate analyses were performed using logistic regression analysis to determine significant predictors of HGPCa. Odd ratios and 95% CIs were determined. The Hosmer-Lemeshow goodness-of-fit test was used to test the quality of the fitted model to the observed data, with a result of $p > 0.05$ considered a good fit. The area under the receiver operating characteristic curve was used to evaluate each predictor and how the model can allow discrimination between patients with and without HGPCa. Area under the curve (AUC) was compared against each other using the DeLong method to determine if a significant difference was present. The statistical analysis was performed using STATA version 9.0 (StataCorp LP, College Station, TX) and Medcalc 15.8 (Medcalc Software bvba, Ostend, Belgium). The nomogram was generated using the R software package (http://www.r-project.org/). An association between the nomogram-based risk-score as well as other parameters with Gleason score (GS) of HGPCa was tested by the Spearman rank correlation analysis. To further evaluate the model's performance, the nomogram-generated probability was calculated for every patient in the validation cohort then compared with pathology outcomes. A $p < 0.05$ was considered to indicate statistical significance.

Results

Patients demographics

For the training cohort, 67 patients (44%) were negative for PCa (benign lesions). Biopsy revealed high-grade PCa in 32 patients (21%) and low-grade PCa in 52 patients (35%). Gleason Score distribution of training cohort was as follows: $3 + 3 = 6$ (52 patients), $3 + 4 = 7$ (6 patients), $4 + 3 = 7$ (8 patients), $4 + 4 = 8$ (6 patients), $4 + 5 = 9$ (4 patients), $5 + 4 = 10$ (4 patients) and $5 + 5 = 10$ (4 patients). For the validation patient cohort, 36 of the 74 (48%) were classified as benign lesions. Biopsy revealed high-grade PCa in 18 patients (24%) and low-grade PCa in 20 patients (28%). Gleason Score distribution of validation cohort was as follows: $3 + 3 = 6$ (20 patients), $3 + 4 = 7$ (4 patients), $4 + 3 = 7$ (3 patients), $4 + 4 = 8$ (3 patients), $4 + 5 = 9$ (4 patients), $5 + 4 = 9$ (2 patients) and $5 + 5 = 9$ (2 patients). Patient characteristics are detailed in Table 1. The baseline characteristics showed no statistically significant differences between both cohorts.

Construction of LR model

The univariate logistic regression analysis showed that patient age, PSA f/t ratio, MRI-based PV, adjusted-PSAD, and PI-RADS v2 score were significant predictors of HGPCa in the training cohort. The multivariate logistic regression analysis revealed that the age, PI-RADS v2 score and adjusted-PSAD were independent predictors of HGPCa (Table 2). The cut-off value of the logit was determined based on the ROC curve in consideration of an appropriate tradeoff between the sensitivity and specificity. At the cut-off value of 0.36, i.e., the estimated present of HGPCa before biopsy in this cohort, sensitivity and specificity were 87.3% and 78.4%, respectively (Fig. 1). In addition, the results of the Hosmer-Lemeshow test, which showed a x^2 value of 2.19 ($p = 0.31$), indicated that the model is almost good fit. For all patients with HGPCa ($n = 50$), adjusted-PSAD and nomogram-based risk-score were positively correlated with the GS of HGPCa ($r = 0.455$, $P = 0.002$ and $r = 0.509$, $P = 0.001$, respectively), while other parameters found no correlation with GS of HGPCa (Fig. 2) in PSA gray zone.

Validation of LR model

The results of ROC-AUC analysis for training set, compare with other parameters are shown in Table 3. The highest AUC for a single risk factor is PI-RADS v2 score (AUC = 0.76). It is notable that in ROC curves, our new model had a larger AUC as compared with other parameters alone. A nomogram was developed using these three independent risk factors (patient age, PI-RADS v2

Table 1 Descriptive characteristics of the study population

Variable	Training cohort	Validation cohort	p value
Patients, n	151	74	NA
Age, yr, (median; IQR)	63.5; 65–74	64.9;62–73	0.26
tPSA, ng/ml, (median; IQR)	5.7; 4.8–6.7	5.3; 4.2–6.6	0.30
fPSA, ng/ml, (median; IQR)	1.12; 0.41–3.39	1.16; 0.32–4.17	0.21
PSA f/t, (median; IQR)	0.13; 0.06–0.44	0.17; 0.09–0.52	0.16
MRI-based PV, cm^3 (median; IQR)	46.2; 36.4–59.4	48.2; 33.7–58.1	0.32
Adjusted PSAD, ng/ml/cm3, mean (median; IQR)	0.17; 0.12–0.53	0.16; 0.06–0.47	0.71
DRE nodules yes/no, n (%)	86 (57) / 65 (43)	44 (59) / 30 (41)	0.46
TRUS, Hypoechoic (positive)/Isoechoic (negative)	81 (53) / 70 (47)	42 (56) / 32 (44)	0.56
PI-RADS v2 scores, mean (± SD)	3.3 (±0.9)	3.1 (±1.0)	0.50
Pathological outcomes, n (%)			
High-grade cancer	32 (21)	18 (24)	0.80
Low-grade cancer	52 (35)	20 (28)	
Benign	67 (44)	36 (48)	

IQR Interquartile range, *SD* Standard deviation, *NA* Not available, *PSA* Prostate-specific antigen, *MRI* Magnetic resonance imaging, *PV* Prostate volume, *PSAD* Prostate-specific antigen density, *DRE* Digital rectal examination, *TRUS* Transrectal ultrasound, *PI-RADS v2* Prostate Imaging Reporting and Data System version 2

score and adjusted-PSAD) to forecast HGPCa (Fig. 3). Sample case of the diagnostic use of the nomogram is given in Fig. 4. In validation set, the AUC of the classifier was 0.82 (95% CI, 0.76–0.89), the sensitivity 85.1% and the specificity 76.3%.

Discussion

In the PSA gray zone there is still the problem of how to separate the patients who have HGPCa from those who don't have it. The positive biopsy rate in the diagnostic gray zone of PSA 4–10 ng/ml has been shown to vary across different ethnic groups and countries [16]. In our study, we also proved that the performance of PSA in predicting HGPCa with PSA 4–10 ng/ml was poor (AUC = 0.54). Notably, in these kinds of patient groups up to 80% of biopsies were unnecessary, and therefore, a better risk prediction method specific to these patients is needed.

MRI became the method of choice for detection and staging of PCa [17]. In response, the European Society of

Table 2 Univariate and multivariate logistic regression analyses to detect clinically significant prostate cancer

Predictor	Univariate analysis		Multivariate analysis	
	OR (95% CI)	p value	OR (95% CI)	p value
Age	1.040 (0.893–2.089)	0.021	1.074 (1.008–1.243)	0.031
tPSA	0.040 (0.012–0.089)	0.238	NA	
fPSA	1.342 (0.712–1.993)	0.413	NA	
PSA f/t	1.772 (0.832–2.116)	0.043	NA NA NA	
MRI-based PV	1.112 (1.069–1.157)	0.011	NA	
Adjusted PSAD	6.433 (4.293–8.140)	<0.001	4.711 (3.704–6.313)	0.013
DRE results	0.547 (0.199–1.639)	0.078	NA	
TRUS results	0.961 (0.370–1.826)	0.069	NA	
PI-RADS v2 scores	3.231 (2.173–6.804)	<0.001	2.171 (1.345–3.504)	<0.001

OR odds ratio, *CI* confidence interval, *NA* Not available, *PSA* Prostate-specific antigen, *MRI* Magnetic resonance imaging, *PV* Prostate volume, *PSAD* Prostate-specific antigen density, *DRE* Digital rectal examination, *TRUS* Transrectal ultrasound, *PI-RADS v2* Prostate Imaging Reporting and Data System version 2

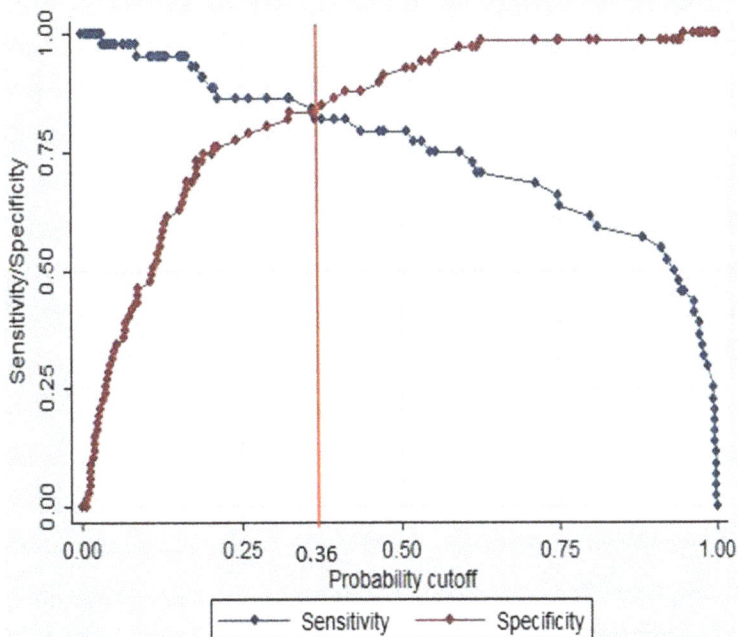

Fig. 1 Plot of sensitivity and specificity for logistic regression model. Plot of sensitivity (*red line*) and specificity (*blue line*) as a function of the probability cut points obtained from the logistic model for diagnosising of high-grade prostate cancer. The optimal probability cutoff point was determined to be 0.36

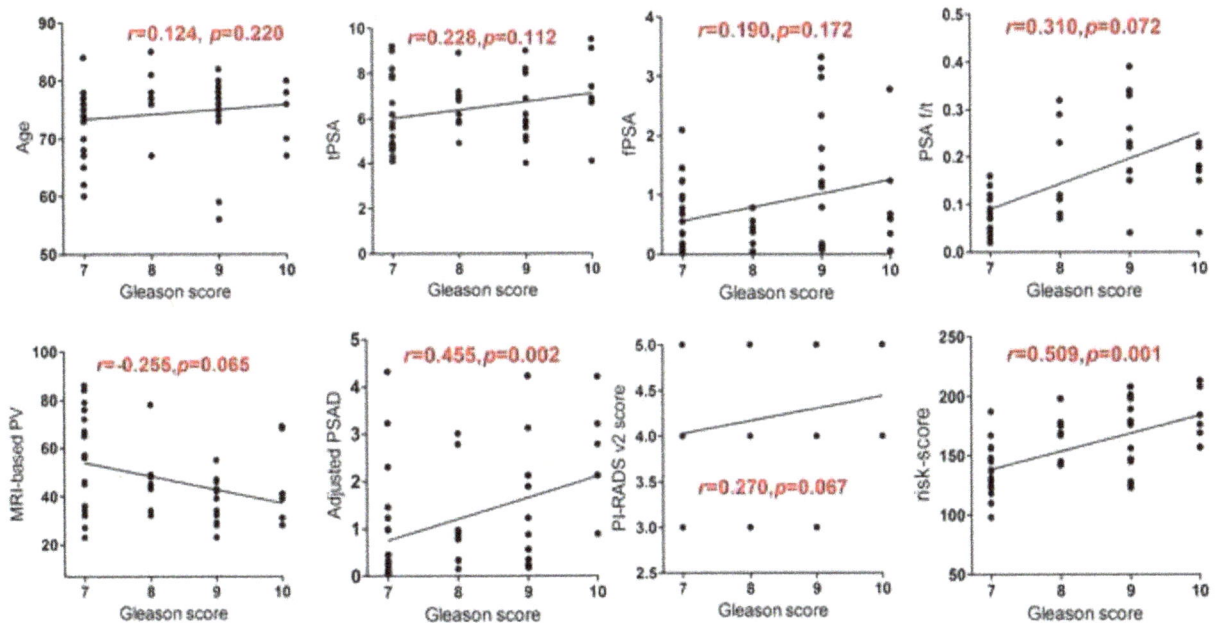

Fig. 2 Relationship between all parameters and Gleason scores. Statistically positive correlation were observed between adjusted-PSAD, nomogram-based risk-score with the GS of HGPCa ($r = 0.455$, $P = 0.002$ and $r = 0.509$, $P = 0.001$, respectively), while other parameters found no correlation with GS of HGPCa in PSA gray zone

Table 3 Diagnostic performance of the LR model with other parameters for predicting high grade prostate cancer

Predictor	Area under the Curve (95% CI)	Threshold	Sensitivity (%)	Specificity (%)	PPV	NPV	p value
LR model	0.85 (0.79–0.90)	>0.36	87.3	78.4	76.3	90.4	(–)
Age (year)	0.63 (0.50–0.67)	>71.2	72.7	59.4	58.4	73.4	<0.001
tPSA (ng/ml)	0.54 (0.48–0.67)	>7.4	61.2	52.9	51.3	63.5	<0.001
fPSA (ng/ml)	0.52 (0.51–0.69)	>2.1	61.7	60.4	59.4	63.4	<0.001
PSA f/t	0.66 (0.61–0.74)	>0.18	61.1	69.9	59.2	72.9	<0.001
MRI-based PV (cm^3)	0.64 (0.54–0.72)	<39.4	70.1	60.9	58.8	72.2	<0.001
Adjusted PSAD (ng/ml/cm^3)	0.74 (0.66–0.79)	>0.16	77.2	60.3	59.3	78.6	0.013
DRE results	0.61 (0.57–0.72)	NA	65.3	59.4	61.5	67.3	<0.001
TRUS results	0.54 (0.51–0.64)	NA	64.1	53.9	51.2	67.9	<0.001
PI-RADS v2 scores	0.76 (0.71–0.84)	>3	78.5	74.2	72.8	79.2	0.018

LR Logistic regression, *PSA* prostate-specific antigen, *MRI* Magnetic resonance imaging, *PV* Prostate volume, *PSAD* Prostate-specific antigen density, *DRE* Digital rectal examination, *TRUS* transrectal ultrasound, *PI-RADS v2* Prostate Imaging Reporting and Data System version 2, *PPV* Positive predictive value, *NPV* Negative predictive value

Urogenital Radiology (ESUR) drafted guidelines, which have been updated to the PI-RADS v2 recently, by a steering committee including the American College of Radiology (ACR), ESUR and the AdMeTech Foundation [18]. This version assesses the likelihood (probability) of HGPCa and maybe useful for suggesting appropriate patients to active surveillance on a 5-point scale [19]. A meta-analysis that assessed the performance of mp-MRI for detecting prostate cancer demonstrated specificity of 0.88 (95% CI, 0.82–0.92), sensitivity of 0.74 (95% CI, 0.66–0.81) and NPV of 0.64–0.94 [20]. Park et al. [10] reported that the use of PI-RADS v2 might help pre-operatively diagnose HGPCa (Sensitivity and specificity were 77.0 and 73.8%, respectively), while, Washino et al. [21] reported that although the PI-RADS score predicts biopsy outcome well, it is difficult to decide which patients

can avoid unnecessary prostate biopsies using only the PI-RADS score because of the relatively low PPV.

Through the result of these studies, a model was developed combining PI-RADS v2 score, PSA level, MRI-based PV, adjusted-PSAD, and PSA-related evolutional markers with other independent risk factors, such as age, DRE and TRUS results, into one logistic regression model. The present study shows the AUC of ROC curve for each univariate variable in predicting a biopsy results. PI-RADS v2 score were relatively more important for forecasting HGPCa and were a significant predictor for HGPCa. Compared with PI-RADS v2 score and adjusted-PSAD alone, our newly developed model enlarged AUC from 0.76, 0.74 to 0.85 separately, showing the accuracy for predicting HGPCa was substantially improved. Notably, Given high NPV (90.4%) in this present study, that is

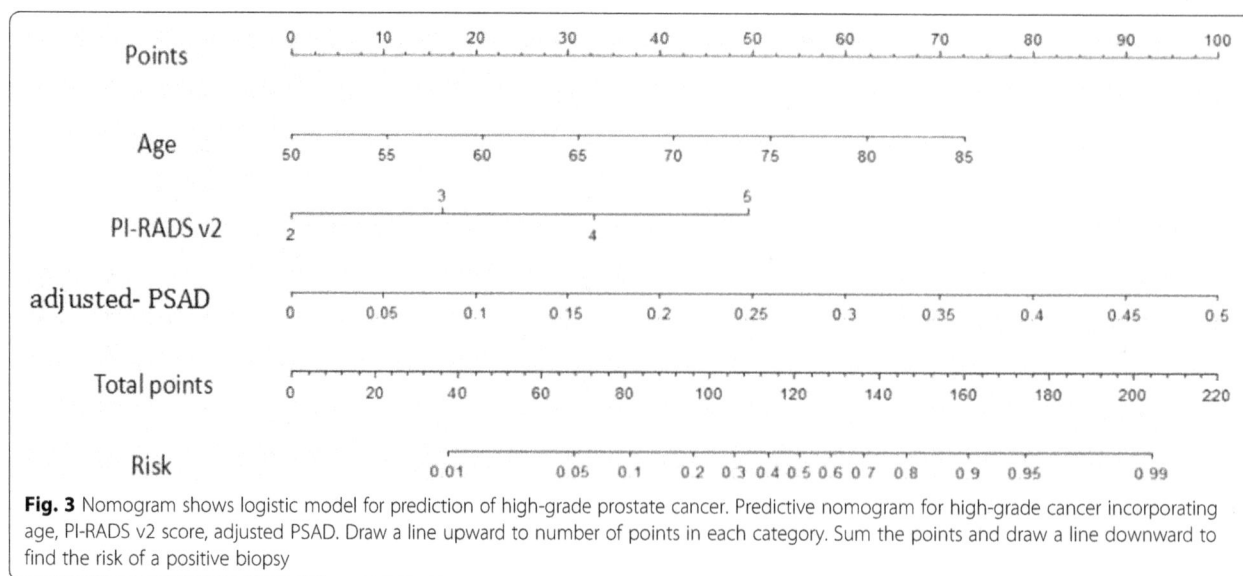

Fig. 3 Nomogram shows logistic model for prediction of high-grade prostate cancer. Predictive nomogram for high-grade cancer incorporating age, PI-RADS v2 score, adjusted PSAD. Draw a line upward to number of points in each category. Sum the points and draw a line downward to find the risk of a positive biopsy

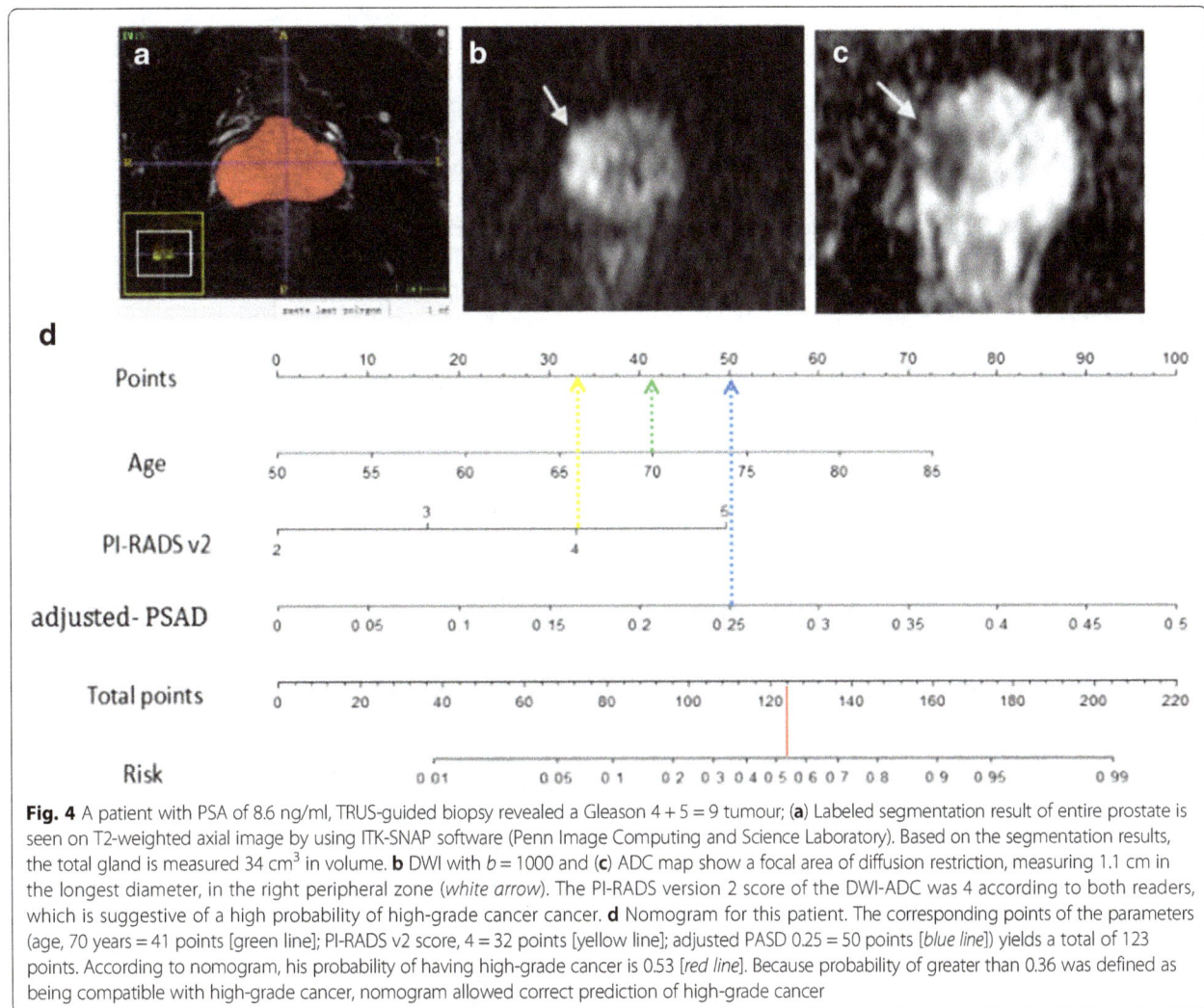

Fig. 4 A patient with PSA of 8.6 ng/ml, TRUS-guided biopsy revealed a Gleason 4 + 5 = 9 tumour; (**a**) Labeled segmentation result of entire prostate is seen on T2-weighted axial image by using ITK-SNAP software (Penn Image Computing and Science Laboratory). Based on the segmentation results, the total gland is measured 34 cm³ in volume. **b** DWI with $b = 1000$ and (**c**) ADC map show a focal area of diffusion restriction, measuring 1.1 cm in the longest diameter, in the right peripheral zone (*white arrow*). The PI-RADS version 2 score of the DWI-ADC was 4 according to both readers, which is suggestive of a high probability of high-grade cancer cancer. **d** Nomogram for this patient. The corresponding points of the parameters (age, 70 years = 41 points [green line]; PI-RADS v2 score, 4 = 32 points [yellow line]; adjusted PASD 0.25 = 50 points [*blue line*]) yields a total of 123 points. According to nomogram, his probability of having high-grade cancer is 0.53 [*red line*]. Because probability of greater than 0.36 was defined as being compatible with high-grade cancer, nomogram allowed correct prediction of high-grade cancer

to say if the patient's LR model risk rate blow 0.36, it could be used to reliably rule out HGPCa, obviating the biopsy procedure.

PSA-related evolutional markers including tPSA, PSA f/t ratio are not sufficiently reliable to allow clinical decision making in individual patients [22], which comparable with our results (AUC for PSA f/t ratio was 0.66). The justification for PSAD evaluation was elaborated in some previous study, where it was stated that such marker is better predictor for PCa then PSA level particularly with 4–10 ng/ml [23, 24]. In contrast, our adjusted-PSAD has higher AUC than previous studies. Traditionally, PSA "density," whereby the PSA value is divided by the prostate volume, estimated from either DRE or TRUS. MRI provides soft-tissue contrast resolution superior to that of transrectal ultrasound so that it can be used for more accurate estimation of prostate volume [25, 26]. Therefore, it is not surprising that the adjusted-PSAD increased the predictive ability of HGPCa and also became a significant predictor for HGPCa.

In current study, although our developed new LR model has achieved high diagnostic performance in detection of HGPCa, the source of false positive and false negative errors should be addressed. Lesion located in PZ, especially central zone (CZ) may not be optimally evaluated using current PZ and TZ criteria. Also, because the CZ commonly exhibits restricted diffusion that is similar in extent to that of tumors, that may potentially yield false-positive or false-negative results. The PZ in men with diffuse prostatitis or marked BPH often exhibits diffusely altered signal characteristics on various sequences, which may pose a diagnostic challenge and yield more false-positive or false-negative results. Furthermore, one particular aspect of PI-RADS v2 for which we have noted particular variability in reader interpretations is scoring of DCE-MRI in PZ of prostate lesions. For example, what exactly constitutes early enhancement and enhancement that is focal and that matches an abnormality on other sequences is unclear. Therefore, once PI-RADS v2 can be applied in a consistent fashion across practices, the system will provide a powerful mechanism for accumulating multicenter data to optimally address these false positive and false negative errors that may change current paradigms for prostate cancer management.

A higher AUC of 0.90 (95% CI, 0.83–0.96) was reported by a study combining traditional clinical risk factors and mRNA levels (HOXC6 and DLX1) to derive a logistic regression model based on a large sample ($n = 905$) [8]. However, to date, only a few biomarkers have reached clinical practice. The main challenge is to validate the performance of the biomarkers in a clinical cohort independently and to demonstrate the clinical utility clearly [27]. Fang et al. [28] developed a 'PAMD' score which based on mp-MRI to categorize patients into three risk groups, and the model showed good predictive accuracy for HGPCa (AUC = 0.824). In their study, the prostate volume was determined by TRUS, and the results was not proved by validation cohort.

Histopathologically, the Gleason grading correlates with patient outcome, with higher Gleason scores (GS) indicating more aggressive PCa [29]. Albertsen et al. [30] showed that men with Gleason score (GS) 8–10 PCa have a relatively high probability of dying from PCa within 10 year (12.1%), whereas this risk is minimal for men with low-grade disease. Therefore, we need to predict tumor aggressiveness non-invasively. Litjens et al. [31] found that use of a normalized ADC significantly improved diagnostic accuracy and prediction of cancer aggressiveness, but their assessment was limited to PZ tumors. The results of this study have demonstrated that patients with HGPCa ($n = 50$), the adjusted-PSAD and nomogram-based risk-score were positively correlated with the GS of HGPCa ($r = 0.455$, $P = 0.002$ and $r = 0.509$, $P = 0.001$, respectively). An accurate noninvasive means of both detecting and potentially grading tumors is appealing as a way to enable more-accurate risk stratification of patients, particularly if different treatment options, such as radical prostatectomy or focal therapy, are being considered. In this regard, our results could provide new tool for predicting the aggressiveness of HGPCa before biopsy procedure, especially, nomogram-based risk-score shows relatively strong correlation with GS of HGPCa in PSA gray zone.

Recently, computer-based medical decision support systems have been applied to clinical use for medical diagnosis, decisions, and patient care. Several models—nomograms, risk groupings, artificial neural networks, support vector machines —have been developed to help predict a positive prostate biopsy in men being evaluated for prostate cancer. Nomograms, artificial neural networks and support vector machines improved the accuracy of prediction compared with the individual factors alone. Nomograms are perfect examples of a predictive application that allows a graphical representation of variable interactions and a depiction of their combined effects. Shariat et al. [32] reported that the nomograms have the highest accuracy and the best discriminating characteristics for predicting outcomes in prostate cancer patients.

Patients whose cancer is not clinically significant may be assigned to active surveillance (the lesion is monitored frequently for signs of progression) instead of treatment. In our clinical practice, there is also great potential benefit in the use of mp-MRI for monitoring AS rather than biopsies. As the process of mp-MRI becomes less invasive, greater acceptance amongst patients may follow. Furthermore, with the reliability of mp-MRI to image the entire prostate, it is feasible that patients will feel further reassured that they did not miss any high-grade cancer.

We acknowledge the following limitations. As with any retrospective study, there is risk for selection bias. On mp-MRI we analysed the index lesion, defined as the largest most likely to be cancerous area, this might have been a source of bias in our results. In addition, as mentioned previously, we haven't compare our new model with other classifiers (e.g., ANN and SVM) in the present study. Finally, our model has not been performed in an external dataset and requires to be tested and verified in more centers with larger samples.

Conclusion

This study found that the nomogram based mp-MRI for forecasting HGPCa is effective, which could reduce unnecessary prostate biopsies in patients with PSA 4–10 ng/ml and nomogram-based risk-score could provide a more robust parameter of assessing the aggressiveness of HGPCa in PSA gray zone. Future research might indicate that additional parameters could further optimize the diagnosis of HGPCa without contributing to the high unnecessary biopsy rate.

Abbreviations

ACR: American College of Radiology; ADC: Apparent diffusion coefficient; AUC: Area under the curve; DCE: Dynamic contrast-enhanced imaging; DRE: Digital rectal examination; DWI: Diffusion weighted imaging; ESUR: European Society of Urogenital Radiology; HGPCa: High-grade prostate cancer; LR: Logistic regression; mp-MRI: Multi-parametric magnetic resonance imaging; MRI: Magnetic resonance imaging; PCa: Prostate cancer; PI-RADS v2: Prostate Imaging Reporting and Data System version 2; PSA: Prostate-specific antigen; PSAD: Prostate-specific antigen density; PV: Prostate volume; ROC: Receiver operating characteristic; T2WI: T2 weighted imaging; TB: Target biopsy; US: Ultra-sonographic

Acknowledgements

We would like to thank radiologist Yang hanfeng of the Department of Radiology, the Affiliated Hospital of Nanchong Medical college, for contributing with expert statistical advice.

Funding

Health and Family planing Commission of Chengdu (Sichuan, china) (grant 2015080) and Youth Innovation Research Fund of Sichuan Medicine (grant Q14004).

Authors' contributions

LJ carried out the conception and design, revised the manuscript, and approved the final version to be published. NXK carried out the design and acquisition of data, analysis and interpretation of data. Das SK participated in the conception and design, drafted and revised the manuscrip. XY participated in the design of the study and performed the statistical analysis. YCB conceived of the study, participated in its design and coordination. PT acquisition of data. All authors read and approved the final manuscript.

Competing interests

The authors declare that they have no competing interests.

Author details

[1]Department of Radiology, Affiliated Hospital of Chengdu University, Chengdu 610081, China. [2]Department of General Surgery, Affiliated Hospital of Chengdu University, No. 82 2nd North Section of Second Ring Road, Chengdu, Sichuan 610081, China. [3]Department of Intervention Radiology, Tenth People's Hospital of Tongji University, Shanghai 200072, China.

References

1. Jemal A, Siegel R, Xu J, Ward E. Cancer statistics, 2010. CA Cancer J Clin. 2010;60:277–300.
2. Schröder FH, Hugosson J, Roobol MJ, et al. Prostate-cancer mortality at 11 years of follow-up. N Engl J Med. 2012;366:981–90.
3. Etzioni R, Penson DF, Legler JM, et al. Overdiagnosis due to prostate-specific antigen screening: lessons from U.S. prostate cancer incidence trends. J Natl Cancer Inst. 2002;94:981–90.
4. Draisma G, Etzioni R, Tsodikov A, et al. Lead time and overdiagnosis in prostate-specific antigen screening: importance of methods and context. J Natl Cancer Inst. 2009;101(6):374–83.
5. Thompson IM, Ankerst DP, Chi C, et al. Operating characteristics of prostate-specific antigen in men with an initial PSA level of 3.0 ng/ml or lower. JAMA. 2005;294:66–70.
6. Vickers AJ, Savage C, O'Brien MF, Lilja H. Systematic review of pretreatment prostate-specific antigen velocity and doubling time as predictors for prostate cancer. J Clin Oncol. 2009;27:398–403.
7. McDonald ML, Parsons JK. 4-Kallikrein test and Kallikrein markers in prostate cancer screening. Urol Clin North Am. 2016;43:39–46.
8. Van Neste L, Hendriks RJ, Dijkstra S, et al. Detection of high-grade prostate cancer using a urinary molecular biomarker-based risk score. Eur Urol. 2016;70:740–8.
9. Junker D, Quentin M, Nagele U, et al. Evaluation of the PI-RADS scoring system for mpMRI of the prostate: a whole-mount step-section analysis. World J Urol. 2015;33:1023–30.
10. Park SY, Jung DC, Oh YT, et al. Prostate cancer: PI-RADS version 2 helps preoperatively predict clinically significant cancers. Radiology. 2016;280:108–16.
11. Karademir I, Shen D, Peng Y, et al. Prostate volumes derived from MRI and volume-adjusted serum prostate-specific antigen: correlation with Gleason score of prostate cancer. AJR Am J Roentgenol. 2013;201:1041–8.
12. Liao S, Gao Y, Lian J, Shen D. Sparse patch-based label propagation for accurate prostate localization in CT images. IEEE Trans Med Imaging. 2013;32:419–34.
13. Barrett T, Turkbey B, Choyke PL. PI-RADS version 2: what you need to know. Clin Radiol. 2015;70:1165–76.
14. Puech P, Rouvière O, Renard-Penna R, et al. Prostate cancer diagnosis: multiparametric MR-targeted biopsy with cognitive and transrectal US-MR fusion guidance versus systematic biopsy–prospective multicenter study. Radiology. 2013;268:461–9.
15. Costa DN, Bloch BN, Yao DF, et al. Diagnosis of relevant prostate cancer using supplementary cores from magnetic resonance imaging-prompted areas following multiple failed biopsies. Magn Reson Imaging. 2013;31:947–52.
16. Vickers AJ, Cronin AM, Roobol MJ, et al. The relationship between prostate-specific antigen and prostate cancer risk: the Prostate Biopsy Collaborative Group. Clin Cancer Res. 2010;16:4374–81.
17. Villers A, Lemaitre L, Haffner J, Puech P. Current status of MRI for the diagnosis, staging and prognosis of prostate cancer: implications for focal therapy and active surveillance. Curr Opin Urol. 2009;19:274–82.
18. Barentsz JO, Weinreb JC, Verma S, et al. Synopsis of the PI-RADS v2 guidelines for multiparametric prostate magnetic resonance imaging and recommendations for use. Eur Urol. 2016;69:41–9.
19. Woo S, Kim SY, Lee J, Kim SH, Cho JY. PI-RADS version 2 for prediction of pathological downgrading after radical prostatectomy: a preliminary study in patients with biopsy-proven Gleason Score 7 (3 + 4) prostate cancer. Eur Radiol. 2016;26:3580–7.
20. de Rooij M, Hamoen EH, Fütterer JJ, Barentsz JO, Rovers MM. Accuracy of multiparametric MRI for prostate cancer detection: a meta-analysis. AJR Am J Roentgenol. 2014;202:343–51.
21. Washino S, Okochi T, Saito K, et al. Combination of prostate imaging reporting and data system (PI-RADS) score and prostate-specific antigen (PSA) density predicts biopsy outcome in prostate biopsy naïve patients. BJU Int. 2017;119:225–33.
22. Tombal B, Querton M, de Nayer P, et al. Free/total PSA ratio does not improve prediction of pathologic stage and biochemical recurrence after radical prostatectomy. Urology. 2002;59:256–60.
23. Saema A, Kochakarn W, Lertsithichai P. PSA density and prostate cancer detection. J Med Assoc Thai. 2012;95:661–6.
24. Zheng XY, Xie LP, Wang YY, et al. The use of prostate specific antigen (PSA) density in detecting prostate cancer in Chinese men with PSA levels of 4–10 ng/mL. J Cancer Res Clin Oncol. 2008;134:1207–10.
25. Lee JS, Chung BH. Transrectal ultrasound versus magnetic resonance imaging in the estimation of prostate volume as compared with radical prostatectomy specimens. Urol Int. 2007;78:323–7.
26. Jeong CW, Park HK, Hong SK, Byun SS, Lee HJ, Lee SE. Comparison of prostate volume measured by transrectal ultrasonography and MRI with the actual prostate volume measured after radical prostatectomy. Urol Int. 2008;81:179–85.
27. Hendriks RJ, Dijkstra S, Jannink SA, et al. Comparative analysis of prostate cancer specific biomarkers PCA3 and ERG in whole urine, urinary sediments and exosomes. Clin Chem Lab Med. 2016;54:483–92.
28. Fang D, Ren D, Zhao C, et al. Prevalence and risk factors of prostate cancer in Chinese Men with PSA 4–10 ng/mL Who underwent TRUS-guided prostate biopsy: the utilization of PAMD score. Biomed Res Int. 2015;2015:596797.
29. Epstein JI. An update of the Gleason grading system. J Urol. 2010;183:433–40.
30. Albertsen PC, Hanley JA, Fine J. 20-year outcomes following conservative management of clinically localized prostate cancer. JAMA. 2005;293:2095–101.
31. Litjens GJ, Hambrock T, Hulsbergen-van de Kaa C, Barentsz JO, Huisman HJ. Interpatient variation in normal peripheral zone apparent diffusion coefficient: effect on the prediction of prostate cancer aggressiveness. Radiology. 2012;265:260–6.
32. Shariat SF, Karakiewicz PI, Suardi N, Kattan MW. Comparison of nomograms with other methods for predicting outcomes in prostate cancer: a critical analysis of the literature. Clin Cancer Res. 2008;14:4400–7.

16

Phase-contrast MRI volume flow – a comparison of breath held and navigator based acquisitions

Charlotta Andersson[1,2], Johan Kihlberg[1,3], Tino Ebbers[1], Lena Lindström[2], Carl-Johan Carlhäll[1,4,5] and Jan E. Engvall[1,4,5*]

Abstract

Background: Magnetic Resonance Imaging (MRI) 2D phase-contrast flow measurement has been regarded as the gold standard in blood flow measurements and can be performed with free breathing or breath held techniques. We hypothesized that the accuracy of flow measurements obtained with segmented phase-contrast during breath holding, and in particular higher number of k-space segments, would be non-inferior compared to navigator phase-contrast. Volumes obtained from anatomic segmentation of cine MRI and Doppler echocardiography were used for additional reference.

Methods: Forty patients, five women and 35 men, mean age 65 years (range 53–80), were randomly selected and consented to the study. All underwent EKG-gated cardiac MRI including breath hold cine, navigator based free-breathing phase-contrast MRI and breath hold phase-contrast MRI using k-space segmentation factors 3 and 5, as well as transthoracic echocardiography within 2 days.

Results: In navigator based free-breathing phase-contrast flow, mean stroke volume and cardiac output were 79.7 ± 17.1 ml and 5071 ± 1192 ml/min, respectively. The duration of the acquisition was 50 ± 6 s. With k-space segmentation factor 3, the corresponding values were 77.7 ml ± 17.5 ml and 4979 ± 1211 ml/min ($p = 0.15$ vs navigator). The duration of the breath hold was 17 ± 2 s. K-space segmentation factor 5 gave mean stroke volume 77.9 ± 16.4 ml, cardiac output 5142 ± 1197 ml/min ($p = 0.33$ vs navigator), and breath hold time 11 ± 1 s. Anatomical segmentation of cine gave mean stroke volume and cardiac output 91.2 ± 20.8 ml and 5963 ± 1452 ml/min, respectively. Echocardiography was reliable in 20 of the 40 patients. The mean diameter of the left ventricular outflow tract was 20.7 ± 1.5 mm, stroke volume 78.3 ml ± 15.2 ml and cardiac output 5164 ± 1249 ml/min.

Conclusions: In forty consecutive patients with coronary heart disease, breath holding and segmented k-space sampling techniques for phase-contrast flow produced stroke volumes and cardiac outputs similar to those obtained with free-breathing navigator based phase-contrast MRI, using less time. The values obtained agreed fairly well with Doppler echocardiography while there was a larger difference when compared with anatomical volume determinations using SSFP (steady state free precession) cine MRI.

Keywords: Phase-contrast flow, Magnetic resonance imaging, Segmentation, 2D Doppler echocardiography

* Correspondence: jan.engvall@regionostergotland.se
[1]Center for Medical Image Science and Visualization, Linkoping University, SE-581 83 Linkoping, Sweden
[4]Department of Medical and Health Sciences, Linkoping University, SE-581 83 Linkoping, Sweden
Full list of author information is available at the end of the article

Background

The generation of cardiovascular flow has been said to be the essence of cardiology [1]. Unfortunately, in clinical practice, the applicability of methods used to determine flow may be restricted by the pre-existing condition of the patient. Various techniques have been favoured and later abandoned such as indicator dilution with indocyanine green, while others, e.g. thermodilution, have withstood the test of time. Completely non-invasive determination of stroke volume with echocardiography and Doppler recording is versatile and readily available at the bedside, but the calculation rests on a number of assumptions such as a circular geometry of the left ventricular outflow tract [2] and a spatially flat flow profile [3]. MRI phase-contrast flow measurement has been regarded as the gold standard since it can address issues of temporally as well as spatially varying flows [4, 5]. However, MRI velocity measurements are sensitive to magnetic field inhomogeneities, concomitant gradient effects, and eddy current effects that are only partly compensated for [6]. Gatehouse suggested that an error of 5 % could be acceptable in clinical practice, which would be equivalent to 4 ml when the stroke volume is 80 ml and 250 ml when cardiac output is 5000 ml/min [7]. Previous work has suggested that the size of the great vessels is the most important factor that determines baseline phase offset [8]. Furthermore, MRI collects flow data from several heart beats and cannot measure beat-by-beat variation, except when using techniques of reduced sampling such as the pencil beam technique for real-time flow velocity [9]. In busy daily practice, sampling is performed during a short breath hold that may introduce some errors due to physiological effects on cardiac filling and effects of averaging when using segmented k-space sampling methods [10–12]. The extent of these effects is influenced by the length of the breath holding, which in its turn depends on heart rate and scanner settings. To avoid the physiological effects of holding breath, the obvious alternative would be sampling during free breathing [13]. However, due to a longer sampling time, this will add a component of temporal averaging.

Patients are at times dyspnoeic and are frequently limited in their capacity to hold their breath which would favour the use of the free breathing technique or an alternative with the shortest breath hold. Since there is no agreement on which MRI phase-contrast technique to prefer, we hypothesized that the accuracy of volume flow measurements obtained with segmented phase-contrast during breath holding, and in particular higher number of k-space segments, would be non-inferior compared to navigator phase-contrast which has potential to become a standard of reference. Volumes obtained from anatomic segmentation of cine MRI and Doppler echocardiography were used for additional reference.

Methods

Forty patients, five women and 35 men, mean age 65 years (range 53–80), were randomly selected and gave written consent to the study (Table 1), which was approved by the Regional Ethics Committee in Linkoping, Dnr M216-09. All were part of the Doppler-cip study and had undergone a cardiac MRI scan and a transthoracic Doppler echocardiography within 2 days [14, 15]. MRI was performed with a Philips Achieva Nova Dual R 3.2, 1.5 T system, with a 5-element phased array cardiac coil (Philips Healthcare, Best, the Netherlands) and Doppler echocardiography with a GE Vivid 7 ultrasound scanner (GE Healthcare, Horten, Norway).

The MR flow slice was positioned transverse to the ascending aorta cranial to the sino-tubular junction where the flow is parallel to the long-axis of the body in order to obtain through-plane flow perpendicular to the slice. The acquisition was retrospectively gated to the EKG using the following parameters: slice thickness 8 mm, field of view (FOV) 320 × 260 mm, acquisition matrix 128 × 104 (reconstructed to 256 × 256), sensitivity encoding (SENSE) factor 2, velocity encoding 200 cm/s, repetition time 4.6 ms and echo time 2.7 ms. The effect on scan duration of using three different k-space segmentation factors (TFE) was studied. Scans with TFE factor of 5 and 3 were acquired in breath hold while free breathing with navigator triggering (6 mm gate and track window, continuous level drift) was used for TFE 1. The number of reconstructed cardiac phases was adjusted to the heart rate and k-space segmentation factor, e.g. from 16 (at TFE 5 and 80 beats/min) to 80 (at TFE 1 and 40 beats/min). Depending on the heart rate, the duration of breath holding could vary between 9 s (TFE 5, 80 beats/min) up to 28 s (TFE 3, 40 beats/min). The navigator scan took from 42 s (TFE 1, 80 beats/min) to 1:24 min (TFE 1, 40 beats/min). All velocity data was corrected for concomitant gradient effects on the scanner as suggested by Bernstein et al [16]. Background offset due to eddy current effects was corrected on the scanner by using the default local phase correction algorithm, which

Table 1 Demographic data for the patients in the study

Demographic data	Age, mean (SD), years	65 (7)
	Female, n (%)	6 (15)
	Body mass index, mean (SD) kg/m2	26.5 (3.7)
Medical history	Diabetes, n (%)	8 (20)
	Hypertension, n (%)	14 (35)
	Myocardial infarction, n (%)	22 (55)
	CABG, n (%)	9 (23)
	PCI, n (%)	18 (45)
	Moderate MR (1) or AR (1) at Doppler	6 (15)

Table 2 Stroke volume and cardiac output results

	Stroke volume (ml)	Scan duration (s)	Heart rate (beats/min)	Cardiac output (ml/min)
Cine segmented	91.2 +/− 20.8		66 +/− 8.8	5964 +/− 1452
Phase contrast TF5	77.9 +/− 16.4	11 +/− 1	66 +/− 9.4	5142 +/− 1197
Phase contrast TFS	77.7 +/− 17.5	17 +/− 2	64 +/− 8.6	4979 +/− 1211
Phase contrast (navigator)	79.7 +/− 17.1	50 +/− 6	64 +/− 7.8	5071 +/− 1192

Mean value and SD (standard deviation) for stroke volume and cardiac output for anatomical calculation from cine MRI and the three phase-contrast techniques

is based on an optimized spatial low pass filter (Philips Healthcare internal white paper April 12, 2012).

In addition to flow, anatomical volume measurements were performed on cine SSFP short axis images covering the left ventricle from base to apex. Slice thickness was 8 mm and slice gap 2 mm. Temporal resolution ranged between 26 and 41 ms (30 acquired phases).

Data analysis was performed on a separate workstation using software from the vendor (Philips Extended MR Workspace, version 2.6.6.3). For flow measurements, an elliptical template covering the aortic perimeter was applied and adapted to the vessel using an active contour-seeking algorithm. After manual correction, the segmentation was migrated to adjacent time frames using the active contour-seeking algorithm until the entire cardiac cycle was covered. Manual corrections were applied whenever necessary. The volume flow was calculated by temporal integration of the velocities within the segmented area, using the antegrade flow component (all forward flow components in the entire heart cycle, without deducting backward flow components) to facilitate a comparison with Doppler echocardiography and cine MRI. Cardiac output was computed as stroke volume multiplied with heart rate. Differences in heart rate between the three flow acquisitions were calculated and the largest individual difference averaged between all patients.

Anatomical MRI-based stroke volume was determined by manually segmenting the stack of short axis images of the left ventricle, in end diastole as well as in end systole. End systole was determined from the smallest ventricular area of a mid-ventricular slice, or, in case of dyssynchrony, from the time point closest to end systole determined from aortic closure in the apical long axis view [17]. The papillary muscles were included in the volume of the left ventricular cavity and the outflow tract was excluded [17]. The measurements were done in duplicate and the mean value was used in the comparisons. The duplicate measurements were used to report intraobserver reproducibility. Interobserver variability was reported from ten studies segmented by a second observer. Further data on reproducibility have been published elsewhere [14].

All patients underwent Doppler echocardiography. Stroke volume was calculated from the area of the left ventricular outflow tract (LVOT), determined from the inner-edge to inner-edge diameter according to recommendations from the European Association of Cardiovascular Imaging [2], and multiplied with the velocity time integral (VTI) determined at the level of the diameter measurement but not requiring the presence of a valve opening artefact. Pulmonary shadowing preventing the delineation of the LVOT was considered a criterion for excluding the measurement as well as excessive VTI due to placement of the sample volume in the aortic annulus. Since the echocardiogram typically was performed two days after the MRI scan, heart rate differed somewhat which necessitated using cardiac output for the comparisons.

Statistical analysis

All measurements were reasonably well normally distributed which allowed Student's t-test to be used for tests of statistical significance. A p-value of <0.05 was considered significant. For differences between methods, analysis according to Bland-Altman and linear regression was used. Percent values were given based on the difference of the averages. Descriptive statistics were reported as mean values with 1 standard deviation (SD).

Table 3 Stroke volume and cardiac output, mean difference between the three phase-contrast techniques

Comparison of methods	Stroke volume (ml) Mean difference, +/−STD	Cardiac output (ml/min) Mean difference, +/− STD
TF5/TF3	0.2	163
	+/− 4.6	+/− 395
	$p = 0.76$	$p = 0.013$
Nav/TF3	2.0	92
	+/− 6.1	+/− 394
	$p = 0.046$	$p = 0.15$
Nav/TF5	1.8	−71
	+/− 6.8	+/− 462
	$p = 0.10$	$p = 0.33$

The mean difference between the phase-contrast based methods. The difference between TF5 (k-space segmentation factor 5) and TF3 (k-space segmentation factor 3) was non-significant ($p = 0.76$) for stroke volume but significant for cardiac output ($p = 0.013$). The difference between navigator vs TF3 as well as navigator vs TF5 was non-significant for cardiac output but barely significant for navigator vs TF3 for stroke volume

Results

Stroke volume and cardiac output from phase-contrast MRI

In navigator based, EKG-gated free-breathing phase-contrast flow, mean stroke volume and cardiac output were 79.7 ± 17.1 ml and 5071 ± 1192 ml/min, respectively (Table 2). The duration of the acquisition was 50 ± 6 s. With TFE 3, the corresponding values were 77.7 ml $\pm$ 17.5 ml and 4979 ± 1211 ml/min. The duration of the breath hold was 17 ± 2 s. Using TFE 5, mean stroke volume, cardiac output and breath hold time was 77.9 ± 16.4 ml, 5142 ± 1197 ml/min, and 11 ± 1 s, Table 2. The mean difference between the three methods is depicted in Table 3 and Figs. 1 and 2 (regression and Bland-Altman). Flow with k-space segmentation factor 5 did not differ from k-space segmentation factor 3 ($p = 0.76$) for stroke volume, but was larger for cardiac output ($p = 0.013$).

Navigator based flow did not differ from TF3 or TF5 for cardiac output, but was barely larger for navigator vs TF3 for stroke volume ($p = 0.046$).

Stroke volume and cardiac output based on left ventricular volumes from cine SSFP MRI

Mean stroke volume and cardiac output were 91.2 ± 20.8 ml and 5963 ± 1452 ml/min, respectively, Table 1. Intraobserver reproducibility expressed as coefficient of variation (SD divided by the mean) was 4 % for LVEDV, 8 % for LVESV and 7 % for stroke volume. The corresponding values for interobserver variability calculated from segmenting 10 patients was 6.4 % for LVEDV, 11.2 % for LVESV and 7.6 % for stroke volume. Interobserver bias and limits of agreement for stroke volume was in this subsample 1.9 ± 13.4 ml.

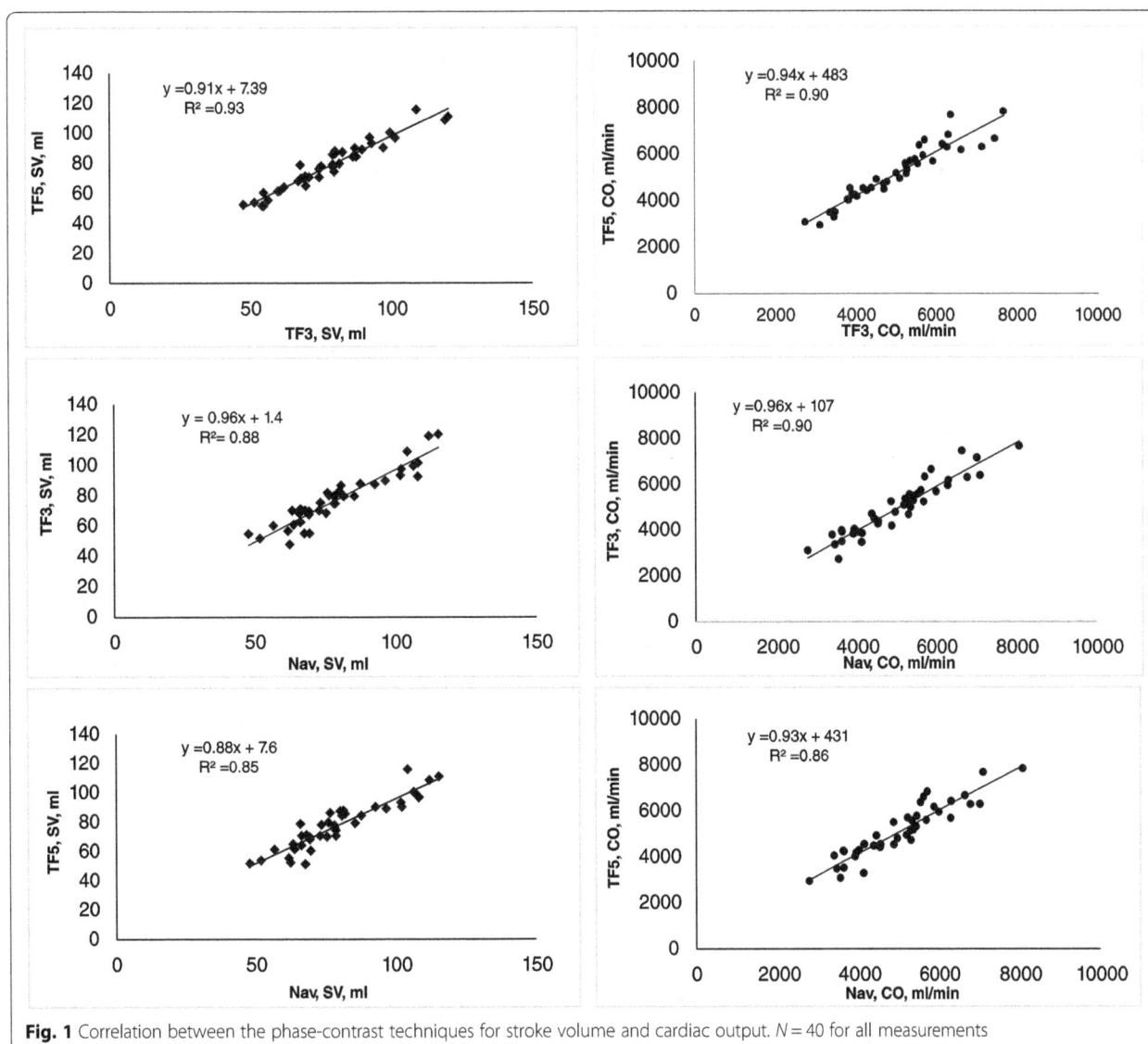

Fig. 1 Correlation between the phase-contrast techniques for stroke volume and cardiac output. $N = 40$ for all measurements

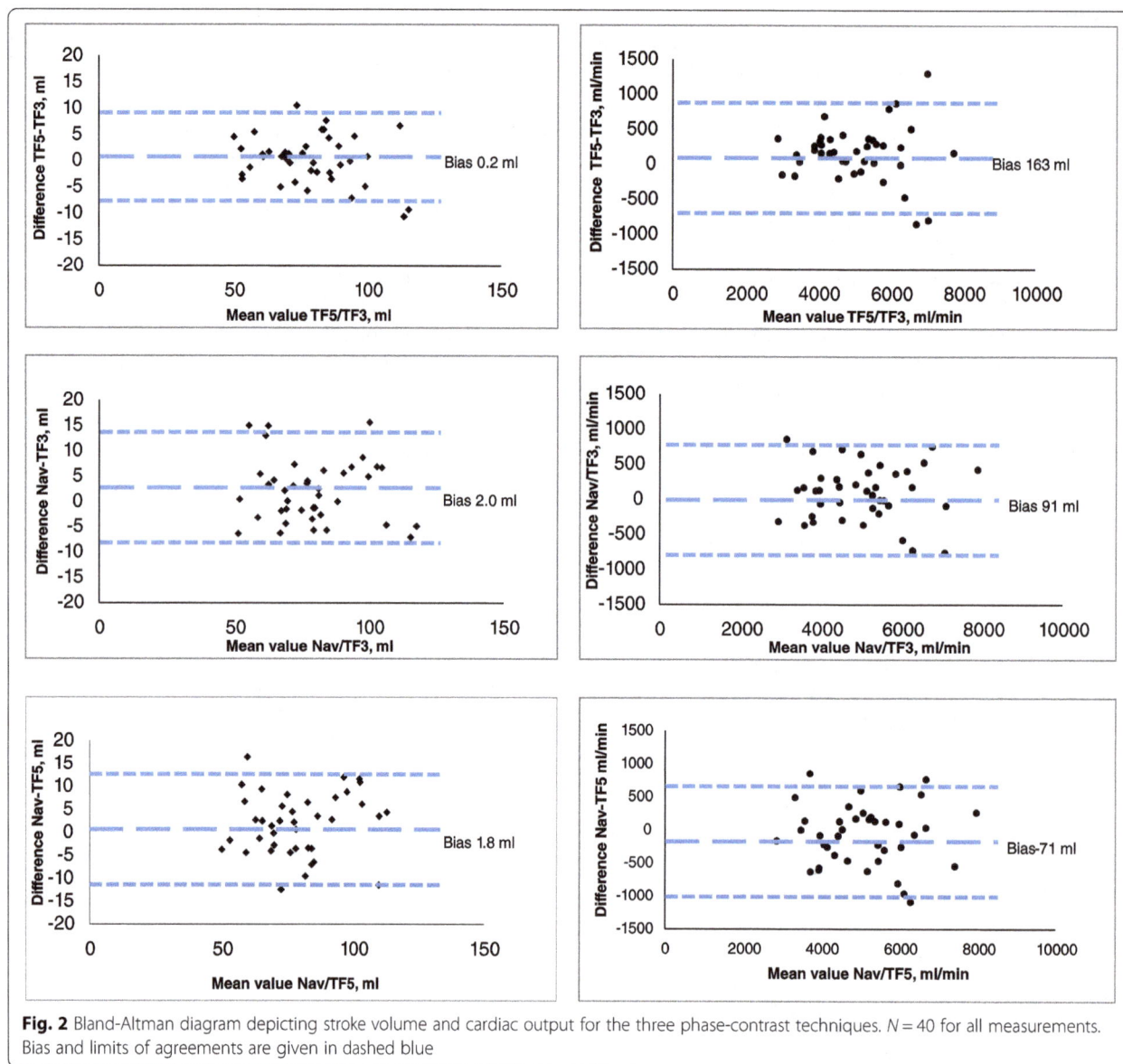

Fig. 2 Bland-Altman diagram depicting stroke volume and cardiac output for the three phase-contrast techniques. $N = 40$ for all measurements. Bias and limits of agreements are given in dashed blue

Doppler Echocardiography for flow measurement

Twenty patients were excluded due to either unreliable diameter measurements of the left ventricular outflow tract or inappropriate placement of the sample volume causing an overestimation of the velocity time integral. In the remaining 20 patients, the mean diameter of the left ventricular outflow tract was 20.7 ± 1.5 mm, stroke volume 78.3 ml ± 15.2 ml and cardiac output 5164 ± 1249 ml/min. A comparison with navigator flow data is given in Fig. 3.

Effects of heart rate

Even over shorter periods of time, heart rate varies with anxiety/arousal of the patient. In this study, individual heart rates differed substantially between the different acquisitions, the largest difference in a particular patient

being 31 beats/min. The lowest difference between any of the acquisitions in one individual was 4 beats/min. The average largest difference for all individuals was 11.3 ± 5.9 beats/min, but in a group-wise comparison, these individual differences are not apparent on the mean values (Table 2).

Discussion

This study shows that measuring aortic flow during short breath holds is feasible, despite concern that breath holding might affect cardiac filling. All measurement methods are prone to biological variation and inherent variation in accuracy and repeatability [18]. Some measurements require the full cooperation of patients, at times exceeding their limits e.g. when holding breath in obstructive pulmonary disease. For a long time, MRI

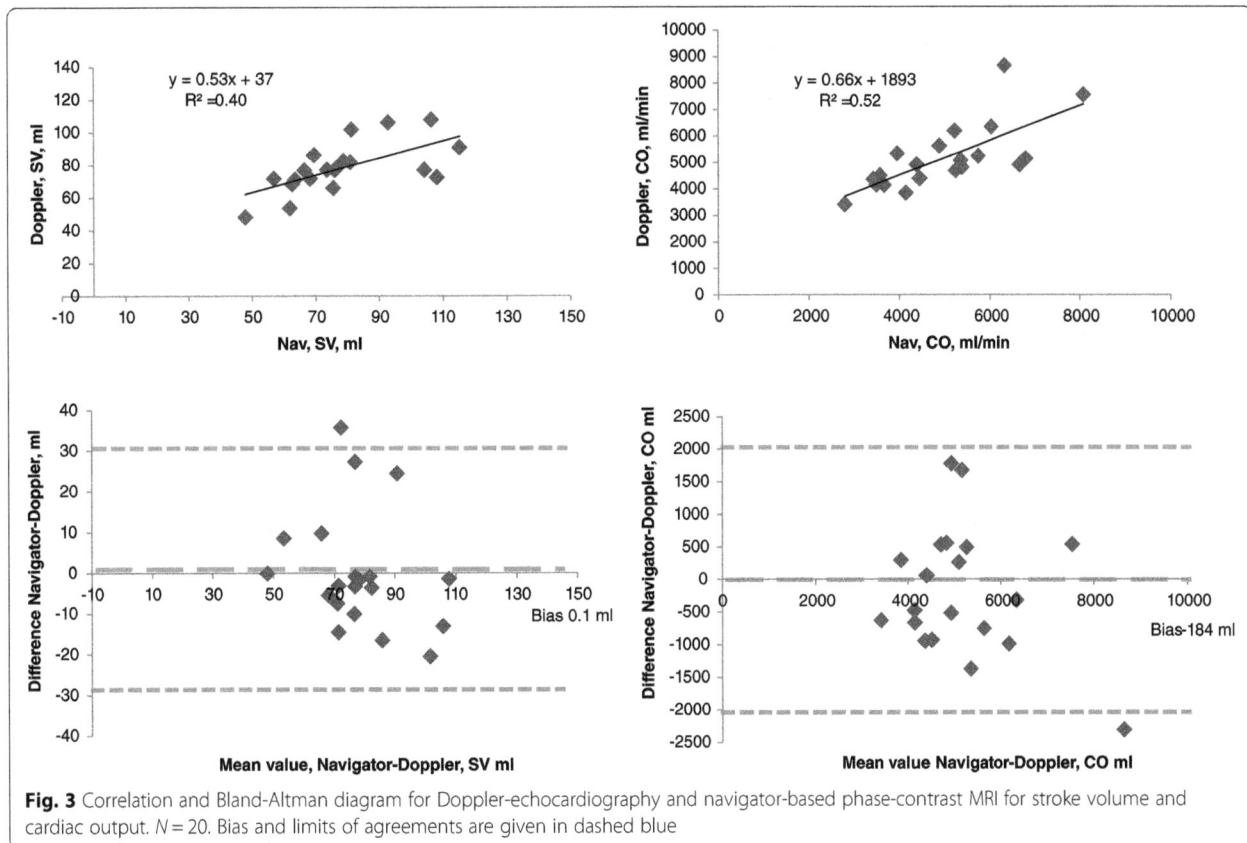

Fig. 3 Correlation and Bland-Altman diagram for Doppler-echocardiography and navigator-based phase-contrast MRI for stroke volume and cardiac output. N = 20. Bias and limits of agreements are given in dashed blue

phase-contrast has been considered the gold standard in the non-invasive determination of stroke volume and cardiac output [19, 20]. However, MRI can be executed in many different ways. In general, methods that shorten the time required for the collection of data are attractive since they ease the demands on the patient thereby facilitating work flow.

In this study comparing free breathing and breath hold recording of aortic flow, we found that the mean difference was below 2 ml (2.5 %) for stroke volume and below 163 ml/min (3.2 %) for cardiac output, which we consider acceptable for everyday clinical practice (Fig. 2, Table 3). Individual differences are also within clinically acceptable levels, with 55–75 % in the interval ±5 ml for stroke volume and 67–82 % ±500 ml/min for cardiac output in Bland-Altman analysis (Fig. 2). Close to one minute acquisition time for the free breathing sequence may seem short, but the breath held techniques are considerably quicker, without significant errors in measurement. When choosing between the two levels of k-space segmentation (TFE factors 3 and 5) TFE 5 was 5 s faster which may seem little, but for an ill patient, holding breath for 11 s is a lot easier than holding breath for 16 s.

All patients provided evaluable phase-contrast flow results, with mean values within 2 % to that from the Doppler echocardiography results when available (Table 3).

However, in Doppler echocardiography an inability to determine the LVOT diameter and a tendency towards overestimation of VTI caused many exclusions. Three-dimensional techniques have demonstrated that the LVOT is elliptical [2] and the spatial flow profile of the LVOT has been demonstrated to be skewed in healthy individuals and in patients with aortic regurgitation [3]. These conditions may have contributed to an inaccurate determination of stroke volume in the present study.

The largest difference found was between the flow based techniques and the anatomically determined MRI flow volume. Few patients in this study (5 MI, 1 AI) had more than trace mitral or aortic regurgitation (Table 1). It has been hypothesized that the combination of coronary blood flow not being included in the phase-contrast aortic sampling and the presence of unrecognized mitral regurgitation may explain a large part of the difference between phase-contrast and anatomic flow values [17, 21].

Relation to earlier studies

In healthy volunteers Polte et al found a bias of 12 ml and limits of agreement of 0–24 ml between anatomic and phase-contrast stroke volumes [22]. Likewise, James et al. found 5–7 ml difference in anatomical vs phase-contrast stroke volume that was attributed to coronary flow [23]. Differences between anatomically based measurements were also found in a recent multi-modality study of LVEDV with smaller 2D- and 3D-echo volumes than those obtained with the goldstandard MRI [23, 24]. Even with the high image quality obtained with SSFP and despite use of a meticulous segmentation technique, there will always be need for training [25] to overcome difficulties in the definition of the most basal slice of the left ventricle and the definition of the endocardial border in the presence of trabeculae. Suinesiaputra et al have recently recommended systematic training on a specific dataset to improve on the result of manual segmentation. However, the reproducibility of segmentation in the Doppler-cip study, of which the data here presented is a subset, has been extensively discussed in a previous publication, with interobserver bias and LOA of 8.2 + 7.7 ml for stroke volume [26]. The recommendations on segmentation are still subject to changes [17].

Conclusions

In forty consecutive patients with coronary heart disease, using breath holding and segmented k-space sampling techniques for phase-contrast flow produced stroke volumes and cardiac outputs similar to those obtained with free breathing navigator based phase-contrast MRI, using less time. The values obtained agreed fairly well with Doppler echocardiography while there was a larger difference when compared with anatomical volume determinations using SSFP MRI.

Abbreviations
LVEDV: left ventricular end diastolic volume; MRI: magnetic resonance imaging; SENSE: sensitivity encoding; SSFP: Steady State Free Precession; TFE: turbo field echo.

Competing interests
The authors declare that they have no competing interests.

Authors' contributions
CA and JE have been involved in conception and design. JE recruited the subjects. JE and JK have been involved in data acquisition. CA and JE have post processed the data. CA, JE, TE and CJC analyzed and interpreted the data. CA has performed the statistical analysis. JE has supervised the study. CA and JE drafted the manuscript. CA, JK, TE, LL, CJC and JE critically revised the manuscript. All authors had full access to the data and take responsibility for its integrity. All authors have read and agree to the manuscript as written.

Acknowledgements
This research was partly funded by the Swedish Heart and Lung Foundation (grants no 20120449 and 20140398), the Region of Östergötland (grant no 281281), the European Union FP 7 (grant no 223615) and the Medical Research Council of Southeast Sweden (grants no 88731 and 157921). The MRI technicians of CMIV and research technician Gunborg Gidby are gratefully acknowledged for performing the patient studies.

Author details
[1]Center for Medical Image Science and Visualization, Linkoping University, SE-581 83 Linkoping, Sweden. [2]Department of Clinical Physiology, Linkoping University, SE-603 79 Norrkoping, Sweden. [3]Department of Diagnostic Radiology, Linkoping University, SE-581 85 Linkoping, Sweden. [4]Department of Medical and Health Sciences, Linkoping University, SE-581 83 Linkoping, Sweden. [5]Department of Clinical Physiology, Linkoping University, SE-581 85 Linkoping, Sweden.

References
1. Richter Y, Edelman ER. Cardiology is flow. Circulation. 2006;113:2679–82.
2. Lang RM, Badano LP, Mor-Avi V, Afilalo J, Armstrong A, Ernande L, Flachskampf FA, Foster E, Goldstein SA, Kuznetsova T, et al. Recommendations for cardiac chamber quantification by echocardiography in adults: an update from the American Society of Echocardiography and the European Association of Cardiovascular Imaging. Eur Heart J Cardiovasc Imaging. 2015;16:233–70.
3. Sjoberg BJ, Ask P, Loyd D, Wranne B. Subaortic flow profiles in aortic valve disease: a two-dimensional color Doppler study. J Am Soc Echocardiogr. 1994;7:276–85.
4. Moran PR. A flow velocity zeugmatographic interlace for NMR imaging in humans. Magn Reson Imaging. 1982;1:197–203.
5. Pelc NJ, Herfkens RJ, Shimakawa A, Enzmann DR. Phase contrast cine magnetic resonance imaging. Magn Reson Q. 1991;7:229–54.
6. Gatehouse PD, Rolf MP, Bloch KM, Graves MJ, Kilner PJ, Firmin DN, Hofman MB. A multi-center inter-manufacturer study of the temporal stability of phase-contrast velocity mapping background offset errors. J Cardiovasc Magn Reson. 2012;14:72.
7. Gatehouse PD, Rolf MP, Graves MJ, Hofman MB, Totman J, Werner B, Quest RA, Liu Y, von Spiczak J, Dieringer M, et al. Flow measurement by cardiovascular magnetic resonance: a multi-centre multi-vendor study of background phase offset errors that can compromise the accuracy of derived regurgitant or shunt flow measurements. J Cardiovasc Magn Reson. 2010;12:5.
8. Chernobelsky A, Shubayev O, Comeau CR, Wolff SD. Baseline correction of phase contrast images improves quantification of blood flow in the great vessels. J Cardiovasc Magn Reson. 2007;9:681–5.
9. Luk Pat GT, Pauly JM, Hu BS, Nishimura DG. One-shot spatially resolved velocity imaging. Magn Reson Med. 1998;40:603–13.
10. Johansson B, Babu-Narayan SV, Kilner PJ. The effects of breath-holding on pulmonary regurgitation measured by cardiovascular magnetic resonance velocity mapping. J Cardiovasc Magn Reson. 2009;11:1.
11. Ley S, Fink C, Puderbach M, Zaporozhan J, Plathow C, Eichinger M, Hosch W, Kreitner KF, Kauczor HU. MRI Measurement of the hemodynamics of the pulmonary and systemic arterial circulation: influence of breathing maneuvers. AJR Am J Roentgenol. 2006;187:439–44.
12. Sakuma H, Kawada N, Kubo H, Nishide Y, Takano K, Kato N, Takeda K. Effect of breath holding on blood flow measurement using fast velocity encoded cine MRI. Magn Reson Med. 2001;45:346–8.
13. Chai P, Mohiaddin R. How we perform cardiovascular magnetic resonance flow assessment using phase-contrast velocity mapping. J Cardiovasc Magn Reson. 2005;7:705–16.
14. Queiros S, Barbosa D, Engvall J, Ebbers T, Nagel E, Sarvari SI, Claus P, Fonseca JC, Vilaca JL, D'Hooge J. Multi-centre validation of an automatic algorithm for fast 4D myocardial segmentation in cine CMR datasets. Eur Heart J Cardiovasc Imaging. 2015. [Epub ahead of print] PMID:26494877.
15. Rademakers F, Engvall J, Edvardsen T, Monaghan M, Sicari R, Nagel E, Zamorano J, Ukkonen H, Ebbers T, Di Bello V, et al. Determining optimal noninvasive parameters for the prediction of left ventricular remodeling in chronic ischemic patients. Scand Cardiovasc J. 2013;47:329–34.
16. Bernstein MA, Zhou XJ, Polzin JA, King KF, Ganin A, Pelc NJ, Glover GH. Concomitant gradient terms in phase contrast MR: analysis and correction. Magn Reson Med. 1998;39:300–8.

17. Schulz-Menger J, Bluemke DA, Bremerich J, Flamm SD, Fogel MA, Friedrich MG, Kim RJ, von Knobelsdorff-Brenkenhoff F, Kramer CM, Pennell DJ, et al. Standardized image interpretation and post processing in cardiovascular magnetic resonance: Society for Cardiovascular Magnetic Resonance (SCMR) board of trustees task force on standardized post processing. J Cardiovasc Magn Reson. 2013;15:35.

18. Douglas GA, Altman J. Practical statistics for medical research. London: Chapman & Hall; 1991. p. 365–95.

19. Gatehouse PD, Keegan J, Crowe LA, Masood S, Mohiaddin RH, Kreitner KF, Firmin DN. Applications of phase-contrast flow and velocity imaging in cardiovascular MRI. Eur Radiol. 2005;15:2172–84.

20. Pennell DJ, Sechtem UP, Higgins CB, Manning WJ, Pohost GM, Rademakers FE, van Rossum AC, Shaw LJ, Yucel EK, Society for Cardiovascular Magnetic R, Working Group on Cardiovascular Magnetic Resonance of the European Society of C. Clinical indications for cardiovascular magnetic resonance (CMR): Consensus Panel report. Eur Heart J. 2004;25:1940–65.

21. Uretsky S, Gillam L, Lang R, Chaudhry FA, Argulian E, Supariwala A, Gurram S, Jain K, Subero M, Jang JJ, et al. Discordance between echocardiography and MRI in the assessment of mitral regurgitation severity: a prospective multicenter trial. J Am Coll Cardiol. 2015;65:1078–88.

22. Polte CL, Bech-Hanssen O, Johnsson AA, Gao SA, Lagerstrand KM. Mitral regurgitation quantification by cardiovascular magnetic resonance: a comparison of indirect quantification methods. Int J Cardiovasc Imaging. 2015;31:1223–31.

23. James SH, Wald R, Wintersperger BJ, Jimenez-Juan L, Deva D, Crean AM, Nguyen E, Paul NS, Ley S. Accuracy of right and left ventricular functional assessment by short-axis vs axial cine steady-state free-precession magnetic resonance imaging: intrapatient correlation with main pulmonary artery and ascending aorta phase-contrast flow measurements. Can Assoc Radiol J. 2013;64:213–9.

24. Greupner J, Zimmermann E, Grohmann A, Dubel HP, Althoff TF, Borges AC, Rutsch W, Schlattmann P, Hamm B, Dewey M. Head-to-head comparison of left ventricular function assessment with 64-row computed tomography, biplane left cineventriculography, and both 2- and 3-dimensional transthoracic echocardiography: comparison with magnetic resonance imaging as the reference standard. J Am Coll Cardiol. 2012;59:1897–907.

25. Karamitsos TD, Hudsmith LE, Selvanayagam JB, Neubauer S, Francis JM. Operator induced variability in left ventricular measurements with cardiovascular magnetic resonance is improved after training. J Cardiovasc Magn Reson. 2007;9:777–83.

26. Suinesiaputra A, Bluemke DA, Cowan BR, Friedrich MG, Kramer CM, Kwong R, Plein S, Schulz-Menger J, Westenberg JJ, Young AA, Nagel E. Quantification of LV function and mass by cardiovascular magnetic resonance: multi-center variability and consensus contours. J Cardiovasc Magn Reson. 2015;17:63.

17

Evaluation of patients with painful total hip arthroplasty using combined single photon emission tomography and conventional computerized tomography (SPECT/CT) – a comparison of semi-quantitative versus 3D volumetric quantitative measurements

Emilienne Barthassat[1,4], Faik Afifi[1], Praveen Konala[2], Helmut Rasch[3] and Michael T. Hirschmann[1,4]*

Abstract

Background: It was the primary purpose of our study to evaluate the inter- and intra-observer reliability of a standardized SPECT/CT algorithm for evaluating patients with painful primary total hip arthroplasty (THA). The secondary purpose was a comparison of semi-quantitative and 3D volumetric quantification method for assessment of bone tracer uptake (BTU) in those patients.

Methods: A novel SPECT/CT localization scheme consisting of 14 femoral and 4 acetabular regions on standardized axial and coronal slices was introduced and evaluated in terms of inter- and intra-observer reliability in 37 consecutive patients with hip pain after THA. BTU for each anatomical region was assessed semi-quantitatively using a color-coded Likert type scale (0-10) and volumetrically quantified using a validated software. Two observers interpreted the SPECT/CT findings in all patients two times with six weeks interval between interpretations in random order. Semi-quantitative and quantitative measurements were compared in terms of reliability. In addition, the values were correlated using Pearson`s correlation. A factorial cluster analysis of BTU was performed to identify clinically relevant regions, which should be grouped and analysed together.

Results: The localization scheme showed high inter- and intra-observer reliabilities for all femoral and acetabular regions independent of the measurement method used (semiquantitative versus 3D volumetric quantitative measurements). A high to moderate correlation between both measurement methods was shown for the distal femur, the proximal femur and the acetabular cup. The factorial cluster analysis showed that the anatomical regions might be summarized into three distinct anatomical regions. These were the proximal femur, the distal femur and the acetabular cup region.

(Continued on next page)

* Correspondence: michael.hirschmann@ksbl.ch;
michael.hirschmann@unibas.ch
[1]Department of Orthopaedic Surgery and Traumatology, Kantonsspital Baselland Bruderholz, Liestal, Laufen, Switzerland
[4]Basel University, Basel, Switzerland
Full list of author information is available at the end of the article

(Continued from previous page)

Conclusions: The SPECT/CT algorithm for assessment of patients with pain after THA is highly reliable independent from the measurement method used. Three clinically relevant anatomical regions (proximal femoral, distal femoral, acetabular) were identified.

Keywords: Hip, SPECT/CT, Total hip arthroplasty, Total hip replacement, Pain, Localization scheme, Bone tracer uptake intensity, Quantification, Three-dimensional

Background

Combined single photon emission computerized tomography and conventional CT (SPECT/CT) promises the combined assessment of anatomical and functional information and hence its value is increasingly recognized in orthopaedics [1–23].

SPECT/CT has been reported to be beneficial in identifying the cause of patients`pain after total knee arthroplasty, patients with chondral or osteochondral lesions, before and after high tibial osteotomy and after ACL reconstruction [1–23]. Although SPECT/CT has also been used in patients with pain after total hip arthroplasty (THA) there is only scarce evidence about the optimal diagnostic algorithm and method of bone tracer uptake (BTU) analysis [24–27].

Due to its specific characteristics SPECT/CT is more sensitive and specific than SPECT and CT alone. Clearly, it is the accurate anatomical localization of the SPECT-tracer uptake using the CT as reference map that promises improved diagnostic confidence, particularly in patients with pain after joint replacement surgery [17, 20, 23]. Detection of mechanical or septic loosening of THA even in early stages might be facilitated. In addition, it could provide the surgeon with information on the position of THA components.

Recently our group has described and validated a standardized diagnostic algorithm using SPECT/CT in patients with pain after total knee arthroplasty including analysis of bone tracer activity and position and alignment of the TKA [14, 17, 20, 23, 28]. However, no such diagnostic algorithm has been reported or validated in patients with pain after THA.

In addition, in clinical practice it is a pertinent question if quantification of BTU in SPECT/CT offers so much more information than formerly semi-quantitative methods to recommend its daily use. There is no current study comparing semi-quantitative and quantitative measurement of BTU in patients with pain after THA.

Hence, it was the primary purpose of our study to evaluate the inter- and intra-observer reliability of a standardized SPECT/CT algorithm for evaluating patients with painful primary THA. The secondary purpose was a comparison of semi-quantitative and 3D volumetric quantification method for assessment of BTU in those patients.

Methods

Patients

A consecutive series of 37 patients (m:f = 16:21, mean age ± standard deviation 71 ± 11 years) presenting with hip pain after primary THA were prospectively collected and retrospectively included in this study. The data from all this patients were collected using our clinical information system (KIS, Erne, Switzerland). All patients had a primary THA with a maximum interval of 6 months from primary THA.

The study was approved by the local ethical committee (EKNZ 205/10). Written informed consent was obtained from all patients.

SPECT/CT was performed using a hybrid system (Symbia T16, Siemens, Erlangen, Germany) with a dual-head gamma camera and an integrated, 16x0.75-mm slice-thickness CT. All patients received a commercial 500–700 MBq Tc-99m-HDP injection (Malinckrodt, Wollerau, Switzerland). Scintigraphic images in anterior-posterior and lateral projection were taken in the perfusion phase (immediately after injection), the soft tissue phase (3–5 min after injection) and the delayed metabolic phase (2–3 h after injection). SPECT/CT was performed with a matrix size of 128x128, an angle step of 32, and a time per frame of 25 s.

The CT protocol was modified according to the Imperial Knee Protocol, which is a low dose CT protocol that includes high-resolution 0.75 mm slices of the knee and 3 mm slices of the hip and ankle joints [29].

The localization of bone tracer activity was recorded on a standardized localization scheme developed for use in patients after primary THA (Fig. 1). This defines biomechanically relevant regions of the femoral shaft and acetabulum around total hip prosthesis on standardized axial, coronal, and sagittal slices to accurately map areas of increased activity. The anatomical area (femur, acetabulum) is indicated with capital letters (F, A). The femur (F) is divided into fourteen zones with regards to the modified Gruen classification [30].

Each femoral zone is represented with a number (1-14). The acetabulum (A) is divided into four zones (superior anterior, superior posterior, inferior anterior, inferior posterior).

The highest activity grading on SPECT/CT for each area of the localization scheme was recorded semiquantitatively

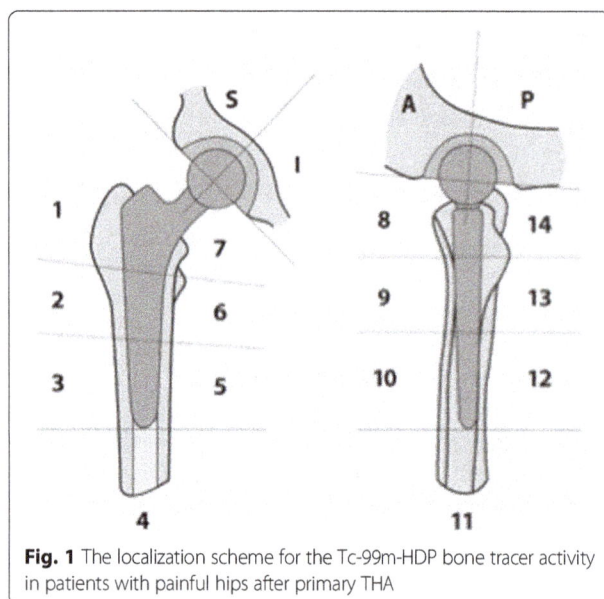

Fig. 1 The localization scheme for the Tc-99m-HDP bone tracer activity in patients with painful hips after primary THA

(0–10). In addition, it was noted whether the area of tracer activity extended to the bone prosthesis interface. In that case an additional "c" was added to the tracer activity value.

In addition, BTU was also quantified in 3D using a voxel based measurement method. For BTU analysis (intensity and anatomical distribution pattern) the 3D reconstructed datasets of the delayed SPECT/CT images were used. The anatomical areas represented by a previously validated localization scheme were 3D volumetrically measured in terms of SPECT/CT tracer uptake values (OrthoImagingSolutions Ltd., London, UK) [4, 9]. The tracer activity was quantified in 3D volumetrically as described in Hirschmann et al. (Figs. 1, 2 and 3) [4]. The maximum intensity values were recorded for each anatomical area.

Two observers interpreted the SPECT/CT findings in all patients two times with six weeks interval between interpretations in random order. Both were blinded to results from previous observations. The inter- and intra-observer reliability of the localization scheme and grading of the tracer activity was determined. Semi-quantitative and quantitative measurements were compared in terms of reliability. In addition, the values were correlated using Pearson`s correlation.

Finally, a factorial cluster analysis of BTU was performed to identify clinically relevant regions, which should be grouped and analysed together.

Statistical analysis

Data were analyzed using SPSS 16.0 (SPSS, Chicago, U.S.A.). Sample size was calculated according to the reported estimates for reliability studies using intraclass correlation coefficients (ICCs) [31].

The median differences in measurements between the two observers (inter-observer) and within the measurements of the first observer (intra-observer) were calculated. The intraclass correlation coefficients for inter- and intra-observer reliability were also calculated. ICC values range from 0 to 1. A value of 1 indicates perfect reliability, 0.81 to 1 very good reliability and 0.61-0.80 good reliability [31]. For all analysis, $p < 0.05$ was considered statistically significant.

Results

The localization scheme showed high inter- and intra-observer reliabilities for all femoral and acetabular regions independent of the measurement methods (semi-quantitative versus 3D volumetric quantitative measurements). Inter- and intra-observer reliability (intra class correlation-ICC) of 99mTc-HDP-SPECT/CT tracer activity using the

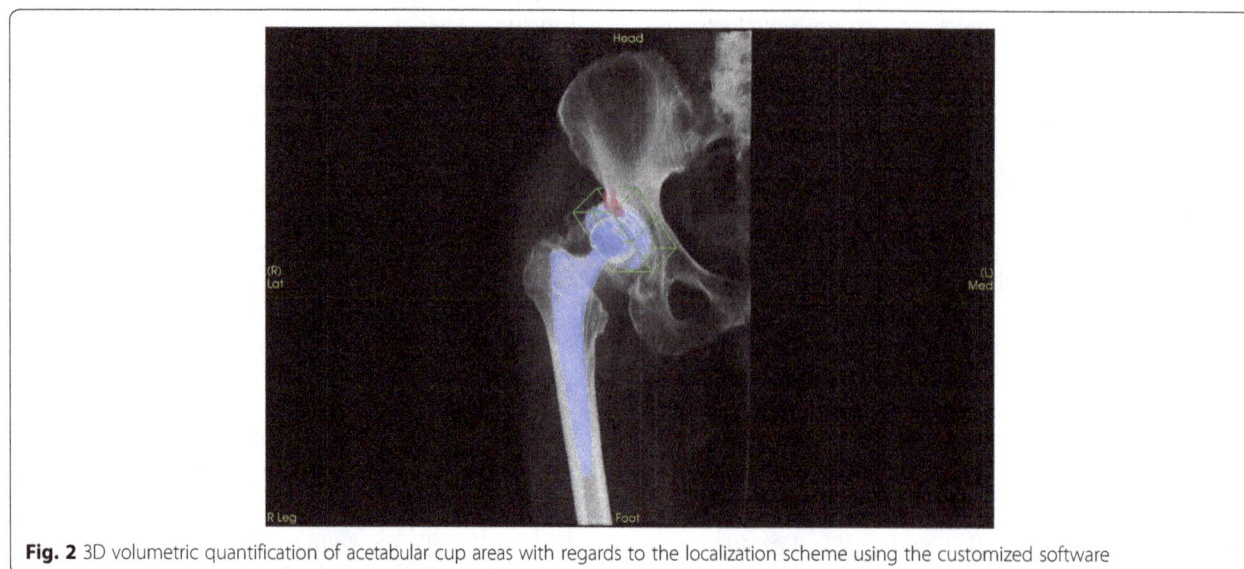

Fig. 2 3D volumetric quantification of acetabular cup areas with regards to the localization scheme using the customized software

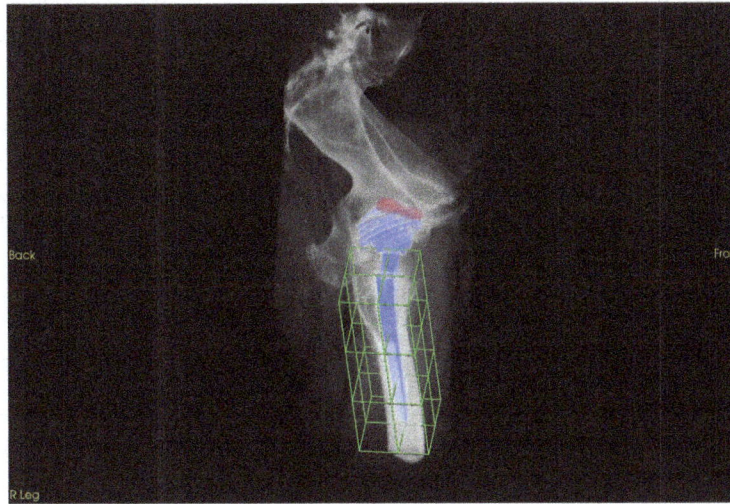

Fig. 3 3D volumetric quantification of femoral areas with regards to the localization scheme using the customized software

localization and semi-quantitative BTU grading scheme for the acetabular and femoral zones (Likert scale 0–10) are presented in Table 1. In mean the femoral regions showed an ICC of 0.981–0.992 for intra-observer reliability and 0.871 for inter-observer-reliability. In mean the acetabular regions showed an ICC of 0.967–0.975 for intra-observer reliability and 0.877 for inter-observer-reliability. The acetabular regions AI and PI showed moderate agreement for intra- (ICC 0.529–0.963) and inter-observer testing (0.401–0.493).

Table 1 Inter- and intra-observer reliability (intra class correlation- ICC) of 99mTc-HDP-BTU activity using the localization and semiquantitative BTU grading scheme for the acetabular and femoral zones (Likert scale 0-10)

| Location | Intra-observer-reliability | | | | Inter-observer- reliability | |
| | Observer 1 | | Observer 2 | | Observer 1-Observer 2 | |
	Mean	95% CI	Mean	95% CI	Mean	95% CI
AS	0.954	0.913–0.976	0.975	0.952–0.987	0.900	0.815–0.947
AI	0.963	0.929–0.981	0.529	0.252–0.726	0.401	0.093–0,639
PS	0.967	0.938–0.983	0.949	0.903–0.973	0.950	0.905–0.974
PI	0.878	0.775–0.935	0.790	0.629–0.886	0.493	0.206–0.703
Z1	0.888	0.794–0.941	0.807	0.656–0.895	0.799	0.643–0.891
Z2	0.882	0.783–0.938	0.692	0.478–0.829	0.703	0.495–0.835
Z3	0.781	0.614–0.881	0.929	0.867–0.963	0.866	0.755–0.928
Z4	0.822	0.680–0.904	0.938	0.883–0.968	0.744	0.557–0.860
Z5	0.884	0.786–0.938	0.975	0.951–0.987	0.829	0.693–0.908
Z6	0.877	0.774–0.935	0.792	0.633–0.887	0.733	0.540–0,853
Z7	0.945	0.895–0.971	0.811	0.663–0.898	0.723	0.524–0.847
Z8	0.955	0.914–0.976	0.923	0.855–0.959	0.864	0.752–0.928
Z9	0.937	0.882–0.967	0.833	0.699–0.910	0.601	0.348–0.773
Z10	0.838	0.708–0.913	0.978	0.958–0.989	0.718	0.517–0.844
Z11	0.878	0.777–0.936	0.955	0.914–0.976	0.681	0.461–0.822
Z12	0.881	0.781–0.937	0.964	0.931–0.981	0.846	0.722–0.918
Z13	0.921	0.852–0.958	0.804	0.651–0.894	0.563	0.296–0.748
Z14	0.889	0.796–0.942	0.876	0.772–0.934	0.819	0.675–0.902
Acetabulum	0.975	0.953–0.987	0.967	0.937–0.983	0.877	0.774–0.935
Femur	0.992	0.984–0.996	0.981	0.963–0.990	0.871	0.764–0.932

Inter- and intra-observer reliability (intra class correlation- ICC) of 99mTc-HDP-SPECT/CT tracer activity using the localization and 3D voxel based quantitative BTU grading scheme for the acetabular and femoral zones were for all regions neary perfect (ICCs > 0.90).

The measured values of BTU activity in SPECT/CT for each anatomical region using the semi-quantitative versus 3D volumetric quantitative method are shown in Table 2. The Pearson`s correlation of both BTU measurement methods is presented in Table 3. A high correlation between both measurement methods was found for the distal femur. A moderate correlation was found for the proximal femur and the acetabular cup regions.

The factorial cluster analysis showed that the anatomical regions might be summarized into three distinct anatomical regions Table 4. These were the proximal femur, the distal femur and the acetabular cup region.

Discussion

The most important findings of the present study were twofold. Firstly, a high inter-observer and intra-observer reliability was found for grading and localization of the BTU activity independent of the investigated region. The localization scheme and BTU grading was reliable and easily applicable, which

would make it understandable by most clinicians. A reliable localization and grading scheme is needed to standardize the evaluation of SPECT/CT data and make those comparable with each other. The Gruen classification is already widely used for assessment of periprosthetic radiolucencies, hence it was decided to adapt this scheme to the biomechanics of the hip reflecting bone remodeling and integration of the prosthetic hip components. It has also been used by others to report BTU findings in SPECT/CT [26, 32].

In a recent pictorial review by Tam et al. dealing with THA the authors reported their SPECT/CT analysis and reporting system, which is in accordance with the one presented in terms of the localization scheme used [26]. However, there only the two-dimensional localization scheme was used. In this study a modified three-dimensional localization scheme was introduced and has proven highly reliable [26, 33]. The localization scheme showed high inter- and intra-observer reliabilities for both femoral and acetabular regions independent of the measurement methods (semi-quantitative versus 3D volumetric quantitative measurements). Clearly, the 3D volumetric quantification has proven to be as reliable as the standard two-dimensional localization and BTU analysis system.

Table 2 Absolute values (mean, SD, median) of BTU for each anatomical area using 3D volumetric voxel based quantification and semi-quantitative measurement methods

Anatomical area	3D volumetric voxel based quantification of BTU			Semiquantitative measurement of BTU		
	Mean	SD	Median	Mean	SD	Median
AS	860.23	425.19	831.00	2.78	1.80	2.50
AI	817.54	422.63	700.00	1.26	0.89	1.50
PS	822.34	427.53	711.00	2.49	1.70	2.00
PI	871.00	589.04	743.00	1.49	1.06	1.50
Z1	1022.54	626.10	897.00	4.40	2.38	4.00
Z2	820.20	498.31	737.00	3.13	2.02	2.50
Z3	841.40	656.74	690.00	3.23	2.61	2.25
Z4	590.76	471.38	494.00	2.92	2.23	2.50
Z5	851.71	598.32	744.00	3.14	2.48	2.75
Z6	927.97	603.05	750.00	2.83	1.98	2.50
Z7	1125.29	832.16	866.00	3.02	1.95	2.75
Z8	1085.48	779.70	877.00	3.97	2.49	3.50
Z9	899.09	580.63	744.00	3.05	2.10	2.50
Z10	854.37	592.66	753.00	3.12	2.37	2.75
Z11	592.29	454.82	530.00	2.74	2.02	2.50
Z12	848.26	621.53	718.00	3.35	2.72	2.50
Z13	799.03	443.21	740.00	3.08	1.91	2.75
Z14	1043.37	692.13	788.00	3.91	2.25	3.50
Hip	877.53	507.60	774.31	2.01	1.27	2.13
Thigh	842.78	428.19	752.50	3.28	1.96	2.80

Table 3 Pearson`s correlations of 99mTc-HDP BTU activity for the acetabular and femoral zones using 3D-quantitative and semi-quantitative methods

	AS Obs	AI Obs	PS Obs	PI Obs	Z1 Obs	Z2 Obs	Z3 Obs	Z4 Obs	Z5 Obs	Z6 Obs	Z7 Obs	Z8 Obs	Z9 Obs	Z10 Obs	Z11 Obs	Z12 Obs	Z13 Obs	Z14 Obs	Hip Obs	Thigh Obs
Voxel AS ratio	0.51	0.29	0.34	0.27	0.19	0.11	0.08	0.08	0.14	0.14	0.17	0.12	0.07	0.17	0.13	0.07	0.17	0.10	0.40	0.14
Voxel AI ratio	0.52	0.29	0.39	0.36	0.12	0.14	0.12	0.16	0.17	0.18	0.17	0.03	0.10	0.19	0.21	0.13	0.22	0.07	0.44	0.16
Voxel PS ratio	0.53	0.29	0.44	0.39	0.19	0.20	0.14	0.22	0.13	0.20	0.24	0.16	0.11	0.17	0.25	0.13	0.30	0.21	0.47	0.21
Voxel PI ratio	0.49	0.42	0.61	0.49	0.01	0.00	0.02	0.07	0.13	0.22	0.18	-0.13	-0.07	0.18	0.11	0.03	0.17	0.08	0.55	0.07
Voxel Z1 ratio	-0.05	-0.01	-0.15	-0.17	0.14	0.26	0.07	0.05	0.09	0.07	0.11	0.10	0.24	0.11	0.09	0.00	0.14	0.09	-0.10	0.12
Voxel Z2 ratio	0.11	0.21	-0.02	-0.01	0.19	0.46	0.37	0.30	0.35	0.29	0.29	0.15	0.41	0.36	0.30	0.32	0.34	0.16	0.07	0.34
Voxel Z3 ratio	0.11	0.28	0.05	0.16	0.25	0.48	0.72	0.63	0.77	0.55	0.46	0.15	0.40	0.77	0.61	0.72	0.49	0.36	0.14	0.60
Voxel Z4 ratio	0.13	0.27	-0.05	0.07	0.16	0.37	0.54	0.62	0.47	0.24	0.22	0.12	0.30	0.42	0.62	0.55	0.22	0.16	0.09	0.40
Voxel Z5 ratio	0.19	0.30	0.12	0.18	0.29	0.50	0.66	0.58	0.77	0.60	0.50	0.19	0.41	0.77	0.58	0.67	0.54	0.43	0.20	0.60
Voxel Z6 ratio	0.13	0.19	0.06	0.04	0.11	0.31	0.37	0.37	0.39	0.41	0.36	0.07	0.30	0.39	0.36	0.33	0.30	0.16	0.11	0.34
Voxel Z7 ratio	-0.03	0.09	-0.06	-0.08	0.05	0.08	0.15	0.15	0.08	0.22	0.25	0.13	0.13	0.14	0.23	0.11	0.13	0.10	-0.03	0.15
Voxel Z8 ratio	-0.07	-0.10	-0.21	-0.19	0.08	0.11	-0.06	0.00	-0.13	-0.06	-0.03	0.14	0.18	-0.14	0.03	-0.11	0.04	-0.02	-0.16	0.00
Voxel z9 ratio	0.25	0.32	0.12	0.19	0.31	0.60	0.51	0.45	0.56	0.51	0.48	0.24	0.61	0.51	0.41	0.49	0.51	0.31	0.23	0.52
Voxel Z10 ratio	0.17	0.30	0.08	0.17	0.21	0.43	0.61	0.57	0.74	0.56	0.46	0.09	0.36	0.73	0.56	0.64	0.48	0.37	0.18	0.55
Voxel Z11 ratio	0.08	0.16	-0.04	0.05	0.14	0.23	0.49	0.57	0.45	0.31	0.25	0.11	0.21	0.40	0.60	0.48	0.24	0.23	0.05	0.38
Voxel Z12 ratio	0.17	0.22	0.04	0.21	0.28	0.48	0.77	0.73	0.77	0.53	0.47	0.20	0.44	0.72	0.70	0.76	0.52	0.38	0.15	0.63
Voxel Z13 ratio	0.14	0.23	0.02	0.03	0.17	0.40	0.37	0.30	0.39	0.33	0.37	0.10	0.36	0.40	0.33	0.32	0.31	0.19	0.10	0.35
Voxel Z14 ratio	0.06	0.12	0.04	0.03	0.19	0.12	0.15	0.18	0.15	0.24	0.34	0.16	0.15	0.17	0.28	0.11	0.19	0.31	0.06	0.22
Voxel Thigh	0.59	0.37	0.51	0.42	0.15	0.13	0.10	0.15	0.16	0.21	0.22	0.05	0.06	0.20	0.20	0.10	0.24	0.13	0.53	0.17
Voxel Hip	0.14	0.26	0.01	0.08	0.25	0.48	0.57	0.55	0.59	0.48	0.45	0.19	0.45	0.58	0.56	0.55	0.45	0.32	0.11	0.52

Table 4 Factorial cluster analysis of 3D voxel based quantified BTU values showing three distinct regions (proximal thigh, distal thigh, acetabular cup)

		Absolute BTU				BTU ratio		
		Distal femur	Proximal femur	Acetabular cup		Distal femur	Proximal femur	Acetabular cup
Distal thigh	Z12	0.93	0.18	0.20	Z3 ratio	0.96	0.10	0.01
	Z3	0.93	0.15	0.22	Z5 ratio	0.93	0.14	0.13
	Z5	0.90	0.22	0.23	Z12 ratio	0.93	0.10	0.06
	Z10	0.87	0.22	0.27	Z10 ratio	0.91	0.11	0.17
	Z11	0.85	0.30	0.09	Z4 ratio	0.71	0.26	-0.06
	Z4	0.83	0.22	-0.04	Z11 ratio	0.71	0.29	-0.02
	Z6	0.73	0.38	0.42	Z6 ratio	0.61	0.56	0.20
	Z13	0.81	0.23	0.41	Z13 ratio	0.60	0.55	0.36
	Z9	0.79	0.32	0.38	Z9 ratio	0.56	0.46	0.14
	Z2	0.77	0.28	0.34	Z2 ratio	0.55	0.62	0.13
Proximal thigh	Z8	0.21	0.94	0.11	Z8 ratio	-0.06	0.90	0.08
	Z7	0.31	0.84	0.33	Z1 ratio	0.24	0.82	0.12
	Z14	0.27	0.78	0.39	Z7 ratio	0.21	0.71	0.11
	Z1	0.42	0.76	0.33	Z14 ratio	0.22	0.44	0.22
Acetabular cup	PI	0.06	0.19	0.91	PI ratio	0.02	-0.01	0.91
	PS	0.23	0.20	0.89	AI ratio	0.13	0.16	0.87
	AI	0.36	0.31	0.84	AS ratio	0.12	0.21	0.86
	AS	0.39	0.35	0.71	PS ratio	0.00	0.22	0.79

In a retrospective study Jin et al. investigated the periprosthetic bone remodeling of THA using SPECT/CT [34]. SPECT/CT was reviewed as three-dimensional multiplanar reconstructions with a slice thickness of 4.4 mm [34]. Two-dimensional regions of interest (ROIs) were generated and placed in specific standardized locations for each dataset [34]. All ROI placements and measurements were performed by a single reader to match standardized locations and with the assistance of a ROI template guide [34]. In agreement with the present study they also normalized the absolute measured values by building ratios of the measured value and a value measured at a specific reference regions [34].

Secondly, a high correlation between both measurement methods was found for the distal femur. A moderate correlation was found for the proximal femur and the acetabular cup regions.

The factorial cluster analysis showed that the anatomical regions might be summarized into three distinct anatomical regions These were the proximal femur, the distal femur and the acetabular cup region. In the study by Jin et al. the ROI analysis was done at five different locations (the greater trochanter, the femoral calcar, the mid-stem of the femur, the femoral stem tip and one acetabular region) [34]. The authors choose these locations for analysis as these appeared to be clinically relevant and highly reproducible [34].

However, Jin et al. questioned the need for routine quantification of BTU in patients with THA [34]. Based on their findings it is possible to distinguish between clearly normal and clearly abnormal SPECT/CT images [34]. In difficult cases semi-quantification might be helpful.

In contrast, we believe that a better understanding of bone remodelling after THA reflected by typical BTU pattern distribution will help to improve the reporting and diagnosis when using SPECT/CT. However, until analysis of BTU activity could lead to a better diagnosis we need to achieve a more profound knowledge of normal and abnormal BTU distribution and activity in native and arthroplasty patients.

Another limitation to gain wider acceptance for quantification methods among clinicians is the utility, availability and simplicity of these analysis methods. Clearly, these have to be robust, reliable and easy to perform.

The study bears a few limitations to be considered. This is a well sized small pilot study aiming to evaluate the analysis algorithm in patients with THA undergoing SPECT/CT. The clinical value of the algorithm needs to be further evaluated in larger, homogenous cohorts. The standard deviations are high, which is due to inter-patient variability. A typical findings in metabolic imaging.

Conclusions

The SPECT/CT algorithm for assessment of patients with pain after THA is highly reliable independent from the measurement method used. Three clinically relevant anatomical regions (proximal femoral, distal femoral, acetabular) were identified.

Abbreviations

BTU: Bone tracer uptake; ICC: Intraclass coefficient; ROI: Region of interest; SPECT/CT: Single photon emission computerized tomography and conventional computerized tomography; THA: Total hip arthroplasty

Acknowledgements

Not applicable.

Funding

There has been no specific grant funding for this study.

Authors' contributions

EB and FA set-up the study, collected the data and helped with drafting of the manuscript. HR and MTH designed the study and performed the data analysis. JH, PK and HR helped with data acquisition and drafting of manuscript. All authors read and approved the final manuscript.

Competing interests

The authors declare that they have no competing interests.

Author details

[1]Department of Orthopaedic Surgery and Traumatology, Kantonsspital Baselland Bruderholz, Liestal, Laufen, Switzerland. [2]Fellow- Musculoskeletal Radiology, The Robert Jones and Agnes Hunt Orthopaedic Hospital NHS Foundation Trust, Oswestry, UK. [3]Institute for Radiology and Nuclear Medicine, Kantonsspital Baselland-Bruderholz, Bruderholz, Switzerland. [4]Basel University, Basel, Switzerland.

References

1. Suter B, Testa E, Stampfli P, Konala P, Rasch H, Friederich NF, Hirschmann MT. A novel standardized algorithm using SPECT/CT evaluating unhappy patients after unicondylar knee arthroplasty–a combined analysis of tracer uptake distribution and component position. BMC Med Imaging. 2015;15:11.
2. Schon SN, Afifi FK, Rasch H, Amsler F, Friederich NF, Arnold MP, Hirschmann MT. Assessment of in vivo loading history of the patellofemoral joint: a study combining patellar position, tilt, alignment and bone SPECT/CT. Knee Surg Sports Traumatol Arthrosc. 2014;22(12):3039–46.
3. Rieger B, Friederich NF, Rasch H, Hirschmann MT. Non-dislocated osteoporotic insufficiency fracture of the medial femoral neck. SPECT/CT makes the diagnostic difference. Unfallchirurg. 2014;117(4):369–73.
4. Rasch H, Falkowski AL, Forrer F, Henckel J, Hirschmann MT. 4D-SPECT/CT in orthopaedics: a new method of combined quantitative volumetric 3D analysis of SPECT/CT tracer uptake and component position measurements in patients after total knee arthroplasty. Skeletal Radiol. 2013;42(9):1215–23.
5. Mucha A, Dordevic M, Testa EA, Rasch H, Hirschmann MT. Assessment of the loading history of patients after high tibial osteotomy using SPECT/CT–a new diagnostic tool and algorithm. J Orthop Surg Res. 2013;8:46.
6. Mucha A, Dordevic M, Hirschmann A, Rasch H, Amsler F, Arnold MP, Hirschmann MT. Effect of high tibial osteotomy on joint loading in symptomatic patients with varus aligned knees: a study using SPECT/CT. Knee Surg Sports Traumatol Arthrosc. 2015;23(8):2315–23.
7. Mathis DT, Rasch H, Hirschmann MT. In vivo bone tunnel remodeling in symptomatic patients after ACL reconstruction: a retrospective comparison of articular and extra-articular fixation. Muscles Ligaments Tendons J. 2015; 5(4):316–24.
8. Konala P, Iranpour F, Kerner A, Rasch H, Friederich NF, Hirschmann MT. Clinical benefit of SPECT/CT for follow-up of surgical treatment of osteochondritis dissecans. Ann Nucl Med. 2010;24(8):621–4.
9. Hirschmann MT, Wagner CR, Rasch H, Henckel J. Standardized volumetric 3D-analysis of SPECT/CT imaging in orthopaedics: overcoming the limitations of qualitative 2D analysis. BMC Med Imaging. 2012;12:5.
10. Hirschmann MT, Schon S, Afifi FK, Amsler F, Rasch H, Friederich NF, Arnold MP. Assessment of loading history of compartments in the knee using bone SPECT/CT: a study combining alignment and 99mTc-HDP tracer uptake/ distribution patterns. J Orthop Res. 2013;31(2):268–74.
11. Hirschmann MT, Schmid R, Dhawan R, Skarvan J, Rasch H, Friederich NF, Emery R. Combined single photon emission computerized tomography and conventional computerized tomography: Clinical value for the shoulder surgeons? Int J Shoulder Surg. 2011;5(3):72–6.
12. Hirschmann MT, Mathis D, Rasch H, Amsler F, Friederich NF, Arnold MP. SPECT/CT tracer uptake is influenced by tunnel orientation and position of the femoral and tibial ACL graft insertion site. Int Orthop. 2013;37(2): 301–9.
13. Hirschmann MT, Mathis D, Afifi FK, Rasch H, Henckel J, Amsler F, Wagner CR, Friederich NF, Arnold MP. Single photon emission computerized tomography and conventional computerized tomography (SPECT/CT) for evaluation of patients after anterior cruciate ligament reconstruction: a novel standardized algorithm combining mechanical and metabolic information. Knee Surg Sports Traumatol Arthrosc. 2013;21(4):965–74.
14. Hirschmann MT, Konala P, Iranpour F, Kerner A, Rasch H, Friederich NF. Clinical value of SPECT/CT for evaluation of patients with painful knees after total knee arthroplasty–a new dimension of diagnostics? BMC Musculoskelet Disord. 2011;12:36.
15. Hirschmann MT, Iranpour F, Konala P, Kerner A, Rasch H, Cobb JP, Friederich NF. A novel standardized algorithm for evaluating patients with painful total knee arthroplasty using combined single photon emission tomography and conventional computerized tomography. Knee Surg Sports Traumatol Arthrosc. 2010;18(7):939–44.
16. Hirschmann MT, Iranpour F, Davda K, Rasch H, Hugli R, Friederich NF. Combined single-photon emission computerized tomography and conventional computerized tomography (SPECT/CT): clinical value for the knee surgeons? Knee Surg Sports Traumatol Arthrosc. 2010;18(3):341–5.
17. Hirschmann MT, Henckel J, Rasch H. SPECT/CT in patients with painful knee arthroplasty-what is the evidence? Skeletal Radiol. 2013;42(9):1201–7.
18. Hirschmann MT, Davda K, Rasch H, Arnold MP, Friederich NF. Clinical value of combined single photon emission computerized tomography and conventional computer tomography (SPECT/CT) in sports medicine. Sports Med Arthrosc. 2011;19(2):174–81.
19. Hirschmann MT, Davda K, Iranpour F, Rasch H, Friederich NF. Combined single photon emission computerised tomography and conventional computerised tomography (SPECT/CT) in patellofemoral disorders: a clinical review. Int Orthop. 2011;35(5):675–80.
20. Hirschmann MT, Amsler F, Rasch H. Clinical value of SPECT/CT in the painful total knee arthroplasty (TKA): a prospective study in a consecutive series of 100 TKA. Eur J Nucl Med Mol Imaging. 2015;42(12):1869–82.
21. Hassink G, Testa EA, Leumann A, Hugle T, Rasch H, Hirschmann MT. Intra- and inter-observer reliability of a new standardized diagnostic method using SPECT/CT in patients with osteochondral lesions of the ankle joint. BMC Med Imaging. 2016;16(1):67.
22. Dordevic M, Hirschmann MT, Rechsteiner J, Falkowski A, Testa E, Hirschmann A. Do Chondral Lesions of the Knee Correlate with Bone Tracer Uptake by Using SPECT/CT? Radiology. 2016;278(1):223–31.
23. Awengen R, Rasch H, Amsler F, Hirschmann MT. Symptomatic versus asymptomatic knees after bilateral total knee arthroplasty: what is the difference in SPECT/CT? Eur J Nucl Med Mol Imaging. 2016;43(4):762–72.

24. Strobel K, Steurer-Dober I, Huellner MW, Veit-Haibach P, Allgayer B. Importance of SPECT/CT for knee and hip joint Prostheses. Radiologe. 2012; 52(7):629–37.

25. Chew CG, Lewis P, Middleton F, van den Wijngaard R, Deshaies A. Radionuclide arthrogram with SPECT/CT for the evaluation of mechanical loosening of hip and knee prostheses. Ann Nucl Med. 2010;24(10):735–43.

26. Tam HH, Bhaludin B, Rahman F, Weller A, Ejindu V, Parthipun A. SPECT-CT in total hip arthroplasty. Clin Radiol. 2014;69(1):82–95.

27. Berber R, Henckel J, Khoo M, Wan S, Hua J, Skinner J, Hart A. Clinical Usefulness of SPECT-CT in Patients with an Unexplained Pain in Metal on Metal (MOM) Total Hip Arthroplasty. J Arthroplasty. 2015;30(4):687–94.

28. Slevin O, Amsler F, Hirschmann MT. No correlation between coronal alignment of total knee arthroplasty and clinical outcomes: a prospective clinical study using 3D-CT. Knee Surg Sports Traumatol Arthrosc. 2016. doi: 10.1007/s00167-016-4400-y.

29. Henckel J, Richards R, Lozhkin K, Harris S, Baena FM, Barrett AR, Cobb JP. Very low-dose computed tomography for planning and outcome measurement in knee replacement. The imperial knee protocol. J Bone Joint Surg (Br). 2006;88(11):1513–8.

30. Gruen TA, McNeice GM, Amstutz HC. "Modes of failure" of cemented stem-type femoral components: a radiographic analysis of loosening. Clin Orthop Relat Res. 1979;141:17–27.

31. Walter SD, Eliasziw M, Donner A. Sample size and optimal designs for reliability studies. Stat Med. 1998;17(1):101–10.

32. Vaz S, Ferreira TC, Salgado L, Paycha F. Bone scan usefulness in patients with painful hip or knee prosthesis: 10 situations that can cause pain, other than loosening and infection. Eur J Orthop Surg Traumatol. 2016;27(2):147-56.

33. Dobrindt O, Amthauer H, Krueger A, Ruf J, Wissel H, Grosser OS, Seidensticker M, Lohmann CH. Hybrid SPECT/CT for the assessment of a painful hip after uncemented total hip arthroplasty. BMC Med Imaging. 2015;15:18.

34. Jin S, Boktor RR, Kc Man K, Pitman AG. Normal range of osteoblastic activity in total hip arthroplasties on single-photon emission computed tomography bone scintigraphy. Nucl Med Commun. 2016;37(9):924–34.

18

Evaluation of the efficacy of amplitude-integrated electroencephalography in the screening of newborns with metabolic disorder admitted to the NICU

Maliheh Kadivar, Ziba Mosayebi, Reza Shervin Badoo, Raziyeh Sangesari, Saeed Jedari Attari, Maryam Saeedi and Elahe Movahedi Moghadam[*]

Abstract

Background: Neonate patients with metabolic disorder show encephalopathy and seizures that may lead to morbidity and mortality. Thus rapid detection and treatment of these patients is necessary. Although Amplitude-integrated electroencephalography (aEEG) has been used for more than a decade in the evaluation of infants with encephalopathy but has not been used in the assessment of neonates suffering from metabolic disorders. In this study, we tried to determine the efficacy of aEEG as an easily available diagnostic tool in the diagnosis of neonates with metabolic diseases.

Methods: All cases which admitted to the Neonatal Intensive Care Unit (NICU) of the Children's Medical Center during a one-year period were enrolled. aEEG recordings were obtained by installing 4 electrodes on the infant's head by a trained nurse and aEEG was recorded for at least 24 h with a description of the whole tracing. Clinical information, final outcome and questionnaires, including patient information: symptoms of the disease, gender, age, duration of hospitalization and the type of the metabolic disease were recorded in details. The obtained data was analyzed with the Spss24 software.

Results: Only 3 (two girl and one boy) out of 29 aEEGs recordings were abnormal; other patients showed normal aEEGs. The most common clinical and neurological manifestations were seizure (34.5%), hypotonia (31%), and mortality rate was 10.3%. There was no significant correlation between aEEG findings and gender, age, type of disease, laboratory tests findings and positive family history.

Conclusions: Although it has been shown that EEG has a diagnostic value in metabolic diseases, there has been no study on the efficacy of aEEG to evaluate neonates with metabolic diseases. But good accessibility and easy of working with aEEG, promote a tendency to use this procedure as screening tool for metabolic diseases.
The current study about aEEG monitoring in these patients, while limited, can be used as a pilot study for further research on this topic.
Therefore, a correct judgment in this field requires administration of aEEG on a larger population of neonates with metabolic diseases.

Keywords: aEEG, Metabolic diseases, Neonates

* Correspondence: elahehmovahedi@protonmail.com
Neonatal Health Research Center, Research Institute for Children Health,
Shahid Beheshti University of Medical Sciences, Tehran, Iran

Background

Inherited metabolic disorders are genetic conditions that result in metabolism problems namely a lowered or deficient activity of an enzyme in a single pathway of intermediary metabolism [1]. Due to the problems in metabolism and homeostasis of sugar, electrolytes, amino acids and ammonia, widespread brain dysfunction may occur in these patients [2].

Metabolic disorders in newborns can ultimately lead to problems such as seizure, mental retardation and even death [3]. Thus screening of metabolic disorders in newborns helps to the earliest possible diagnosis and management of the affected newborns, which in turn prevents the morbidity, mortality, and disabilities associated with the metabolic disorders [1].

Metabolic disorders screening is usually performed by means of various clinical analysis on blood and urine samples as well as imaging evaluations [4]. On the other hand, metabolic disorders are not symptomatic immediately after the birth and they can even manifest slowly with progressive encephalopathy [5]. Thus accurate diagnostic evaluation of neural function in newborns with a possible metabolic disorder is very important [4].

Electroencephalography (EEG) is one of the required tests in order to diagnose and assess the clinical condition of metabolic disorders through the abnormalities in brain electrical activity [6]. Although EEG is a non-invasive test that helps to determine metabolic diseases, the complexity of the equipment and the need for specialized staff to apply the numerous electrodes make it difficult to use.

In contrast, an appropriate alternative to solve this problem in Neonatal Intensive Care Units (NICUs) is the amplitude integrated electroencephalography (aEEG). According to previous studies, in order to generate an aEEG, one or two-channel EEG tracings are obtained, filtered, rectified and compress in time to provide a global overview of brain cerebral activity [7, 8]. Notably, frontal leads are less commonly used to detect seizures because, according to the literature, it is possible to miss more pathologies over frontal region. The 2-channel aEEG from channel C3 to P3 and C4 to P4 (named by the 10–20 system) is able to identify unilateral pathologies in brain activity. Additionally, more pathologies can be missed with a 1-channel aEEG as compared to the 2-channel method [9]. Applying the aEEG is inexpensive, easy and affordable procedure that could be carried out by NICU staff after a fairly short training period [7]. Today, aEEG is used routinely in an increasing number of NICUs, as a quantitative predictor and provides a global overview of brain cerebral activity [8, 10].

Studies in the current literature show that aEEG could help to diagnose and follow up the newborns with neonatal encephalopathy [6, 11, 12]. Although studies show the benefits of EEG for initial evaluation and management of patients with metabolic disorder [6, 13], no study has been conducted to assess the efficiency of aEEG for the assessment of newborns with metabolic diseases.

Therefore, in this study, we tried to determine aEEG performance in the diagnosis of neonates with metabolic diseases through diagnosing abnormalities in electrical brain activity.

Methods

The present study was conducted over a one-year period (April, 2017-April, 2018) on neonates with suspicious metabolic disorders who were admitted to the NICU of the Children's Medical Center, Tehran, Iran.

The study proposal was approved in the local ethics committee and informed consents were obtained from parents of neonates who fulfilled the inclusion criteria. Inclusion criteria included neonates with:

Laboratory criteria

- Ammonia > 150 µg/dl
- Lactate > 30 mmol/l
- Blood Sugar (BS) < 40 mg/dl
- High-anion gap acidosis resistant to treatment, and Base Excess (BE) < – 10
- HPLC (High-performance liquid chromatography) results that indicates metabolic disorder
- Glycine of cerebrospinal fluid /serum > 0.08
- Urine findings: Organic urine acid, regenerative materials and positive ketones
- Electrolyte disorders: hypo / hypernatremia, hyper / hypoglycemia, hyper / hypocalcaemia and hypomania

Clinical criteria

- Neurological symptoms: seizure, hypertonia, decreased consciousness
- Gastrointestinal symptoms: prolong jaundice, hepatosplenomegaly
- Cardiovascular Symptoms: Cardiomyopathy, hypotension
- Systemic Symptoms: Unwillingness to eat milk, tachypnea, acidosis, especially in cases of familial marriage
- Hydrops
- Positive family history of metabolic disease (previous child)
- Death without known cause
- Failure to justify the above with common diseases (sepsis)

Table 1 Relationship between different metabolic diseases and aEEG/EEG results

Metabolic diseases	EEG			aEEG		
	Abnormal No (%)	Normal No (%)	P.value	Abnormal No (%)	Normal No (%)	P.value
Hypoglycemia	1 (14.3)	6 (85.7)	0.016	0(0)	7(100.0)	0.839
Urea cyclic disorder	1(16.7)	5(83.3)		1(16.6)	5(83.3)	
Galactosemia	0(0)	3(100.0)		0(0)	3(100.0)	
MSUD	3(100.0)	0(0)		1(33.3)	2 (66.7)	
NKH	4(80.0)	1(20.0)		1(20.0)	4 (80.0)	
Familial hypercalciuria hypomagnesemia	0(0)	1(100.0)		0(0)	1(100.0)	
Zellweger	0 (0)	1 (100.0)		0(0)	1(100.0)	
Glycine deficiency	1 (100.0)	0(0)		0(0)	1(100.0)	
Tyrosinemia	2 (100.0)	0(0)		0(0)	2(100.0)	
Total	12 (41.4)	17 (58.6)		3 (10.34)	26 (89.65)	

Exclusion criteria included neonates with asphyxia diagnosis, death before aEEG acquisition and parent dissatisfaction.

The aEEG evaluations were done through installing 4 electrodes on the infant's head (on c3, c4, p3, p4) by a trained nurse and recorded for at least 24 h with a description of the whole tracing. Patients' diagnoses and relevant clinical information were also recorded. The obtained aEEG recordings were collected and interpreted by both pediatrician and neurologist subspecialist clinicians carefully.

Findings were recorded using questionnaires, including patient information: symptoms of the disease, gender, age, duration of hospitalization and type of metabolic disease.

The final outcome was determined by the length of hospitalization, the response to treatment, discharge from NICU or death.

Statistical analyses

Descriptive analyses of the data were performed using McNemar test. Pearson's chi-squared test and independent

sample t-test were used to evaluate the relationship aEEG abnormality and different metabolic disorders and the differences between neonates with normal and abnormal aEEG, respectively. The analyses were performed using SPSS software version 24 and a $P < 0.05$ was considered statistically significant.

Results

A total of 29 patients in NICU department were enrolled in the present study. Of the neonates, 15 (51.7%) were boy and 14 (48.3%) were girl. The mean age of neonates was 10.62 (±5.6) days. Also the mean of gestational age was 37.8 weeks (±0.88).

The most common neurological manifestations were seizure (34.5%), hypotonia (31%), and the mortality rate was 10.3%.

In this study, the most common metabolic diseases in the neonates included hypoglycemia (24.1%), urea cycle (20.7%), and NKH (Nonketotic hyperglycinemia) (17.2%) and the least common were glycine deficiency (3.4%), Zellweger (3.4%) and familial hypercalciuria hypomagnesemia (3.4%).

The results show no significant correlation between aEEG findings (normal and abnormal) and different metabolic diseases ($p = 0.839$) (Table 1). There was no relation between age, familial relation, final outcome,

Table 2 Relationship between EEG and aEEG results with seizure manifestations of the studied neonates

	Seizure manifestations		Total	Pearson chi-square	P.value Fisher's exact test
	YES	NO			
			EEG		
Abnormal	9	3	11	0.367	0.449
Normal	10	7	17		
Total	19	10	29		
			aEEG		
Abnormal	2	1	3	0.965	1
Normal	17	9	27		
Total	19	10	29		

Table 3 Relationship between EEG results with aEEG results of the studied neonates

	EEG		Total	Pearson chi-square	P.value Fisher' sexact test
	Abnormal	Normal			
			aEEG		
Abnormal	2	1	3	0.348	0.553
Normal	10	16	26		
Total	12	17	29		

Table 4 Agreement measure between pediatricians and neurologists based on aEEG finding

	Neonatologist			Total	Measure of agreement Kappa	P. value
	Continuous normal voltage	Discontinuous normal voltage	Burst suppression			
Neurologist						
Continuous normal voltage	24	0	0	24	0.713	0.003
Discontinuous normal voltage	2	1	0	3		
Burst suppression	0	0	2	2		
Total	26	1	2	29		

ultrasound result, MS MS result, HPLC result, Ammonia, lactate, ABG amount with aEEG findings.

However, as shown in the Table 1, there is a significant statistical relationship between EEG findings and the type of metabolic disease in newborns ($p = 0.016$, $_x2 = 18.7$). There was no relation between age, familial relation, final outcome, ultrasound result, MS MS result, HPLC result, Ammonia, lactate, ABG amount with EEG findings.

As shown in Table 2, none of the patients' clinical characteristics (with or without seizure) were significantly associated with aEEG ($p = 1$) and EEG ($p = 0.449$) results.

In this study, we also investigated the relationship between aEEG and EEG in neonates with metabolic diseases. The results showed that none of aEEG findings were significantly associated with EEG results ($p = 0.553$) (Table 3).

Finally, the measure of agreement between pediatric neurologists and neonatologist reports based on aEEG findings was 0.724 (strong) and statistically significant ($p = 0.003$) (Table 4).

Discussion

In this study we obtained of the 24 h-length aEEG tracings of 29 patients with different metabolic disorders. Among 29 neonates, 41.4% had abnormal EEG and 6.89% showed abnormal aEEG. The findings of aEEG were abnormal in two girls and one boy, and normal in 14 boys and 12 girls. Thus, there was no significant correlation between the findings of aEEG (normal and abnormal) and gender.

In this study, we examined the difference between the type of neonatal metabolic disease and aEEG. Our results showed no significant relation between aEEG finding and type of disease. However, given the sample size and the number of patients in different metabolic disease in this pilot study, we do not expect a meaningful association between aEEG finding and type of disease. Thus it seems that aEEG abnormalities help to monitor brain function in neonates with metabolic disorder rather than diagnostic performance towards the type of metabolic disorder [13]. Our results are in accordance with the results reported by Olischar et al. who showed that aEEG is not 'diagnostic' in IEM (Inborn error of

metabolism) but it could help in assessing the severity of encephalopathy and seizure [13]. This valuable use of aEEG has been reported by Theda et al. [7] where encephalopathy and seizure were found in IEM patients by aEEG monitoring. Also in another study on a case of hyperammonemic coma, the response to the treatment was assessed by aEEG successfully [11].

In this study, normal EEG results were consistent with normal aEEG in some diseases. For example, normal EEG in urea cycle disorder was found in 100% of cases, which was in accordance with 100% normal aEEG finding. Similarly, in the galactosemia, zellweger and Familial hypercalciuria hypomagnesemia, EEG findings were similar to aEEG findings.

As reported there was no relation between age, familial relation of the parents, final outcome, ultrasound results, MS MS result, HPLC result, Ammonia, lactate, ABG amount and aEEG and EEG findings.

We have also found a significant agreement between pediatric neurologists and neonatologist on the aEEG report. Considering the 93.1% agreement between pediatric neurologists and neonatologist in reading and reporting aEEG, and simplicity of using aEEG by other specialists, it seems that this device could be a good procedure for screening seizure problems in NICUs.

Other studies also reported that aEEG has high sensitivity and specificity in predicting neurodevelopmental outcome for screening of asphyxiated full-term infants [14–17].

Conclusion

Although finding of this study showed no relation between aEEG and different metabolic disorder, this procedure can provide valuable information about brain activity, especially during metabolic crisis. In regard to the low number of patients in this study, more studies with larger population are needed to determine the amplitude-integrated efficacy of EEG in neonates with metabolic disorder. However, inspite of the above-mentioned limitations, the current study appears to be a promising avenue to perform further projects in this field.

Abbreviations

aEEG: Amplitude-integrated electroencephalography; BE: Base Excess; BS: Blood Sugar; HPLC: High-performance liquid chromatography; NICU: Neonatal Intensive Care Unit; NKH: Nonketotic hyperglycinemia

Acknowledgements

We acknowledge the staff of NICU ward of Neonatal Health Research Center, Research Institute for Children Health, Shahid Beheshti University of Medical Sciences. We thank Mrs. Saeeedi for performing aEEG. We also thank Dr. Mahboobel Sadat Modaresi doing statistical analysis. We also thank Mofid research center and Neourology research center. The authors would like to thank Dr. Mohammad Taghi Ashtiani and Mr. Khatami.

Authors' contributions

MK and EMM: has made substantial contributions to conception and design, or acquisition of data, or analysis and interpretation of data; ZM, SJA and RSB: has been involved in performing the work, Collecting information from questionnaire and drafting the manuscript or revising it critically for important intellectual content; and RS: involved in literature review, preparing the questionnaire and has given final approval of the version to be published. EMM: has made substantial contributions to conception and design, or acquisition of data, or analysis and interpretation of data; MS has been involved in literature review and drafting the manuscript or revising it critically for important intellectual content. All authors have read and approved the manuscript.

Competing interests

The authors declare that they have no competing interests.

References

1. Pourfarzam M, Zadhoush F. Newborn screening for inherited metabolic disorders; news and views. J Res Med Sci. 2013;18:801.
2. Lin C. EEG manifestations in metabolic encephalopathy. Acta Neurol Taiwanica. 2005;14:151.
3. Yu JY, Pearl PL. Metabolic causes of epileptic encephalopathy. Epilepsy Res Treat. 2013;2013:124934.
4. Faigle R, Sutter R, Kaplan PW. Electroencephalography of encephalopathy in patients with endocrine and metabolic disorders. J Clin Neurophysiol. 2013; 30:505–516. https://doi.org/10.1097/WNP.0b013e3182a73db9, http://www.ncbi.nlm.nih.gov/pubmed/24084183.
5. Karimzadeh P, Taghdiri MM, Abasi E, Amouzadeh MH, Naghavi Z, Ghazavi A, et al. Metabolic screening in children with neurodevelopmental delay, seizure and/or regression. Iran J Child Neurol. 2017;11:42.
6. Demir AB, Bora I, Kaygili E, Ocakoglu G. The assessment of basic features of electroencephalography in metabolic encephalopathies. J Neurol Res. 2014; 4:101–9.
7. Theda C. Use of amplitude integrated electroencephalography (aEEG) in patients with inborn errors of metabolism - a new tool for the metabolic geneticist. Mol Genet Metab. 2010;100 Suppl 1:S42–S48. https://doi.org/10.1016/j.ymgme.2010.02.013, http://www.ncbi.nlm.nih.gov/pubmed/20303809.
8. Sanchez Fernandez I, Loddenkemper T. aEEG and cEEG: two complementary techniques to assess seizures and encephalopathy in neonates: editorial on "amplitude-integrated EEG for detection of neonatal seizures: a systematic review" by Rakshasbhuvankar et al. Seizure. 2015;33:88–89. https://doi.org/10.1016/j.seizure.2015.10.010, http://www.ncbi.nlm.nih.gov/pubmed/26560180.
9. Lavery S, Shah DK, Filan PM, Doyle LW, Inder TE. Single versus bihemispheric amplitude-integrated electroencephalography in relation to cerebral injury and outcome in the term encephalopathic infant. J Paediatr Child Health. 2008;44(5):285–90.
10. Spitzmiller RE, Phillips T, Meinzen-Derr J, Hoath SB. Amplitude-integrated EEG is useful in predicting neurodevelopmental outcome in full-term infants with hypoxic-ischemic encephalopathy: a meta-analysis. J Child Neurol. 2007;22:1069–1078. https://doi.org/10.1177/0883073807306258, http://www.ncbi.nlm.nih.gov/pubmed/17890403.
11. Whitelaw A, Bridges S, Leaf A, Evans D. Emergency treatment of neonatal hyperammonaemic coma with mild systemic hypothermia. Lancet. 2001; 358:36–38. https://doi.org/10.1016/S0140-6736(00)05269-7, http://www.ncbi.nlm.nih.gov/pubmed/11454378.
12. Olischar M, Theda C, Lavery S, Coleman L, Hunt RW. Amplitude-integrated EEG abnormalities in two neonates with encephalopathy due to mitochondrial dysfunction (respiratory chain complex I deficiency). J Pediatr Neurol. 2009;7:285–92.
13. Olischar M, Shany E, Aygun C, Azzopardi D, Hunt RW, Toet MC, et al. Amplitude-integrated electroencephalography in newborns with inborn errors of metabolism. Neonatology. 2012;102:203–211. https://doi.org/10.1159/000339567, http://www.ncbi.nlm.nih.gov/pubmed/22797054.
14. Glass HC. Advancing neurologic care in the intensive care nursery. NeoReviews. 2015;16:e519–e25.
15. Kliegman RM, Behrman RE, Jenson HB, Stanton BM. Nelson textbook of pediatrics e-book: Elsevier Health Sciences; 2007.
16. Lu WY, Chen JY, Chang CF, Weng WC, Lee WT, Shieh JS. Multiscale entropy of electroencephalogram as a potential predictor for the prognosis of neonatal seizures. PLoS One. 2015;10:e0144732. https://doi.org/10.1371/journal.pone.0144732, http://www.ncbi.nlm.nih.gov/pubmed/26658680.
17. Sisman J, Campbell DE, Brion LP. Amplitude-integrated EEG in preterm infants: maturation of background pattern and amplitude voltage with postmenstrual age and gestational age. J Perinatol. 2005;25:391–396. https://doi.org/10.1038/sj.jp.7211291, http://www.ncbi.nlm.nih.gov/pubmed/15815708.

19

The diagnostic performance of ^{18}F-FAMT PET and ^{18}F-FDG PET for malignancy detection

Arifudin Achmad[1,2]* ⓘ, Anu Bhattarai[1], Ryan Yudistiro[1,3], Yusri Dwi Heryanto[1], Tetsuya Higuchi[1] and Yoshito Tsushima[1]

Abstract

Background: This meta-analysis aims to compare the diagnostic performance of L-3-^{18}F-α-methyl tyrosine (^{18}F-FAMT) positron emission tomography (PET) and 2-deoxy-2-[^{18}F]fluoro-D-glucose (^{18}F-FDG) PET for malignancy detection.

Methods: The workflow of this study follows Cochrane Collaboration Guidelines of a systematic review of diagnostic test accuracy studies. An electronic search was performed for clinical diagnostic studies directly comparing ^{18}F-FAMT and ^{18}F-FDG PET for malignant tumors. Study quality, the risks of bias and sources of variation among studies were assessed using the QUADAS (Quality Assessment of Diagnostic Accuracy Studies) assessment tool. A separate meta-analysis was performed for diagnostic performance based on visual assessment and diagnostic cut-off values. Whenever possible, a bivariate random-effect model was used for analysis and pooling of diagnostic measures across studies.

Results: Electronic search revealed 56 peer-reviewed basic science investigations and clinical studies. Six eligible studies (272 patients) of various type of cancer were meta-analyzed. The ^{18}F-FAMT diagnostic accuracy for malignancy was higher than ^{18}F-FDG based on both visual assessment (diagnostic odd ratio (DOR): 8.90, 95% confidence interval (CI) [2.4, 32.5]) vs 4.63, 95% CI [1.8, 12.2], area under curve (AUC): 77.4% vs 72.8%) and diagnostic cut-off (DOR: 13.83, 95% CI [6.3, 30.6] vs 7.85, 95% CI [3.7, 16.8], AUC: 85.6% vs 80.2%), respectively. While the average sensitivity and specificity of ^{18}F-FAMT and ^{18}F-FDG based on visual assessment were similar, ^{18}F-FAMT was significantly more specific than ^{18}F-FDG ($p < 0.05$) based on diagnostic cut-off values.

Conclusions: ^{18}F-FAMT is more specific for malignancy than ^{18}F-FDG, while their sensitivity is comparable. ^{18}F-FAMT PET is equal to ^{18}F-FDG PET in diagnostic performance for malignancy detection in several cancer types.

Keywords: ^{18}F-FAMT, ^{18}F-FDG, Malignancy, Meta-analysis, Diagnostic accuracy

Background

Since its introduction as a positron emission tomography (PET) tracer back in the early 1970's, [^{18}F]-fluoro-deoxyglucose (^{18}F-FDG) has been widely utilized and now comprises more than 96% of PET studies worldwide [1]. Even though ^{18}F-FDG is mainly a radiotracer for

oncology, it is not a tumor-specific PET tracer, since it is essentially based on the presence of elevated glucose uptake [2]. Many malignant lesions, in fact, are poorly imaged with ^{18}F-FDG; some due to their slow growth or low metabolic nature, and others due to their location within highly metabolic organs such as the brain and liver [3]. Various alternative PET tracers have been synthesized and evaluated over the last decade to overcome the limitations of ^{18}F-FDG, including tracers based on amino acid metabolism such as L-3-^{18}F-α-methyl tyrosine (^{18}F-FAMT) [1, 4].

^{18}F-FAMT has been validated in several clinical studies to be useful for the prediction of cancer prognosis and

---

* Correspondence: aachmad@gunma-u.ac.jp; m09702036@gunma-u.ac.jp
[1]Department of Diagnostic Radiology and Nuclear Medicine, Gunma University Graduate School of Medicine, 3-39-22 Showa-machi, Maebashi, Gunma 371-8511, Japan
[2]Department of Nuclear Medicine and Molecular Imaging, Faculty of Medicine, Padjadjaran University, Jl. Professor Eyckman No.38, Bandung, West Java 40161, Indonesia
Full list of author information is available at the end of the article

to rule out benign lesions from malignant neoplasms [5–13]. The tumor accumulation of ^{18}F-FAMT is exclusively facilitated by the L-type amino acid transporter 1 (LAT1), which is highly upregulated in malignant cells [14]. Unlike other amino acid PET tracers that are not specific to a single amino acid transporter, ^{18}F-FAMT has a α-methyl moiety that allows it to be transported only by LAT1, making it highly specific for malignancies [15]. Although a handful of clinical studies have investigated its potential in malignant tumor detection, the overall diagnostic performance of ^{18}F-FAMT remains unknown. The present meta-analysis aimed to determine the diagnostic performance of ^{18}F-FAMT PET for detection and evaluation of malignant lesions in a direct side-by-side comparison to ^{18}F-FDG PET.

Methods
Search strategy and study selection
The design of this study followed the current recommendations for systematic review of diagnostic test accuracy studies from the Cochrane Collaboration [16, 17]. Studies evaluating ^{18}F-FAMT PET or PET/CT as a diagnostic tool for evaluation of malignancy were electronically searched in Pubmed/MEDLINE, Web of Science, ScienceDirect, and Google Scholar databases from the inception of ^{18}F-FAMT to December 2016 without language restriction. The search algorithm was based on a combination of the following terms: ^{18}F-FAMT or ^{18}F-FMT or "alpha-methyltyrosine." To find more potential studies, we also screened references of the retrieved studies. Articles without raw clinical data such as reviews, conference abstracts, editorial, comments, preclinical, animal and non-radiopharmaceutical studies, or clinical studies with fewer than ten patients were excluded. The following information was extracted: first author's name, year of publication, study design, study population, types/subtypes of malignancies, injected dose, imaging parameters, cut-off values of quantitative parameters, study and follow-up period, final diagnosis, and the reference standard.

The clinical studies obtained were subject to inclusion criteria for further analysis: (a) both ^{18}F-FAMT and ^{18}F-FDG were used to differentiate malignant tumors from benign lesions, (b) histopathological analysis and/or close clinical and imaging follow-up were used as reference standards, (c) when data or subsets of data were presented in more than one article, the article with the most detailed/recent data was chosen, and (d) only articles in which at least 10 of the 14 questions in the QUADAS (Quality Assessment Tool for Diagnostic Accuracy Studies) questionnaire were answered 'yes' were included [18]. Studies were screened for eligibility, the risk of bias, and source of variations by three authors

(AA, AB, RY) independently. Disagreements regarding the eligibility of a study were resolved by consensus.

Meta-analysis
Meta-analysis of the diagnostic performance of ^{18}F-FAMT and ^{18}F-FDG in recognizing malignancies was performed following the current recommendations [17] and was conducted separately for two diagnostic methods: 1) by visual assessment, and 2) by diagnostic cut-off values applied in each study. From each study included, the number of true positives, false positives, true negatives, and false negatives were extracted to construct a 2 × 2 contingency table. If studies lacked clear data to produce such tables, the first authors were contacted when possible. This main data were described on forest plots of specificity and sensitivity.

Heterogeneity and between-study variability were evaluated, and subgroup study (meta-regression analysis) was used to investigate the source, if any. A Higgins' inconsistency I^2 up to 30% was considered little evidence of heterogeneity. To determine whether different thresholds were used to define positive and negative test results (either explicitly or implicitly), the Spearman ρ between the logit of sensitivity and logit of 1 – specificity was calculated to assess the presence of a threshold effect. A strong positive correlation (Spearman $\rho > 0.6$) would suggest the presence of a threshold effect. Whenever possible, a bivariate random-effect model meta-analysis method was used to obtain summary estimates of sensitivity and specificity across studies instead of univariate approaches.

The hierarchical summary of the receiver operating characteristic (HSROC) curve was plotted following the method of Rücker and Schumacher [19]. The area under the curve (AUC), which is the average true-positive rate over the entire range of false-positive rate, serves as a global measure of test performance, while the diagnostic odd ratio (DOR) is calculated to describe the diagnostic value [20]. Note that the DOR is a single overall indicator of diagnostic performance and is, unlike sensitivity and specificity, independent of any threshold value. Meta-analysis was performed using the 'mada' (Meta-Analysis of Diagnostic Accuracy) package in R statistical software version 3.2.2 [21, 22].

Results
Literature search
The systematic search was performed to collect diagnostic test studies using ^{18}F-FAMT and ^{18}F-FDG PET for malignancy detection. The search yielded 65 studies involving ^{18}F-FAMT as PET radiotracer in basic science investigations and clinical studies. There were three radiochemistry studies, nine in vitro and animal studies, four review articles, and 49 clinical studies. Thirty

studies among these 49 clinical studies were original articles in which both PET radiotracers were employed. Figure 1 summarizes the systematic study selection.

Study eligibility, quality, and risk of bias

Nine eligible studies according to the inclusion criteria (Table 1) were further evaluated with QUADAS tool. All were prospective studies of good quality (QUADAS Scores >10) involving at least 19 patients (patient number range: 19–74) and 21 lesions (lesion number range: 21–75). Overall, the nine eligible studies had a low risk of bias, except in blinding from the index test results (Additional file 1: Table S1). Blinding from the index test results was sometimes unavoidable in the clinical workflow, since histopathological diagnosis is established after the primary surgery or biopsy, while PET imaging is an early step in workups to establish the clinical diagnosis. In one study, the histopathology (biopsy) diagnosis was known before the PET study was performed [7]. However, this study was later excluded from the meta-analysis (Table 1). The other important potential source of bias was the use of other imaging studies (CT, MRI or bone scans) and close clinical monitoring as verification methods in one study [5]. However, in this study, only two patients (from 19 patients, total 57 lesions) had their lesions diagnosed without any histological examination:

one had malignant melanoma in the foot (single lesion), and the other had diffuse malignant melanoma (lesions in the brain and spinal cord).

Six studies were included in the final meta-analysis due to the availability of individual patient data to construct 2×2 contingency tables (Table 1 and Additional file 1: Table S2). All studies employed maximum standardized uptake value (SUV_{max}) for quantitative interpretation of the PET images. Four explicitly described SUVmax cut-off value for discrimination between malignant and benign lesions. The SUVmax cut-offs of ^{18}F-FAMT studies ranged from 1 to 1.45 while in ^{18}F-FDG studies, they ranged from 0.81 to 4.72. Six studies with a total sample size of 272 patients (278 lesions) with malignancy from musculoskeletal [12, 23], fatty tumors [11], maxillofacial tumors [9], lung cancer [24], and several different tumors [5] were included.

Descriptive statistics

Figure 2 described the paired sensitivity and specificity of ^{18}F-FAMT and ^{18}F-FDG of each study in forest plots. The sensitivity of both radiotracers was homogeneous either based on the visual assessment or diagnostic cut-off values. Their specificity was heterogeneous based on visual assessment. The Spearman correlation (ρ) between sensitivity and the logit of 1-specificity suggest that

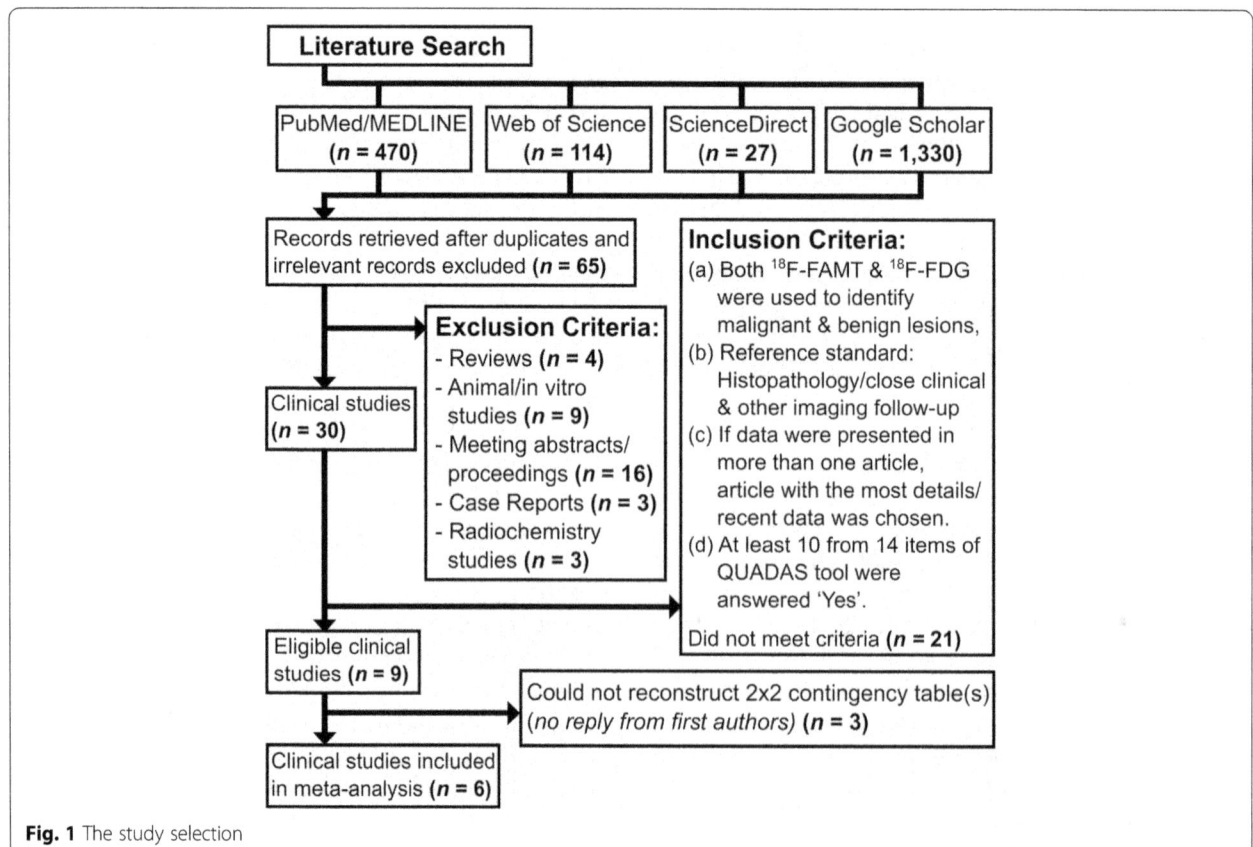

Fig. 1 The study selection

Table 1 Characteristics of Diagnostic Comparison Studies of ^{18}F-FAMT and ^{18}F-FDG

Study (year) [Ref]	N	Mean/ Median Age (range)	Sex (M/F)	Tumour & other pathology examined	No. of lesions	^{18}F-FAMT dose	^{18}F-FDG dose	PET studies interval	Follow-up period	Gold Standard & verification	Study design	Study Period	QUADAS Score[b]
Inoue (1999) [6]	20	41 ± 21 (–71)	8/12	Brain tumour	23	185 MBq	200 MBq	Within 1 wk.	> 4 mo.	H (16), Img & Cln (4)	Pro	ND	12 (6,11)
Watanabe (2000) [12][a]	74	44 (12–83)	37/38	Musculoskeletal tumours: 24 bone, 48 soft tissue	22 mlg, 53 bgn	185–350 MBq	185–350 MBq	ND	> 1 y.	H	Pro	2/'98–6/'99	13 (11)
Inoue (2001) [5][a]	19	58 (20–84)	13/6	Lung cancer (10), mlg myeloma (2), Chondrosarcoma (1), Prostate (1), mlg lymphoma (1), mlg of unknown origin (1), Schwannoma (1), Sarcoidosis (2)	57	200–370 MBq	200–370 MBq	Within 1 wk.	> 8 mo.	H (31), Img & Cln (26)	Pro	ND	10 (1,6,7,11)
Sato (2003) [13]	14	Gliomatosis: 45 (15–60) Non-neoplastic: 41.2 (23–76)	4/4 5/1	- Gliomatosis cerebri (8): Anaplastic (1), grade II astrocytoma (4) grade III astrocytoma (3) - Non-neoplastic diseases (6)	ND	185 MBq	ND	1–5 wk. (detailed)	ND	H (8) for gliomatosis Img & Cln for non-neoplasms	Pro	ND	12 (6,11)
Suzuki (2005) [11][a]	57	58.1 (27–87)	29/28	Fatty tissue tumour	32 lipoma, 25 liposarcoma	185–350 MBq	185–350 MBq	ND	ND	H (57)	Pro	9/'97–12/'03	12 (11,4Un)
Kaira (2007) [7]	41	61 (45–82) 43 (20–73)	13/4 9/15	Lung cancer (17) Sarcoidosis (24)	9 AC, 6 SQC, 2 NSCLC, 16 LNM, 24 sarcoidosis	4–5 MBq/kg	5–6 MBq/kg	ND for lung cancer. Sarcoidosis: 1 wk. after diagnosis established.	> 2 y.	H (41)	Pro	Sarcoidosis: 9/'98–8/'05	12 (10,12)
Miyakubo (2007) [9] [a]	43	ND (31–90) ND (32–81)	16/20 5/2	Maxillofacial tumours: mlg. (36), bgn. (7) and LNM (14)	34 SQC, 1 rhabdomyosarcoma, 1 mucoepidermoid carcinoma, 14 LNM, 7 bgn	5–6 MBq/kg	5–6 MBq/kg	2 wk.	> 6 mo.	H (43)	Pro	5/'99–7/'06	13 (11)
Kaira (2009) [24][a]	43	67 (41–79)	33/10	Thoracic tumours: mlg. (37), bgn. (6)	19 AC, 9 SQC, 1 LCC, 2 atypical SQC, 3 Bronchoalveolar carci-noma, 1 carcinoid, 6 bgn	ND	5 MBq/kg	1–14 d. (mean: 4 d.)	ND	H (43)	Pro	5/'07–3/'08	12 (11,12)
Tian (2011) [23][a]	36	ND (11–84)	22/14	Musculoskeletal tumour	13 mlg, 23 bgn	260 MBq	320 MBq	Maximum 2 wk.	ND	H, Img & Cln (36)	Pro	ND	13 (11)

Abbreviations: MBq/kg (MegaBecquerel/kg), d. Days, wk. Weeks, mo. Months, y. Year, H Histopathology, Img Imaging, Cln Clinical follow-up, Pro Prospective, Retro Retrospective, mlg malignant, bgn benign, LNM lymph node metastases, AC adenocarcinoma, SQC squamous cell carcinoma, NSCLC non-small cell lung cancer, LCC large cell carcinoma, ND not determined
[a]Studies included in the meta-analysis
[b]QUADAS Score was presented as 'total score (item number which answered 'No' or 'Unclear' (Un)'. QUADAS tool items were described in Tablze S1

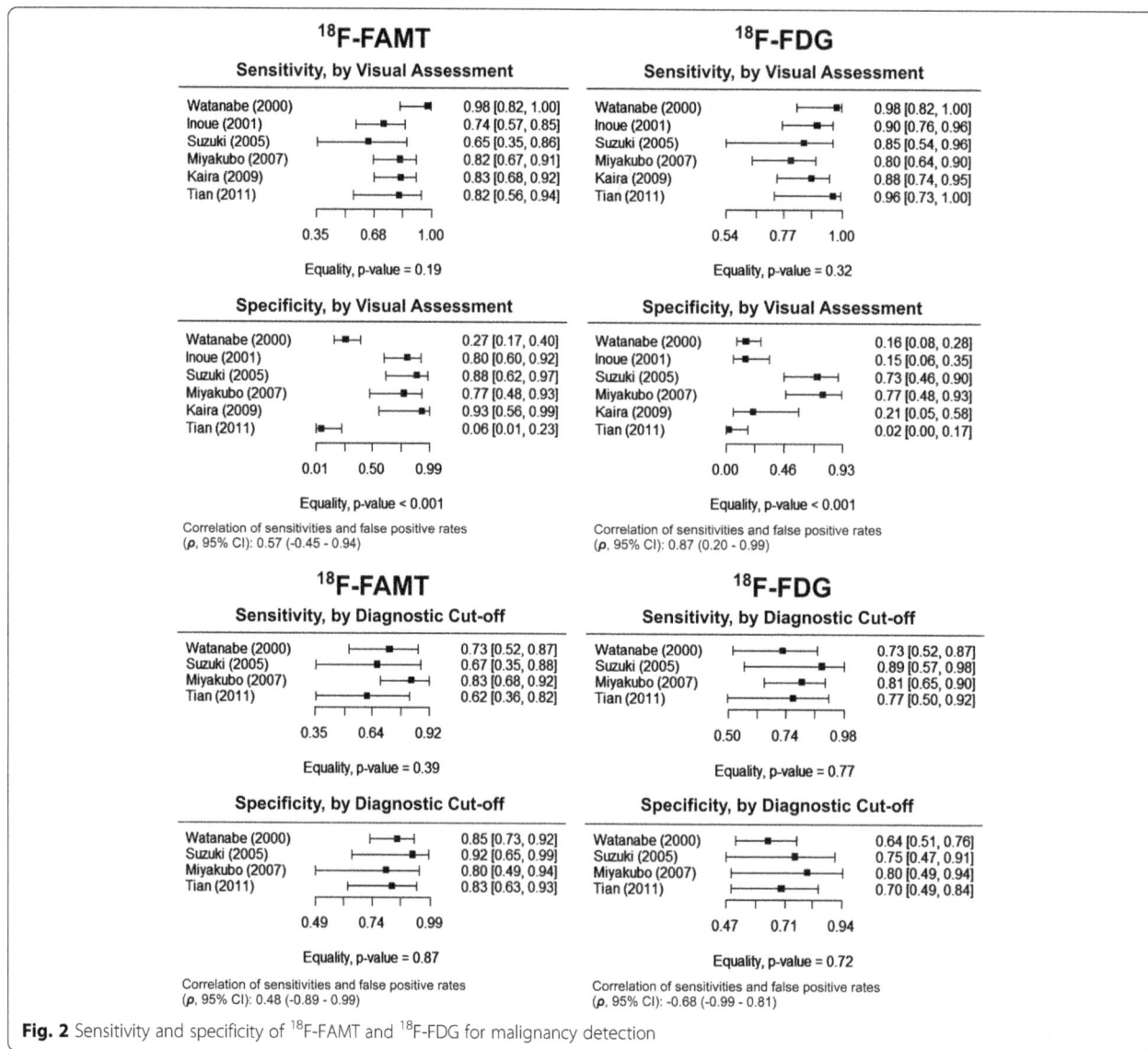

Fig. 2 Sensitivity and specificity of ^{18}F-FAMT and ^{18}F-FDG for malignancy detection

accuracy of both radiotracers based on visual assessment may be influenced by threshold effects ($\geq$ 0.6). However, their accuracy was less affected by threshold effect when the diagnostic cut-off value was implemented.

Meta-analysis

Due to the small number of studies included, both univariate and bivariate approach meta-analysis was performed. The bivariate approach is the method currently recommended; however, it cannot handle small sample sizes [17]. Meta-regression or subgroup analysis (to explore the source of heterogeneity) was also irrelevant due to the limited number of studies.

Table 2 described the summary estimates from the random effects univariate analysis. DOR of ^{18}F-FAMT and ^{18}F-FDG based on visual assessment were 8.90 and

4.63, while those based on diagnostic cut-off were 13.83 and 7.85, respectively. The heterogeneity between studies as well as inter-study was observed only mildly on ^{18}F-FAMT studies based on visual assessment (Higgins' I^2: 11.76%, τ^2: 1.46) while it was not observed in other studies.

Table 2 Summary estimates from univariate meta-analysis

Summary estimates (95% CI)	Based on visual assessment		Based on diagnostic cut-off	
	^{18}F-FAMT	^{18}F-FDG	^{18}F-FAMT	^{18}F-FDG
Between-study heterogeneity	I^2: 11.76%	I^2: 0%	I^2: 0%	I^2: 0%
Inter-study heterogeneity	τ^2: 1.46	τ^2: 0.30	τ^2: 0.00	τ^2: 0.00
DOR	8.90 (2.4–32.5)	4.63 (1.8–12.2)	13.83 (6.3–30.6)	7.85 (3.7–16.8)

The summary estimate measures of the random effects bivariate model are described in Table 3. There was no significant difference in average sensitivity and specificity between ^{18}F-FAMT and ^{18}F-FDG based on visual assessment ($p = 0.181$ and 0.207, respectively). However, ^{18}F-FAMT was significantly more specific than ^{18}F-FDG ($p < 0.01$) based on diagnostic cut-off values. DOR of ^{18}F-FAMT and ^{18}F-FDG based on visual assessment were 8.33 and 3.88 while based on diagnostic cut-off were 16.70 and 8.17, respectively.

The HSROC curves of diagnostic performance comparison are shown in Fig. 3. The AUC of diagnostic performance of ^{18}F-FAMT and ^{18}F-FDG based on visual assessment was 77.4% and 72.8%, while those based on diagnostic cut-off were 85.6% and 80.2%, respectively. The estimated SROC curves from the bivariate model (Rutter-Gatsonis method) were also plotted as a reference (Fig. 3, *dashed lines*). The summary operating points of ^{18}F-FAMT were on the left side of those of ^{18}F-FDG in both HSROC curves comparison, which indicated that ^{18}F-FAMT provided more specificity. Meanwhile, their similar heights of the summary operating points on the Y-axis showed that their sensitivities were comparable.

Discussion

This meta-analysis summarized the diagnostic performance of ^{18}F-FAMT PET for detection of various malignancies in six studies with total 278 patients. Overall, the included studies have a low risk of bias with good methodological quality based on QUADAS tool. Our results demonstrated that ^{18}F-FAMT is comparable with ^{18}F-FDG for its diagnostic performance in detecting

malignancies by either visual assessments or diagnostic cut-off values. Moreover, ^{18}F-FAMT capability is coherent in several types of tumors, where all individual diagnostic test studies directly compared the two radiotracers on the same patients in a prospective study design. Additionally, the potential for selection bias can be safely ignored due to the sufficient number of lesions evaluated in each study included ($n > 20$). Another strength of this meta-analysis is that even though the study number is limited, heterogeneity was not substantial. The source of observed mild heterogeneity was likely due to threshold effects, which was found in studies based on visual assessment. However, other potential sources of heterogeneity should not be neglected since subgroup analysis was not applicable [25]. Publication bias is an important consideration in any meta-analysis. However, DOR heterogeneity observed in our results precludes the necessity for a funnel plot asymmetry test [26].

In the current recommendation for meta-analysis of diagnostic test accuracy from The Cochrane Collaboration, bivariate approach meta-analysis is preferred over the traditional univariate meta-analysis [17]. However, guidance for determining methodological approaches for meta-analysis with small numbers of studies is currently lacking. In this case, Doebler et al. and Takwoingi et al. encouraged the use of univariate approaches excluding pooling sensitivities and specificities [21, 27]. Eventually, both univariate and bivariate methods were conducted in the current study, and the diagnostic performance of ^{18}F-FAMT against ^{18}F-FDG was consistent under both approaches. The more conservative approach for HSROC estimation (Rücker-Schumacher's method) also showed a similar tendency to the traditional HSROC parametrization (Rutter-Gatsonis's method) [19].

Despite the limited number of studies included, results of our meta-analysis reflect the natural characteristics of both radiotracers that assess malignant lesions via different metabolic processes. The key feature of ^{18}F-FDG is its superior capability to depict increased metabolic activity reflected by cell glucose consumption. The price of this high sensitivity is the detection accuracy that is prone to being obscured by normal physiological uptake, inflammation, and active benign tumors [2]. In a recent large-size meta-analysis, ^{18}F-FDG PET failed to maintain its diagnostic accuracy for lung cancer in populations with endemic infectious lung disease [28]. ^{18}F-FDG PET was also only moderately accurate for differentiating benign from malignant pleural effusions [29].

In another meta-analysis, whole-body ^{18}F-FDG PET/ CT remained superior to conventional imaging in the detection of distant malignancies, regardless of the primary tumor site and type [30]. However, the diagnostic accuracy of a PET radiotracer for lesions in the thorax and abdomen, where most primary lesions are located, is

Table 3 Summary estimates from bivariate meta-analysis

Summary estimates (95% CI)	Based on visual assessment		Based on diagnostic cut-off	
	^{18}F-FAMT	^{18}F-FDG	^{18}F-FAMT	^{18}F-FDG
Average Sensitivity	80.7% (72.4–87.0%)	88.8% (80.2–93.9%)	74.1% (63.0–82.7%)	78.3% (67.8–86.1%)
p values	0.181		0.542	
Average Specificity	60.7% (25.3–87.6%)	29.2% (9.2–62.5%)	84.4% (75.7–90.4%)	68.1% (58.1–76.6%)
p values	0.207		0.009	
Positive Likelihood	2.46 (1.11–6.23)	1.34 (1.00–2.25)	4.90 (2.96–7.92)	2.48 (1.81–3.44)
Negative Likelihood	0.36 (0.20–0.70)	0.44 (0.20–0.98)	0.31 (0.20–0.45)	0.33 (0.20–0.49)
DOR	8.33 (1.60–20.10)	3.88 (1.02–10.40)	16.70 (7.25–33.40)	8.19 (3.86–15.40)
AUC[a]	77.4%	72.8%	85.6%	80.2%
λ (mean accuracy)	3.81	3.08	3.44	2.99

[a]approximated following Rucker-Schumacher's method [19]

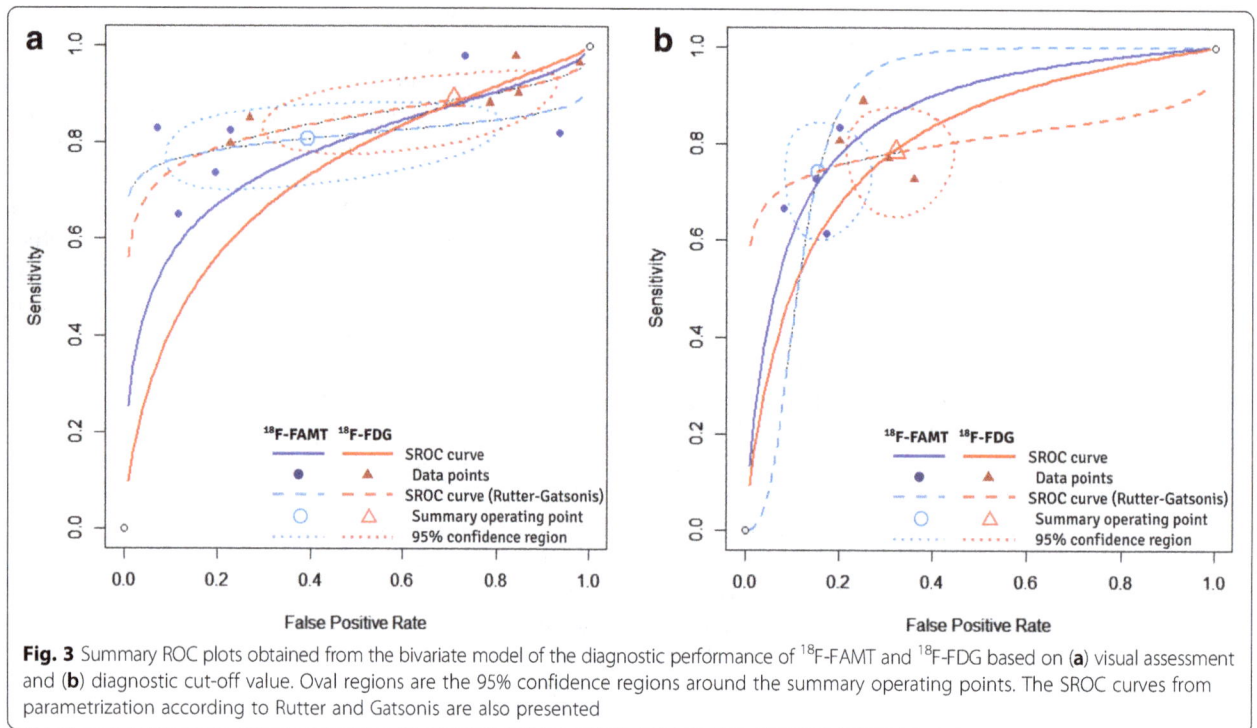

Fig. 3 Summary ROC plots obtained from the bivariate model of the diagnostic performance of ^{18}F-FAMT and ^{18}F-FDG based on (**a**) visual assessment and (**b**) diagnostic cut-off value. Oval regions are the 95% confidence regions around the summary operating points. The SROC curves from parametrization according to Rutter and Gatsonis are also presented

essential. It is well known that the role of ^{18}F-FDG PET in oncology is often mitigated by many pitfalls, including background physiological uptake of major organs [31].

On the other hand, ^{18}F-FAMT specific uptake depicted the actual malignant process. ^{18}F-FAMT uptake reflects excessive transport of amino acids via LAT1, which is absent in normal cells and pathology other than malignancy [15]. However, the trade-off of ^{18}F-FAMT's high specificity is the relatively small absolute uptake in tumor cells, as a consequence of the nature of the LAT1 transporter. The influx of one amino acid substrate into tumor cells via LAT1 is mandatoryly coupled to the efflux of another amino acid substrate, resulting in ^{18}F-FAMT's relatively fast clearance from the tumor [14]. Nonetheless, the advantage of ^{18}F-FAMT is the minimal background uptake in all organs except kidney and urinary tracts, allowing one to obtain high contrast images clearly depicting various types of malignancy including brain tumors [6, 13].

Meta-analyses evaluating the diagnostic performance of ^{18}F-FDG PET in malignancy detection were mostly limited to a particular cancer type, or in comparison with conventional imaging (CT or MRI) or hybrid imaging (PET/CT or PET/MRI). Currently, only a few tumor-specific PET radiotracers are continuously investigated in a clinical setting for various type of cancers [32]. ^{18}F-FET is probably the closest to ^{18}F-FAMT in terms of chemical compound, radiochemistry, and clinical applicability. While ^{18}F-FET has higher diagnostic accuracy than ^{18}F-FDG, its effectiveness is

limited for brain tumors [33]. L-[methyl-^{11}C]-methionine (^{11}C-MET), the most popular amino acid-based PET radiotracer to date, also has excellent diagnostic accuracy for glioma compared to ^{18}F-FDG [34]. However, both ^{18}F-FET and ^{11}C-MET are also substrates for LAT2 transporters, which is also expressed in normal cells [14, 35]. The low kidney uptake PET tracer *anti*-1-amino-3-^{18}F-fluorocyclobutane-1-carboxylic acid (^{18}F-FACBC) has recently been meta-analyzed for its accuracy in prostate cancer recurrence detection. However, the specificity of ^{18}F-FACBC is lower than ^{11}C-choline PET and even T2-weighted MRI [36]. Therefore, ^{18}F-FAMT probably the most versatile oncologic PET radiotracer currently available.

However, there a few limitations in this study and also in ^{18}F-FAMT itself. First, all studies were from a single institution, which was potentially affected by publication bias despite the authors of each study belonging to various departments and evaluating different types of tumors. Even though studies by Watanabe et al. and Tian et al. focused on musculoskeletal tumors, they were separated by more than a decade, eliminating the possibility of overlapping patients [12, 23]. A study of various tumors by Inoue et al., however, included two patients with chondrosarcoma and schwannoma that might also be involved in the Watanabe et al. study, since these studies were from the same period [5, 12]. Unfortunately, this is difficult to confirm. Second, not all types of malignancies were evaluated; in particular, lymphoma, melanoma, pancreas and thyroid cancer, which are tumor types for which ^{18}F-FDG PET is recommended to improve diagnostic accuracy [3]. Tumors in the pelvic area and abdomen were also poorly represented in this study.

Another drawback of the current ^{18}F-FAMT studies is the absence of dynamic PET data. Currently ^{18}F-FAMT PET scan is performed at 40–60 min post injection. However, phases as early as 5–15 min post injection might show higher tumor detection accuracy for any amino acid PET tracer considering the two-way-directional characteristic of amino acid uptake by their transporters [37]. A dynamic ^{18}F-FAMT PET study in an animal tumor model showed that tumor-to-muscle uptake ratio is highest at 20 min and remains high at 60 min [38]. However, clinical dynamic PET studies are necessary to obtain optimal scan times.

Our current findings emphasize the need for prospective multicenter studies to overcome limitations of the single center report. This can only be achieved when the ^{18}F-FAMT synthesis method is optimized and becomes widely used. The current ^{18}F-FAMT radiofluorination method yields a low radioactivity that is only enough for PET scans for a mere three to four patients in each radiosynthesis [39]. Recently, a modified method of ^{18}F-FAMT synthesis allows production to achieve high radioactivity for routine use [40]. However, a more practical approach is warranted. The twenty years of anticipation might soon be realized with the recent rapid development of fluorination methods. Of particular interest are the so-called late-stage fluorination methods which allow optimized synthesis of previously inaccessible PET radiotracers [41]. These novel radiofluorination approaches which make possible large-scale synthesis allow reconsideration of promising but underutilized radiotracers, like ^{18}F-FAMT. Hence, revisiting the diagnostic performance of ^{18}F-FAMT is a major step in the quest for an ideal general oncology PET tracer. Once these impediments are resolved, which we foresee shortly, the future may bring increased clinical impact of ^{18}F-FAMT in oncology.

Conclusion

^{18}F-FAMT has diagnostic performance equal to or perhaps even better than ^{18}F-FDG for malignancy detection in several cancer types. Future development in ^{18}F-FAMT radiosynthesis might allow this tracer to be evaluated in other tumor types.

Abbreviations
[11]C-MET: L-[methyl-^{11}C] methionine; ^{18}F-FACBC: anti-1-amino-3-^{18}F-fluorocyclobutane-1-carboxylic acid; ^{18}F-FAMT: L-3-^{18}F-α-methyl tyrosine; ^{18}F-FDG: 2-deoxy-2-[^{18}F]fluoro-D-glucose; ^{18}F-FET: O-(2-[^{18}F]fluoroethyl)-L-tyrosine; DOR: Diagnostic odds ratio; LAT(1–4): L-type amino acid transporter (1–4); PET: Positron emission tomography; QUADAS: Quality Assessment of Diagnostic Accuracy Studies; SPECT: Single-photon emission computed tomography; SROC: Summary receiver operating characteristics; SUV$_{max}$: Maximum standardized uptake value

Acknowledgements
We are very grateful to Dr. Ayako Taketomi-Takahashi for her assistance in improving the English in this manuscript.

Funding
Not applicable.

Authors' contributions
AA designed the study, selected articles for inclusion, performed data extraction, assessed study quality, undertook meta-analysis, and wrote the paper. AB and RY selected articles for inclusion, assisted with data extraction, and assessed study quality. YDH performed additional statistical analysis. TH and YT edited and reviewed the final manuscript. All authors contributed during manuscript preparation, and read and approved the final manuscript.

Competing interests
Authors are educational staffs (AA, TH, YT) and graduate students (AB, RY, YDH) at the academic institution where the ^{18}F-FAMT is developed. None of the authors are among the first authors of the studies included in this meta-analysis.

Author details
[1]Department of Diagnostic Radiology and Nuclear Medicine, Gunma University Graduate School of Medicine, 3-39-22 Showa-machi, Maebashi, Gunma 371-8511, Japan. [2]Department of Nuclear Medicine and Molecular Imaging, Faculty of Medicine, Padjadjaran University, Jl. Professor Eyckman No.38, Bandung, West Java 40161, Indonesia. [3]Department of Nuclear Medicine, Mochtar Riady Comprehensive Cancer Center, Jl. Garnisun Dalam No. 2–3, Semanggi, Jakarta 12930, Indonesia.

References
1. Farwell MD, Pryma DA, Mankoff DA. PET/CT imaging in cancer: current applications and future directions. Cancer. 2014;120:3433–45.
2. Gillies RJ, Robey I, Gatenby RA. Causes and consequences of increased glucose metabolism of cancers. J Nucl Med. 2008;49(Suppl 2):24S–42S.
3. Fletcher JW, Djulbegovic B, Soares HP, Siegel BA, Lowe VJ, Lyman GH, et al. Recommendations on the use of F-18-FDG PET in oncology. J Nucl Med. 2008;49:480–508.
4. Huang C, McConathy J. Radiolabeled amino acids for oncologic imaging. J Nucl Med. 2013;54:1007–10.
5. Inoue T, Koyama K, Oriuchi N, Alyafei S, Yuan Z, Suzuki H, et al. Detection of malignant tumors: whole-body PET with fluorine 18 alpha-methyl tyrosine versus FDG - preliminary study. Radiology. 2001;220:54–62.
6. Inoue T, Shibasaki T, Oriuchi N, Aoyagi K, Tomiyoshi K, Amano S, et al. F-18 alpha-methyl tyrosine PET studies in patients with brain tumors. J Nucl Med. 1999;40:399–405.
7. Kaira K, Oriuchi N, Otani Y, Yanagitani N, Sunaga N, Hisada T, et al. Diagnostic usefulness of fluorine-18-alpha-methyltyrosine positron emission tomography in combination with F-18-fluorodeoxyglucose in sarcoidosis patients. Chest. 2007;131:1019–27.
8. Kaira K, Oriuchi N, Shimizu K, Tominaga H, Yanagitani N, Sunaga N, et al. F-18-FMT uptake seen within primary cancer on PET helps predict outcome of non-small cell lung cancer. J Nucl Med. 2009;50:1770–6.
9. Miyakubo M, Oriuchi N, Tsushima Y, Higuchi T, Koyama K, Arai K, et al. Diagnosis of maxillofacial tumor with L-3-[F-18]-fluoro-alpha-methyltyrosine (FMT) PET: a comparative study with FDG-PET. Ann Nucl Med. 2007;21:129–35.
10. Sohda M, Sakai M, Honjyo H, Hara K, Ozawa D, Suzuki S, et al. Use of pre-treatment F-18-FAMT PET to predict patient survival in Squamous cell carcinoma of the esophagus treated by curative surgery. Anticancer Res. 2014;34(7):3623–8.
11. Suzuki R, Watanabe H, Yanagawa T, Sato J, Shinozaki T, Suzuki H, et al. PET evaluation of fatty tumors in the extremity: possibility of using the standardized uptake value (SUV) to differentiate benign tumors from liposarcoma. Ann Nucl Med. 2005;19:661–70.
12. Watanabe H, Inoue T, Shinozaki T, Yanagawa T, Ahmed AR, Tomiyoshi K, et al. PET imaging of musculoskeletal tumours with fluorine-18 alpha-methyltyrosine: comparison with fluorine-18 fluorodeoxyglucose PET. Eur J Nucl Med. 2000;27:1509–17.

13. Sato N, Inoue T, Tomiyoshi K, Aoki J, Oriuchi N, Takahashi A, et al. Gliomatosis cerebri evaluated by F-18 alpha-methyl tyrosine positron-emission tomography. Neuroradiology. 2003;45:700–7.

14. Wiriyasermkul P, Nagamori S, Tominaga H, Oriuchi N, Kaira K, Nakao H, et al. Transport of 3-Fluoro-L-alpha-methyl-tyrosine by tumor-Upregulated L-type amino acid transporter 1: a cause of the tumor uptake in PET. J Nucl Med. 2012;53:1253–61.

15. Wei L, Tominaga H, Ohgaki R, Wiriyasermkul P, Hagiwara K, Okuda S, et al. Specific transport of 3-fluoro-l-α-methyl-tyrosine by LAT1 explains its specificity to malignant tumors in imaging. Cancer Sci. 2016;107: 347–52.

16. Reitsma JB, Moons KGM, Bossuyt PMM, Linnet K. Systematic reviews of studies quantifying the accuracy of diagnostic tests and markers. Clin Chem. 2012;58:1534–45.

17. Macaskill P, Gatsonis C, Deeks J, Harbord R, Takwoingi Y. Chapter 10: Analysing and Presenting Results. In: Cochrane Handbook for Systematic Reviews of Diagnostic Test Accuracy Version 1. Deeks J, Bossuyt P, Gatsonis C, editors. The Cochrane Collaboration. 2010. http://methods.cochrane.org/sdt/handbook-dta-reviews. Accessed 15 Dec 2015.

18. Whiting PF, Rutjes AW, Westwood ME, Mallett S, Deeks JJ, Reitsma JB, et al. QUADAS-2: a revised tool for the quality assessment of diagnostic accuracy studies. Ann Intern Med. 2011;155:529–36.

19. Rücker G, Schumacher M. Summary ROC curve based on a weighted Youden index for selecting an optimal cutpoint in meta-analysis of diagnostic accuracy. Stat Med. 2010;29:3069–78.

20. Glas AS, Lijmer JG, Prins MH, Bonsel GJ, Bossuyt PMM. The diagnostic odds ratio: a single indicator of test performance. J Clin Epidemiol. 2003;56:1129–35.

21. Doebler P. Mada: meta-analysis of diagnostic accuracy. R package version 0. 5.7. 2015.

22. R-Core-Team. R: a language and environment for statistical computing. Vienna: R Foundation for Statistical Computing; 2015.

23. Tian M, Zhang H, Endo K. Comparison of cell proliferation, protein, and glucose metabolism in musculoskeletal tumors in a PET study. J Biomed Biotechnol. 2011; 10.1155/2011/807929.

24. Kaira K, Oriuchi N, Shimizu K, Ishikita T, Higuchi T, Imai H, et al. Evaluation of thoracic tumors with F-18-FMT and F-18-FDG PET-CT: a clinicopathological study. Int J Cancer. 2009;124:1152–60.

25. Lijmer JG, Bossuyt PMM, Heisterkamp SH. Exploring sources of heterogeneity in systematic reviews of diagnostic tests. Stat Med. 2002;21:1525–37.

26. Bürkner P-C, Doebler P. Testing for publication bias in diagnostic meta-analysis: a simulation study. Stat Med. 2014;33:3061–77.

27. Takwoingi Y, Guo B, Riley RD, Deeks JJ. Performance of methods for meta-analysis of diagnostic test accuracy with few studies or sparse data. Stat Methods Med Res. 2015; 10.1177/0962280215592269.

28. Deppen SA, Blume JD, Kensinger CD, Morgan AM, Aldrich MC, Massion PP, et al. Accuracy of FDG-PET to diagnose lung cancer in areas with infectious lung disease a meta-analysis. JAMA. 2014;312:1227–36.

29. Porcel JM, Hernandez P, Martinez-Alonso M, Bielsa S, Salud A. Accuracy of Fluorodeoxyglucose-PET imaging for differentiating benign from malignant pleural effusions a meta-analysis. Chest. 2015;147:502–12.

30. Xu G, Zhao L, He Z. Performance of whole-body PET/CT for the detection of distant malignancies in various cancers: a systematic review and meta-analysis. J Nucl Med. 2012;53:1847–54.

31. Corrigan AJG, Schleyer PJ, Cook GJ. Pitfalls and artifacts in the use of PET/CT in oncology imaging. Semin Nucl Med. 2015;45:481–99.

32. Rice SL, Roney CA, Daumar P, Lewis JS. The next generation of positron emission tomography radiopharmaceuticals in oncology. Semin Nucl Med. 2011;41:265–82.

33. Dunet V, Rossier C, Buck A, Stupp R, Prior JO. Performance of F-18-Fluoro-ethyl-tyrosine (F-18-FET) PET for the differential diagnosis of primary brain tumor: a systematic review and Metaanalysis. J Nucl Med. 2012;53:207–14.

34. Zhao C, Zhang Y, Wang J. A meta-analysis on the diagnostic performance of ^{18}F-FDG and ^{11}C-methionine PET for differentiating brain tumors. AJNR Am J Neuroradiol. 2014;35:1058–65.

35. Habermeier A, Graf J, Sandhofer BF, Boissel JP, Roesch F, Closs EI. System L amino acid transporter LAT1 accumulates O-(2-fluoroethyl)-L-tyrosine (FET). Amino Acids. 2015;47:335–44.

36. Ren J, Yuan L, Wen G, Yang J. The value of anti-1-amino-3-^{18}F-fluorocyclobutane-1-carboxylic acid PET/CT in the diagnosis of recurrent prostate carcinoma: a meta-analysis. Acta Radiol. 2016;57:487–93.

37. Kameyama M, Umeda-Kameyama Y. Strategy based on kinetics of O-(2-[^{18}F]fluoroethyl)-L-tyrosine ([^{18}F] FET). Eur J Nucl Med Mol Imaging. 2016;43: 2267–8.

38. Yamaguchi A, Hanaoka H, Fujisawa Y, Zhao S, Suzue K, Morita A, et al. Differentiation of malignant tumours from granuloma by using dynamic [^{18}F]-fluoro-L-α-methyltyrosine positron emission tomography. EJNMMI Res. 2015;5:29.

39. Tomiyoshi K, Amed K, Muhammad S, Higuchi T, Inoue T, Endo K, et al. Synthesis of isomers of ^{18}F-labelled amino acid radiopharmaceutical: position 2- and 3-L-^{18}F-α-methyltyrosine using a separation and purification system. Nucl Med Commun. 1997;18:169–75.

40. Meleán JC, Humpert S, Ermert J, Coenen HH. Stereoselective radiosynthesis of L- and D-3-[F-18]fluoro-alpha-methyltyrosine. J Fluor Chem. 2015;178: 202–7.

41. Preshlock S, Tredwell M, Gouverneur V. ^{18}F-labeling of Arenes and Heteroarenes for applications in positron emission tomography. Chem Rev. 2016;116:719–66.

20

A prospective study to evaluate the intra-individual reproducibility of bone scans for quantitative assessment in patients with metastatic prostate cancer

Mariana Reza[1,2], Reza Kaboteh[3], May Sadik[3], Anders Bjartell[2,4], Per Wollmer[1,2] and Elin Trägårdh[1,2]*

Abstract

Background: The Bone Scan Index (BSI) is used to quantitatively assess the total tumour burden in bone scans of patients with metastatic prostate cancer. The clinical utility of BSI has recently been validated as a prognostic imaging biomarker. However, the clinical utility of the on-treatment change in BSI is dependent on the reproducibility of bone scans. The objective of this prospective study is to evaluate the intra-patient reproducibility of two bone scan procedures performed at a one-week interval.

Methods: We prospectively studied prostate cancer patients who were referred for bone scintigraphy at our centres according to clinical routine. All patients underwent two whole-body bone scans: one for clinical routine purposes and a second one as a repeated scan after approximately one week. BSI values were obtained for each bone scintigraph using EXINI bone[BSI] software.

Results: A total of 20 patients were enrolled. There was no statistical difference between the BSI values of the first (median = 0.66, range 0–40.77) and second (median = 0.63, range 0–22.98) bone scans ($p = 0.41$). The median difference in BSI between the clinical routine and repeated scans was − 0.005 (range − 17.79 to 0). The 95% confidence interval for the median value was − 0.1 to 0. A separate analysis was performed for patients with BSI ≤ 10 ($n = 17$). Differences in BSI were smaller for patients with BSI ≤ 10 compared to the whole cohort (median − 0.1, range − 2.2-0, 95% confidence interval − 0.1 to 0).

Conclusions: The automated BSI demonstrated high intra-individual reproducibility for BSI ≤ 10 in the two repeated bone scans of patients with prostate cancer. The study supports the use of BSI as a quantitative parameter to evaluate the change in total tumour burden in bone scans.

Keywords: Reproducibility, Prostate cancer, Bone metastasis, Bone scan quantitative analysis, Bone scan index

Background

Bone metastases cause much of the morbidity and mortality associated with prostate cancer and lead to complications that include pathologic fractures and severe pain [1, 2]. Therefore, bone-targeted therapies are important and in continuous development. Over the last few years, several novel agents have been approved by the US Food and Drug Administration for use in advanced prostate cancer [3]. Despite the advances, several areas of urgent need remain. In the context of medical imaging more objective methods are needed for the evaluation of bone metastasis, staging, and response measures. Advances in this area would be valuable in clinical routine and clinical trials.

Bone scan examination remains the most widely used and recommended method for assessing metastatic spread to the bone when progression of the disease is suspected in patients with prostate cancer [4]. However, there is still no standardisation of bone scan

* Correspondence: Elin.tragardh@med.lu.se
[1]Department of Clinical Physiology and Nuclear Medicine, Skåne University Hospital, Inga Marie Nilssons gata 49, SE-205 02 Malmö, Sweden
[2]Department of Translational Medicine, Lund University, Malmö, Sweden
Full list of author information is available at the end of the article

interpretation. The current methods used in clinical routine are based on traditional visual analysis, which is qualitative and mainly focuses on merely whether or not metastatic lesions are present in the bone [4]. However, several studies have shown that the degree of tumour extension in the bone is a more accurate approach for prognostic evaluation. Nevertheless, in clinical practice, estimating the degree of tumour extension is also subjective and highly dependent on the interpreter [5]. Therefore, automatic quantitative analysis of the images could be useful for reducing intra- and inter-observer variability [6].

The Bone Scan Index (BSI) was developed and later automated to obtain more information from bone scans [7]. The index represents the percentage of bone affected by tumours and is calculated from bone scan images. BSI has been proposed as a pre- and post-treatment prognostic imaging biomarker as a complement to traditional clinical prognostic parameters to improve the stratification of patients [8, 9]. Several studies also discuss the possibility of using this biomarker as a predictive marker for treatment response since changes in BSI after follow-up have been related to survival and other outcomes [10, 11].

However, knowledge is needed about the degree of reproducibility of BSI measurements for the reliable detection of changes over time. Before BSI can be applied for therapy monitoring in clinical practice and clinical trials, the accuracy and precision of the measurement method and the spontaneous variability of the biological signal should be determined. BSI quantification shows robust reproducibility when analysing the same image [12], but the intra-patient variability when the patient is examined at different times is currently unknown (i.e. the variability of repeated measurements after re-injection of the compound within the same week) [13]. To our knowledge, test-retest data has not been published for the variability of BSI in patients with prostate cancer. Such an evaluation would clarify the biological reproducibility of BSI within each individual. Thus, the aim of this study is to assess the intra-individual reproducibility of automatically obtained BSI when measuring tumour burden in the bones of prostate cancer patients. The ultimate goal is to fully validate the automated BSI method as a clinical applicable biomarker.

Methods
Patients
The study participants were recruited from all prostate cancer patients who underwent bone scintigraphy at Sahlgrenska University Hospital in Gothenburg, Sweden, from March to October 2015 and at Skåne University Hospital, Sweden, from November 2015 to March 2016. The eligibility criteria for participating in the study

Table 1 Basic characteristics of patients and scans

Age, year, median (range)	76 (70–86)
Time between bone scans, days, median (range)	6 (1–9)
1st Bone Scan: Time from injection to image acquisition, min (SD)	210 (25)
2nd Bone Scan: Time from injection to image acquisition, min (SD)	201 (30)

included a documented prostate cancer diagnosis and age older than 70 years. The exclusion criteria included planned radiotherapy during the week after the first scan.

Those who met the inclusion criteria were asked to contribute an additional whole-body bone scan examination one week after the first bone scan examination. Due to the limited availability for performing additional examinations, patients were only asked to participate when a free camera time slot was available. The study was performed in accordance with the Declaration of Helsinki and was approved by the Regional Ethical Review Boards at Lund University, Sweden and the Regional Radiation Protection Committees at Skåne University Hospital and Sahlgrenska University Hospital. The patients gave written consent to participate.

Bone scintigraphy
All patients were scanned according to the same standards used in clinical routine, as indicated in the current procedure guidelines for tumour imaging of the European Association of Nuclear Medicine [14]. Each participating patient underwent two whole-body bone scans: one performed as part of the clinical routine and a repeated bone scan performed approximately one week after. The bone scans were performed approximately three hours after intravenous injection of 600 MBq of technetium-99 m hydroxyethylene diphosphonate (Malmö) or technetium-99 m 2,3-dicarboxypropane-1,1-disphosphonate (Gothenburg). Anterior- and posterior-view whole-body images were obtained using one of four different gamma cameras: a Tandem Discovery 670 (GE Healthcare); Infinia (GE Healthcare); IRIX (Marconi Medical Systems), or Symbia (Siemens Healthcare).

Table 2 Median and range for BSI measurements from the first and the second bone scans

All patients (n = 20)			
First BSI	Second BSI	BSI difference	p
0.66 (0–40.77)	0.63 (0–22.98)	−0.005 (−17.99–0)	0.41 (NS)
Patients with BSI ≤10 (n = 17)			
First BSI	Second BSI	BSI difference	p
0.24 (0–5.41)	0.14 (0–5.28)	−0.1 (−2.2–0)	0.11 (NS)

BSI Bone Scan Index, *NS* Not significant

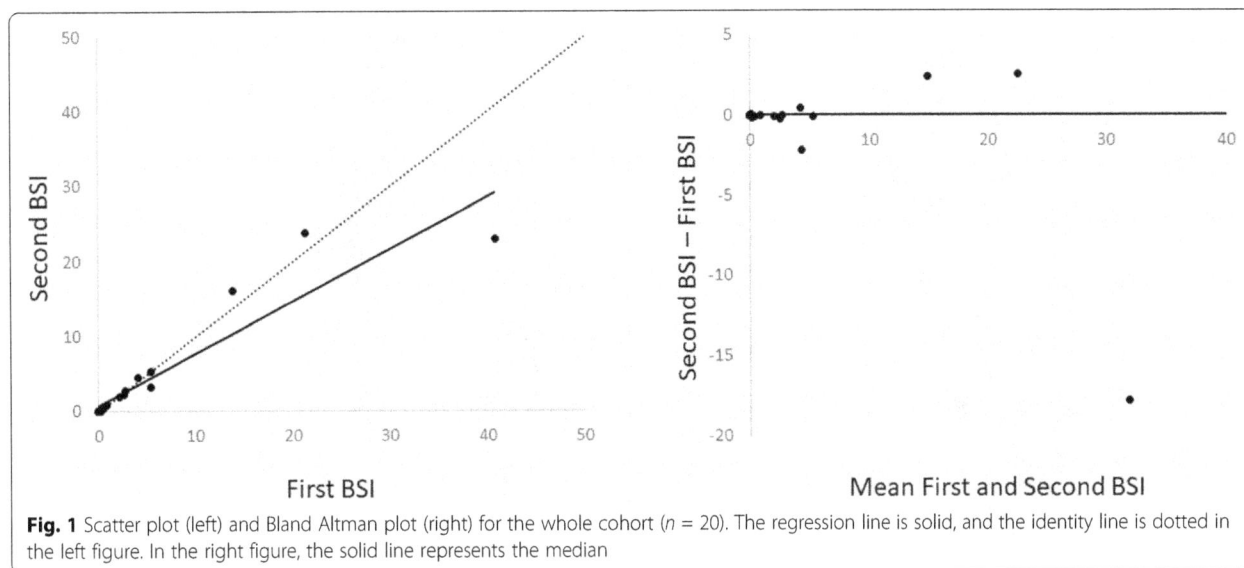

Fig. 1 Scatter plot (left) and Bland Altman plot (right) for the whole cohort (*n* = 20). The regression line is solid, and the identity line is dotted in the left figure. In the right figure, the solid line represents the median

The first three gamma cameras were used in Gothenburg, and the last one was used in Malmö. We aimed to use the same camera to examine the patients both times. All gamma cameras were equipped with low-energy, high-resolution, parallel-hole collimators with a scan rate of 10 cm/min and a 256 × 1024 matrix. Energy discrimination was provided by a 20% window for the first two cameras and 15% for the second two cameras. For all cameras, the energy discrimination was centred at 140 keV for Tc-99 m. All the resulting bone scan images showed the same quality level and were appropriate for further analysis.

BSI analysis

BSI was calculated using the commercially available software EXINI bone^{BSI} version 2 (EXINI Diagnostics AB, Lund Sweden). The automated method of calculating BSI has been described in detail elsewhere [7] and was analytically validated in a recent study [12]. In summary, different anatomical regions of the skeleton were segmented, and hotspots were detected and classified as metastatic lesions or not. The mass fraction of the skeleton was calculated for each metastatic hotspot, and the BSI was finally calculated as the sum of all fractions. Only minimal manual corrections were made in cases of misclassification of the urine bladder or catheters as hotpots according to the manufacturer's instructions.

Statistical analysis

The intra-individual reproducibility of the repeated BSI measurements was tested using the Wilcoxon signed-rank test based on the bone scan measurements. The Bland-Altman method was used to detect systematic differences between the test-retest BSI measurements and to identify possible outliers. A linear regression procedure was performed to determine the presence of proportional bias.

Previous studies indicated high variability in comparisons of manual versus automatic BSI measurements in patients with extensive bone disease (BSI > 10) [7]. Therefore, we performed a second series of reproducibility analyses that included only patients who showed BSI < 10 in the clinical routine scan. Statistical significance was set at 0.05 for the tests performed. All statistical analyses were performed using IBM SPSS for Windows version 23.

Results

A total of 20 patients were included (13 in Gothenburg and 7 in Malmö). The median age was 76 years (range 70 to 86 years). Table 1 provides the basic characteristics of the patients, the time between bone scans, and the time from injection to image acquisition.

The BSI values for the whole cohort had a median value of 0.66 (range 0 to 40.77) for the first BSI measurement and 0.63 (range 0 to 22.98) for the second BSI measurement. There was no significant difference between the routine and repeated BSI measurements (*p* = 0.41). The median difference in BSI for the whole cohort (*n* = 20) was – 0.005 (range – 17.99 to 0) with a 95% confidence interval (CI) of – 0.1 to 0 (Table 2). The scatter and Bland-Altman plots are presented in Fig. 1. For five of the patients, BSI was identical in both examinations. Eight patients showed an absolute difference in BSI of > 0 to 0.1, two patients had an absolute difference of > 0.1 to 0.5, and four patients had an absolute difference of > 1. Figure 2 shows a patient with similar BSI at the two examinations, and Fig. 3 shows a patient with a large difference in BSI between the two different examinations. The largest difference in BSI between the first and second bone scan was found in the patient with highest BSI (Fig. 4).

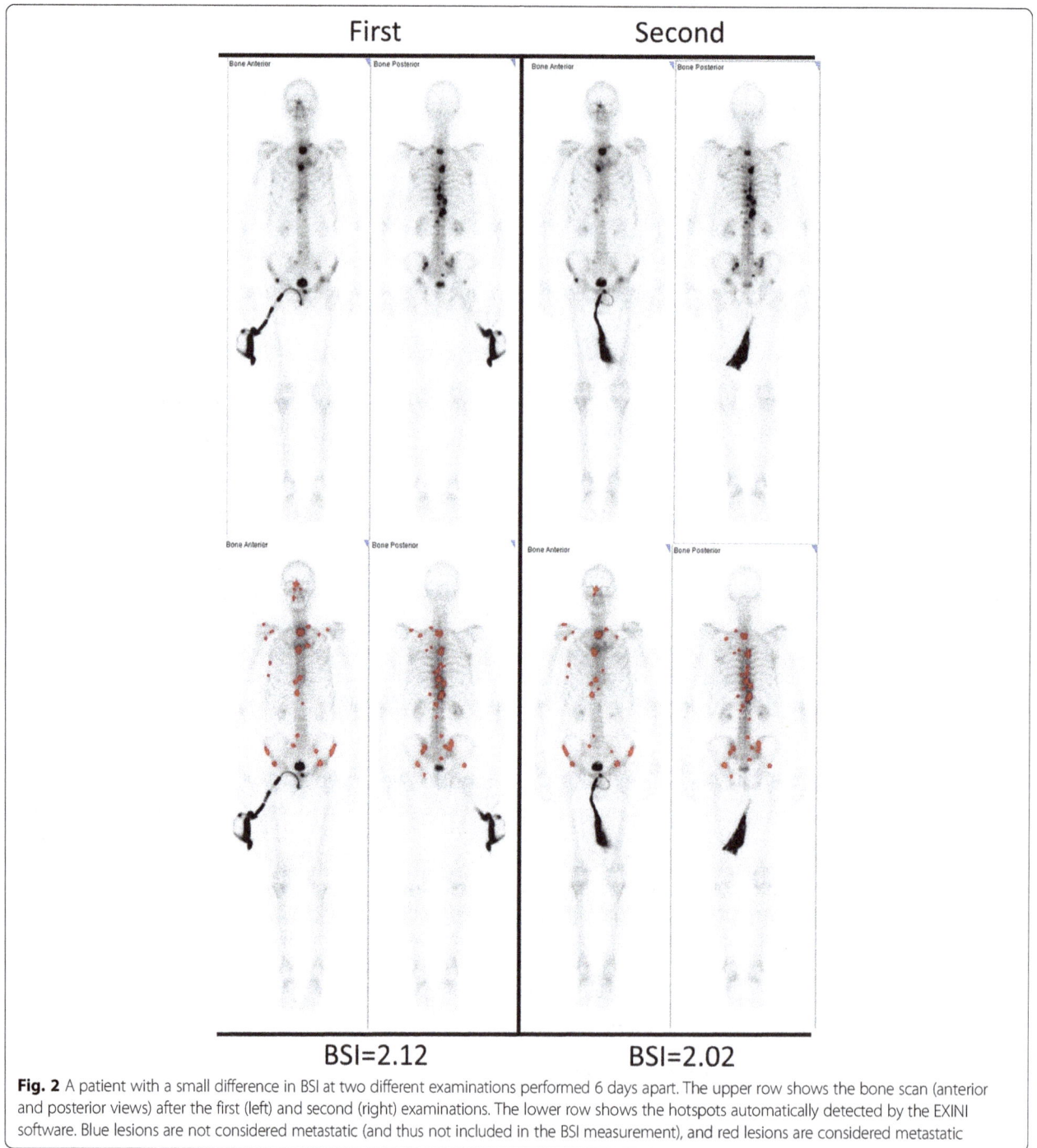

Fig. 2 A patient with a small difference in BSI at two different examinations performed 6 days apart. The upper row shows the bone scan (anterior and posterior views) after the first (left) and second (right) examinations. The lower row shows the hotspots automatically detected by the EXINI software. Blue lesions are not considered metastatic (and thus not included in the BSI measurement), and red lesions are considered metastatic

The calculations were also performed for patients with BSI ≤ 10 at the first examination (Table 2). A total of 3 of the 20 patients were therefore excluded from the second series of analyses, leading to a sub-cohort of 17 patients. All three excluded patients had a difference > 1 between the first and second BSI. The BSI values for this sub-cohort had median values of 0.24 (range 0 to 5.41) for the first BSI measurement and 0.14 (range 0 to 5.28) for the second BSI measurement. There was no

significant difference between the routine and repeated BSI measurements ($p = 0.11$). The median difference in BSI for the sub-cohort was − 0.01 (range − 2.2 to 0) with a 95% CI of − 0.1 to 0. The scatter and Bland-Altman plots are presented in Fig. 5.

Discussion

This study shows high intra-individual reproducibility in the BSI values calculated from bone scans with only

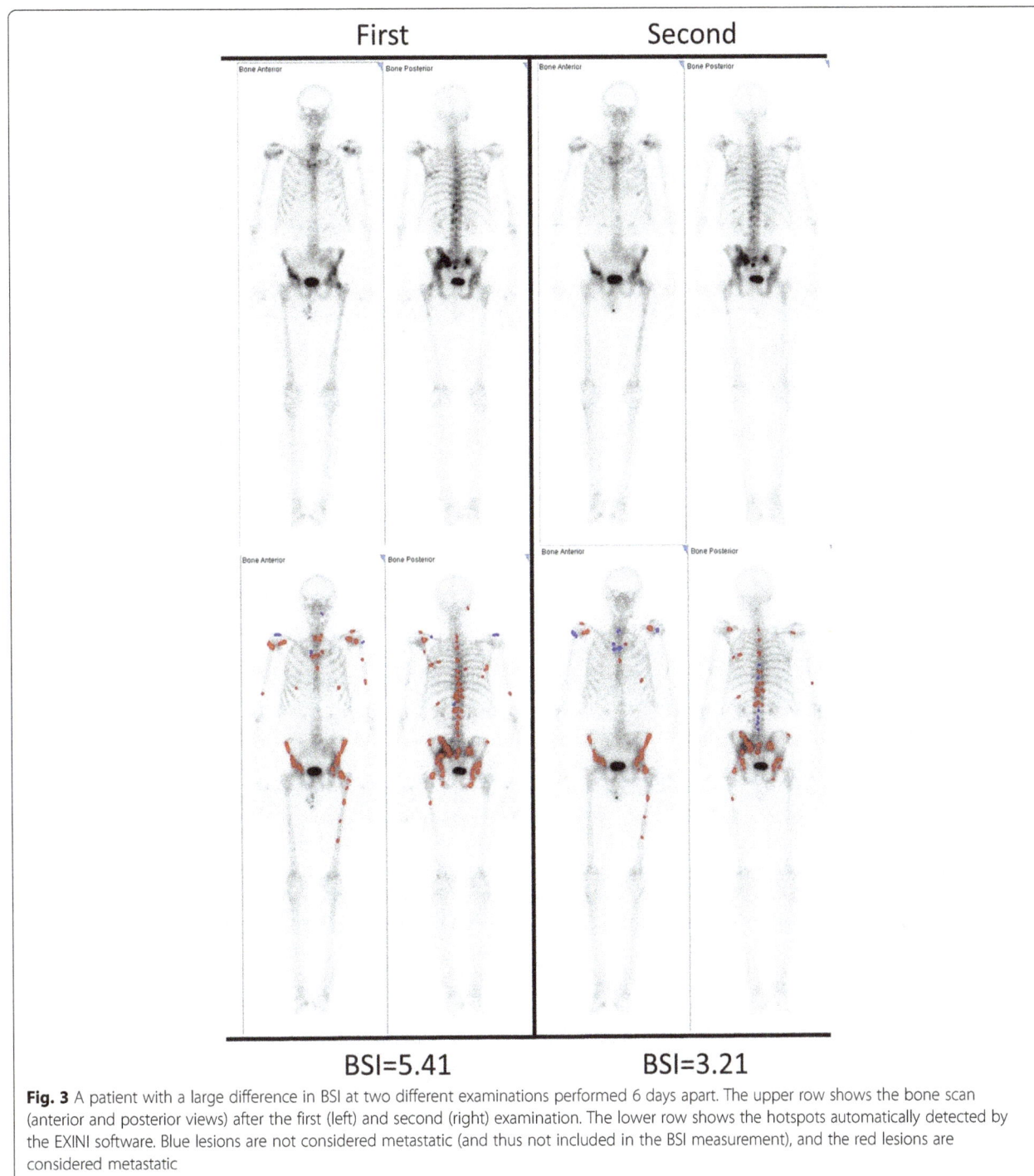

Fig. 3 A patient with a large difference in BSI at two different examinations performed 6 days apart. The upper row shows the bone scan (anterior and posterior views) after the first (left) and second (right) examination. The lower row shows the hotspots automatically detected by the EXINI software. Blue lesions are not considered metastatic (and thus not included in the BSI measurement), and the red lesions are considered metastatic

minimal manual intervention for different bone scans taken one week apart, especially for patients with BSI ≤ 10. The median difference in BSI for the whole cohort was – 0.005 with a 95% CI of – 0.1 to 0. These results show that the automated BSI is a consistent measure of tumour burden in the bones of prostate cancer patients. For patients with a high BSI the method is less reproducible. As seen in Fig. 4, small differences in

hotspot delineation in a patient with a highly metastasised skeleton lead to a vast difference in BSI.

The clinical implications of these results are related to the utility of using BSI difference measurements when analysing follow-up bone scans to describe significant changes in bone status in a quantitative and more objective manner. This information could be useful as a complement to traditional visual analysis of bone scans

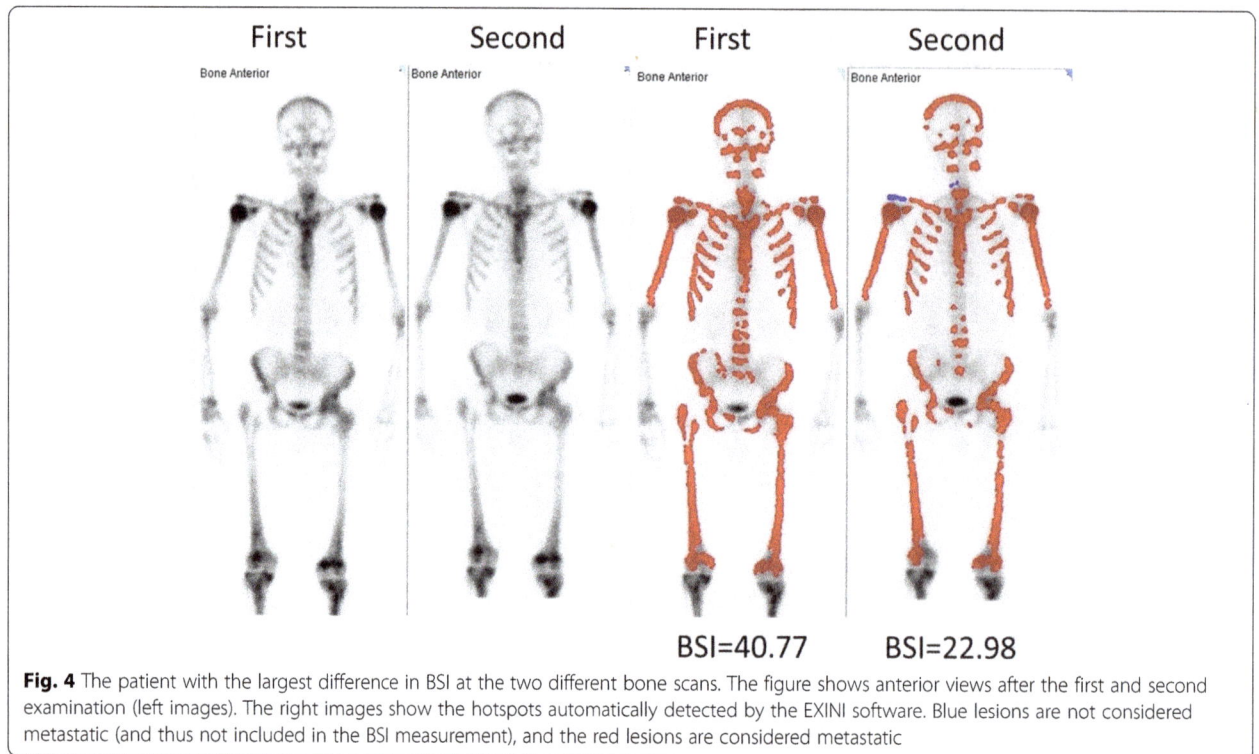

Fig. 4 The patient with the largest difference in BSI at the two different bone scans. The figure shows anterior views after the first and second examination (left images). The right images show the hotspots automatically detected by the EXINI software. Blue lesions are not considered metastatic (and thus not included in the BSI measurement), and the red lesions are considered metastatic

to produce more objective reports regarding possible stabilisation or progression of bone disease. This type of evaluation would be valuable when monitoring patients undergoing specific therapies for prostate cancer to support physicians on decisions to adjust treatment when necessary.

A recent meta-analysis examined the prognostic value of BSI as an imaging biomarker in prostate cancer [15]. The analysis included 14 high-quality studies involving 1295 patients. The pooled results indicated that a high baseline BSI and high change in BSI over time were significantly predictive of poor overall survival and that BSI could improve predictive models. The conclusion was that BSI may be beneficial as a predictive imaging biomarker in patients with metastatic prostate cancer.

Previous studies have explored the reproducibility of BSI when analysing bone scans performed at different times after injection [16]. Other studies showed robust reproducibility when analysing the same image [12], but the intra-patient variability is currently unknown (i.e. the

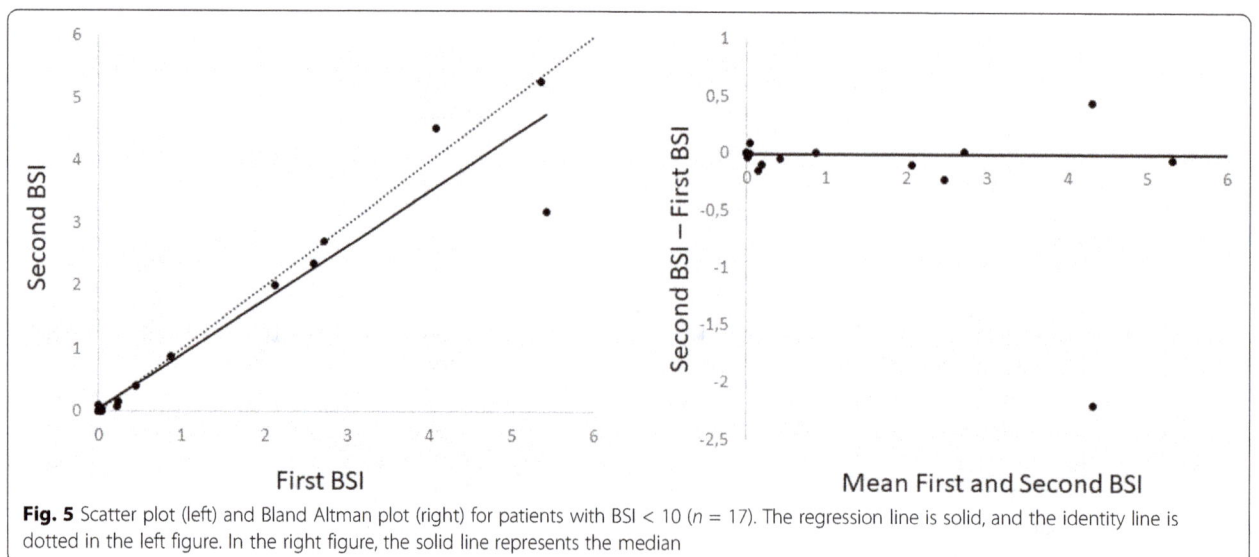

Fig. 5 Scatter plot (left) and Bland Altman plot (right) for patients with BSI < 10 ($n = 17$). The regression line is solid, and the identity line is dotted in the left figure. In the right figure, the solid line represents the median

variability of a repeated measurement after re-injection of the compound within the same week). Therefore, the design of the present study included a completely new bone scan examination conducted approximately one week after to explore the intra-individual reproducibility of automated BSI.

Among the limitations of this study are those of the bone scan technique itself and those related to daily clinical work. One example is the impossibility of performing the repeated bone scans using exactly the same gamma camera in some cases, which occurred for three patients. However, Anand et al. [17] did not find any significant difference in BSI in simulated phantom data for gamma cameras from different vendors. Considering the high variability between manual and automated BSI measurements in patients with BSI values > 10 [7], we included a second series of analyses for such patients. The difference between the first and second BSI was higher for patients with BSI > 10.

Despite the small scale of this prospective study, we have presented important evidence in support of the hypothesis of high intra-individual reproducibility of the automated BSI measurement method. Reproducibility studies are rare in the field of nuclear medicine, partly due to the need for an extra dose of radiation to obtain subsequent imaging studies. In this study, the risks associated with extra radiation are minimal, considering the patients' age. This examination was needed for further standardisation for evaluating changes in BSI change [13, 18, 19]. The results also indicate the possibility of using this method as a clinically applicable biomarker in patients with prostate cancer.

Conclusions

Automated BSI demonstrated high intra-individual reproducibility for BSI ≤ 10 in the two repeated bone scans of prostate cancer patients. The study supports the use of BSI as a quantitative assessment to evaluate changes in total tumour burden in bone scans.

Abbreviations
BSI: Bone Scan Index; CI: Confidence interval

Acknowledgements
The authors would like to acknowledge the staff at the Department of Clinical Physiology and Nuclear Medicine, Skåne University hospital, and at the Department of Clinical Physiology, Sahlgrenska University Hospital, for help with data collection.

Funding
This study was funded by government grants from the National Health Services and the Skåne University Hospital Cancer Foundation.

Authors' contributions
All authors participated in the design of the study, interpretation of the data and drafting of the manuscript. All authors read and approved the final version of the manuscript. MR, RK, and MS collected clinical data. MR and ET carried out the statistical analysis and collected nuclear medicine data for the BSI analysis.

Competing interests
AB received honoraria as a consultant to EXINI Diagnostics. The other authors declare that they have no competing interests.

Author details
[1]Department of Clinical Physiology and Nuclear Medicine, Skåne University Hospital, Inga Marie Nilssons gata 49, SE-205 02 Malmö, Sweden. [2]Department of Translational Medicine, Lund University, Malmö, Sweden. [3]Department of Molecular and Clinical Medicine, Sahlgrenska University Hospital, Gothenburg, Sweden. [4]Department of Urology, Skåne University Hospital, Malmö, Sweden.

References
1. Macherey S, Monsef I, Jahn F, Jordan K, Yuen KK, Heidenreich A, Skoetz N. Bisphosphonates for advanced prostate cancer. Cochrane Database Syst Rev. 2017;12:CD006250.
2. Wong KW, Ma WK, Wong CW, Wong MH, Tsang CF, Tsu HL, Ho KL, Yiu MK. Impact of skeletal-related events on survival in patients with metastatic prostate cancer prescribed androgen deprivation therapy. Hong Kong Med J. 2016;22(2):106–15.
3. Suzman DL, Boikos SA, Carducci MA. Bone-targeting agents in prostate cancer. Cancer Metastasis Rev. 2014;33(2–3):619–28.
4. Heidenreich A, Bastian PJ, Bellmunt J, Bolla M, Joniau S, van der Kwast T, Mason M, Matveev V, Wiegel T, Zattoni F, et al. EAU guidelines on prostate cancer. Part II: treatment of advanced, relapsing, and castration-resistant prostate cancer. Eur Urol. 2014;65(2):467–79.
5. Bombardieri E, Aktolun C, Baum RP, Bishof-Delaloye A, Buscombe J, Chatal JF, Maffioli L, Moncayo R, Mortelmans L, Reske SN. Bone scintigraphy: procedure guidelines for tumour imaging. Eur J Nucl Med Mol Imaging. 2003;30(12):BP99–106.
6. Sadik M, Suurkula M, Hoglund P, Jarund A, Edenbrandt L. Improved classifications of planar whole-body bone scans using a computer-assisted diagnosis system: a multicenter, multiple-reader, multiple-case study. J Nucl Med. 2009;50(3):368–75.
7. Ulmert D, Kaboteh R, Fox JJ, Savage C, Evans MJ, Lilja H, Abrahamsson PA, Bjork T, Gerdtsson A, Bjartell A, et al. A novel automated platform for quantifying the extent of skeletal tumour involvement in prostate cancer patients using the bone scan index. Eur Urol. 2012;62(1):78–84.
8. Kaboteh R, Damber JE, Gjertsson P, Hoglund P, Lomsky M, Ohlsson M, Edenbrandt L. Bone scan index: a prognostic imaging biomarker for high-risk prostate cancer patients receiving primary hormonal therapy. EJNMMI Res. 2013;3(1):9.
9. Kaboteh R, Gjertsson P, Leek H, Lomsky M, Ohlsson M, Sjostrand K, Edenbrandt L. Progression of bone metastases in patients with prostate cancer - automated detection of new lesions and calculation of bone scan index. EJNMMI Res. 2013;3(1):64.
10. Mitsui Y, Shiina H, Yamamoto Y, Haramoto M, Arichi N, Yasumoto H, Kitagaki H, Igawa M. Prediction of survival benefit using an automated bone scan index in patients with castration-resistant prostate cancer. BJU Int. 2012; 110(11 Pt B):E628–34.
11. Dennis ER, Jia X, Mezheritskiy IS, Stephenson RD, Schoder H, Fox JJ, Heller G, Scher HI, Larson SM, Morris MJ. Bone scan index: a quantitative treatment response biomarker for castration-resistant metastatic prostate cancer. J Clin Oncol. 2012;30(5):519–24.
12. Anand A, Morris MJ, Kaboteh R, Bath L, Sadik M, Gjertsson P, Lomsky M, Edenbrandt L, Minarik D, Bjartell A. Analytical validation of the automated bone scan index as an imaging biomarker to standardize the quantitative changes in bone scans of patients with metastatic prostate Cancer. J Nucl Med. 2015;
13. Ulmert D, Solnes L, Thorek D. Contemporary approaches for imaging skeletal metastasis. Bone Res. 2015;3:15024.
14. Van den Wyngaert T, Strobel K, Kampen WU, Kuwert T, van der Bruggen W, Mohan HK, Gnanasegaran G, Delgado-Bolton R, Weber WA, Beheshti M,

et al. The EANM practice guidelines for bone scintigraphy. Eur J Nucl Med Mol Imaging. 2016;43(9):1723–38.

15.   Li D, Lv H, Hao X, Dong Y, Dai H, Song Y. Prognostic value of bone scan index as an imaging biomarker in metastatic prostate cancer: a meta-analysis. Oncotarget. 2017;8(48):84449–58.

16.   Shintawati R, Achmad A, Higuchi T, Shimada H, Hirasawa H, Arisaka Y, Takahashi A, Nakajima T, Tsushima Y. Evaluation of bone scan index change over time on automated calculation in bone scintigraphy. Ann Nucl Med. 2015;29(10):911–20.

17.   Anand A, Morris MJ, Kaboteh R, Reza M, Tragardh E, Matsunaga N, Edenbrandt L, Bjartell A, Larson SM, Minarik D. A Preanalytic validation study of automated bone scan index: effect on accuracy and reproducibility due to the procedural variabilities in bone scan image acquisition. J Nucl Med. 2016;57(12):1865–71.

18.   Reza M, Jones R, Aspegren J, Massard C, Mattila L, Mustonen M, Wollmer P, Tragardh E, Bondesson E, Edenbrandt L, et al. Bone scan index and progression-free survival data for progressive metastatic castration-resistant prostate Cancer patients who received ODM-201 in the ARADES multicentre study. Eur Urol Focus. 2016;2(5):547–52.

19.   Reza M, Ohlsson M, Kaboteh R, Anand A, Franck-Lissbrant I, Damber JE, Widmark A, Thellenberg-Karlsson C, Budaus L, Steuber T, et al. Bone scan index as an imaging biomarker in metastatic castration-resistant prostate Cancer: a multicentre study based on patients treated with Abiraterone acetate (Zytiga) in clinical practice. Eur Urol Focus. 2016;2(5):540–6.

21

A pilot study on adjunctive use of parametric colour-coded digital subtraction angiography in endovascular interventions of haemodialysis access

Ru Yu Tan[1*] (ORCID), Tze Tec Chong[2], Fu Chieh Tsai[3], Suh Chien Pang[1], Kian Guan Lee[1], Apoorva Gogna[3], Alicia Huiying Ong[4] and Chieh Suai Tan[1]

Abstract

Background: Two-dimensional digital subtraction angiography (DSA) is the gold standard for angiographic evaluation of dysfunctional haemodialysis access. We aim to investigate the utility of parametric colour coded DSA in providing hemodynamic analysis during haemodialysis access interventions.

Methods: We retrospectively studied 20 patients who underwent access intervention and applied parametric colour-coding on selected DSA acquisitions before and after percutaneous transluminal angioplasty (PTA). The difference in time to peak (dTTP) contrast enhancement and time attenuation curve (TAC) of pre- and post-stenotic regions of interest (ROIs) were obtained and compared after treatment.

Results: Improvements were seen in mean percent of stenosis after PTA ($p < 0.0001$) for all cases. Median dTTP improved from 0.52 (IQR 0.26, 0.8) to 0.25 (IQR 0, 0.26) seconds ($p = 0.001$). Median 50% contrast washout time improved from 0.77 (IQR 0.39, 1.17) to 0.42 (IQR 0.23, 0.59) seconds ($p = 0.031$). Significant correlation was seen for dTTP vs. percent of stenosis ($r = 0.723$, $p = 0.043$) pre-PTA and for change in dTTP vs. percent change in stenosis post-PTA ($r = 0.786$, $p = 0.021$) for inflow lesions. Such correlation was however not seen in outflow lesions.

Conclusions: Adjunctive use of parametric colour-coded DSA may provide potentially useful hemodynamic information during vascular access interventions. Larger prospective studies are needed to validate our findings.

Keywords: Colour-coded, Digital subtraction angiography, Haemodialysis, Vascular access, Endovascular intervention

Background

Vascular access dysfunction remains a major contributor of morbidity and hospitalization in end stage renal failure (ESRF) patients on hemodialysis [1]. Stenosis secondary to neointimal hyperplasia can occur within the dialysis access, resulting in stenosis and thrombosis [2, 3]. Percutaneous transluminal angioplasty (PTA) of stenosis is the current standard of care as it is effective and less invasive when compared to open surgical techniques [4]. In carefully selected patients, some of these interventions can be performed in an outpatient setting [5].

Two-dimensional digital subtraction angiography (DSA) is the gold standard imaging modality during percutaneous assessment and intervention of vascular access [6]. Propagation of contrast agent through vessels or grafts during angiographic sequences is used to assess the patency of the vascular access visually, followed by determination of severity of stenosis and percutaneous intervention if required.

Anatomic measurement of luminal narrowing has been widely used to determine the severity of vascular access stenosis. Any stenosis causing greater than 50% luminal reduction should be treated [4]. Anatomic reduction of vessel diameter however may not be hemodynamically or clinically significant. Overzealous treatment of inflow stenosis especially on upper arm

* Correspondence: tan.ru.yu@singhealth.com.sg
[1]Department of Renal Medicine, Singapore General Hospital, Singapore, Singapore
Full list of author information is available at the end of the article

access may precipitate steal syndrome and increase risk of rupture [7]. Conversely, inadequate dilatation of stenosis may result in early or repeated recurrence of stenosis. Combination of anatomic with hemodynamic or clinical criteria is therefore recommended for assessment of disease severity during dialysis access interventions [8].

Using enhanced technology, DSA sequences can be post-processed to enable hemodynamic assessment of vasculature patency to aid planning of intervention during PTA. Parametric colour coding can be applied using computer software to convert conventional DSA sequences into colour images and automate quantitative hemodynamic analysis. The temporal evolution of the contrast agent at a fixed position can be recorded in a pixel-specific time-intensity curve, computed mathematically and visualized as a parametric image. The flow of contrast captured by DSA in multiple sequences will be combined into one single colour coded image which is used for hemodynamic quantification.

Parametric colour coding of DSA has been successfully used in angiographic assessment and treatment of neuroendovascular procedures and peripheral arterial disease [9–12]. However, limited information is available on adjunctive use of parametric colour coded DSA during percutaneous treatment of hemodialysis vascular access. We hypothesize that parametric colour coded DSA enables quantification of hemodynamic changes during PTA of hemodialysis vascular access. This pilot study was performed to examine the feasibility of using the difference in time to peak (dTTP) contrast enhancement and time attenuation curve (TAC) derived from colour-coded DSA to assess hemodynamic changes of stenosis in relation to anatomical changes before and after angioplasty.

Methods
Case selection, procedures, DSA acquisitions and post-processing
This is a single center retrospective study involving interventions performed for dysfunctional hemodialysis accesses. DSAs during the procedures were acquired as per standard hospital protocol for hemodialysis access interventions. In general, procedures were performed under local anaesthesia with aseptic preparation using a single plane angiography system (Artis one, Healthcare Sector, Siemens AG, Forchheim Germany). Prior to the intervention, bedside ultrasound was performed to determine the site of the lesions. For patients with only inflow stenosis, a vascular sheath was placed in the peripheral outflow vein in a retrograde direction and a catheter and a guidewire were advanced into the feeding artery. DSA was acquired with contrast injection via the catheter situated in the feeding artery to document the severity of the lesion. Following treatment with balloon

angioplasty, post-intervention DSA was acquired with the catheter at a similar position to document the results. For patients with outflow stenosis, a vascular sheath was placed in an antegrade direction and DSA was acquired with contrast injection through the sheath. A catheter and a guidewire were then advanced centrally via the sheath. Following intervention with balloon angioplasty, post-intervention DSA was acquired with contrast injection through the same sheath. For patients with both inflow and outflow lesions, the outflow lesions were treated prior to inflow lesions. All DSA acquisitions were done with hand-injection of contrast. The angiographic data and images of each patient were stored in a dedicated work station within the centre, running software for both standard angiography and parametric colour-coded DSA.

Cases were selected by the following criteria: the procedure must be performed by the same operator throughout to exclude inter-operator variability during contrast injection, DSA sequences on intervened segment must have identical projection, and magnification and similar catheter positions in the pre- and post-PTA studies. Contrast injection must also be with catheter in proximity to the stenotic lesion. Given that the presence of multiple stenoses may interfere with interpretation of hemodynamic parameters, only DSA sequences of the last treated lesions were used for hemodynamic assessment. Procedures complicated by rupture of vessels and deployment of vascular stents were excluded in the study.

Of the 20 patients studied, 15 patients have arteriovenous fistula (AVF) and 5 have arteriovenous graft (AVG). The baseline demographics and characteristics of the patients were obtained from electronic medical records.

Anatomic evaluation using conventional DSA acquisition (Fig. 1)
Anatomic measure of disease severity and treatment success was determined using the measurement and magnification tools on the workstation.

Pre-treatment evaluation
Diameters of the most stenotic ($D_{stenosis}$) and normal (D_{normal}) segments of the vessels/grafts were obtained

$$\text{Percent of Stenosis}_{pre-angioplasty} = [1-(D_{stenosis}/D_{normal})] \times 100$$

Post-treatment evaluation
Diameters of the residual stenosis ($D_{residual}$) and normal (D_{normal}) segments of the vessels/grafts were obtained

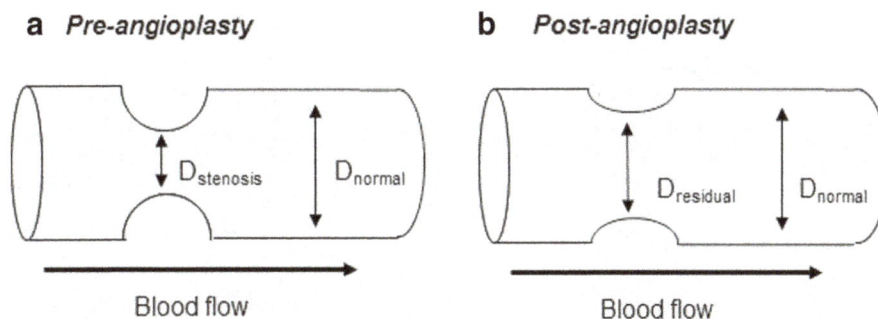

Fig. 1 Anatomic measure of disease severity and residual stenosis. (**a**): Diameter of stenotic and normal segment were measured to estimate the percent of stenosis pre-angioplasty. (**b**): Diameter of residual stenosis and normal segment were measured to estimate the percent of stenosis post-angioplasty

$$\text{Percent of Stenosis}_{\text{post-angioplasty}} = [1-(D_{\text{residual}}/D_{\text{normal}})] \times 100$$

Evaluation of treatment success

Change in Percent of Stenosis:

$$[(\text{Percent of Stenosis}_{\text{pre-angioplasty}} - \text{Percent of Stenosis}_{\text{post-angioplasty}})$$

$$/\text{Percent of Stenosis}_{\text{pre-angioplasty}}] \times 100$$

Hemodynamic evaluation using parametric colour-coded DSA

Difference in time to peak contrast density (dTTP) (Fig. 2)

Pre- and post-PTA sequences were post-processed and converted into colour images. For each image, one region of interest (ROI) was chosen pre- and post-stenosis. Time to peak (TTP) contrast enhancement or time at which each pixel reached its peak intensity was computed for each ROI. The difference in time to peak (dTTP) contrast density between these 2 ROIs pre- and post-PTA provides information on hemodynamic changes and were compared before and after intervention.

Quantification of contrast wash out (Fig. 3)

Time attenuation curves (TAC) pre- and post-treatment were generated using opacity data per ROI per time point calculated by the software. 50% contrast wash out time or time taken for 50% attenuation in contrast density after the peak intensity was obtained and compared pre- and post-PTA.

Statistical analysis

Data was presented as frequency (percentage) for categorical variable; mean (standard deviation) for normally distributed or median (interquartile range (IQR)) for non-normally distributed continuous

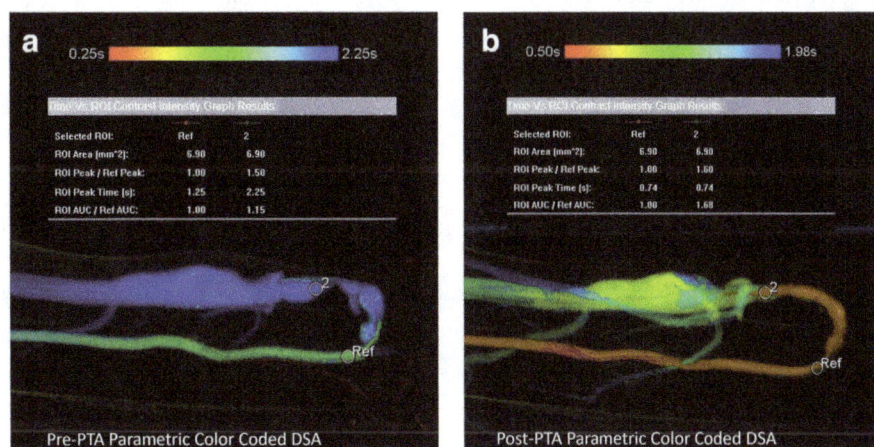

Fig. 2 Pre- and post-PTA parametric colour-coded DSA with region of interests (ROI) of the same AVF shown in Fig. 6. DSA sequences were post-processed and parametric colour-coded DSA was generated. ROIs were chosen pre- and post-stenosis. The differences of TTP (dTTP) values between these 2 ROIs pre- and post-PTA were generated. (**a**) Pre-PTA dTTP was 1 s. (**b**) Post-PTA dTTP was 0, indicating contrast flow was faster after intervention

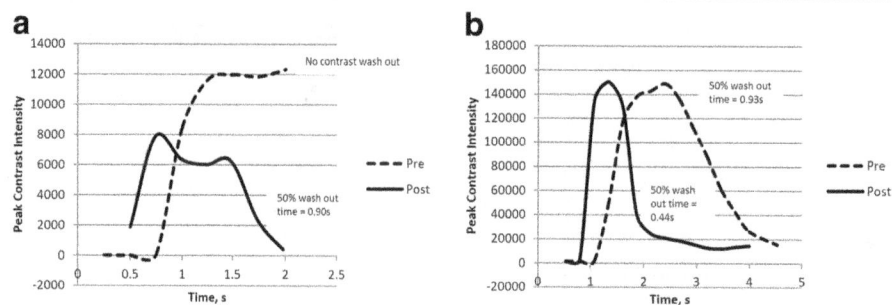

Fig. 3 Quantification of contrast wash out time using time attenuation curve (TAC). (**a**) Time vs. contrast intensity curve of the AVF shown in Fig. 6. Pre-PTA TAC showed no contrast washout during the entire DSA captured, indicating slow flow. Post-PTA TAC exhibited contrast wash out over time and the time taken for 50% contrast wash out was 0.9 s. (**b**) Time vs. contrast intensity curve of an AVG treatment showing contrast wash out over time in both pre- and post-PTA TAC. The time taken for 50% contrast wash improved from 0.93 to 0.44 s

variables. Percent of stenosis, dTTP and 50% contrast washout time were compared using paired sample t-test or Wilcoxon signed-rank test depending on data type. Correlations between pre-PTA percent of stenosis vs. dTTP and post-PTA change in percent of stenosis vs. change in dTTP were obtained using Spearman's rank correlation test. Data analyses were performed using SPSS Statistics for Windows, Version 21 (Armonk, NY:IBM Corp).

Results

The baseline demographics and characteristics of the patients is summarized in Table 1. The study subjects have a mean age of 66.6 ± 9.3 years. AVF was the predominant vascular access (75%) with median access age of 3.1 (IQR 0.7, 5.3) years. Two third of the lesions studied were outflow stenosis (60%).

Information on each vascular access, location of lesions, anatomic and hemodynamic parameters obtained, and patency is summarized on Table 2. All inflow lesions were located at the juxta-anastomotic segment. Conversely, outflow lesions were located at various anatomical sites including peripheral vein, cephalic arch, graft vein junctions and central veins. (Table 2) All cases demonstrated variable anatomical improvements following angioplasty. Improvements in dTTP were observed in 15 patients. Lack of improvement in dTTP was noted in 5 patients. Of which, 3 of the patients have inflow lesions with less than 50% stenosis. The remaining 2 patients had outflow stenoses with more than 50% anatomical improvement. Pre-PTA TAC of 8 out of 20 patients did not show attenuation in contrast density due to high resistance in contrast flow caused by severe stenosis. Contrast washout was exhibited in all patients post-PTA. (Fig. 3) Comparison of 50% contrast washout time pre- and post-PTA was only possible for 12 patients. Of which, 10 patients exhibited improvement in 50% contrast washout time while 2 patients did not. All

patients underwent successful haemodialysis through the index vascular access with blood flow of at least 200mls/min after intervention. 18 patients have recurrent stenosis requiring repeat interventions at the time of patency measurement. The median primary patency was 3.9 (IQR 2.5, 10.3) months. (Table 2).

Anatomical and hemodynamic assessments (Table 3)

Mean percent of stenosis improved from 64.85 ± 21.39 to 24.73 ± 17.03% after PTA ($p < 0.0001$). Median dTTP

Table 1 Baseline Demographics of Patients

Demographics	Mean ± standard deviation or Median (IQR) or n (%)
Age, years	66.6 ± 9.3
Female, n (%)	12 (60)
Age of Access, years	3.1 (0.7, 5.3)
Reason for Intervention, n (%)	
Decreased access flow	7 (35)
High venous pressure	5 (25)
Weak thrill	3 (15)
Arm swelling	4(20)
Thrombosis	1 (5)
Access Type, n (%)	
Arteriovenous fistula (AVF)	15 (75)
Radiocephalic	4 (20)
Brachiocephalic	8 (40)
Brachiobasillic	3 (15)
Arteriovenous graft (AVG)	5 (25)
Brachiobasillic	2 (10)
Femoral-artery-vein	3 (15)
Number of lesions, n (%)	
1	16 (80)
2	4 (20)

Table 2 Characteristics of Vascular Access, Anatomical and Hemodynamic Parameters

Cases	Access	Anastomosis	Number of Stenosis	Anatomical site assessed	Anatomical Parameters, %		Hemodynamic Parameters, s			Time to Next PTA, months
					% of stenosis	Change in % of Stenosis	dTTP	Improvement in dTTP	Improvement in 50% Contrast Wash Out Time	
1	AVF	Brachio-cephalic	1	Cephalic arch	74.76	50.15	0.25	0.80	0.97	Nil[c]
2	AVF	Brachio-cephalic	2[a]	Juxta-anastomosis	20.69	33.55	0.26	−0.01	0.14	11.27
3	AVF	Radio-cephalic	1	Juxta- anastomosis	50.86	66.33	0.80	0.01	0.61	5.29
4	AVF	Radio-cephalic	1	Juxta- anastomosis	68.89	92.20	0.51	0.80	No wash out	3.91
5	AVF	Brachio-cephalic	2[a]	Juxta- anastomosis	44.10	56.30	3.72	0.25	0.38	2.46
6	AVF	Radio-cephalic	1	Juxta- anastomosis	45.47	92.78	0.25	3.47	No wash out	Nil[c]
7	AVF	Brachio-cephalic	2[a]	Juxta- anastomosis	42.04	19.07	0.26	0	−0.14	15.87
8	AVF	Brachio-cephalic	1	Juxta- anastomosis	30.96	33.82	1.00	−0.01	0.34	11.96
9	AVF	Brachio-basillic	1	Draining vein	72.37	83.06	0.80	0.53	No wash out	1.64
10	AVF	Radio-cephalic	1	Juxta- anastomosis	75.93	60.41	0.53	1.00	No wash out	7.33
11	AVG	Brachio-basillic	1	Graft vein junction	74.57	95.93	0.53	0.27	0.49	0.59
12	AVG	Brachio-basillic	2[b]	Draining vein	83.63	54.42	1.06	0.81	No wash out	3.19
13	AVG	Femoral artery-vein	1	Graft vein junction	56.56	71.63	0.26	0	No wash out	3.58
14	AVG	Femoral artery-vein	1	Graft vein junction	52.86	86.59	0.54	0.28	0.94	4.63
15	AVG	Femoral artery-vein	1	Graft vein junction	60.12	81.49	0.25	0.25	No wash out	3.91
16	AVF	Brachio-basillic	1	Brachiocephalic vein	100.00	50.08	0.54	0.54	0.12	2.46
17	AVF	Brachio-cephalic	1	Brachiocephalic vein	91.47	32.59	0.27	0.01	No wash out	2.76
18	AVF	Brachio-cephalic	1	Subclavian vein	77.98	41.22	0.80	0.51	0.06	2.07
19	AVF	Brachio-cephalic	1	Subclavian vein	89.33	51.25	0.27	0	−0.37	1.91
20	AVF	Brachio-basillic	1	Brachiocephalic vein	84.34	69.86	0.26	0.26	0.12	7.56

[a]Proximal lesions were treated before distal lesions, therefore anatomical and hemodynamic parameters of the distal lesions were obtained for comparison
[b]Both lesions were treated simultaneously
[c]Intervention free at last follow-up

improved from 0.52 (IQR 0.26, 0.8) to 0.25 (IQR 0, 0.26) seconds ($p = 0.001$). Median 50% contrast washout time also improved from 0.77 (IQR 0.39, 1.17) to 0.42 (IQR 0.23, 0.59) seconds ($p = 0.031$).

Table 3 Pre- and Post-percutaneous Angioplasty Comparison of Anatomic and Hemodynamic Parameters

Parameters, $n = 20$	Mean ± standard deviation or Median (IQR)	P – value
Percent of Stenosis, %		< 0.0001
Pre-PTA	64.85 ± 21.39	
Post-PTA	24.73 ± 17.03	
dTTP, s		0.001
Pre-PTA	0.52 (0.26, 0.8)	
Post-PTA	0.25 (0, 0.26)	
50% Contrast Washout Time, s		0.031
Pre-PTA	0.77 (0.39, 1.17)	
Post-PTA	0.42 (0.23, 0.59)	

Scatter plot diagrams and correlation analysis

Scatter plot diagrams of dTTP vs. percent of stenosis (Fig. 4) and change in dTTP vs. change in percent of stenosis (Fig. 5) were obtained. Correlation analysis revealed no significant correlation for pre-PTA dTTP vs. percent of stenosis ($r = 0.409$, $p = 0.073$) and post-PTA change in dTTP vs. change in percent of stenosis ($r = 0.399$, $p = 0.082$). However, when the lesions were subdivided into inflow and outflow lesions, significant correlation was seen for dTTP vs. percent of stenosis for inflow stenosis ($n = 8$, $r = 0.723$, $p = 0.043$) but not for outflow stenosis ($n = 12$, $r = 0.158$, $p = 0.623$). Similarly, there was significant correlation for post-PTA change in dTTP vs. percent change in stenosis for inflow lesions ($r = 0.786$, $p = 0.021$) but not for outflow lesions ($r = -0.161$, $p = 0.681$).

Discussions

In this study, we have explored the use of parametric colour coded DSA in the management of dysfunctional dialysis access. The hallmark of successful interventions in dialysis access has always been successful effacement

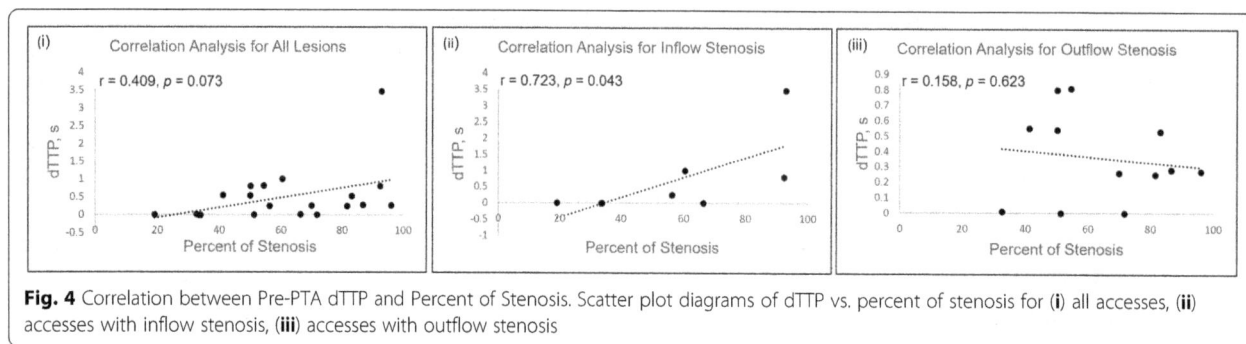

Fig. 4 Correlation between Pre-PTA dTTP and Percent of Stenosis. Scatter plot diagrams of dTTP vs. percent of stenosis for (**i**) all accesses, (**ii**) accesses with inflow stenosis, (**iii**) accesses with outflow stenosis

of stenosis (Fig. 6). However, the functional aspect is equally important, and we hypothesize that parametric colour-coded DSA will provide a quantitative assessment of interventional outcome. We demonstrated significant improvements in dTTP and time taken for 50% contrast attenuation post-PTA as surrogates for improvement in access flow after PTA and significant correlations of anatomical vs. hemodynamic assessments pre- and post PTA. This information might be potentially useful for assessing the significance of lesion and adequacy of treatment during percutaneous intervention of haemodialysis vascular access.

Maintaining sufficient access flow is crucial for adequate hemodialysis [13]. Secondary patency of vascular access after PTA however remains dismal, with re-stenosis and re-intervention rates reported to be up to 60% at 6 months [14, 15]. Visual analysis of conventional two-dimensional DSA sequences typically requires viewing a series images and evaluating the differences in images which the contrast medium creates as it passes through the obstructions in the vessels. Browsing through the entire black and white filling sequences frame by frame during the procedure can be time consuming and is subjected to interpersonal variability. Lack of correlation between angiographic visual assessment and hemodynamic performance of vascular access has been demonstrated in many previous studies [16, 17]. Hence, risk of poor long-term outcome despite successful intervention if treatment adequacy is relied solely on angiographic visual assessment.

Several techniques for assessment of vascular stenosis and intra-procedural real-time hemodynamic assessments in hemodialysis accesses have been described. Magnetic resonance angiography (MRA) and computed tomography angiography (CTA) have been reported to provide high quality diagnostic images for vascular stenosis [3, 18–21]. Time resolved MRA could be a useful screening tool as it is non-invasive and is able to detect vascular stenosis with smaller dose of contrast [20, 21]. Catheter based thermodilution on the other hand is a method to extrapolate intra-access blood flow from thermodilution equation and the thermal properties of blood and saline [17, 22]. It was reported to correlate well with the current gold standard of ultrasound dilution method but the major drawbacks were high cost and high technical failure rates as correct placement of catheter may not always be possible [22]. Ultrasound Doppler flow measurement is another method which is readily available in most interventional radiology suite. However, it is operator dependent and its precision is limited by uncertainties in the measure of vessel diameter, Doppler angle and blood velocity determination. Utility of intra-access static pressure was also investigated and found to be a simple and potentially useful hemodynamic indicator during PTA. An elevated static pressure which declined to normal represented adequately treated outflow stenosis while restoration of a negative static pressure PTA to normal reading could represent adequately treated inflow stenosis [23]. Unfortunately, static pressure may be normal when there is

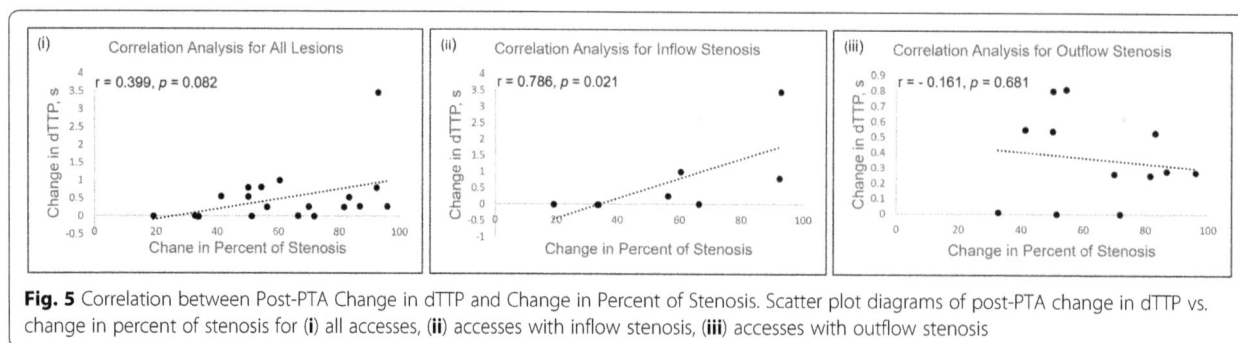

Fig. 5 Correlation between Post-PTA Change in dTTP and Change in Percent of Stenosis. Scatter plot diagrams of post-PTA change in dTTP vs. change in percent of stenosis for (**i**) all accesses, (**ii**) accesses with inflow stenosis, (**iii**) accesses with outflow stenosis

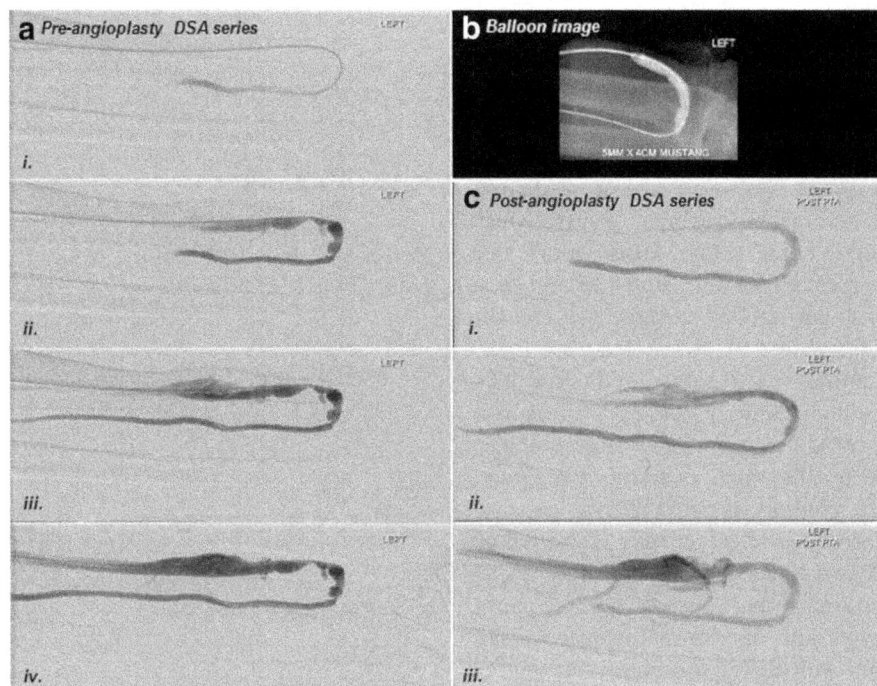

Fig. 6 Images of a left radio-cephalic arterio-venous fistula (AVF) with stenosis along juxta-anastomosis segment. (**i**): Frame by frame black and white images showing juxta-anastomotic segment stenosis pre-PTA. (**ii**): An angioplasty balloon was used to treat the stenosis, complete effacement of the balloon was seen. (**iii**): Frame by frame black and white images showing interval improvement of the juxta-anastomotic segment stenosis with more prominent opacification of collaterals from outflow vein after PTA

co-existing inflow and outflow stenosis exerting opposing hemodynamic effects of equal magnitude, making hemodynamic assessment impossible as there will not be a change in static pressure after treatment [23].

Parametric colour-coded DSA provides an alternative method for hemodynamic assessment. It is easy to use, non-invasive and does not involve use of additional expensive equipment. More importantly, hemodynamic parameters can be instantly generated during the procedure to enable real-time therapeutic planning. Vascular access with multifocal stenosis is not uncommonly encountered during interventional procedures. The approach of treating all encountered lesions has not been shown to improve access patency [24]. Determining whether a visible lesion is clinically indicated for treatment may be challenging on table. Hemodynamic parameters from colour-coded DSA could therefore be a useful adjunctive tool to help determine the necessity and adequacy of treatment of every lesion seen on venography, resulting in potential cost saving and reduction in radiation exposure.

Although pre-PTA 50% contrast washout times were not available in 8 cases, the TACs of these cases still provided some insight on the hemodynamic parameters of the accesses. In these cases, stenosis was likely hemodynamically significant as resistant to contrast flow has resulted in slow contrast attenuation below 50% during the entire DSA sequences captured (Fig. 3). The delay in contrast attenuation was also congruent with anatomical assessment as 7 out of 8 of these patients have lesions with more than 50% stenosis.

Significant correlations were noted between anatomic and hemodynamic parameters pre- and post-PTA for inflow stenosis but not outflow stenosis. We postulated that this could be due to the different vascular characteristics of the different outflow components. For example, size, elasticity and curvature are different in central veins compared to peripheral veins [25]. Furthermore, when the access has more than one outflow such as in a radio-cephalic fistula, the quantity, size and location of the outflow veins may also result in inaccuracy during hemodynamic assessment.

Although the effect of colour was not evaluated in our study, previous studies on colour-coded DSA have suggested that colour coding provided images of high quality that were not impaired by motion artefact [10]. Furthermore, colour is known to improve visual search and identification performance [26]. The display of colour can be used to enhance human perception of medical information and has been successfully used in computed tomography, magnetic resonance imaging and sonograms. As human eyes perceive colour differentiation over a wide

172   Handbook of Medical imaging

range, changes in signal intensity can be easily distinguishable with the naked eye [27]. Evaluation of vascular access with parametric colour coding could therefore be easier and more accurate than conventional black and white DSA [9].

We acknowledge that there were several limitations of this study. The major limitation of our study was the small sample size from a single centre which limits its power and generalizability. Furthermore, due to the retrospective nature of this study where hand injection of contrast during DSA acquisition was the standard of care, differences in pressure during injection, volume of contrast used before and after PTA may affect the hemodynamic parameters measured. However, contrast injections for all the cases included in the study were by the same operator throughout the procedure. Our method of retrospective case selection may also introduce selection bias. Although all PTA were deemed successful clinically and radiologically, we did not examine the effect of hemodynamic parameters on resolution of clinical symptoms nor correlate the results with direct flow measurement or indirect pressure measurement. Estimation of percentage of luminal stenosis using diameter measurement is not the most ideal as this calculation is a one-dimensional view. Vessels are circular or elliptical, and the stenoses are frequently asymmetric when viewed in cross section. Estimating the luminal stenosis using one plane in this study may therefore result in inaccuracy. Additionally, although there was statistical improvement in the TTP and contrast wash out time post angioplasty, we are unable to determine the cut off values to define success or adequacy of angioplasty due to the small sample size. Nevertheless, within the limits of the study, we have demonstrated that parametric colour-coded DSA may be able to provide potentially useful quantitative information on hemodynamic changes in vascular access during PTA, especially for inflow lesions. This is relevant to clinical practice as the aim of PTA is to restore sufficient flow within the dialysis access for hemodialysis.

Conclusions

This pilot study suggests that adjunctive use of parametric colour-coded DSA may have positive impact in haemodialysis vascular access interventions. We proposed that a larger prospective study using standardized contrast injection rate with correlation of hemodynamic parameters with the gold standard ultrasound dilution technique of intra-access flow should be performed to further evaluate the effectiveness and reliability of colour-coded DSA in haemodynamic assessment of haemodialysis vascular access.

Abbreviations

AVF: Arteriovenous fistula; AVG: Arteriovenous graft; DSA: Digital subtraction angiography; dTTP: Difference in time to peak; ESRF: End stage renal failure; PTA: Percutaneous transluminal angioplasty; ROI: Regions of interest; TAC: Time attenuation curve

Authors' contributions

RYT, AG, TTC and CST conceptualized this study. RYT, FCT, SCP, KGL and AHO recruited the patients, analyzed the images and performed statistical analysis of the data. RYT, AHO and CST prepared the manuscript. All authors read and approved the final manuscript.

Competing interests

The authors declare that they have no competing interests.

Author details

[1]Department of Renal Medicine, Singapore General Hospital, Singapore, Singapore. [2]Department of Vascular Surgery, Singapore General Hospital, Singapore, Singapore. [3]Department of Vascular and Interventional Radiology, Singapore General Hospital, Singapore, Singapore. [4]Duke-NUS Medical School, Singapore, Singapore.

References

1. Schinstock CA, Albright RC, Williams AW, Dillon JJ, Bergstralh EJ, Jenson BM, et al. Outcomes of arteriovenous fistula creation after the fistula first initiative. Clin J Am Soc Nephrol. 2011;6(8):1996–2002.
2. Roy-Chaudhury P, Sukhatme VP, Cheung AK. Hemodialysis vascular access dysfunction: a cellular and molecular viewpoint. J Am Soc Nephrol. 2006; 17(4):1112–27.
3. Razek AA, Saad E, Soliman N, Elatta HA. Assessment of vascular disorders of the upper extremity with contrast-enhanced magnetic resonance angiography: pictorial review. Jpn J Radiol. 2010;28(2):87–94.
4. NKF-DOQI. Clinical Practice Guidelines for Vascular Access. Am J Kidney Dis. 2006;48:S176–247.
5. Mishler R, Sands JJ, Ofsthun NJ, Teng M, Schon D, Lazarus JM. Dedicated outpatient vascular access center decreases hospitalization and missed outpatient dialysis treatments. Kidney Int. 2006;69(2):393–8.
6. Doelman C, Duijm LEM, Liem YS, Froger CL, Tielbeek AV, Donkers-van Rossum AB, et al. Stenosis detection in failing hemodialysis access fistulas and grafts: comparison of color Doppler ultrasonography, contrast-enhanced magnetic resonance angiography, and digital subtraction angiography. J Vasc Surg. 2005;42(4):739–46.
7. Leontiev O, Mondschein JI, Dagli MS, Clark TWI, Soulen MC, Stavropoulos SW, et al. Catheter-based Intraaccess blood flow measurement as a problem-solving tool in hemodialysis access intervention. J Vasc Interv Radiol. 2013;24(5):717–21.
8. Gray RJ, Sacks D, Martin LG, Trerotola SO. Reporting standards for percutaneous interventions in dialysis access. J Vasc Interv Radiol. 2003;14(9 Pt 2):S433–42.
9. Strother CM, Bender F, Deuerling-Zheng Y, Royalty K, Pulfer KA, Baumgart J, et al. Parametric color coding of digital subtraction angiography. AJNR Am J Neuroradiol. 2010;31(5):919–24.
10. Golitz P, Struffert T, Lucking H, Rosch J, Knossalla F, Ganslandt O, et al. Parametric color coding of digital subtraction angiography in the evaluation of carotid cavernous fistulas. Clin Neuroradiol. 2013;23(2):113–20.
11. Lin CJ, Hung SC, Guo WY, Chang FC, Luo CB, Beilner J, et al. Monitoring peri-therapeutic cerebral circulation time: a feasibility study using color-coded quantitative DSA in patients with steno-occlusive arterial disease. AJNR Am J Neuroradiol. 2012;33(9):1685–90.
12. Su H, Lou W, Gu J. Clinical values of hemodynamics assessment by parametric color coding of digital subtraction angiography before and after endovascular therapy for critical limb ischaemia. Zhonghua Yi Xue Za Zhi. 2015;95(37):3036–40.
13. Whittier WL. Surveillance of hemodialysis vascular access. Semin Interv Radiol. 2009;26(2):130–8.

14. Kim WS, Pyun WB, Kang BC. The primary patency of percutaneous Transluminal angioplasty in hemodialysis patients with vascular access failure. Korean Circ J. 2011;41(9):512–7.

15. Agarwal SK, Nadkarni GN, Yacoub R, Patel AA, Jenkins JS, Collins TJ, et al. Comparison of cutting balloon angioplasty and percutaneous balloon angioplasty of Arteriovenous fistula stenosis: a meta-analysis and systematic review of randomized clinical trials. J Interv Cardiol. 2015;28(3):288–95.

16. Ahya SN, Windus DW, Vesely TM. Flow in hemodialysis grafts after angioplasty: do radiologic criteria predict success? Kidney Int. 2001;59(5):1974–8.

17. Goyal A, Orth RC, Parekh RS, Wolfson T, Gamst A, Kuo MD. Endpoints for hemodialysis access procedures: correlation between fistulography and intraaccess blood flow measurements. J Vasc Interv Radiol. 2011;22(12):1733–9.

18. Abdel Razek AAK, Denewer AT, Hegazy MAF, Hafez MTA. Role of computed tomography angiography in the diagnosis of vascular stenosis in head and neck microvascular free flap reconstruction. Int J Oral Maxillofac Surg. 2014;43(7):811–5.

19. Lin YP, Wu MH, Ng YY, Lee RC, Liou JK, Yang WC, et al. Spiral computed tomographic angiography--a new technique for evaluation of vascular access in hemodialysis patients. Am J Nephrol. 1998;18(2):117–22.

20. Razek AA, Gaballa G, Megahed AS, Elmogy E. Time resolved imaging of contrast kinetics (TRICKS) MR angiography of arteriovenous malformations of head and neck. Eur J Radiol. 2013;82(11):1885–91.

21. Zhang J, Hecht EM, Maldonado T, Lee VS. Time-resolved 3D MR angiography with parallel imaging for evaluation of hemodialysis fistulas and grafts: initial experience. AJR Am J Roentgenol. 2006;186(5):1436–42.

22. Heerwagen ST, Hansen MA, Schroeder TV, Ladefoged SD, Lonn L. Blood flow measurements during hemodialysis vascular access interventions–catheter-based thermodilution or Doppler ultrasound? J Vasc Access. 2012;13(2):145–51.

23. Asif A, Besarab A, Gadalean F, Merrill D, Rismeyer AE, Contreras G, et al. Utility of static pressure ratio recording during angioplasty of arteriovenous graft stenosis. Semin Dial. 2006;19(6):551–6.

24. Leontiev O, Shlansky-Goldberg RD, Stavropoulos SW, Mondschein JI, Itkin M, Clark TWI, et al. Should all inflow Stenoses be treated in failing autogenous hemodialysis fistulae? J Vasc Interv Radiol. 2014;25(4):542–7.

25. Agarwal AK. Endovascular interventions for central vein stenosis. Kidney Res Clin Pract. 2015;34(4):228–32.

26. Cole BL, Maddocks JD, Sharpe K. Visual search and the conspicuity of coloured targets for colour vision normal and colour vision deficient observers. Clin Exp Optom. 2004;87(4–5):294–304.

27. Benndorf G. Color-coded digital subtraction angiography: the end of a monochromatic era? AJNR Am J Neuroradiol. 2010;31(5):925–7.

22

Follow-up of iatrogenic aorto-coronary "Dunning" dissections by cardiac computed tomography imaging

Stefan Baumann[1†], Michael Behnes[1*†], Benjamin Sartorius[1], Tobias Becher[1], Ibrahim El-Battrawy[1], Christian Fastner[1], Uzair Ansari[1], Dirk Loßnitzer[1], Kambis Mashayekhi[2], Thomas Henzler[3], Stefan O. Schoenberg[3], Martin Borggrefe[1] and Ibrahim Akin[1]

Abstract

Background: Iatrogenic aorto-coronary dissections following percutaneous coronary interventions (PCI) represent a rare but potentially life threatening complication. This restrospective and observational study aims to describe our in-house experience for timely diagnostics and therapy including cardiovascular imaging to follow-up securely high-risk patients with Dunning dissections.

Methods: Dunning dissections (DD) occurred during clinical routine PCIs, which were indicated according to current ESC guidelines. Diagnostic assessment, treatment and follow-up were based on coronary angiography with PCI or conservative treatment and cardiac computed tomography (cCTA) imaging.

Results: A total of eight patients with iatrogenic DD were included. Median age was 69 years (IQR 65.8–74.5). Patients revealed a coronary multi-vessel-disease in 75% with a median SYNTAX-II-score of 35.3 (IQR 30.2–41.2). The most common type of DD was type III (50%), followed by type I (38%) and type II (13%). In most patients (88%) the DD involved the right coronary arterial ostium. 63% were treated by PCI, the remaining patients were treated conservatively. 88% of patients received at least one cCTA within 2 days, 50% were additionally followed-up by cCTA within a median of 6 months (range: 4–8 months) without any residual.

Conclusion: Independently of the type of DD (I-III) it was demonstrated that cCTA represents a valuable imaging modality for detection and follow-up of patients with DDs.

Keywords: Aortocoronary dissection, Coronary computed tomography, Complication, Dunning, Percutaneous coronary intervention

Background

Iatrogenic aorto-coronary dissections following percutaneous coronary interventions (PCI) represent rare but potentially life threatening complications [1]. The overall incidence is estimated around 0.02% and more common in patients with acute myocardial infarction compared to elective PCI [2]. Dunning et al. classified these dissections into three groups, where the local involvement of the ipsilateral cusp was defined as class I, the extension along the ascending aorta of less than 40 mm as class II and more than 40 mm as class III [2]. Patients with limited aortic involvement (class I and II) were described to be managed successfully by a "wait-and-see" strategy or PCI with implantation of a stent at the coronary dissection entry [2]. In contrast, Dunning dissections (DD) of type III require treatment by cardiovascular surgery [2]. While surgical treatment is still under debate, it is still under ongoing debate whether PCI with implantation of drug eluting stents (DES) at the aorto-ostial dissection might represent a valuable treatment alternative even in extensive dissections [3]. Nonetheless, large-scaled randomized controlled studies evaluating the best treatment choice in patients with DD are not available and the

* Correspondence: michael.behnes@umm.de

†Equal contributors

[1]First Department of Medicine, University Medical Centre Mannheim, Theodor-Kutzer-Ufer 1-3, 68167 Mannheim, Germany

Full list of author information is available at the end of the article

current scientific knowledge is limited to single case series [2].

Because patients suffering from DD underlie an increased risk of death, they may ultimately profit from an accurate diagnostic follow-up to guarantee best medical treatment [4]. However, no cCTA imaging algorithm for follow-up was yet developed in order to ensure an accurate treatment of this rare disease entity. Therefore, this study aims to describe our institutional experience to follow-up these high-risk patients.

Methods

Study population and patient recruitment

This monocentric, retrospective and observational study evaluates diagnostic and therapeutic regimens including imaging examples of patients developing iatrogenic aorto-coronary DD during clinical routine care. Identification of the patients was performed retrospectively by reviewing our in-hospital electronic documentation system, while the initial diagnostic assessment was always performed within coronary angiography at index PCI. The classification of DD was described recently by Dunning et al. [2] (Fig. 1).

A total of eight patients with iatrogenic aorto-coronary DDs occurring during PCI were included during routine clinical care. PCI was indicated according to current European guidelines [5] and were performed at the First Department of Medicine, University Medical Centre Mannheim (UMM), Germany, in between October 2013 and September 2016. The study was carried out according to the principles of the declaration of Helsinki and was approved by the local ethics committee of the University Medical Centre Mannheim (ethical approval number 2016-864R-MA). All participants provided verbal informed consent.

Coronary computed tomography angiography (cCTA)

All cCTA examinations were performed by using dual-source CT scanners with a minimum of 64 detector rows (Somatom Definition or Force, Siemens Healthcare Sector, Forchheim, Germany). Our standardized imaging protocol included a single phase ECG-gated 100 kV CTA study (320 reference mAs, 0.6 mm slice collimation, rotation speed 330 ms) from the thoracic inlet to the inguinal region. Vessel enhancement was achieved via injection of 90 mL iodinated contrast medium (Iomeprol 400, Bracco, Italy) with a flow rate of 5 cm^3/s. Automatic tube current modulation in x, y and z-direction as well as ECG-dependent tube current modulation (20–80% RR-interval) was used in all patients. All CT data acquisitions were acquired during an inspiratory breath-hold. Analysis of the cCTA images were performed on a separate workstation with a predefined high resolution screen.

PCI of aorto-coronary dissections

Type of treatment of DD was performed according to the operator's discretion and considered either conservatively with a "wait-and-see" strategy, interventional with PCI and sealing of the coronary dissection entry or surgical treatment.

A conservative treatment of a DD was chosen as an adequate treatment option only, when imaging results by coronary angiography or cCTA revealed limited or no further progress of the DD after the index procedure. Additionally, hemodynamic stability was required in conservatively treated patients.

PCI of DD aimed to seal appropriately the entry of the aorto-coronary dissection by implantation of DES. PCI was usually performed immediately within the index coronary angiography. An overlap of up to 3–5 mm into the ascending aorta was regarded as being sufficient to guarantee adequate sealing. An interdisciplinary discussion of all cases within a heart team was performed in all cases [5].

Results

Study population

A total of eight patients with iatrogenic aorto-coronary DD were included. At our institution, we have performed 3600 PCI in the study period, resulting to an incidence of 0.22%. Baseline characteristics are shown in Table 1. The median

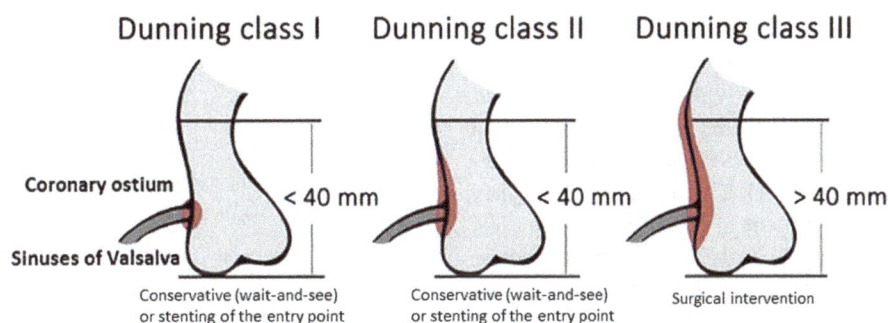

Fig. 1 Classification of aortocoronary dissection based upon the extent of aortic involvement according to Dunning et al. [2] Class I (left), involves only the coronary cusp. Class II (middle), extends up the aortic wall, but remains under 40 mm. Class III (right), contrast media extends over 40 mm up to the aortic wall

Table 1 Baseline characteristics of patients with Dunning dissections. *IQR* interquartile range

Age, median (IQR)	69.0 (65.8–74.5)
Male gender, n (%)	4 (50)
Height (cm), median (IQR)	164.0 (160.0–169.5)
Weight (kg), median (IQR)	72.5 (70.0–78.0)
Body mass index (kg/m^2), median (IQR)	27.3 (26.8–29.3)
Cardiovascular risk factors, n (%)	
Diabetes mellitus	4 (50)
Arterial hypertension	7 (88)
Smoking	5 (63)
Dyslipidaemia	4 (50)
Prior medical history, n (%)	
Coronary artery disease	
1-vessel	1 (13)
2-vessel	1 (13)
3-vessel	5 (63)
Myocardial infarction	3 (38)
Bypass surgery	1 (13)
Percutaneous coronary intervention	6 (75)
Heart failure	3 (38)
Chronic kidney disease	0 (0)
Stroke	2 (25)
Chronic obstructive pulmonary disease	0 (0)
LVEF (%), median (IQR)	60.0 (48.8–60.0)
SYNTAX-II-Score, median (IQR)	35.3 (30.2–41.2)
Laboratory values, median (IQR)	
Creatinine (mg/dl)	1.2 (0.9–1.3)
Glomerular filtration rate (ml/min)	60.0 (57.5–60.0)
Haemoglobin (g/dl)	12.3 (11.2–13.4)
International Normalized Ratio	1.0 (0.9–1.5)
Antithrombotic medication, n (%)	
Acetylsalicylacid	8 (100)
Clopidogrel	5 (63)
Prasugrel	2 (25)
Vitamin K antagonists	2 (25)

Procedural data of patients with DD

As shown in Table 2, the most common type of DD was of type III (50%), followed by type I (38%) and type II (13%). DD occurred mostly during PCI of the right coronary artery (RCA) (88%), followed by the left anterior

Table 2 Procedural data of patients with Dunning dissections treated by percutaneous coronary intervention. [a]elective CTO with puncture of two vessels. *CTO* chronic total occlusion, *F* french, *SD* standard deviation

Dunning dissections, n (%)	
Type I	3 (38)
Type II	1 (13)
Type III	4 (50)
Revascularized vessel, n (%)	
Left main trunk (LMT) and Left anterior descending (LAD)	1 (13)
Right coronary artery (RCA)	7 (88)
Multivessel disease	8 (100)
Chronic total occlusion CTO	3 (38)
Arterial access, n (%)	
6 F	7 (88)
7 F	1 (13)
Radial	1 (13)
Brachial[a]	2 (25)
Femoral[a]	6 (75)
Antithrombotic treatment, n (%)	
Acetylsalicylacid	8 (100)
Heparin	8 (100)
Clopidogrel	6 (75)
Prasugrel	2 (25)
Abciximab	2 (25)
Vitamin K antagonists	2 (25)
Non compliant (NC) balloon, n (%)	3 (38)
Procedural data, median (IQR)	
Maximum dilation pressure (atm)	18.0 (17.0–20.0)
Maximum balloon diameter (mm)	3.0 (3.0–3.5)
Maximum balloon length (mm)	15.0 (15.0–16.3)
Total stent length (mm)	30.5 (24.8–59.5)
Coronary angiography data, median (IQR)	
Procedure time (min)	80.5 (63.5–108.3)
Total fluoroscopy time (min)	19.4 (12.6–30.3)
Total contrast volume (ml)	255.0 (158.5–341.3)
Total radiation exposure (Gycm^2)	62.0 (42.3–177.3)
CT-data, median (IQR)	
Radiation-Dose (mSV)	1.9 (1.7–2.0)
Dose length product (mGy x cm)	133.2 (121.0–142.3)
Total contrast volume (ml)	90 (90.0–90.0)

age of patients was 69.0 years (IQR 65.8–74.5), and 50% were of male gender. Most patients revealed an increased cardiovascular risk profile (up to 88%) with at least one cardiovascular risk factor (Table 1). The presence of coronary multi-vessel-disease was present in 75%. Six patients (75%) had underwent previous coronary angiography, whereas only one patient had a history of coronary artery bypass grafting (CABG). A history of heart failure was present in 38% with a median left ventricular ejection fraction (LVEF) of 60% (IQR 48.8–60.0). The median SYNTAX-II-score was 35.2 (30.2–41.2) (Table 1).

descending (LAD) and left main trunk (LMT) (13%). Arterial access-site was mostly of 6 French (88%) using femoral arterial access (75%) with a median implanted stent length of 30.5 mm (IQR 24.8–59.5). A mother in child catheter was used in 4 of 8 patients (Guideliner). The total procedural length was 80.5 min (IQR 63.5–108.3) accompanied by a total radiation exposure of 62 Gycm^2 (IQR 42.3–177.3) and contrast volume of 255 ml (IQR 158.5–341.3). The median dose length product (DLP) of cCTA examinations was 113.2 mGy × cm (IQR 121.0–142.3), which corresponds to an estimated median radiation dose of 1.9 mSv (IQR 1.7–2.0).

Analysis of individual patients´ data sets

Usually patients presented with symptoms of acute chest pain during DD complicating PCI. As outlined in Table 3, index PCI were mostly performed using at least 6 French (F) arterial access sheaths, either using femoral access (75%) compared to radial/brachial access (38%). PCI were performed in most cases as an elective complex PCI of chronic total occlusions (CTO) (38%) or PCI with rotablation of heavily calcified lesions (13%) as shown in Table 3. DD mostly occurred as a consequence of a too deep intubation of coronary arteries with the guiding catheter (63%), and rarely during sub-intimal wire tracking during wire externalization of a CTO. The most commonly used type of guiding catheter was an Amplatz left (AL 1) (50%).

Diagnostics and therapy treatment of DDs

Table 3 outlines data sets of cases with DD, specifically regarding target vessel and treatment by PCI. 63% of patients were treated by PCI, whereas 38% of patients were treated conservatively. Initial diagnostic assessment was visualized during index coronary angiography in 88% of the patients, while in one case the DD was detected only by cCTA. Interventional treatment by PCI was performed according to the following steps: positioning of 2nd or 3rd generation DES with an intra-aortal overlap and subsequent high pressure PCI/DES implantation. However, the respective treatment of the DD was at the discretion of the responsible operator and based on an individual decision, in consideration of the patient condition.

Follow-up CTA was not performed at predefined fixed intervals; nonetheless, the majority of the patients (88%) received at least one cCTA within the first two days after index event and 50% were additionally followed-up by cCTA within a median of 6 months (range: 4–8 months). Fifty percent of patients did not present back to our clinic, because of subjective improvement of symptoms and stable cardiopulmonary status, and therefore clinical re-assessment by cCTA was not necessary in these patients, as being decided by clinicians during routine clinical care. The follow-up of patients as well as the treatment of DD patients totally relied on the physicians being involved in clinical routine care. Their decisions were based on clinical considerations implementing a stable course with until complete healing without further re-evaluation by cCTA. In case of more severe stages of DD and as well-being based on clinical decision-making cCTA was planned and re-investigated during follow-up.

Imaging examples according to the different types of DD

As shown in Fig. 2, this DD type I occurred in a patient with progredient typical angina (Canadian cardiovascular society (CCS) class III), who was planned for an elective PCI of a chronic total occlusion (CTO) of the RCA. During guiding catheter (AL 1) intubation and contrast injection of the RCA a local DD occurred at the RCA ostium (Fig. 2a). Figure. 2b shows positioning of the DES (Promus 4.0/16 mm) overlapping into the aorta in order to seal the entry. One day after index PCI, cCTA revealed a circular intramural hematoma (Fig. 2c. cCTA at 4 months of follow-up demonstrates complete regression of DD without any residual hematoma as well as adequate positioning of the DES (Fig. 2d).

Figure 3 illustrates follow-up of a patient with multi-vessel coronary artery disease and initially successful PCI of the LAD and posterlateral branch of the circumflex . After switch to the RCA and intubation with an AL1 the vessel showed a spiral winded DD II (Fig. 3a). The instantly performed axial contrast-enhanced cCTA confirmed the extensive intramural hematoma (Fig. 3b). Due to failed re-wiring the patient underwent a conservative wait and see approach with closed meshed cCTA with four consecutive cCTA (<24 h, day 1, 5 and 9) and showed final satisfactory result after 9 days (Fig. 3c) and control coronary angiography after 5 months (Fig. 3d).

An even more extended dissection was seen in a 76-year-old-female patient initially presenting with Non–ST-Segment Elevation Myocardial Infarction (NSTEMI) in the chest pain unit. Complex intubation of the RCA ostium with AR2 results in a very extensive DD of type 3 reaching from the ascending aorta to the brachiocephalic trunc (Fig. 4a). Immediate PCI with implantation of a covered stent (Graftmaster 3.5/16 mm) lead to a sufficient sealing of the dissection entry without further progress. One day after the index PCI an extensive dissection was confirmed by cCTA (Fig. 4b). The invasive follow-up 6 days later showed good result of sealing, with subsequent successful complex multi-vessel Re-PCI with implantation of multiple DES at the RCA and LMT (Fig. 4c). The mid-term follow-up cCTA confirms complete resolution at 5 months after index PCI (Fig. 4d).

A final patient was planned for complex PCI with planned revascularization of a CTO of the RCA. After assessing coronary angiography the SYNTAX-II-Score

Table 3 Data sets of patients with Dunning dissections. *HS* hockey stick, *EBU* extra back-up, *AL* Amplatz left, *RCB* right coronary bypass, *AR* Amplatz right, *BMW* balance middleweight

Patient	Type of Dunning dissection	Access	Catheter type	Guidewire	Syntax-II-score	Procedure	Dissection-associated procedure	Type of treatment	Number and type of implanted stents	CTA post intervention time intervall (days)	Follow-Up CTA (Time interval in months)
1	III	Femoral, 7F	HS	Mailman	30.5	RCA, elective rotablation, CTO	Intubation/Engagement Guiding catheter	Ostial PCI with sealing	3 (Xience Pro 2.25/18; 2.25/15; 2.5/15 mm)	1, 2, 5	8
2	I	Femoral, 6F	EBU	BMW	29.4	LMT/LAD, elective PCI, CCS class III	Engagement of guiding catheter in ostial LMT stenosis	Conservative, wait and see	2 [Xience Pro 2.75/15; 4.0/12 mm]	x	8
3	III	Brachial, 6F	AL 1	Fielder XT	36.4	RCA, elective PCI, CCS class III	Intubation/Engagement Guiding catheter	Ostial PCI with sealing	1 [Integrity 3.5/12 mm]	2	X
4	I	Femoral, 6F	RCB	PT2	34.1	RCA, elective PCI, CCS class III	Inadequate PCI of the ostial RCA without aortic overlap	Ostial PCI with sealing	1 [Integrity 3.5/18 mm]	<24 h	X
5	III	Femoral, 6F	AL 1	Pilot 50	51.7	Cardiogenic shock, complete revascularisation of RCA-CTO and LMT/RIVA/CX in one session	Unknown, postinterventional pericardial hemorrhage (1550 ml)	Conservative, protamin	6 [Xience Pro 2.75/18; 3.0/23; 2.75/23; 3.0/23; 3.5/18; 2.75/18 mm]	<24 h, 1	X
6	II	Femoral, 6F	AL 1	Whisper	37.7	RCA, elective PCI, CCS class III	Intubation/Engagement Guiding catheter	Failed rewiring, Conservative, wait and see	2 [Resolute 2.5/28 mm, Promus 3.0/20 mm]	<24 h, 1, 5, 9	X
7	III	Radial 6F	AR 2	Whisper	52.6	LMT, LAD, RCA Unstable angina	Intubation/Engagement Guiding catheter	Ostial PCI with sealing	2 [Promus 3.0/12 mm, Graftmaster 3.5/16 mm]	1, 2	6
8	I	Brachial, 6F Femoral, 6F	AL 1	Whisper	20.2	RCA, elective CTO, CCS class III	Retrograde subintimal wire tracking externalization	Ostial PCI with sealing	4 [Promus 2.75/20; 3.0/38, 3.5/20, 4.0/16 mm]	1	4

HS hockey stick; *EBU* extra back-up; *AL* Amplatz left; *RCB* right coronary bypass; *AR* Amplatz right; *BMW* balance middleweight

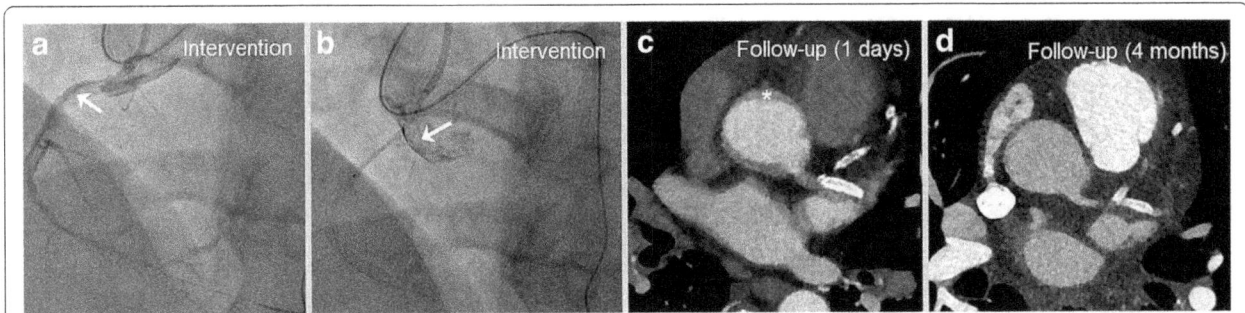

Fig. 2 Dunning Dissection type I. Patient with CCS III and elective CTO of the RCA resulting in aortocoronary dissection. Illustration before (a) and after aorto-ostial sealing (b), c The cCTA the following day showed a slight intramural hematoma with d complete recovery after 4 months

was 36.4%. During CTO-PCI of the RCA (Fig. 5a) a DD of type III occurred during sub-intimal wire tracking with a Fielder XT CTO wire being supported by a micro catheter and final wire externalization. The lesion was successfully sealed with an aorto-ostial PCI/DES implantation (Integrity 3.5/12 mm) overlapping into the ascending aorta (Fig. 5b). Coronal cCTA images of the ascending aorta 1 day after the index procedure confirmed extensive DD type III as well as optimal sealing of the dissection entry by the DES (Fig. 5c).

Discussion

The present retrospective and observational study outlines clinically relevant aspects about the timely diagnosis, treatment and imaging follow-up of patients suffering from iatrogenic aorto-coronary dissections i.e. Dunning dissection (DD) as a consequence of PCI during routine clinical care.

Modern interventional cardiology allows the chance of treating most complex and technically challenging coronary lesions by PCI [6]. The most important advantage from the patient's perspective represents the minimally invasive treatment approach compared to open-heart

surgery. As reported by Dunning et al. the rate of iatrogenic aorto-coronary dissections is higher during PCI of patients suffering from an acute myocardial infarction (0.19%) or of elective patients (0.03%) compared to conventional diagnostic coronary angiographies (<0.01%) [2]. Within the present cohort DD occurred mostly during elective and planned complex PCI and in one patient suffering from NSTEMI with subsequent cardiogenic shock. The most frequent causes of dissection occurred during interventions of the RCA (88%) and CTOs (38%). All PCIs were complex interventions being affirmed by a median SYNTAX-II-score of 35.3. After high-risk PCIs such as a PCI of a CTO close-meshed follow-up and clinical assessment is mandatory to ensure a successful outcome, because the risk of aorto-coronary dissections was markedly increased by 1.8% [7].

The vast majority occurred during PCI of the RCA, while the exact underlying pathomechanism still remains unclear [1, 8]. Within the present study the most important risk factors for Dunning dissections as being estimated by the PCI-operator contain a too deep intubation and engagement with the catheter (50%), use of an AL 1 catheter (50%), use of a mother in child

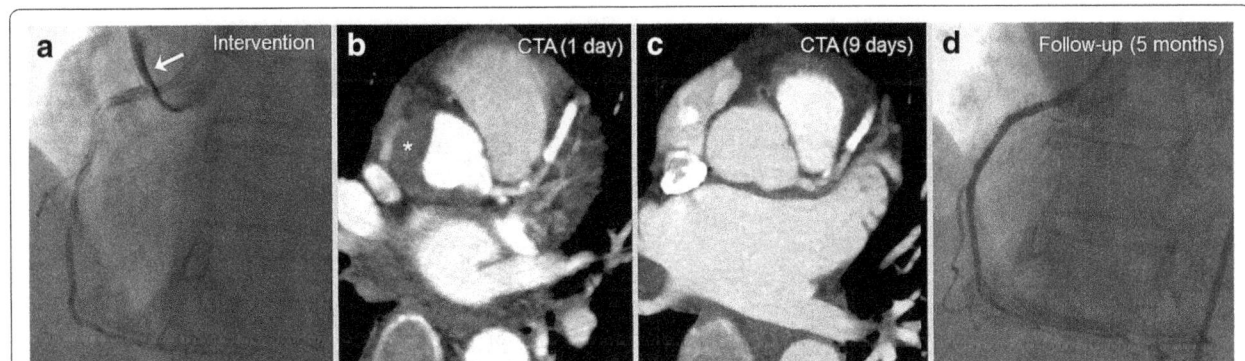

Fig. 3 Dunning Dissection type II. Patient with 3-vessel coronary artery disease and PCI of the LAD and 90% long-segment stenoses of the RCA. a After intubation of the RCA with an AL1 a spiral winded DD occurred with failed rewiring. b cCTA confirmed the extensive haematoma. c The patient underwent a conservative wait and see with closed meshed cCTA with four cCTA within 9 days and d final satisfactory result. cCTA, coronary CT angiography; PCI, percutaneous coronary intervention; RCA; right coronary artery

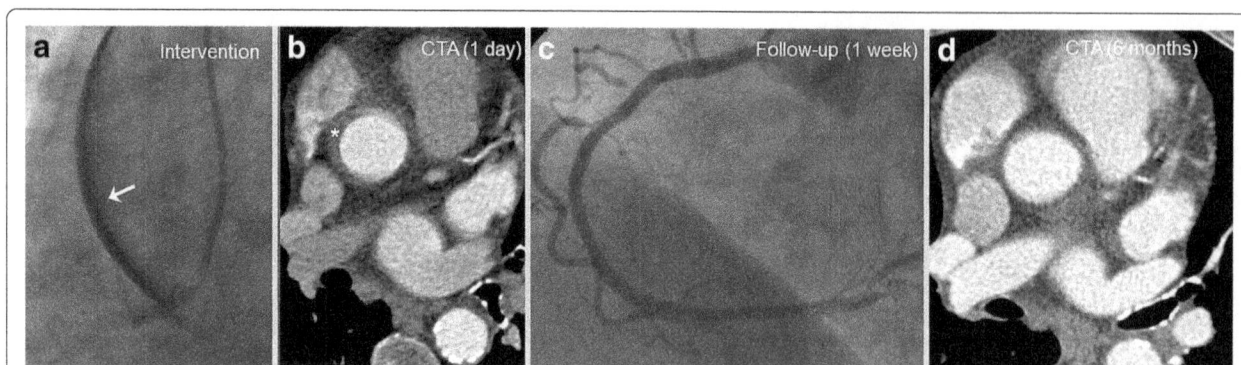

Fig. 4 Dunning Dissection type III. Patient presenting with unstable angina in the chest pain unit. **a** Complex intubation of the RCA ostium with AR2 results in a Dunning Typ 3 dissection (arrow) with emergency sealing (Graftmaster 3.5/16 mm) without further progress of the dissection. **b** One day after the initial intervention CT confirmed an extensive dissection. **c** The invasive follow-up 9 days later showed good result, with subsequent successful re-intervention of the RCA and the LMT. **d** The follow-up cCTA confirms complete recovery after a follow-up period of 6 months. cCTA, coronary CT angiography; RCA; right coronary artery

catheter (50%) and subintimal wire tracking or wire externalization (13%). According to the literature, further potential risk factors seem to be the tortuous anatomy and smaller size auf the RCA, the degree of calcification mainly the aortic root, the type and manipulation of used guiding catheters, heavy coronary calcification and wires during the intervention [4, 9, 10].

Aorto-coronary dissections extending into the aortic root as described in this study were treated with central ostial PCI/DES implantation being positioned by an overlap into the ascending aorta after diagnostic confirmation by angiography. If interventional entry sealing could not perform rapidly, a conservative wait-and-see approach has a high risk of uncontrollable dissections with consecutive major vascular complications [3]. Therefore, the exact extension of the dissection is mandatory to know, while coronary angiography often underestimates the extent of the dissection due to inadequate contrast opacification. Some authors recommend intravascular ultrasound (IVUS) guided coronary stenting to ensure complete coverage of the DD and exact placement of the stent to entirely cover the ostium [11, 12]. Furthermore, only slight and few contrast should be injected carefully and directly over the guiding catheter in order not to sustain or even increase the dissection entry. IVUS or CTA may be applied instead of these direct contrast injections at coronary ostia via catheters.

The technical advances in ECG-gated CTA scanner technologies with low-radiation dose and high resolution images allow to show progression or regression of the dissection [13]. Novel technical developments allow to reduce the noise and residual artifacts with simultaneous detail preservation even in low-dose cCTA images [14, 15].

Therefore, CTA is ideally suited to confirm the presence of residual aortocoronary dissection and evaluation of its exact extent and later noninvasive follow-up. Tansie et al. investigated retrospectively eight patients with DD and described their CTA findings. Similar to our population the main side of the dissection was the

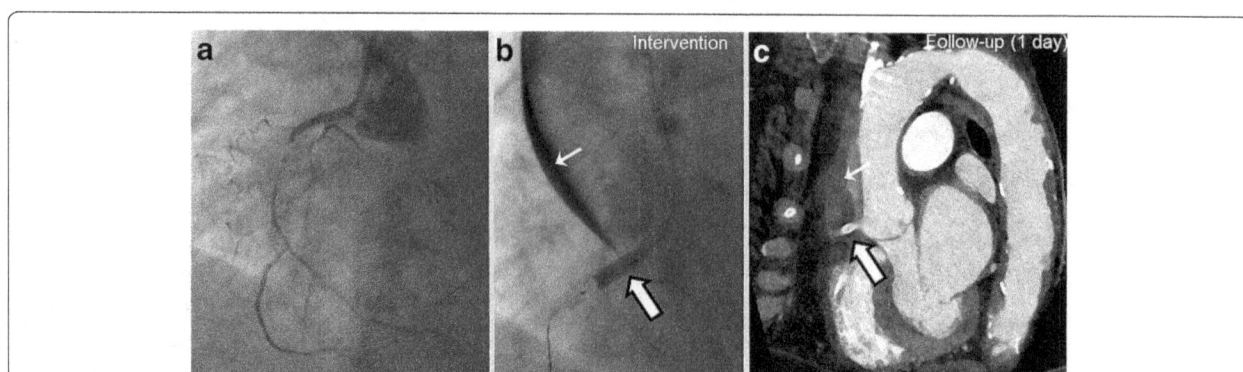

Fig. 5 Dunning Dissection type III. **a** Angiographic findings of a patient initially admitted with CCS class II and complex coronary artery disease (SYNTAX-II-Score 36.4%) undergoing PCI of a CTO of the RCA. **b** The lesion was successfully treated with an aorto-ostial PCI/DES implantation (Integrity 3.5/12 mm) overlapping into the ascending aorta (broad arrow). **c** cCTA at day 1 confirms the extensive dissection from the RCA ostium up to the ascending aorta (slim arrow). PCI, percutaneous coronary intervention; RCA, right coronary artery

ostium of the RCA (88%), but in their case series the majority of the DD occurred during conventional coronary angiography (62.5%) [16].

As DD are rare and need immediate treatment, thus randomized multicenter clinical trials are missing and even in the future will be difficult to realize. This single center experience emphasizes the use of CTAs at follow-up in order to control the exact extension of the dissection as soon as the patient is hemodynamically stable, before discharge and after a follow-up period of 3 to 6 months.

Conclusions

DD are rare but serious complications of coronary interventions, while the extent of the dissection is defined at angiography. This study demonstrates that cCTA plays a valuable role for detection and follow-up of patients with DD. While using high-resolution scanners, cCTA can be helpful to provide precious information about the origin and extent of the dissection and is therefore a helpful tool for non-invasive follow-up.

Abbreviations

CABG: coronary artery bypass grafting; cCTA: coronary computed tomography angiography; CTO: chronic total occlusion; DD: Dunning dissections; DES: drug eluting stents; F: French; IQR: interquartile ranges; IVUS: intravascular ultrasound; LAD: left anterior descending; LMT: left main trunk; LVEF: left ventricular ejection fraction; PCI: percutaneous coronary interventions; RCA: right coronary artery; SD: standard deviation

Acknowledgements

We acknowledge financial support by Deutsche Forschungsgemeinschaft and Ruprecht-Karls-Universität Heidelberg within the funding programme Open Access Publishing.

Funding

None.

Authors' contributions

SB 1) has made substantial contributions to conception and design, or acquisition of data, or analysis and interpretation of data; 2) has been involved in drafting the manuscript or revising it critically for important intellectual content; and 3) has given final approval of the version to be published. MBe (corresponding author) 1) has made substantial contributions to conception and design, or acquisition of data, or analysis and interpretation of data; 2) has been involved in drafting the manuscript or revising it critically for important intellectual content; and 3) has given final approval of the version to be published. BS 1) has made substantial contributions to acquisition of data; 2) has been involved in drafting the manuscript; and 3) has given final approval of the version to be published. TB 1) has been involved in revising the manuscript critically for important intellectual content; and 3) has given final approval of the version to be published. IEB 1) has been involved in revising it critically for important intellectual content; and 2) has given final approval of the version to be published. CF 1) has made substantial contributions to acquisition of data; 2) has been involved in drafting the manuscript or revising it critically for important intellectual content; and 3) has given final approval of the version to be published. UA 1) has been involved in revising it critically (linguistic revision) for important intellectual content; and 2) has given final approval of the version to be published. DL 1) has been involved in revising it critically for important intellectual content; and 2) has given final approval of the

version to be published. KM 1) has made substantial contributions to conception and design analysis and interpretation of data; 2) has been involved in revising it critically for important intellectual content; and 3) has given final approval of the version to be published. TH 1) has made substantial contributions to analysis of data; 2) has been involved in revising it critically for important intellectual content; and 3) has given final approval of the version to be published. SOS 1) has been involved in revising it critically for important intellectual content; and 2) has given final approval of the version to be published. MB 1) has made substantial contributions to conception and design; 2) has been involved in revising it critically for important intellectual content; and 3) has given final approval of the version to be published. IA 1) has made substantial contributions to conception and design, or acquisition of data, or analysis and interpretation of data; 2) has been involved in drafting the manuscript or revising it critically for important intellectual content; and 3) has given final approval of the version to be published.

Competing interests

The authors declare that they have no competing interests.

Author details

[1]First Department of Medicine, University Medical Centre Mannheim, Theodor-Kutzer-Ufer 1-3, 68167 Mannheim, Germany. [2]Division of Cardiology and Angiology II, University Heart Center Freiburg-Bad Krozingen, Bad Krozingen, Germany. [3]Institute of Clinical Radiology and Nuclear Medicine, University Medical Center Mannheim, Medical Faculty Mannheim, Heidelberg University, Mannheim, Germany.

References

1. Perez-Castellano N, et al. Dissection of the aortic sinus of Valsalva complicating coronary catheterization: cause, mechanism, evolution, and management. Catheter Cardiovasc Diagn. 1998;43(3):273–9.
2. Dunning DW, et al. Iatrogenic coronary artery dissections extending into and involving the aortic root. Catheter Cardiovasc Interv. 2000;51(4):387–93.
3. Carstensen S, Ward MR. Iatrogenic aortocoronary dissection: the case for immediate aortoostial stenting. Heart Lung Circ. 2008;17(4):325–9.
4. Gomez-Moreno S, et al. Iatrogenic dissection of the ascending aorta following heart catheterisation: incidence, management and outcome. EuroIntervention. 2006;2(2):197–202.
5. Authors/Task Force, m, et al. ESC/EACTS guidelines on myocardial revascularization: the task force on myocardial revascularization of the European Society of Cardiology (ESC) and the European Association for Cardio-Thoracic Surgery (EACTS)developed with the special contribution of the European Association of Percutaneous Cardiovascular Interventions (EAPCI). Eur Heart J. 2014;35(37):2541–619.
6. Behan MW, et al. Coronary bifurcation lesions treated with simple or complex stenting: 5-year survival from patient-level pooled analysis of the Nordic bifurcation study and the British bifurcation coronary study. Eur Heart J. 2016;37(24):1923–8.
7. Shorrock D, et al. Frequency and outcomes of aortocoronary dissection during percutaneous coronary intervention of chronic total occlusions: a case series and systematic review of the literature. Catheter Cardiovasc Interv. 2014;84(4):670–5.
8. Yip HK, et al. Unusual complication of retrograde dissection to the coronary sinus of valsalva during percutaneous revascularization: a single-center experience and literature review. Chest. 2001;119(2):493–501.
9. Santos M, et al. Aortocoronary dissection complicating percutaneous angioplasty. Rev Port Cardiol. 2011;30(9):745–7.
10. Boyle AJ, et al. Catheter-induced coronary artery dissection: risk factors, prevention and management. J Invasive Cardiol. 2006;18(10):500–3.
11. Abdou SM, Wu CJ. Treatment of aortocoronary dissection complicating anomalous origin right coronary artery and chronic total intervention with intravascular ultrasound guided stenting. Catheter Cardiovasc Interv. 2011; 78(6):914–9.
12. Oda H, et al. Aortocoronary dissection resolved by coronary stenting guided by intracoronary ultrasound. Circ J. 2004;68(4):389–91.

23

Apparent diffusion coefficient as an effective index for the therapeutic efficiency of brain chemoradiotherapy for brain metastases from lung cancer

Kai Liu, Zenglin Ma[*] and Lili Feng

Abstract

Background: The potential of apparent diffusion coefficient (ADC) value alteration before and after chemoradiotherapy as a potential monitor for therapeutic efficiency of treatment for brain metastases from lung cancer were discussed.

Method: Thirty lung cancer patients with brain metastases, conventional magnetic resonance imaging (MRI) examination and diffusion weighted imaging (DWI) were performed one week before chemoradiotherapy and after one treatment cycle and two treatment cycles. 43 tumor lesions were divided into effective group and invalid group according to the changes of the tumor size. The differences in ADC values at different time points before and after treatment in each treatment group were analyzed.

Result: The maximum diameter of the tumor was no difference after one treatment cycle, but decreased after two treatment cycles. ADC values significantly increased after both one and two treatment cycles. In effective group, the ADC values were significantly increased after one and two treatment cycles. While, there are no difference in invalid group after one treatment cycle but decreased after two treatment cycles. ΔADC values in effective group after one and two treatment cycles were both significantly higher than those in the invalid group. ROC curve analysis then revealed that the area under the curve (AUC) of ΔADC after one treatment was 0.872.

Conclusion: ADC values in brain metastases from lung cancer can help monitor and dynamically observe the therapeutic efficiency of whole brain chemoradiotherapy.

Keywords: Apparent diffusion coefficient (ADC), Magnetic resonance imaging (MRI), Brain metastases, Therapeutic efficiency

Background

Brain metastases from are an increasingly common problem with an incidence ten times that of primary brain tumors and the diagnosis is often made by general radiologists [1, 2]. Cumulative incidence of brain metastases is noted to be particularly high for patients with locally advanced lung cancer and HER2 positive metastatic breast cancer, with figures of up to 30–60% reported [3–5].

Traditionally, magnetic resonance imaging (MRI) has been regarded as a gold standard for detection of brain metastases and used for assessing the site and number of metastases, planning for surgery or radiosurgery and assessing the response to therapy [6, 7]. However, the differentiation of high-grade gliomas from brain metastases represents a common differential diagnosis problem since both tumors may display similar imaging characteristics and contrast enhancement patters on conventional MRI [8]. Besides, it is not universally given to cancer patients who lack neurological symptoms at presentation. Even in patients with a normal MRI brain scan at diagnosis and limited-stage small cell lung cancer, a recent study found that 32.5% subsequently developed MRI evidence of brain metastases by the end of chemotherapy, before receiving prophylactic cranial irradiation [5]. In the course of radiotherapy for brain

* Correspondence: zenglinma@163.com
Department of Radiology, The Third Affiliated Hospital of Beijing University of Chinese Medicine, No. 51 Xiaoguan Street, Andingmenwai, Chaoyang District, Beijing, People's Republic of China

metastases from lung cancer, the changes of the tumor size exist significantly behind changes in biological and molecular levels. Thus, developing early biological indicators to measure radiotherapy efficacy has become an urgent need.

Newer MRI techniques have been applied to help diagnosis and prognosis. Diffusion-weighted magnetic resonance (MR) imaging detects the water mobility to reflect the morphologic and physiologic changes in tissues which was wildly applied in chest tumors characterization [9, 10]. tThe apparent diffusion coefficient (ADC) of the lesion but these readings have more recently been suggested to have some prognostic value as well as diagnostic in brain metastases cancers [11, 12]. An inverse relationship was observed between ADC values and tumor cellularity [8]. Previous studies had shown that ADC values can be used in differentiating between certain types of cerebral tumors [13–15]. However, the efficiency of the ADC values as an index of brain metastases, and its advantages over MRI remain controversial.

In the present study, we attempted to analyze the dynamic trends of maximal tumor diameter and ADC values at different time points after chemotherapy and whole-brain radiotherapy in patients with brain metastasis from lung cancer, to predict and to monitor the efficacy of ΔADC values as an index for brain metastasis from lung cancer after brain radiation therapy.

Methods

Patients

Institutional review board approval was obtained for this study. All the subjects were informed of the contents of the test and signed the informed consent voluntarily. From October 2013 to August 2016, 30 patients diagnosed with brain metastasis from lung cancer by pathology or clinical follow-up and clinical imaging tests were involved in the present study. The clinical characteristics of the 30 patients were shown in Table 1.

Case inclusion criteria: 1. Patients who were pathologically diagnosed with brain metastases from lung cancer, no limitation of gender and ethnicity; 2. Patients who were receiving radiotherapy and chemotherapy for the first time to ensure the uniformity of the initial state; 3. Patients with at least one measurable lesion (necrosis and cystic lesions not included) in the parenchyma of the brain, lesion diameter > 10 mm.

Case exclusion criteria: 1. Patients who could not complete the entire treatment plan, the radiochemotherapy and Chinese medicine treatment were terminated in advance; 2. Patients who received pacemaker implantation, coronary intervention, and Coronary Artery Bypass Grafting (CABG), thus contraindicated to MRI; 3. Patients who were unable to cooperate with MRI examinations.

Table 1 The clinical characteristics of enrolled patients

Clinical characteristics	Case number
Lesion number	43
Mean age	63.6 (45–85)
Gender	Female 18: Male 12
Pathological type	
Squamous carcinoma	12
Adenocarcinoma	11
Small cell lung cancer	3
Undifferentiated carcinoma	4
Location of brain metastasis	
Frontal lobe	9
Parietal lobe	11
Occipital lobe	12
Basal ganglia	4
Opisthencephalon	4
Temporal lobe	2
Brainstem	1

Treatment protocols

Chemotherapy: oral administration of drugs that can pass through the blood-brain barrier, such as CCNU or me-CCNU, simultaneously supplemented by intramuscular injection of dexamethasone (MTX) once a week, 4 times as a treatment course, and the dehydration agent. Systemic chemotherapy is based on the patient's condition, the primary lesion and the cellular type of the cancer: for adenocarcinoma, CMF regimen (cyclophosphamide (CTX), MTX, fluorouracil (5-FU)) or CAF regimen (CTX, M (ADM), 5-FU] was used; for squamous carcinoma, DAV regimen (cisplatin (DDP), ADM, vincristine (VCR)) was used; for undifferentiated cancer, CVA regimen (CTX, VCR, ADM) was used. The above treatment was conducted once every 4 weeks, each time as a treatment cycle. Radiotherapy: Cobalt-60 bilateral whole brain irradiation was conducted, the dosage was 4000-5000Gy, supplemented by mannitol dehydration or hormone therapy to reduce the radiotherapy response. Chinese traditional medicine: dialectical therapy.

Examination protocols

All examinations were performed on Achieva 1.5 T SE MRI systems with an NV-8 combined coil for head and neck (Philips Healthcare, Amsterdam, Netherlands). The examinations were conducted with a gradient set of strength of 33 mT/m and a gradient switching rate of 122 mT/m/ms. Conventional sequences, including T1-weighted images (T1WI), T2-weighted images (T2WI), DWI, FLAIR images, and transverse, coronal and sagittal T1WI contrast-enhanced MRI were obtained. MRI parameters are shown in Table 2.

Table 2 Description of MRI parameters for Philips Achieva 1.5 T SE MRI systems

	T1WI	T2WI	FLAIR	DWI	Contrast-enhanced[*]
TR (ms)	488	4748	8000	3090	156
TE (ms)	15	110	120	102	2.4
TI (ms)	–	–	2200	–	–
Slice thickness (mm)	6	6	6	6	6
Slice gap (mm)	1	1	1	1	1
Slice number of scanning (layers)	18	18	18	18	20
Scanning time (s)	24	42	24	36	22
NSA	1	2	2	1	2
Field of view (mm^2)	230 × 201	230 × 201	230 × 183	230 × 201	230 × 199
Matrix	256 × 256	256 × 256	256 × 512	152 × 256	388 × 640

[*]The Contrast-enhanced scan was performed by rapid bolus injection of gadopentate glucosamine (Gd-DTPA) at a dose of 0.1 mmol/kg through the cubital vein at a flow rate of 2.5 ml/s. After bolus injection, 20 mL of saline was intravenously injected. B-values for DWI are 0 s/mm^2 and 1000 s/mm^2

Image and data processing

All measurements were performed on a Philips station. ADC maps were generated from the DWI sequence using Philips station. Image interpretation was done by two radiologists (five years of experience). The investigators were unaware of the patients' clinical and pathologic information.

The maximum diameter of the lesion was measured on the enhanced images combined with T2WI, T1WI, DWI and ADC images. In the tumor parenchyma region, the region of interest (ROI) was manually selected on the ADC map corresponding to the area of marked enhancement in the contrast-enhanced scan sequence. The ROI was placed in the lesion to select the region significantly enhanced in the contrast-enhanced scan sequence according to T1WI. Adjacent large blood vessels, cystic necrosis, and bleeding areas were avoided. Each lesion was measured three times, and ADC values were the average of 3 measurements. The cystic area after treatment should be included. ADC measurements were performed one week before comprehensive treatment, after one treatment cycle and two treatment cycles. The rates of ADC changes in effective and ineffective groups after one treatment cycle were calculated: ΔADC = (post-treatment ADC-pre-treatment ADC)/pre-treatment ADC × 100%. To measure the maximum diameter of the lesion, we measured the maximum cross-section of the lesion in the contrast-enhanced MRI and expressed it as a mean value of three measurements. If there were controversies between investigators, an average value for ADC was chosen by consensus.

RECIST

Patients with brain metastases underwent conventional MRI and contrast-enhanced MRI examinations at 1 week before treatment, one treatment cycle and two treatment cycles later. Treatment protocols are listed below. The

layer with the maximum tumor diameter was selected; the maximum diameter or the maximum diameter summation of the tumor was measured and used as a grouping standard of the patients. Then the maximum diameters of the tumors 1 week before treatment and two treatment cycles later were compared. According to RECIST criteria, the evaluation of the target lesion is:

Complete remission (CR): the disappearance of almost all target lesions.

Partial remission (PR): the lesions were significantly reduced, and the summation of the maximum baseline diameter was reduced by ≥30%.

Progression (PD): the summation of the maximum baseline diameter increased by ≥20% or new lesions appeared.

Stable (SD): the summation of the maximum baseline diameter reduced but did not reach PR or increased but did not reach PD.

The lesions that met with the CR and PR criteria were identified as effective groups, and the lesions that met the SD and PD criteria were classified as invalid groups.

Statistical analysis

The data was analyzed by SPSS20.0 software. The measurement data were expressed as mean ± standard deviation (mean ± S.D.). Normal distribution and homogeneity of variance tests were performed on different groups, and the data were in normal distribution. Paired t-test was used for comparison between paired samples. The ADC values pre-treatment and one treatment cycle after between the ineffective group and the effective group were compared using the independent sample t-test. The receiver operating characteristic (ROC) curve analysis was performed on the degree of change in the average ADC values of the patients treated for one cycle. $P < 0.05$ indicates that the difference was statistically significant.

Result

ADC values indicate the tumor progression more sensitively than MRI in brain metastases from lung cancer

The maximum diameters of tumors and ADC values of brain metastases from lung cancer patients one week before treatment, one treatment cycle and two treatment cycles later were examined. The results showed that the maximum diameter of the tumor was no difference after one treatment cycle ($p = 0.092$); the maximum diameter of the tumor was significantly decreased after two treatment cycles ($p < 0.001$) (Fig. 1a, Table 3). However, ADC values increased significantly after one and two treatments cycles (Fig. 1b, Table 3), suggesting that ADC values indicate tumor progression more sensitively than the maximum diameters of tumors, especially after one treatment cycle.

ΔADC is a potential monitor of therapeutic efficacy on brain metastases from lung cancer

Tumor lesions from patients were divided into two groups, effective group ($n = 22$) and invalid group (21), according to RECIST standard (details were shown in Fig. 2), and the ADC was examined. As Table 4 shown, before and after treatment cycles, the ADC values were no statistical difference between the effective group and invalid group. In the effective group, the ADC values were significantly increased after one and two treatment cycles. In the invalid group, the ADC values are not different after one treatment cycle, but decreased after two treatment cycles.

Then, ΔADC was calculated. As Table 5 shown, after one and two treatment cycles, ΔADC values in effective

group were significantly higher than those in the invalid group. ROC curve analysis then revealed that the area under the curve (AUC) of ΔADC after one treatment cycle was 0.872 (sensitivity = 81.8%, specificity = 85.7%, 95% CI: 0.805–0.992) (Fig. 3). These data indicating the potential of ΔADC as a novel index for brain metastasis progression and might help with monitoring therapeutic efficacy and distinguishing effective and invalid groups.

Discussion

Brain metastases from lung cancer are common intracranial tumors in adults and the incidence rate is about 20% [16]. With the continuous development of clinical examination methods, the increase in the incidence of lung cancer, and the prolongation of survival after radiotherapy and chemotherapy, the incidence of brain metastases from lung cancer has increased. In the past decades, the whole brain radiation therapy is still the standard treatment for brain metastasis from lung cancer [16], especially for lung cancer with multiple brain metastases.

Nowadays, clinicians commonly evaluate the therapeutic effect of brain metastasis from lung cancer by comparing the reduction of tumor size before and after treatment via CT or MRI [17]. Evaluating the therapeutic effect is critical to the further treatment of the patient. In the process of tumor treatment, establishing a method that can evaluate the treatment effect early and objectively becomes a considerable challenge. However, during the course of tumor treatment, the changes of tumor size exist significantly behind the changes in the biological and molecular levels [18, 19]. Due to the different components of the tumor, it is unlikely that different types of tumors will

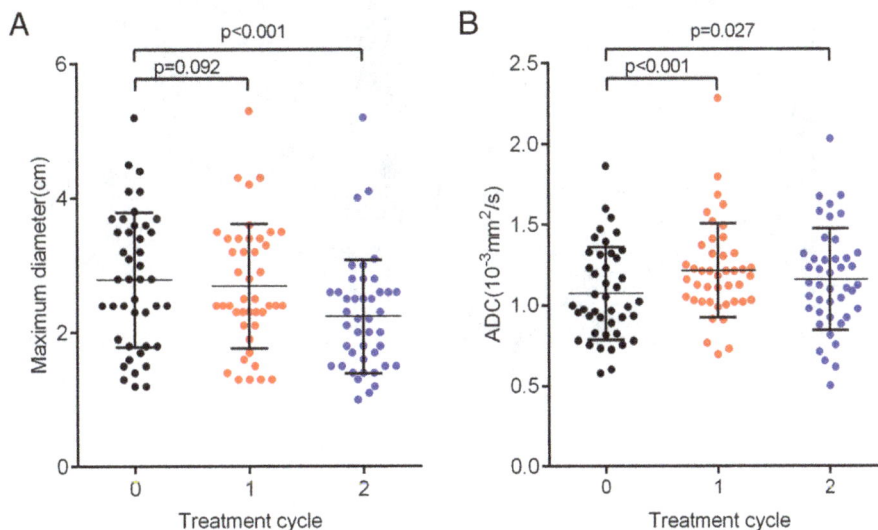

Fig. 1 ADC values indicate the tumor progression more sensitively than MRI (**a**) The maximum diameters of tumors for brain metastases from lung cancer before and after treatments. **b** ADC values of brain metastases from lung cancer before and after treatments. $n = 43$, $p < 0.05$ statistical significance compared to one week before treatment

Table 3 The maximum diameters of tumors and ADC values for brain metastases from lung cancer ($n = 43$)

Treatment	The maximum diameters of tumors (cm)	ADC values (10^{-3} mm^2/s)
One week before treatment	2.78 ± 0.15	1.07 ± 0.29
One treatment cycle	2.69 ± 0.14	1.21 ± 0.29**
Two treatment cycles	2.24 ± 0.13**	1.16 ± 0.32*

*$p < 0.05$, **$p < 0.01$, compared to one week before treatment

respond to the same treatment [20]. Unreasonable treatment may even accelerate the growth of tumors and causes tumor resistance. Developing the early measurement of biological indicators of therapeutic effectiveness has become an urgent need which can stop ineffective treatment in an early stage and reduce unnecessary toxicity and medical expenses.

Several imaging modalities were wildly applied in cancer diagnosis and assessment of therapy outcome. The tumor vascular physiology and hemodynamics could be measured by perfusion CT (PCT). The PCT parameters were considered as independent predictor of radiation therapy failure in head and neck cancer [21]. Diffusion tensor imaging (DTI) is valuable in diagnosing of idiopathic intracranial hypertension, differentiating gliomas grades and and residual head and neck cancer from post-radiation changes [22–24]. Moreover, combination with arterial spin labeling (ASL) perfusion increased the accuracy of MRI in

distinguishing residual/recurrent gliomas from postradiation change [25]. DWI has changed the traditional diagnostic imaging model based on the anatomy and structural changes and led imaging diagnostics to a microscopic molecular level. It is currently the only non-invasive detection of water molecules free diffusion movement in vivo. The ADC value of the water molecules is determined by the viscosity of the molecules, the permeability of the cell membrane, the direction of the tissue, and the structure of the cells that impede the movement of the water molecules [26, 27]. Therefore, the ADC values can distinguish tumor cells from non-cellular regions, cystic regions from solid regions, and the critical issues at the cellular level during tumor therapy. Recently, both animal and cell models have demonstrated that ADC values are of great importance in prognosis and the early monitoring of tumor therapeutic efficiency [28–30]. For example, lower ADC values were associated with greater tumor size and highly aggressive in cerebral cancers [31]. In addition, there are few human studies in this area, including gliomas [32], breast tumors [33], hepatic tumors [34], and rectal tumors [35], and all obtained the similar results.

Previous studies revealed that a higher ADC mean showed a longer overall survival regardless of adjuvant therapies in non-small cell lung cancer cerebral metastasis [36]. In the present study, we revealed that the significant increase of ADC values was appeared after one treatment cycle, which was earlier than the presence of

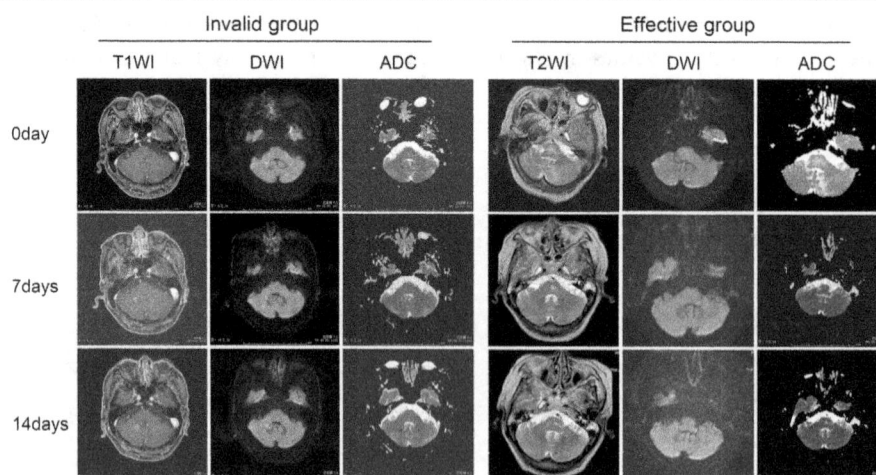

Fig. 2 Two cases were shown below for example the group division: Case 1: Pathologically diagnosed as brain metastases from right lung adenocarcinoma. The maximum diameter of the lesion was 10 mm one week before treatment and the ADC value was 0.653×10^{-3} mm^2/s; the maximum diameter of the lesion was 12 mm and the ADC value was 0.733×10^{-3} mm^2/s after one treatment cycle; the maximum diameter of the lesion was 14 mm and the ADC value was 0.706×10^{-3} mm^2/s after two treatment cycles. According to RECIST criteria, the patient belonged to the invalid group. Case 2: pathologically diagnosed as brain metastases from lung cancer. The lesions on the right occipital lobe were nodular with slightly higher signal intensity on T2WI, slightly lower signal intensity on T1WI, high signal intensity on DWI, and obviously enhanced lesions on contrast-enhanced T1WI. The maximum diameter was 17 mm before treatment and the ADC value was 0.759×10^{-3} mm^2/s; after one treatment cycle, the maximum diameter of the lesion was reduced to about 16 mm, and the ADC value was 1.05×10^{-3} mm^2/s; after two treatment cycles, the enhanced part of the lesion was obviously reduced, with a diameter of 3 mm, and the ADC value was 1.10×10^{-3} mm^2/s, suggesting that the treatment was effective. According to RECIST criteria, this patient belongs to the effective group.

Table 4 The change of ADC values after one and two treatment cycles in effective group and invalid group

Treatment	ADC values of effective group (10^{-3} mm^2/s)	ADC values of invalid group (10^{-3} mm^2/s)
One week before treatment	0.97 ± 0.05	1.17 ± 0.06
One treatment cycle	1.21 ± 0.04**	1.20 ± 0.08
Two treatment cycles	1.20 ± 0.05**	1.10 ± 0.08*

*$p < 0.05$, **$p < 0.01$, compared to before treatment, no difference of ADC value between effective group and invalid group under different treatment cycles

tumor maximum diameter alterations (after two treatment cycles). Effective anti-tumor therapy results in necrosis of tumor cells, reduced cell density, the disappearance of cell membrane integrity, increased extracellular space, and thus increased ADC values which can be sensitively detected by DWI [37]. Therefore, by observing the movement of water molecules in the tumor, the ADC value can be used as an early indicator to evaluate the effect of tumor treatment in brain metastasis from lung cancer.

Tumors with higher ADC values often contain more necrotic tissue and/or damaged cell membranes, with a poorer blood perfusion, and are relatively insensitive to radiotherapy [38], indicating that pre-radiotherapy ADC values can predict radiotherapy effects to a certain extent and can be used by clinicians to assess the sensitivity of tumors before radiotherapy. However, in the present study, no statistical difference was noted between effective group ADC values and invalid group ADC values before treatment cycle. In addition, we demonstrated that the ΔADC values were significantly higher in effective group than those in the invalid group. The AUC of ΔADC is 0.898 with 81.8% sensitivity and 85.7% specificity. These results demonstrated that ΔADC values have a potential to monitor therapeutic efficacy and distinguish chemoradiotherpy sensitive and insensitive brain metastasis from lung cancer.

There are a few limitations of this study. First, the small number of patients might limit the statistical results of the cases. Second, there is lack of long time follow-up of patients after treatment. The correlation of ADC with the overall survival in patients with brain metastasis from lung cancer is needed in the further studies.

Table 5 Comparison of ΔADC values in effective group and invalid group

Treatment	ΔADC values of effective group (%)	ΔADC values of invalid group (%)
One treatment cycle	28.23 ± 3.97*	2.5 ± 2.27
Two treatment cycle	27.56 ± 5.16*	−7.44 ± 2.62

*$p < 0.05$, compared to invalid group

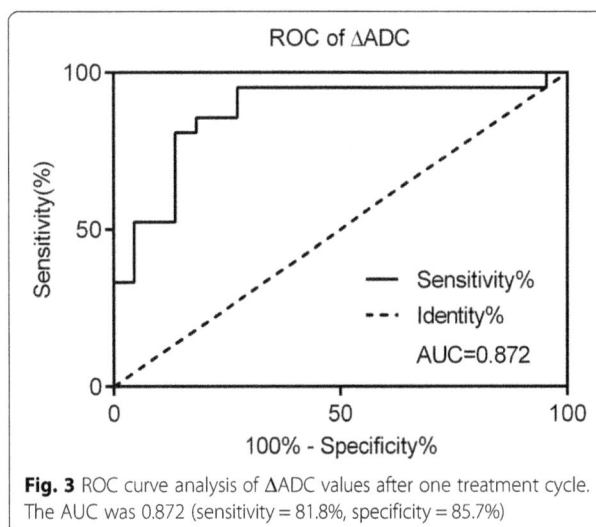

Fig. 3 ROC curve analysis of ΔADC values after one treatment cycle. The AUC was 0.872 (sensitivity = 81.8%, specificity = 85.7%)

Conclusions

In summary, ADC value examination during the chemoraidotherapy treatment cycles can help early monitoring and dynamic observation of therapeutic efficacy in brain metastases from lung cancer. It is possible for clinicians to quickly, accurately and non-invasively predict and monitor the responses of tumors before and during treatment, to stop ineffective treatment early and to reduce unnecessary toxicity and medical expenses.

Abbreviations
ADC: Apparent diffusion coefficient; ASL: Arterial spin labeling; AUC: The area under the curve; CABG: Coronary Artery Bypass Grafting; CR: Complete remission; DTI: Diffusion tensor imaging; DWI: Diffusion weighted imaging; PCT: Perfusion CT; PR: Partial remission; ROC: The receiver operating characteristic; T1WI: T1-weighted images; T2WI: T2-weighted images

Funding
The study was supported by Independent topic selection of Beijing University of Chinese Medicine in 2016 (Young and Middle-aged Teachers Project),No. 2016-JYB-JSMS-066.

Authors' contributions
KL the mainly writer of the article, conceived and designed the experiments. LF Data analysis and statistical analysis. ZM Experimental guidance, conceived and designed the experiments, data verification. All authors have read and approved the manuscript.

Competing interests
The authors declare that they have no competing interest.

References

1. Jenkinson MD, Haylock B, Shenoy A, Husband D, Javadpour M. Management of cerebral metastasis: evidence-based approach for surgery, stereotactic radiosurgery and radiotherapy. Eur J Cancer. 2011;47(5):649–55.

2. Nussbaum ES, Djalilian HR, Cho KH, Hall WA. Brain metastases. Histology, multiplicity, surgery, and survival. Cancer. 1996;78(8):1781–8.

3. Auperin A, Arriagada R, Pignon JP, Le Pechoux C, Gregor A, Stephens RJ, Kristjansen PE, Johnson BE, Ueoka H, Wagner H, et al. Prophylactic cranial irradiation for patients with small-cell lung cancer in complete remission. Prophylactic cranial irradiation overview collaborative group. N Engl J Med. 1999;341(7):476–84.

4. Gore EM, Bae K, Wong SJ, Sun A, Bonner JA, Schild SE, Gaspar LE, Bogart JA, Werner-Wasik M, Choy H. Phase III comparison of prophylactic cranial irradiation versus observation in patients with locally advanced non-small-cell lung cancer: primary analysis of radiation therapy oncology group study RTOG 0214. J Clin Oncol. 2011;29(3):272–8.

5. Brufsky AM, Mayer M, Rugo HS, Kaufman PA, Tan-Chiu E, Tripathy D, Tudor IC, Wang LI, Brammer MG, Shing M, et al. Central nervous system metastases in patients with HER2-positive metastatic breast cancer: incidence, treatment, and survival in patients from registHER. Clin Cancer Res. 2011;17(14):4834–43.

6. Fink KR, Fink JR. Imaging of brain metastases. Surg Neurol Int. 2013;4(Suppl 4):S209–19.

7. Young RJ, Sills AK, Brem S, Knopp EA: Neuroimaging of metastatic brain disease. Neurosurgery 2005, 57(5 Suppl):S10–S23; discusssion S11–14.

8. Chen L, Liu M, Bao J, Xia Y, Zhang J, Zhang L, Huang X, Wang J. The correlation between apparent diffusion coefficient and tumor cellularity in patients: a meta-analysis. PLoS One. 2013;8(11):e79008.

9. Razek AA. Diffusion magnetic resonance imaging of chest tumors. Cancer Imaging. 2012;12(3):452.

10. Abdel Razek AA, Gaballa G, Denewer A, Tawakol I. Diffusion weighted MR imaging of the breast. Acad Radiol. 2010;17(3):382–6.

11. Kim YJ, Chang KH, Song IC, Kim HD, Seong SO, Kim YH, Han MH. Brain abscess and necrotic or cystic brain tumor: discrimination with signal intensity on diffusion-weighted MR imaging. AJR Am J Roentgenol. 1998; 171(6):1487–90.

12. Berghoff AS, Spanberger T, Ilhan-Mutlu A, Magerle M, Hutterer M, Woehrer A, Hackl M, Widhalm G, Dieckmann K, Marosi C, et al. Preoperative diffusion-weighted imaging of single brain metastases correlates with patient survival times. PLoS One. 2013;8(2):e55464.

13. Surov A, Ginat DT, Sanverdi E, Lim CC, Hakyemez B, Yogi A, Cabada T, Wienke A. Use of diffusion weighted imaging in differentiating between Maligant and benign Meningiomas. A multicenter analysis. World Neurosurg. 2016;88:598–602.

14. Kono K, Inoue Y, Nakayama K, Shakudo M, Morino M, Ohata K, Wakasa K, Yamada R. The role of diffusion-weighted imaging in patients with brain tumors. AJNR Am J Neuroradiol. 2001;22(6):1081–8.

15. Svolos P, Tsolaki E, Kapsalaki E, Theodorou K, Fountas K, Fezoulidis I, Tsougos I. Investigating brain tumor differentiation with diffusion and perfusion metrics at 3T MRI using pattern recognition techniques. Magn Reson Imaging. 2013;31(9):1567–77.

16. Kawabe T, Phi JH, Yamamoto M, Kim DG, Barfod BE, Urakawa Y. Treatment of brain metastasis from lung cancer. Prog Neurol Surg. 2012;25:148–55.

17. Binder D, Temmesfeld-Wollbruck B, Wurm R, Woiciechowsky C, Schaper C, Schurmann D, Suttorp N, Beinert T. brain metastases of lung cancer. Dtsch Med Wochenschr. 2006;131(4):165–71.

18. Pickles MD, Gibbs P, Lowry M, Turnbull LW. Diffusion changes precede size reduction in neoadjuvant treatment of breast cancer. Magn Reson Imaging. 2006;24(7):843–7.

19. Koh DM, Padhani AR. Diffusion-weighted MRI: a new functional clinical technique for tumour imaging. Br J Radiol. 2006;79(944):633–5.

20. Heppner GH, Miller FR. The cellular basis of tumor progression. Int Rev Cytol. 1998;177:1–56.

21. Razek AA, Tawfik AM, Elsorogy LG, Soliman NY. Perfusion CT of head and neck cancer. Eur J Radiol. 2014;83(3):537–44.

22. El-Serougy L, Abdel Razek AA, Ezzat A, Eldawoody H, El-Morsy A. Assessment of diffusion tensor imaging metrics in differentiating low-grade from high-grade gliomas. Neuroradiol J. 2016;29(5):400.

23. Razek AAKA, Batouty N, Fathy W, Bassiouny R. Diffusion tensor imaging of the optic disc in idiopathic intracranial hypertension. Neuroradiology. 2018:1–8.

24. Razek AAKA. Diffusion tensor imaging in differentiation of residual head and neck squamous cell carcinoma from post-radiation changes. Magn Reson Imaging. 2018.

25. Razek AAKA, El-Serougy L, Abdelsalam M, Gaballa G, Talaat M. Differentiation of residual/recurrent gliomas from postradiation necrosis with arterial spin labeling and diffusion tensor magnetic resonance imaging-derived metrics. Neuroradiology. 2018;60(2):169–77.

26. Razek AAKA. Routine and advanced diffusion imaging modules of the salivary glands. Neuroimaging Clin N Am. 2018;28(2):245–54.

27. Kauppinen RA. Monitoring cytotoxic tumour treatment response by diffusion magnetic resonance imaging and proton spectroscopy. NMR Biomed. 2002;15(1):6–17.

28. Moffat BA, Hall DE, Stojanovska J, McConville PJ, Moody JB, Chenevert TL, Rehemtulla A, Ross BD. Diffusion imaging for evaluation of tumor therapies in preclinical animal models. MAGMA. 2004;17(3–6):249–59.

29. Jennings D, Hatton BN, Guo J, Galons JP, Trouard TP, Raghunand N, Marshall J, Gillies RJ. Early response of prostate carcinoma xenografts to docetaxel chemotherapy monitored with diffusion MRI. Neoplasia. 2002;4(3):255–62.

30. Galons JP, Altbach MI, Paine-Murrieta GD, Taylor CW, Gillies RJ. Early increases in breast tumor xenograft water mobility in response to paclitaxel therapy detected by non-invasive diffusion magnetic resonance imaging. Neoplasia. 1999;1(2):113–7.

31. Razek AA, Nada N. Correlation of choline/Creatine and apparent diffusion coefficient values with the prognostic parameters of head and neck squamous cell carcinoma. NMR Biomed. 2016;29(4):483–9.

32. Hamstra DA, Chenevert TL, Moffat BA, Johnson TD, Meyer CR, Mukherji SK, Quint DJ, Gebarski SS, Fan X, Tsien CI, et al. Evaluation of the functional diffusion map as an early biomarker of time-to-progression and overall survival in high-grade glioma. Proc Natl Acad Sci U S A. 2005;102(46):16759–64.

33. Buijs M, Kamel IR, Vossen JA, Georgiades CS, Hong K, Geschwind JF. Assessment of metastatic breast cancer response to chemoembolization with contrast agent enhanced and diffusion-weighted MR imaging. J Vasc Interv Radiol. 2007;18(8):957–63.

34. Cui Y, Zhang XP, Sun YS, Tang L, Shen L. Apparent diffusion coefficient: potential imaging biomarker for prediction and early detection of response to chemotherapy in hepatic metastases. Radiology. 2008;248(3):894–900.

35. DeVries AF, Kremser C, Hein PA, Griebel J, Krezcy A, Ofner D, Pfeiffer KP, Lukas P, Judmaier W. Tumor microcirculation and diffusion predict therapy outcome for primary rectal carcinoma. Int J Radiat Oncol Biol Phys. 2003; 56(4):958–65.

36. Zakaria R, Das K, Radon M, Bhojak M, Rudland PR, Sluming V, Jenkinson MD. Diffusion-weighted MRI characteristics of the cerebral metastasis to brain boundary predicts patient outcomes. BMC Med Imaging. 2014; 14(1):26.

37. Lee KC, Moffat BA, Schott AF, Layman R, Ellingworth S, Juliar R, Khan AP, Helvie M, Meyer CR, Chenevert TL, et al. Prospective early response imaging biomarker for neoadjuvant breast cancer chemotherapy. Clin Cancer Res. 2007;13(2 Pt 1):443–50.

38. Koh DM, Scurr E, Collins D, Kanber B, Norman A, Leach MO, Husband JE. Predicting response of colorectal hepatic metastasis: value of pretreatment apparent diffusion coefficients. AJR Am J Roentgenol. 2007;188(4):1001–8.

24

Significance of arterial spin labeling perfusion and susceptibility weighted imaging changes in patients with transient ischemic attack

Inger Havsteen[1]* [iD], Lasse Willer[2], Christian Ovesen[2], Janus Damm Nybing[1], Karen Ægidius[2], Jacob Marstrand[2], Per Meden[2], Sverre Rosenbaum[2], Marie Norsker Folke[2], Hanne Christensen[2] and Anders Christensen[1]

Abstract

Background: In a prospective cohort of patients with transient ischemic attack (TIA), we investigated usefulness and feasibility of arterial spin labeling (ASL) perfusion and susceptibility weighted imaging (SWI) alone and in combination with standard diffusion weighted (DWI) imaging in subacute diagnostic work-up. We investigated rates of ASL and SWI changes and their potential correlation to lasting infarction 8 weeks after ictus.

Methods: Patients with TIA underwent 3T-MRI including DWI, ASL and SWI within 72 h of symptom onset. We defined lasting infarction as presence of 8-week MRI T2-fluid attenuated inversion recovery (FLAIR) hyperintensity or atrophy in the area of initial DWI-lesion.

Results: We included 116 patients. Diffusion and perfusion together identified more patients with ischemia than either alone (59% vs. 40%, $p < 0.0001$). The presence of both diffusion and perfusion lesions had the highest rate of 8-week gliosis scars, 65% ($p < 0.0001$). In white matter, DWI-restriction was the determinant factor for scar development. However, in cortical gray matter half of lesions with perfusion deficit left a scar, while lesions without perfusion change rarely resulted in scars (56% versus 21%, $p = 0.03$). SWI lesions were rare (6%) and a subset of perfusion lesions. SWI-lesions with DWI-lesions were all located in cortical gray matter and showed high scar rate.

Conclusions: ASL perfusion increased ischemia detection in patients with TIA, and was most useful in conjunction with DWI. ASL was fast, robust and useful in a subacute clinical diagnostic setting. SWI had few positive findings and did not add information.

Trial Registration.: http://www.clinicaltrials.gov. Unique Identifier NCT01531946, prospectively registered February 9, 2012.

Keywords: Transient ischemic attack, Cerebral cortex, Arterial spin labeling

Background

Diagnosing a patient with transient ischemic attack (TIA) clinically and evaluating the stroke risk hereafter [1] is a challenge even to experienced stroke neurologists [2]. The addition of noninvasive arterial spin labeling (ASL) perfusion imaging to standard TIA-MRI protocol has been shown to significantly increase the MRI detection [3] of ischemic findings. Increased reliability, [4] accessibility and automatization of post-processing have turned ASL perfusion into a clinically applicable tool [5] in stroke [6–9] and TIA [3, 10–12]. Focal ASL changes in cerebral blood flow (CBF), [13, 14] and arterial transit time, [12, 15, 16] are well described in TIA populations. [3, 10, 14] Based on ASL, lesions are estimated to occur in 35–56% [3, 17] of patients with TIA. In patients with no diffusion lesions, contrast-enhanced dynamic susceptibility contrast (DSC) perfusion imaging detects abnormalities in 16–32% [18, 19] and in 18–46% [3, 17] with both

* Correspondence: Inger.birgitte.havsteen@regionh.dk
[1]Department of Radiology, Copenhagen University Hospital Bispebjerg, Bispebjerg Bakke 23, 2400 Copenhagen, NV, Denmark
Full list of author information is available at the end of the article

DSC and ASL. Also, perfusion changes in diffusion negative patients with clinical TIA are associated with higher rates of new diffusion weighted imaging (DWI) lesions on 3-day follow-up [20, 21]. It is conceivable that originally hypoperfused areas may progress to critical ischemia indicated by new DWI or T2-FLAIR lesions on follow-up [11, 19]. In addition, perfusion changes might also hold predictive power towards risk for de-novo future ischemic events. Consequently, the usefulness of ASL as standard add-on sequence to DWI in a subacute clinical setting without off-line post-processing is an open question.

Findings of asymmetric veins based on T2* and susceptibility weighted imaging (SWI) have also been described in stroke populations and correspond approximately to DSC hypoperfusion areas [22–25] and infarct volume at 72-h follow-up [26]. To our knowledge, SWI and findings in TIA are not described in literature. As the ischemic event in TIA is transitory and presumably less profound than in stroke, SWI may supplement ASL, reflecting venous output from ischemic tissues and indicating the depth of perfusion disturbance.

Optimizing the diagnostic yield of the various sequences included in the TIA work-up protocol is important, as since prolonged scan time decreases the quality of diagnostic evaluation due to the increased incidence of motion artefacts. Motion artefacts increase with increasing scan time, [27, 28] presence of pathology [29] and in acute settings [30].

Consequently, we aimed to investigate if standard DWI plus ASL and SWI compared to DWI alone increases the neuroradiological detection of ischemia in patients with TIA in a subacute clinical setting. In addition, we tested if ASL and SWI added to the prediction of 8-week infarction signs and recurrent cerebrovascular events after TIA.

Methods

We studied a prospective cohort of patients with TIA admitted February 2012 – December 2014 to our comprehensive stroke center. Patients were included after own written informed consent within 72 h of symptom onset. The study was approved by the National Committee of Biomedical Research Ethics (H-1-2011-75, ClinicalTrials.gov Identifier NCT01531946).

Clinical assessment

Senior consultant stroke neurologists clinically evaluated patients. Inclusion criteria were admission with acute focal neurological symptoms believed to be of vascular origin. Exclusion criteria were MRI contraindications, non-TIA discharge diagnosis, and severe comorbidity. We defined TIA as acutely appearing focal neurological deficit with resolution within 24 h. Resolution was defined as National Institute of Health Stroke Scale (NIHSS) 0.

Patients were treated in accordance with European and national guidelines. In this study an ischemic event was defined based on either radiological signs of ischemia or clinical judgment in imaging negative patients.

Recurrent ischemic events were defined as new TIA or stroke diagnosis with clear temporal separation from the index event. We performed long-term follow-up by national electronic patient files.

Study procedures

All patients included in this study underwent the baseline sub-acute MRI during their admission at the stroke unit. The second MRI was obtained after 8 weeks as an outpatient procedure.

Imaging

Imaging was performed at 3T (Siemens Magnetom Verio, Siemens, Erlangen, Germany) with a 32-channel head coil (Siemens, Erlangen, Germany). The baseline imaging protocol consisted of ASL, SWI, and DWI and T2-FLAIR used in our routine TIA protocol. At 8-week follow-up MRI, we scanned only DWI and T2-FLAIR.

We used Siemens' 3D background suppressed ep2d pulsed ASL sequence, TR 2500 ms, TE 11 ms, 192-mm FOV, FA 90, voxel size $3 \times 3 \times 6$ mm^3, TI1 = 700 ms, TI2 = 1800 ms, acceleration factor $R = 2$, acquisition time 4:22 min:s. Perfusion weighted images, motion corrected relative CBF and the intrinsic motion correction series were sent to PACS. The SWI protocol was TR 27 ms, TE 20 ms, 240-mm FOV, FA 15, matrix 243×256, $1.0 \times 0.9 \times 1.5$ mm^3 voxel size, 80 slices, acquisition time 5:18 min:s. ASL and SWI-postprocessing were fully automated as provided by the vendor.

The DWI was single-shot spin-echo diffusion echoplanar imaging with 220-mm FOV, 25 4-mm axial slices with 0-mm gap, b-value 0,1000 s/mm^2 along 3 orthogonal axes; TR 6600 ms, TE 100 ms, acceleration factor R = 2, matrix 192×192. ADC maps were automatically generated as provided by the vendor.

For T2-FLAIR we used 240-mm FOV, 27 4-mm axial slices with 0-mm gap, TR 6500 ms, TE 133 ms, TI 2134 ms, acceleration factor R = 2, matrix 256×256.

Image analysis

In this study we used only the PACS and no external software. Between sequences and MRIs performed at baseline and 8-weeks we identified lesions through their location, describing their position with two orthogonal intrathecal diameters. To provide a standardized description we developed a case report form (CRF) and literature-based image template with defined scoring categories. We validated CRF and template on 50 randomly chosen cases from the cohort with two blinded board-certified consultant neuroradiologists (AC, IH) reading first independently and then jointly establishing final consensus on the reading tools. Hereafter one reader (IH), blinded to clinical information except for the referral information, systematically assessed all baseline and 8-week imaging sequences in accordance with the predefined CRF for ASL perfusion changes, DWI-lesions, SWI asymmetric veins and missing flow voids and lesion visibility on T2-FLAIR (Fig. 1). We scored ASL, SWI and DWI images separately to avoid bias. We categorized lesion location according to vascular territory and as hemispheric left-, right, bilateral or infratentorial. For quality control we calculated intraobserver variability for two CRF readings, except for area measurements, at 3 months' interval in a 10% sample (patients born 4th, 14th and 24th day in any month) and found substantial agreement (Cohen's kappa = 0.80).

As motion artefacts may compromise ASL interpretation, we defined the threshold for permissible motion as motion in one plane, usually physiological motion in cranio-caudal direction, and motion presence in less than 2/3 of the whole brain series' images. ASL image quality assessment is detailed in Additional files 1 and 2.

The arterial transit artefact (ATA) depicts areas where CBF may be normal, but where arterial transit time is increased, and is seen as vivid serpiginous high signal of labeled blood stagnated in precapillary cortical vessels [15, 16, 31]. We deemed ASL positive, when at least one of the following was present: focal low CBF, ATA or focal hyperperfusion (Fig. 1). SWI asymmetric

prominent veins were defined as regions of multiple hypointense vessels [25] and dichotomized into presence and absence. We accepted newfound focal gliosis or atrophy on 8-week follow-up MRI as marker for scar tissue after neuronal death and thus critical ischemic depth [32].

We investigated lesions' tissue localization stratifying lesions after their DWI location into white matter (WM), cortical gray matter (cGM) and deep gray matter (dGM).

After finalized clinical and radiological data collection, radiological lesion localization was compared with clinical symptoms for consistency under supervision of a senior neurological consultant (HC).

Statistical analysis

Categorical data were analyzed using Fisher's exact test. Differences in continuous and ordinal data were analyzed using Mann-Whitney U test, and for differences between proportions we used McNemar-test. Linear relations between variables and a dichotomous outcome were tested using bivariate logistic regression. Un-adjusted survival analysis for recurrent cerebrovascular event was conducted using Kaplan-Meier curves and log-rank test. Relation between imaging findings and recurrent cerebrovascular event was analyzed using Cox Proportional Hazard Model adjusting for other risk factors. Data were presented as frequencies, medians with interquartile range (IQR), odds ratios (OR) or hazard ratios (HR) with 95%

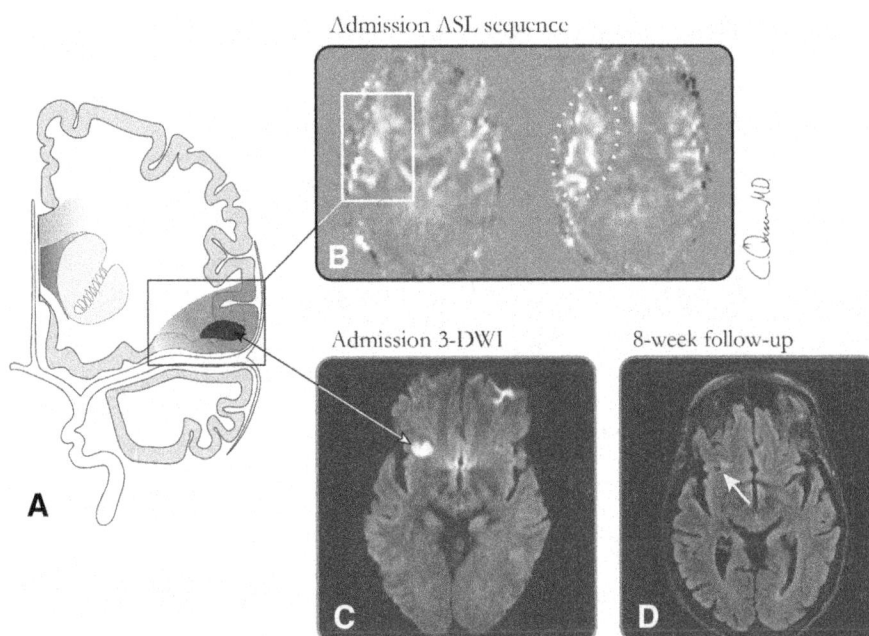

Fig. 1 Subacute diffusion and ASL perfusion lesion and 8-week lasting infarction. Panel **a** displays a schematic illustration of infarct core with surrounding penumbra zone of perfusion restriction. Panel **b** illustrates the larger area of arterial spin labeling lesion with vivid cortical serpiginous hyperintensities (arterial transit artefact), surrounding a smaller DWI lesion (**c**). Panel **d** illustrates the permanent infarction lesion on the 8-week follow-up T2-FLAIR appearing in the same area as the DWI lesion

confidence intervals (CI) as appropriate. *P*-values less than 0.05 were considered significant. Statistical analysis was performed with RStudio (Version 0.97.168) 2012 RStudio Inc., Boston, MA, USA and SPSS (version 20) statistical software (IBM Corp, Armonk, New York, USA).

Results

Population

Patient flow is described in (Fig. 2). Median (IQR) age was 65 (54–71) years, 43% were female, and median (IQR) ABCD2 was 4 (3–5). Table 1 shows detailed patient characteristics. The median (IQR) time from ictus to initial MRI was 38 (24–58) hours. Scans from 4 patients had unacceptable motion artifacts, and 2 patients had no ASL done due to a technical error, these were excluded from the analysis. ASL and SWI with 8-week follow-up MRI were consequently available for 116 patients with 148 clinical or radiological events, hereof were 100 visible ischemic lesions on at least one sequence. We differentiated between patients and lesions, as patients may have multiple lesions in several vascular territories and not all foci showed perfusion changes.

Among patients 46 (40%) had at least one DWI lesion and 46 (40%) showed ASL abnormalities, 24 patients were both DWI and ASL positive (Table 1). Including both DWI and ASL as diagnostic markers of ischemia increased ischemia detection from 46 (40%) to 68 (59%) of 116 patients ($p < 0.0001$). In the cohort 148 acute clinical or radiological events were detected. Of these, 79 (53%) were DWI positive and 68 (46%) were ASL positive lesions. Diffusion and perfusion were both positive in 47 (32%) lesions and 21 lesions (14%) were ASL-

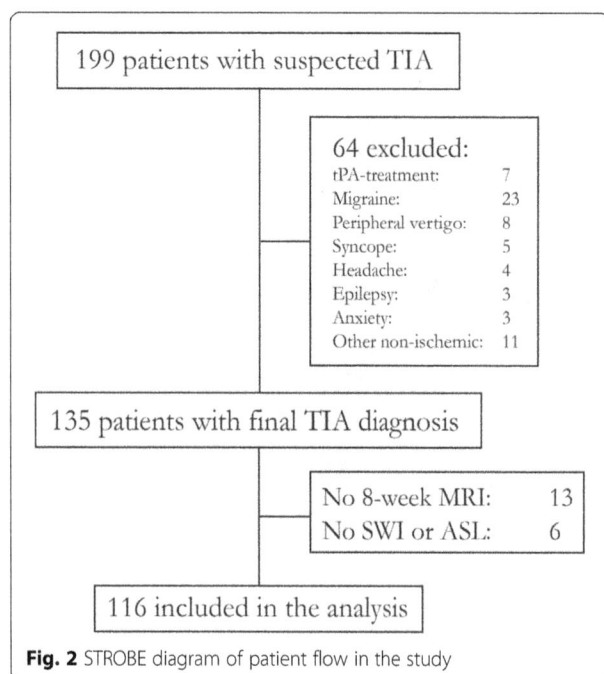

Fig. 2 STROBE diagram of patient flow in the study

Table 1 Patient characteristics

All patients	116
Female sex	50 (43%)
Age, median (IQR)	65 (54–71)
Medical history:	
Prior stroke	21 (17%)
Prior TIA	10 (9%)
Prior MI	9 (8%)
Atrial fibrillation	12 (10%)
Hypertension	57 (49%)
Diabetes	15 (13%)
Depression	11 (10%)
Current smoking	40 (35%)
Alcohol overuse	10 (9%)
Antiplatelet use	38 (33%)
Warfarin use	0 (0%)
Index stroke:	
ABCD2, median (IQR)	4 (3–5)
Duration of symptoms:	
< 60 min	56 (48%)
> 60 min	60 (52%)
TOAST etiology:	
Small vessels	47 (41%)
Large vessels	26 (22%)
Cardiogenic	18 (16%)
Multiple possible etiologies	25 (22%)
TTS, median (IQR)	38 (24–58)
TTF, median (IQR)	56 (55–60)
Radiological findings:	
DWI positive patients	46 (40%)
Lesions, n.	79
ASL positive patients	46 (40%)
Hypoperfusion lesions, n.	38
Hyperperfusion lesions, n.	22
ATA, n.	28
SWI positive patients	5 (4%)
SWI lesions, n.	6

Numbers are frequency (%) unless otherwise indicated. *IQR* interquartile range, *TIA* transient ischemic attack, *MI* myocardial infarction, *NA* not applicable, *TTS* time to scan, *TTF* time to follow-up, *ATA* arterial transit artefact

positive and DWI-negative. Diffusion and ASL findings in patients are detailed in Fig. 3. Among the 68 perfusion lesions in 46 patients, ATA was present in 24 (52%, $p < 0.0001$) patients with perfusion changes and in relation to 20 (53%, $p < 0.0001$) hypoperfusion lesions. One patient with several lesions showed foci with hypoperfusion-ATA combination and foci with

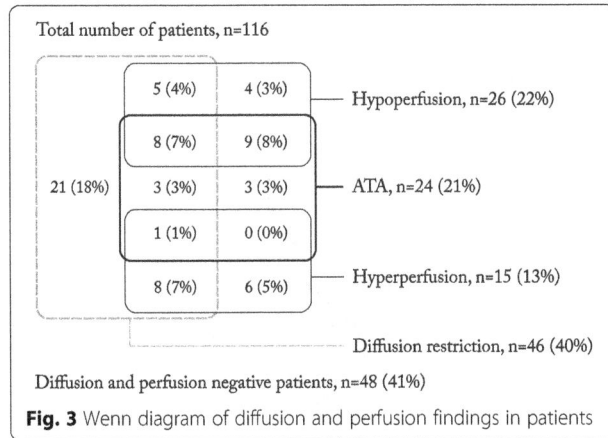

Total number of patients, n=116

5 (4%)   4 (3%) — Hypoperfusion, n=26 (22%)

8 (7%)   9 (8%)

21 (18%)   3 (3%)   3 (3%) — ATA, n=24 (21%)

1 (1%)   0 (0%)

8 (7%)   6 (5%) — Hyperperfusion, n=15 (13%)

Diffusion restriction, n=46 (40%)

Diffusion and perfusion negative patients, n=48 (41%)

Fig. 3 Wenn diagram of diffusion and perfusion findings in patients

hyperperfusion (Fig. 3). There were no distinct lesions with discernible combinations of ATA and hyperperfusion or of hypo- and hyperperfusion.

Characteristics of patients with 8-week infarction signs

In patients with DWI-lesions, a subsequent scarring was observed in 85% at 8 weeks. There was a significant difference between the different TOAST categories and the probability of ASL-lesion with small vessel etiology yielding the lowest probability of ASL-lesion (19%), and large vessel etiology yielding the highest probability (65%, $p < 0.001$). Adjusted for the presence of a DWI lesion, large vessel (OR 8.08, 95% CI 2.66–24.52) and multiple possible etiologies (OR 5.27, 95% CI 1.76–15.75) yielded a higher probability of ASL-lesion than either small vessel etiology (reference category) or cardiogenic etiology (OR 1.97, 95% CI 0.57–6.84). Detailed large vessel findings are shown in Additional file 1: Table S2. Adding ASL to initial DWI does not increase diagnostic accuracy of permanent infarction development (Table 2).

During the median (IQR) follow-up period of 1237 (771–1536) days, 17 patients suffered a recurrent

Table 2 Diagnostic accuracies of DWI and ASL findings for 8-week infarction in patients and lesions

Patients	sensitivity	specificity	PPV	NPV	accuracy
DWI+	0.98	0.91	0.85	0.99	0.93
ASL+	0.58	0.68	0.49	0.75	0.65
DWI+, ASL+	0.98	0.62	0.57	0.98	0.74
DWI+, ASL-	0.40	0.93	0.76	0.75	0.75
DWI-, ASL+	0	0.71	0	0.57	0.47
Lesions					
DWI+	0.98	0.71	0.65	0.99	0.80
ASL+	0.60	0.61	0.46	0.61	0.61
DWI+, ASL+	0.60	0.83	0.66	0.79	0.75
DWI+, ASL-	0.38	0.88	0.63	0.72	0.72
DWI-, ASL+	0	0.78	0	0.59	0.51

cerebrovascular event. Patients with initial ASL lesion (Fig. 4) did not show a higher risk of recurrent cerebrovascular event (HR 1.87, 95% CI 0.70–4.97) after adjusting for presence of DWI-lesion and ABCD2.

Characteristics of lesions with 8-week infarction signs

A total of 65% of DWI-lesions and 45% of ASL-lesions subsequently developed a scar on 8-week MRI. We found the scar-rate to be highest in lesions showing both diffusion restriction and altered perfusion (65%), however only slightly, and non-significantly higher than DWI positive and ASL negative patients (64%). The type of perfusion finding, e.g. ATA, showed no effect on the odds for persistent infarction sign development (Additional file 1: Table S3).

In WM DWI lesions had a high probability of scarring independent of the presence of perfusion abnormalities (94% vs. 92%, $p = 0.765$). In cGM DWI lesions were significantly more likely to develop subsequent infarction after 8 weeks if the lesions was ASL positive (56% vs. 21%, $p = 0.029$). The median (IQR) size of the DWI lesions located in the cGM was not significantly larger than those located in the WM (28.0 (14.0–51.0) vs. 24.5 (9.0–59.0) mm^2; $p = 0.463$). There was a significant correlation between the size of the DWI lesion and probability of surrounding ASL lesion (OR 1.02, 95% CI 1.01–1.03 per additional mm^2).

We had too few ($n = 4$) deep gray matter lesions to conduct a meaningful analysis.

SWI findings

As a subset of patients with ASL abnormalities, we found 5 patients (with 6 lesions) with SWI abnormalities. In only one patient no corresponding DWI lesion was found to the ASL and SWI abnormality; this lesion did not show any scarring at the 8-week MRI. All 5 diffusion positive lesions were located in the cortical gray matter, and 4 (80%) lesions were followed by 8-week gliosis scars; this scar rate was higher than the 52% scar-rate in patients with cGM lesions with ASL abnormalities without SWI findings, though not statistically significant ($p = 0.355$). SWI abnormalities occurred both in focal hypoperfusion (2/6), ATA (2/6) and hyperperfusion (3/6).

Discussion

This study showed that using both diffusion and ASL perfusion imaging identified significantly more patients as MRI-imaging positive for acute vascular findings than DWI alone in a subacute clinical setting without external software. DWI-lesion presence seemed to be the decisive factor for determining lasting infarct changes after TIA, especially in white matter. DWI lesions in cortical gray matter without perfusion change developed few scars,

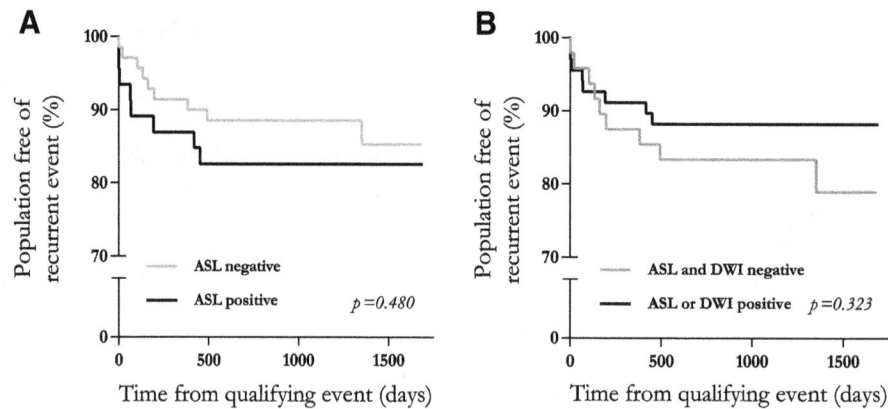

Fig. 4 Event recurrence stratified by lesion characteristics. Two Kaplan-Meier curves showing recurrent cerebrovascular event in the TIA population stratified by MRI-sequence positivity. Panel **a** shows that patients with ASL perfusion lesions do not experience a higher risk of recurrent cerebrovascular events compared to TIA patients displaying no perfusion lesion. Panel **b**: shows that radiological evidence of acute ischemia (either restricted perfusion or diffusion) does not identify patients in higher risk of recurrent event

while half of lesions with perfusion change left a scar. SWI did not add to detection of ischemia in TIA, but may indicate profound perfusion disturbance.

Our study has a high frequency of lesions, most likely because of inclusion of well-defined patients and subsequent exclusion of patients with other final diagnoses than TIA. This hampers generalizability to less selected emergency room patients concerning lesion frequency, however not regarding the natural MRI history of ischemic lesions after TIA. The rates of DWI lesions are reported to vary between 25 and 50% [3, 17, 18, 33–36] and to be halved in populations with high stroke awareness and easy-access high-volume TIA clinics [37].

Other potential limitations are: Motion artifacts increase with scan time [27, 28, 38] and may compromise perfusion parameter estimates [5]. We had too few deep gray matter lesions and SWI positives for meaningful subgroup analysis. Our SWI positive lesions were a subset of perfusion positives that with concomitant DWI lesions showed high scarring rate. This may indicate that visible venous congestion serves as marker for focal ischemic depth, exploration would need more data.

We confirmed that the combination of diffusion and ASL perfusion identifies significantly more lesions than either sequence alone in TIA, [3, 14] from 40% up to nearly 60% of TIA patients in our subacute clinical setting. Roughly half of white matter lesions showed perfusion change compared to three quarters of cortical lesions: This presumably reflects the local vascularity with rich collaterals cortically and fewer in deeper tissue, relying on perforants, [39–41] and the longer and more heterogeneous transit times of white matter [42, 43] decreasing ASL's sensitivity to focal changes. This also explains the lower probability of ASL changes in patients with small vessel etiology. Larger cortical lesions may also show

signs of venous congestion, their frequency in our TIA population was scarce compared to stroke populations [25].

In our small population positive image findings did not influence the post-TIA stroke risk, nor did anyone among the 22 patients with perfusion deficits only develop infarction signs at 8-week follow-up, perhaps due to small sample size.

In our clinical setting without external post-processing software the speed and accessibility of diffusion and ASL perfusion imaging enabled us to increase ischemia detection in comparison to diffusion imaging alone. This may aid in identification of high-risk patients with TIA with imaging abnormalities. Our standard vendor pulsed ASL sequence proved robust and identified perfusion changes larger than diffusion lesions and showed perfusion change in DWI-negative patients. ATA often bordered hypoperfused areas and served as an easily identifiable pointer useful in the clinical situation, and we deemed it worth the extra scan time.

Conclusions

Ischemia detection is improved by adding ASL to the TIA protocol, and the standard sequence proved feasible and robust in a clinical setting. SWI did not add critical information in subacute diagnostic work-up for TIA. Localization and underlying local vascularity seem to be key factors in the morphologic development of ischemia lesion depth and long-term traces.

Abbreviations
ASL: Arterial spin labeling; ATA: Arterial transit artefact; CBF: Cerebral blood flow; cGM: Cortical gray matter; CI: Confidence interval; CRF: Case report form; dGM: Deep gray matter; DSC: Dynamic susceptibility contrast; DWI: Diffusion weighted imaging; FLAIR: Fluid attenuated inversion recovery; HR: Hazard ratio;

IQR: Interquartile range; MRI: Magnetic resonance imaging; NIHSS: National Institutes of Health Stroke Scale; OR: Odds ratio; SWI: Susceptibility weighted imaging; TIA: Transient ischemic attack; TOAST: Trial of ORG 10172 in acute stroke treatment; WM: White matter

Funding
CO holds research grants from the Velux-foundation, Bispebjerg University Hospital, University of Copenhagen, Axel Muusfeldts Foundation and Danish Medical Association. None were designated for this study.

Authors' contributions
IH, HC, AC conceived and designed the study. All authors were involved in data acquisition. KÆ, JM, PM, SR, MF, HC were involved in patient inclusion. LW performed the clinical follow-up and provided critical feed-back in the manuscript writing. IH, CO, JD, AC, HC analyzed and interpreted data. IH wrote the first draft. All authors reviewed and edited the manuscript and approved the final version of the manuscript.

Competing interests
The authors declare that they have no competing interests.

Author details
[1]Department of Radiology, Copenhagen University Hospital Bispebjerg, Bispebjerg Bakke 23, 2400 Copenhagen, NV, Denmark. [2]Department of Neurology, Copenhagen University Hospital Bispebjerg, Bispebjerg Bakke 23, 2400 Copenhagen, NV, Denmark.

References
1. Amarenco P, Lavallée PC, Labreuche J, Albers GW, Bornstein NM, Canhão P, et al. One-year risk of stroke after transient ischemic attack or minor stroke. N Engl J Med. 2016;374:1533–42.
2. Castle J, Mlynash M, Lee K, Caulfield AF, Wolford C, Kemp S, et al. Agreement regarding diagnosis of transient ischemic attack fairly low among stroke-trained neurologists. Stroke. 2010;41:1367–70.
3. Zaharchuk G, Olivot J-M, Fischbein NJ, Bammer R, Straka M, Kleinman JT, et al. Arterial spin labeling imaging findings in transient ischemic attack patients: comparison with diffusion- and bolus perfusion-weighted imaging. Cerebrovasc Dis. 2012;34:221–8.
4. Chen Y, Wang DJ, Detre JA. Test-retest reliability of arterial spin labeling with common labeling strategies. J Magn Reson Imaging. 2011;33:940–9.
5. Deibler AR, Pollock JM, Kraft RA, Tan H, Burdette JH, Maldjian JA. Arterial spin-labeling in routine clinical practice, part 1: technique and artifacts. AJNR Am J Neuroradiol. 2008;29:1228–34.
6. Viallon M, Altrichter S, Pereira VM, Nguyen D, Sekoranja L, Federspiel A, et al. Combined use of pulsed arterial spin-labeling and susceptibility-weighted imaging in stroke at 3T. Eur Neurol. 2010;64:286–96.
7. Hernandez DA, Bokkers RPH, Mirasol RV, Luby M, Henning EC, Merino JG, et al. Pseudo-continuous arterial spin labeling quantifies relative cerebral blood flow in acute stroke. Stroke. 2012;43:753–8.
8. Zaharchuk G, El Mogy IS, Fischbein NJ, Albers GW. Comparison of arterial spin labeling and bolus perfusion-weighted imaging for detecting mismatch in acute stroke. Stroke. 2012;43:1843–8.
9. Wang DJ, Alger JR, Qiao JX, Hao Q, Hou S, Fiaz R, et al. The value of arterial spin-labeled perfusion imaging in acute ischemic stroke - comparison with dynamic susceptibility contrast enhanced MRI. Stroke. 2012;43:1018–24.
10. MacIntosh BJ, Lindsay AC, Kylintireas I, Kuker W, Günther M, Robson MD, et al. Multiple inflow pulsed arterial spin-labeling reveals delays in the arterial arrival time in minor stroke and transient ischemic attack. AJNR Am J Neuroradiol. 2010;31:1892–4.
11. Asdaghi N, Hameed B, Saini M, Jeerakathil T, Emery D, Butcher K. Acute perfusion and diffusion abnormalities predict early new MRI lesions 1 week after minor stroke and transient ischemic attack. Stroke. 2011;42:2191–5.
12. Zaharchuk G, Bammer R, Straka M, Shankaranarayan A, Alsop DC, Fischbein NJ, et al. Arterial spin-label imaging in patients with normal bolus perfusion-weighted MR imaging findings: pilot identification of the Borderzone sign. Radiology. 2009;252:797–807.
13. Deibler AR, Pollock JM, Kraft RA, Tan H, Burdette JH, Maldjian JA. Arterial spin-labeling in routine clinical practice, part 2: Hypoperfusion patterns. AJNR Am J Neuroradiol. 2008;29:1235–41.
14. Qiao XJ, Salamon N, Wang DJ, He R, Linetsky M, Ellingson BM, et al. Perfusion deficits detected by arterial spin labeling (ASL) in TIA patients with negative diffusion and vascular imaging. AJNR Am J Neuroradiol. 2013;34:2125–30.
15. Chalela JA, Alsop DC, Gonzalez-Atavales JB, Maldjian JA, Kasner SE, Detre JA. Magnetic resonance perfusion imaging in acute ischemic stroke using continuous arterial spin labeling. Stroke. 2000;31:680–7.
16. Wolf RL, Alsop DC, McGarvey ML, Maldjian JA, Wang J, Detre JA. Susceptibility contrast and arterial spin labeled perfusion MRI in cerebrovascular disease. J Neuroimaging. 2003;13:17–27.
17. Kleinman JT, Zaharchuk G, Mlynash M, Ogdie AA, Straka M, Lansberg MG, et al. Automated perfusion imaging for the evaluation of transient ischemic attack. Stroke. 2012;43:1556–60.
18. Mlynash M, Olivot J-M, Tong DC, Lansberg MG, Eyngorn I, Kemp S, et al. Yield of combined perfusion and diffusion MR imaging in hemispheric TIA. Neurology. 2009;72:1127–33.
19. Tong T, Yao Z, Feng X. Combined diffusion- and perfusion-weighted imaging: a new way for the assessment of hemispheric transient ischemic attack patients. Int J Dev Neurosci. 2011;29:63–9.
20. Nah H-W, Kwon SU, Kang D-W, Lee D-H, Kim JS. Diagnostic and prognostic value of multimodal MRI in transient ischemic attack. Int. J. Stroke off. J Int Stroke Soc. 2014;9:895–901.
21. Lee SH, Nah HW, Kim BJ, Ahn SH, Kim JS, Kang DW, et al. Role of perfusion-weighted imaging in a diffusion-weighted-imaging-negative transient ischemic attack. J Clin Neurol. 2017;13:129–37.
22. Mittal S, Wu Z, Neelavalli J, Haacke EM. Susceptibility-weighted imaging: technical aspects and clinical applications, part 2. AJNR Am J Neuroradiol. 2009;30:232–52.
23. Kesavadas C, Thomas B, Pendharakar H, Sylaja PN. Susceptibility weighted imaging: does it give information similar to perfusion weighted imaging in acute stroke? J Neurol. 2011;258:932–4.
24. Baik SK, Choi W, Oh SJ, Park K-P, Park M-G, Yang TI, et al. Change in cortical vessel signs on susceptibility-weighted images after full recanalization in Hyperacute ischemic stroke. Cerebrovasc Dis. 2012;34:206–12.
25. Jensen-Kondering U, Bohm R. Asymmetrically hypointense veins on T2*w imaging and susceptibility-weighted imaging in ischemic stroke. World J Radiol. 2013;5:156–65.
26. Kaya D, Dinçer A, Yildiz ME, Çizmeli MO, Erzen C. Acute ischemic infarction defined by a region of multiple Hypointense vessels on gradient-Echo T2* MR imaging at 3T. AJNR Am J Neuroradiol. 2009;30:1227–32.
27. Qin L, van Gelderen P, Derbyshire JA, Jin F, Lee J, de Zwart JA, et al. Prospective head-movement correction for high-resolution MRI using an in-bore optical tracking system. Magn Reson Med. 2009;62:924–34.
28. Kober T, Gruetter R, Krueger G. Prospective and retrospective motion correction in diffusion magnetic resonance imaging of the human brain. NeuroImage. 2012;59:389–98.
29. Dold C, Zaitsev M, Speck O, Firle EA, Hennig J, Sakas G. Prospective head motion compensation for MRI by updating the gradients and radio frequency during data acquisition. Med Image Comput Comput Assist Interv. 2005;8:482–9.
30. Andre JB, Bresnahan BW, Mossa-Basha M, Hoff MN, Smith CP, Anzai Y, et al. Toward quantifying the prevalence, severity, and cost associated with patient motion during clinical MR examinations. J Am Coll Radiol. 2015; 12:689–95.
31. Detre JA, Samuels OB, Alsop DC, Gonzalez-At JB, Kasner SE, Raps EC. Noninvasive magnetic resonance imaging evaluation of cerebral blood flow with acetazolamide challenge in patients with cerebrovascular stenosis. J Magn Reson Imaging. 1999;10:870–5.
32. Asdaghi N, Campbell BCV, Butcher KS, Coulter JI, Modi J, Qazi A, et al. DWI reversal is associated with small infarct volume in patients with TIA and Minor stroke. AJNR Am J Neuroradiol. 2014;35:660–6.
33. Merwick A, Albers GW, Amarenco P, Arsava EM, Ay H, Calvet D, et al. Addition of brain and carotid imaging to the ABCD[2] score to identify patients at early risk of stroke after transient ischaemic attack: a multicentre observational study. Lancet Neurol. 2010;9:1060–9.
34. Purroy F, Begué R, Quílez A, Piñol-Ripoll G, Sanahuja J, Brieva L, et al. The California, ABCD, and unified ABCD2 risk scores and the presence of acute ischemic lesions on diffusion-weighted imaging in TIA patients. Stroke. 2009;40:2229–32.

35.   Ay H, Arsava EM, Johnston SC, Vangel M, Schwamm LH, Furie KL, et al. Clinical- and imaging-based prediction of stroke risk after transient ischemic attack the CIP model. Stroke. 2009;40:181–6.

36.   Giles MF, Albers GW, Amarenco P, Arsava EM, Asimos AW, Ay H, et al. Early stroke risk and ABCD2 score performance in tissue- vs time-defined TIA. Neurology. 2011;77:1222–8.

37.   Lavallée PC, Meseguer E, Abboud H, Cabrejo L, Olivot J-M, Simon O, et al. A transient ischaemic attack clinic with round-the-clock access (SOS-TIA): feasibility and effects. Lancet Neurol. 2007;6:953–60.

38.   Zaitsev M, Maclaren J, Herbst M. Motion artifacts in MRI: a complex problem with many partial solutions. J Magn Reson Imaging. 2015;42:887–901.

39.   Cho HJ, Yang JH, Jung YH, Kim YD, Choi H-Y, Nam HS, et al. Cortex-sparing infarctions in patients with occlusion of the middle cerebral artery. J Neurol Neurosurg Psychiatry. 2010;81:859–63.

40.   Brozici M, van der Zwan A, Hillen B. Anatomy and functionality of Leptomeningeal anastomoses a review. Stroke. 2003;34:2750–62.

41.   Schwamm LH, Koroshetz WJ, Sorensen AG, Wang B, Copen WA, Budzik R, et al. Time course of lesion development in patients with acute stroke serial diffusion- and hemodynamic-weighted magnetic resonance imaging. Stroke. 1998;29:2268–76.

42.   van Gelderen P, de Zwart JA, Duyn JH. Pittfalls of MRI measurement of white matter perfusion based on arterial spin labeling. Magn Reson Med. 2008;59:788–95.

43.   van Osch MJ, Teeuwisse WM, van Walderveen MAA, Hendrikse J, Kies DA, van Buchem MA. Can arterial spin labeling detect white matter perfusion signal? Magn Reson Med. 2009;62:165–73.

25

Dual-phase whole-heart imaging using image navigation in congenital heart disease

Danielle M. Moyé[1,2,6*] ⓘ, Tarique Hussain[1,2,3], Rene M. Botnar[4,5], Animesh Tandon[1,2,3], Gerald F. Greil[1,2,3], Adrian K. Dyer[1,2] and Markus Henningsson[4]

Abstract

Background: Dual-phase 3-dimensional whole-heart acquisition allows simultaneous imaging during systole and diastole. Respiratory navigator gating and tracking of the diaphragm is used with limited accuracy. Prolonged scan time is common, and navigation often fails in patients with erratic breathing. Image-navigation (iNAV) tracks movement of the heart itself and is feasible in single phase whole heart imaging. To evaluate its diagnostic ability in congenital heart disease, we sought to apply iNAV to dual-phase sequencing.

Methods: Healthy volunteers and patients with congenital heart disease underwent dual-phase imaging using the conventional diaphragmatic-navigation (dNAV) and iNAV. Acquisition time was recorded and image quality assessed. Sharpness and length of the right coronary (RCA), left anterior descending (LAD), and circumflex (LCx) arteries were measured in both cardiac phases for both approaches. Qualitative and quantitative analyses were performed in a blinded and randomized fashion.

Results: In volunteers, there was no significant difference in vessel sharpness between approaches ($p > 0.05$). In patients, analysis showed equal vessel sharpness for LAD and RCA ($p > 0.05$). LCx sharpness was greater with dNAV ($p < 0.05$). Visualized length with iNAV was 0.5 ± 0.4 cm greater than that with dNAV for LCx in diastole ($p < 0.05$), 1.0 ± 0.3 cm greater than dNAV for LAD in diastole ($p < 0.05$), and 0.8 ± 0.7 cm greater than dNAV for RCA in systole ($p < 0.05$). Qualitative scores were similar between modalities ($p = 0.71$). Mean iNAV scan time was $5:18 \pm 2:12$ min shorter than mean dNAV scan time in volunteers ($p = 0.0001$) and $3:16 \pm 1:12$ min shorter in patients ($p = 0.0001$).

Conclusions: Image quality of iNAV and dNAV was similar with better distal vessel visualization with iNAV. iNAV acquisition time was significantly shorter. Complete cardiac diagnosis was achieved. Shortened acquisition time will improve clinical applicability and patient comfort.

Keywords: Steady-state free precession MRI, Congenital heart disease, Dual phase imaging, Respiratory motion correction

Background

Three-dimensional (3D) whole-heart imaging for assessment of morphology in congenital heart disease has revolutionized how images have been obtained in the last decade [1, 2]. Sørensen et al. [3] evaluated the diagnostic ability and utility of 3D whole heart balanced steady-state free precession (3D WH bSSFP) MRI for morphology in congenital heart disease with single-phase imaging. All images were acquired in end diastole and scanning was performed during free breathing with a pencil beam navigator (dNAV) on the right hemi-diaphragm. They showed the 3D WH bSSFP to be reliable and accurate in the assessment of morphology in congenital heart disease. This showed that 3D, single phase imaging with the conventional navigational technique (dNAV) was superior to the two-dimensional (2D) scanning that was being done at that time. Uribe et al.

* Correspondence: dmoye@stanfordalumni.org
[1]Department of Pediatrics, Division of Cardiology, UT Southwestern Medical Center Dallas, Dallas, TX, USA
[2]Department of Pediatrics, Division of Cardiology, Children's Health, Children's Medical Center Dallas, Dallas, TX, USA
Full list of author information is available at the end of the article

[4] extended this analysis to dual phase imaging with dNAV in an attempt to determine optimal coronary artery imaging timing. They found that optimal timing (systolic versus diastolic rest period) was patient dependent and different for each coronary artery segment, favoring dual phase whole heart imaging to allow for optimal coronary artery visualization by retrospectively selecting the optimal imaging rest period. Furthermore, in previous work by Hussain et al. [5], it was shown that images obtained during the systolic rest period offer better clarity for many cardiac segments in congenital heart disease, including all four cardiac chambers and pulmonary veins in particular. Diastolic imaging, however, was preferable when imaging the aorta and branch pulmonary arteries. This finding of some cardiac structures imaging better during the systolic rest period while other structures image better during the diastolic rest period led to the thought that dual phase imaging would be superior in diagnostic quality when compared with either single phase alone, which they illustrated.

Technically, dual-phase 3D WH bSSFP is an extension of conventional 3D WH bSSFP, which is acquired in either systole or diastole, and uses T2 preparation [6] and fat suppression pre-pulses to improve contrast. To compensate for respiratory motion, a one-dimensional navigator is typically used, positioned over the right hemi-diaphragm and measures respiratory motion in the foot-head (FH) direction [7]. This pencil beam diaphragmatic navigator signal is used to gate the 3D WH bSSFP scan to end-expiration using a narrow gating window, typically 5 mm, resulting in a scan efficiency of approximately 30–50%. Additionally, the dNAV can be used to correct for the translational respiratory FH motion of the heart using an estimated correction factor to convert translational motion of the diaphragm to that of the heart. For dual-phase 3D WH bSSFP, a dNAV acquisition is performed for both the systolic and diastolic rest phases where each dNAV has a separate 5 mm gating window. Systolic and diastolic 3D WH bSSFP data for any given cardiac cycle, however, are only accepted if both the systolic and diastolic dNAV are within their individual gating windows [8]. This further lowers the scan efficiency, extending the total dual-phase 3D WH bSSFP scan time. Furthermore, although dNAV can adequately suppress respiratory motion artifact for 3D WH bSSFP in most patients, for some patients respiratory artifacts remain, leading to lower diagnostic yield [9]. Additionally, the dNAV navigator often fails in cases of erratic breathing patterns, resulting in the inability to acquire necessary images.

In recent years, image-based navigation (iNAV) has been proposed for single-phase whole heart bSSFP to enable direct measurement and respiratory motion correction of the heart itself rather than the diaphragm [10–13]. With this approach, 2D or 3D real-time images are acquired, which allow localization of the heart and differentiation from surrounding structures. One approach to iNAV acquisition involves adding phase encoding gradients to the start-up echoes of a bSSFP sequence to generate a 2D image. Although this results in low spatial resolution in the phase encoding direction and projection of the field-of-view (FOV) in the slice encoding direction, it is sufficient to track the respiratory motion of the heart provided that the acquisition is oriented with readout along FH direction (high spatial resolution). In addition to correcting for translational respiratory motion of the heart, gating has been implemented for iNAV, using either respiratory bellows [14] or more recently the Constant Respiratory efficiency UsIng Single End-expiratory threshold (CRUISE) technique [15]. The CRUISE algorithm predefines a 50% gating efficiency whereby k-space is fully acquired during the first half of the 3D WH bSSFP scan and the most motion corrupted data are discarded and re-acquired in the second half. A challenge of extending iNAV to dual-phase 3D WH bSSFP is the different cardiac motion states between systole and diastole, which precludes the use of a common navigator for both phases, as cardiac motion may be interpreted as respiratory motion. This issue can be addressed by using separate iNAV reference frames for systole and diastole. Further, the use of separate systolic and diastolic iNAVs using CRUISE gating may improve dual-phase 3D WH bSSFP gating efficiency as the CRUISE algorithm does not require both systolic and diastolic navigators to be within a pre-defined gating window for a given cardiac cycle.

The purpose of this study was to implement and evaluate the diagnostic ability of a new iNAV approach for dual-phase 3D WH bSSFP in healthy volunteers and patients with congenital heart disease, using separate systolic and diastolic image navigators with CRUISE gating.

Methods

Approval was obtained from the University of Texas Southwestern Institutional Review board and the local ethics committee before initiation of the study. All participants provided written informed consent and all data were collected per standard of care at Children's Health Children's Medical Center Dallas and the University of Texas Southwestern Medical Center. All experiments were performed on a 1.5 T clinical scanner (Ingenia, Philips Healthcare, Best, The Netherlands) using a 32-channel cardiac coil.

Dual-phase 3D WH bSSFP with iNAV motion compensation

The proposed iNAV motion correction strategy for dual-phase 3D WH bSSFP is shown in Fig. 1. The iNAVs were acquired by adding phase encoding gradients to 10 startup echoes of the bSSFP pulse sequence as previously described [10]. To account for differences in each cardiac motion state, separate iNAV references were acquired for the systolic and diastolic rest phase. The iNAV references were defined as the first acquired iNAV in each cardiac phase. Each subsequent iNAV for a given phase was registered to its corresponding iNAV reference using normalized cross-correlation. Translational motion correction was performed in FH and left-right (LR) direction. Additionally, respiratory gating was implemented using the CRUISE algorithm, where a predefined gating efficiency of 50% was used. This gating efficiency has been shown to have an equivalent dNAV gating window of 5 mm and had a similar, if not slightly superior efficiency. The details of this CRUISE algorithm have recently been described [15]. For the dual-phase implementation of CRUISE, the systolic and diastolic iNAVs were separately gated to end-expiration, as shown in Fig. 2. The iNAV motion correction and gating were implemented in real-time on the scanner and no post-processing of the 3D WH bSSFP was required.

MRI experiments

All subjects underwent dual-phase 3D WH bSSFP with dNAV and independent systolic and diastolic iNAV correction and CRUISE gating. For comparison, a dual-phase scan was acquired using dNAV with a 0.6 tracking factor and a 5 mm gating window. As previously outlined, the dual phase implementation of dNAV gating required both systolic and diastolic navigators to be within the 5 mm gating window for the k-space segment of a particular cardiac cycle to be accepted. The 3D WH bSSFP sequence had the following image parameters: FOV = $300 \times 300 \times 100$ mm (coronal orientation), $\Delta x = 1.5 \times 1.5 \times 1.5$ mm^3, $\alpha = 70°$, echo time 1.7 ms, repetition time 3.4 ms, SENSE factor = 2.5 (phase encoding direction). Fat suppression and T2-preparation pulses were used to improve contrast (T2 prep time = 50 ms) [16]. ECG-triggering using subject-specific delay times were determined using high temporal resolution cine 4 chamber scans to coincide with the systolic and diastolic rest periods. The systolic and diastolic data acquisition windows were identical and defined as the shortest rest period of the two cardiac phases, typically approximately 90 msec. With these imaging parameters and a heart-rate of 70 beats-per-minute the nominal scan time was 3 min and 26 s (i.e. assuming 100% navigator efficiency). Acquisition time was recorded for each sequence.

Healthy volunteers

Nineteen healthy subjects participated in the study and underwent dual-phase 3D WH bSSFP with both dNAV and iNAV motion compensation. The scans were

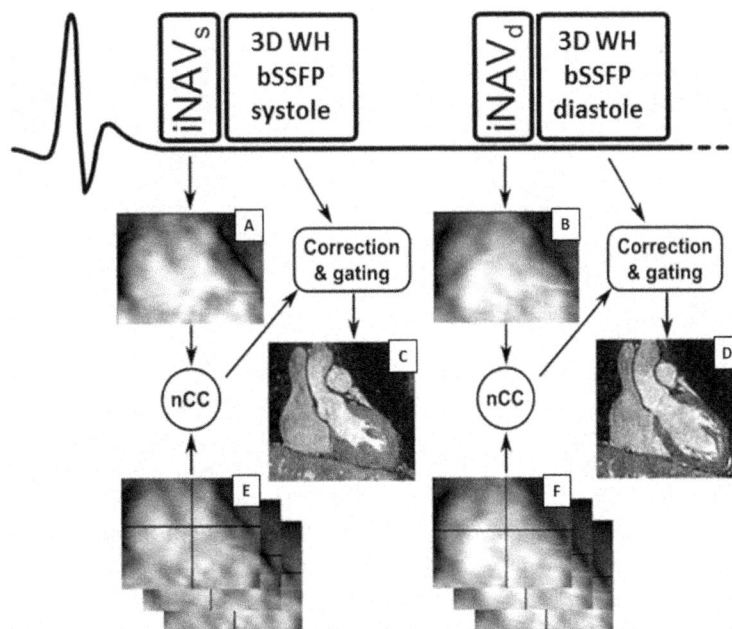

Fig. 1 This describes the schematics of iNAV respiratory motion correction when applied to dual-phase 3D WH bSSFP. A separate iNAV reference (iNAV REF) was used for systole (**a**) and diastole (**b**). All subsequent systolic and diastolic iNAVs (**e** and **f**) were registered to their respective reference iNAV (**a** and **b** respectively) using normalized cross-correlation (nCC). Images **c** and **d** show the reconstructed images obtained

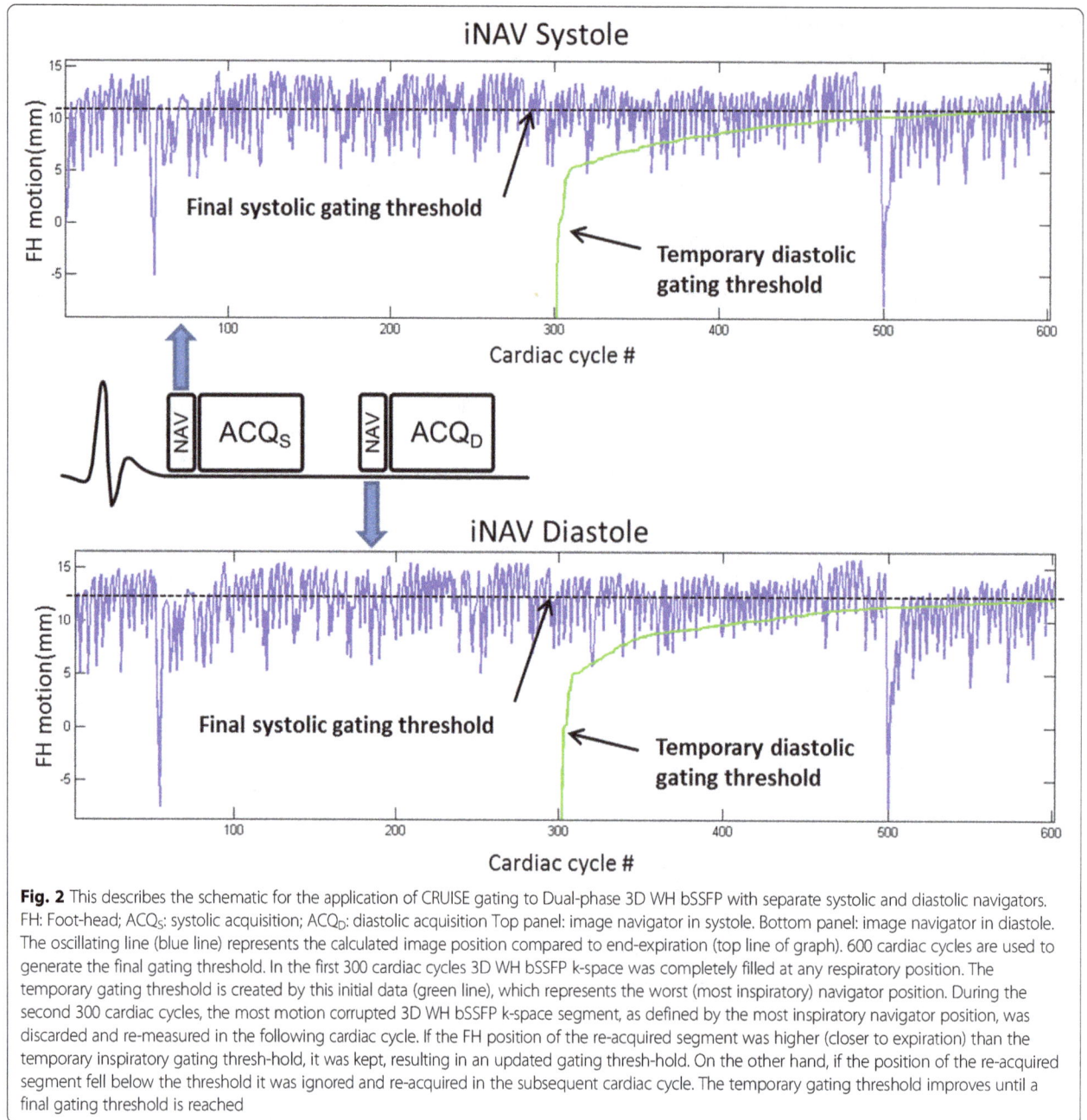

Fig. 2 This describes the schematic for the application of CRUISE gating to Dual-phase 3D WH bSSFP with separate systolic and diastolic navigators. FH: Foot-head; ACQ$_S$: systolic acquisition; ACQ$_D$: diastolic acquisition Top panel: image navigator in systole. Bottom panel: image navigator in diastole. The oscillating line (blue line) represents the calculated image position compared to end-expiration (top line of graph). 600 cardiac cycles are used to generate the final gating threshold. In the first 300 cardiac cycles 3D WH bSSFP k-space was completely filled at any respiratory position. The temporary gating threshold is created by this initial data (green line), which represents the worst (most inspiratory) navigator position. During the second 300 cardiac cycles, the most motion corrupted 3D WH bSSFP k-space segment, as defined by the most inspiratory navigator position, was discarded and re-measured in the following cardiac cycle. If the FH position of the re-acquired segment was higher (closer to expiration) than the temporary inspiratory gating thresh-hold, it was kept, resulting in an updated gating thresh-hold. On the other hand, if the position of the re-acquired segment fell below the threshold it was ignored and re-acquired in the subsequent cardiac cycle. The temporary gating threshold improves until a final gating threshold is reached

acquired in a randomized order. Interim analysis of the volunteer data was performed to evaluate for potential benefit prior to starting patient recruitment.

Patients

Thirty patients undergoing a non-sedated clinically indicated cardiac MRI for congenital or pediatric heart disease were included in the study. The dual phase 3D WH bSSFP scans with both dNAV and iNAV motion compensation were acquired in a randomized order at the end of each patient's clinically indicated study. Gadobutrol contrast was used in 28/30 (93%) patients

and contrast agent was administered as part of the clinically indicated study, prior to study image acquisition. For all patients receiving gadolinium, the first whole-heart sequence was started from 4 to 8 min post dose. No patient, by study design, was scanned under anesthesia. Patient demographics and clinical indications for cardiac MRI are shown in Table 1.

Data and statistical analysis

The dual phase 3D WH bSSFP datasets were reformatted using dedicated software (Soap-bubble software tool [Release 5.1 for PRIDE, Philips Healthcare, Best the

Table 1 Patient Demographics and Clinical Indications for cardiac MRI

Age, (years, mean ± standard deviation):	16.7 ± 5.1
Male gender, N (%)	13 (43%)
Ethnicity, N (%)	
• Caucasian	22 (73%)
• Hispanic	5 (17%)
• Asian	2 (7%)
• African American	1 (3%)
Clinical indications for cardiac MRI, N (%)	
• Congenital heart disease post-surgical repair	16 (53%)
Underlying cardiac disease:	
○ Tetralogy of Fallot	
○ Tetralogy of Fallot, absent pulmonary valve	
○ Total anomalous pulmonary venous return	
○ DORV, D-TGA, VSD, pulmonary stenosis	
○ DORV, D-TGA, VSD, aortic stenosis	
○ Coarctation of the aorta	
○ Coarctation of the aorta, VSD, bicuspid aortic valve	
○ Turner syndrome, partial anomalous pulmonary venous return	
○ Unbalanced AVCD, DORV, L-TGA, pulmonary stenosis	
○ AVCD, pulmonary stenosis, pulmonary regurgitation	
○ Ebstein's malformation of the tricuspid valve	
○ Pulmonary atresia, intact ventricular septum	
○ Pulmonary valve regurgitation	
○ Pulmonary stenosis, sinus venosus defect	
○ Shone's complex	
○ Partial anomalous pulmonary venous return, Atrial septal defect	
• Hypertrophic cardiomyopathy	4 (13%)
• Evaluation for arrhythmogenic right ventricular cardiomyopathy/dysplasia	2 (7%
• Bicuspid aortic valve; evaluation of aortic dilation	3 (10%)
• Loeys-Dietz syndrome	1 (3%)
• Evaluation for myocarditis	1 (3%)
• Suspected abnormal left coronary artery origin	1 (3%)
• Kawasaki disease with giant aneurysms	1 (3%)
• Ectopic atrial tachycardia; evaluate cardiac anatomy	1 (3%)

DORV Double outlet right ventricle, *TGA* transposition of the great arteries, *VSD* ventricular septal defect, *AVCD* Atrioventricular canal defect

Netherlands]) [17] to visualize the right coronary artery (RCA), left anterior descending (LAD) artery and left circumflex (LCx) artery. Vessel sharpness and visualized length were measured for the RCA, LAD and LCx for both cardiac rest phases and for both motion correction navigation methods according to previously validated techniques [4, 14]. All variables were tested for normality of distribution using a one-sample Kolmogorov-Smirnov Test. Descriptive statistics such as mean and standard deviation were used for normally distributed variables. Median and range are used for variables with a non-parametric distribution and variables are compared using a Wilcoxon-signed rank test. The 95% confidence intervals of normally distributed measurements were reported and a paired t-test was employed to assess the difference between them. All statistical analyses were performed using SAS 9.4 (SAS Institute, Cary, NC). Qualitative analysis was performed using a previously described and validated visual score [7, 10] on reformatted images of each coronary artery in a blinded and randomized fashion by two readers (AT and AD, with three and 5 years of experience in cardiovascular MR imaging respectively). The scoring was performed using a consensus agreement as previously described [5]. Additionally, each cardiac or great vessel structure was scored as to whether its connection was visualized with diagnostic adequacy. Adequate visualization was defined by the structure being adequately defined without severe blurring (i.e. score ≥ 3 out of 5, using a previously described scoring system [18]). A generalized linear model was used to determine the effect on coronary artery, systolic or diastolic phase and navigator type on image quality score.

Results

Healthy volunteers

Dual phase 3D WH bSSFP was successfully obtained in all nineteen volunteers (7 male, age (mean ± standard deviation): 33.1 ± 8.4 years) using iNAV and dNAV motion compensation. The mean scan time using iNAV was 5:33 ± 1:50 min (min), was significantly shorter than that of dNAV which was 9:51 ± 4:02 min ($p = 0.0001$). In 17 out of 19 volunteers, the scan time was longer using dNAV and in one case, the dNAV method resulted in excessively long scan duration of more than 22 min. In contrast, the longest observed scan time using iNAV was 9:30 min. Reformatted dual phase 3D WH bSSFP images using iNAV and dNAV in both systole and diastole from two volunteers are shown in Fig. 3.

The vessel sharpness for systole and diastole of the RCA, LAD and LCx using iNAV and dNAV, averaged across all 19 healthy subjects are shown in Fig. 4. There was no statistically significant difference in vessel sharpness between images obtained with iNAV compared to those obtained with dNAV for either cardiac phase. The iNAV RCA sharpness (mean ± standard deviation) during systole was 52.69% ± 15.10% versus 54.79% ± 12.99% with dNAV ($p = 0.17$). The iNAV RCA sharpness during diastole was 53.45 ± 17.37% with iNAV 53.69% ± 12.67% with dNAV ($p = 0.92$). The LAD sharpness (mean ± standard deviation) was 48.28% ± 15.36% in systole with

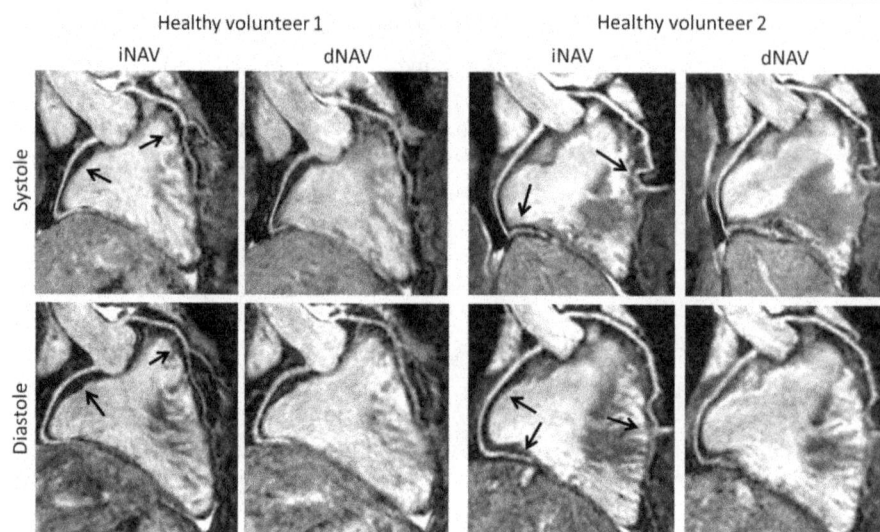

Fig. 3 Reformatted dual-phase 3D WH bSSFP data from two healthy subjects in systole and diastole. This figure shows that in some subjects with poor dNav gating, excessively long scan times can result in worse image quality. iNAV = image-navigator; dNAV = diaphragmatic 1D pencil beam navigator. Arrows highlight coronary segments with improved sharpness using iNAV compared to dNAV

iNAV versus 49.49% ± 11.83% with dNAV ($p = 0.39$) and 49.55% ± 14.80% in diastole with iNAV versus 50.57% ± 12.27% with dNAV ($p = 0.52$). The LCx sharpness (mean ± standard deviation) during systole was 45.69% ± 15.56% with iNAV versus 48.42% ± 11.40% with dNAV ($p = 0.23$) and 45.56% ± 15.69% during diastole with iNAV versus 47.25% ± 13.23% with dNAV ($p = 0.25$).

Patients

Thirty-two patients underwent dual phase 3D WH bSSFP imaging. Two patients failed dNAV imaging due to erratic breathing patterns resulting in extremely low gating efficiency, and were excluded from analysis.

Representative pictures of reformatted dual phase 3D WH bSSFP images using iNAV and dNAV in both systole and diastole from one patient are shown in Fig. 5.

Vessel sharpness was similar for the LAD and RCA in both systole (LAD mean sharpness of 38.4% ± 7.0% with iNAV versus 39.4% ± 8.9% with dNAV, $p = 0.51$; RCA mean sharpness of 39.4% ± 8.5% with iNAV versus 41.4% ± 8.2% with dNAV, $p = 0.11$) and diastole (LAD mean sharpness of 40.5% ± 9.8% with iNAV versus 41.1% ± 9.5% with dNAV, $p = 0.61$; RCA mean sharpness of 37.6% ± 8.7% with iNAV versus 40.3% ± 10.7% with dNAV, $p = 0.13$) between the two modalities. Vessel sharpness of the LCx was statistically higher with dNAV

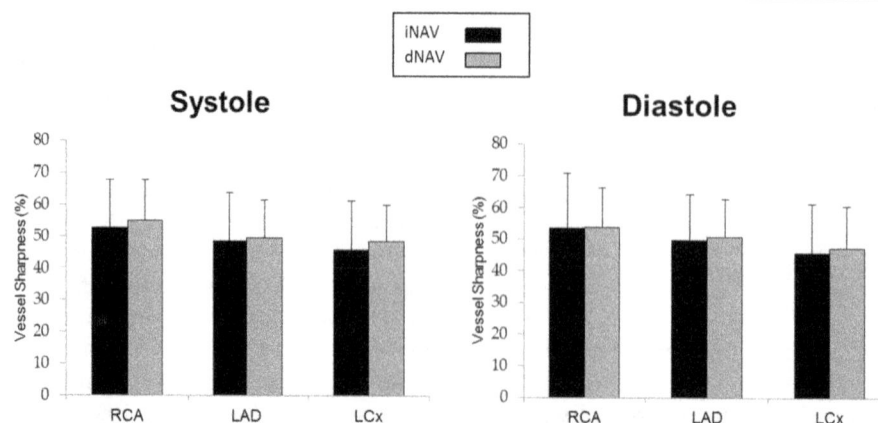

Fig. 4 Coronary Vessel Sharpness in Volunteers. Graphical depiction of average coronary vessel sharpness for all 19 healthy subjects for systolic and diastolic 3D WH bSSFP using iNAV (black bars) and dNAV (grey bars) for motion correction. This shows equivalent sharpness for the two sequences. iNAV = image-navigator; dNAV = diaphragmatic 1D pencil beam navigator; RCA = right coronary artery; LAD = left anterior descending artery; LCx = circumflex artery

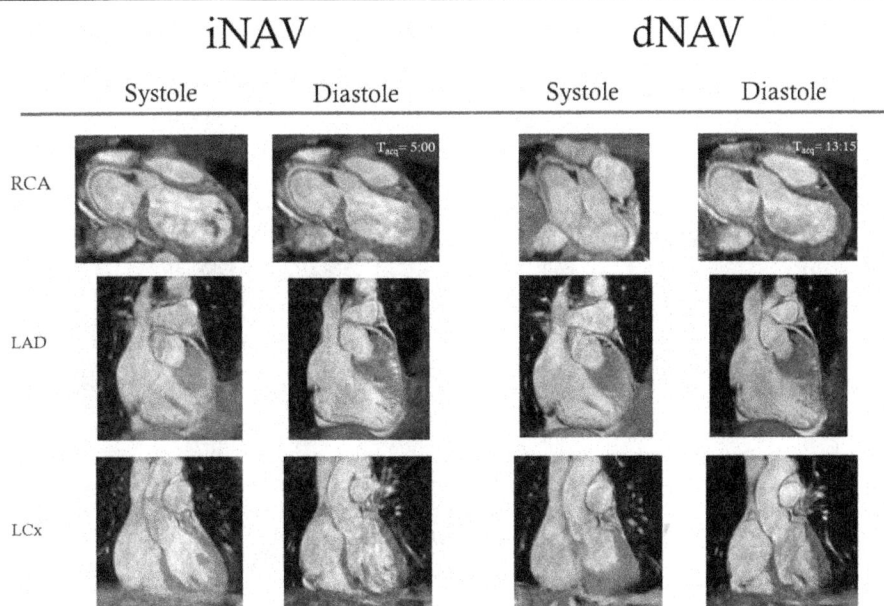

Fig. 5 This figure shows representative reformatted dual-phase 3D WH bSSFP data from one patient obtained with both techniques using "Soapbubble" reformatting [17]. These were the images used for consensus scoring. iNAV = image-navigator; dNAV = diaphragmatic 1D pencil beam navigator; T_{acq} = acquisition time RCA = right coronary artery; LAD = left anterior descending artery; LCx = circumflex artery

for both systole (iNAV mean sharpness of 36.8% ± 9.8% versus 41.0% ± 9.6% with dNAV, $p = 0.007$) and diastole (iNAV mean sharpness of 38.3% ± 9.5% versus 41.7% ± 10.5% with dNAV, $p = 0.04$) (Fig. 6). Visualized length, however, was significantly greater with iNAV for LCx in diastole (mean length of 2.2 ± 1.7 mm with iNAV versus 1.7 ± 1.3 mm with dNAV; $p = 0.04$), LAD in diastole (6.2 ± 3.4 mm with iNAV versus 5.2 ± 3.1 mm with dNAV; $p = 0.02$) and RCA in systole (5.0 ± 3.0 mm with iNAV versus 4.2 ± 2.3 mm with dNAV; $p = 0.01$) (Fig. 7).

There was no statistically significant effect on qualitative image score according to the type of respiratory motion compensation (PB versus iNav. OR = 0.85, 95%CI 0.60, 1.20; $p = 0.36$ phase (systole or diastole) or according to phase imaged (systole vs diastole, OR = 0.94, 95% CI 0.66, 1.32; $p = 0.71$).

In assessing cardiac anatomy, iNAV allowed complete morphological diagnosis in 27/30 patients: there were two failures due to an inability in visualizing the right subclavian artery and one failure due to inability to visualize the left upper pulmonary vein. Representative images from two patients are shown in Fig. 8. These findings are similar when assessing cardiac images obtained with dNAV, where there was a complete morphological diagnosis in 27/30 patients. Two failures were secondary to inability to visualize a pulmonary vein (1 right lower pulmonary vein and 1 right upper pulmonary vein) and one failure secondary to inability to visualize the left subclavian artery. There was overlap of one patient whose images obtained with iNAV did not allow

visualization of the right subclavian artery while images obtained with dNAV did not show the right upper pulmonary vein.

The mean scan time using iNAV was 6:41 ± 2:17 min and 9:57 ± 3:29 min using dNAV, a difference that was statistically significant ($p = 0.0001$). In 24 out of the 30 patients, the scan time was longer using dNAV with the longest scan time using pencil beam lasting 18 min. In contrast, the longest scan time using iNAV was 11:20 min. A comparison of mean scan times for both volunteers and patients between iNAV and dNAV is shown in Fig. 9.

Discussion

The main finding of this study is that the proposed iNAV motion compensation technique for dual phase 3D WH bSSFP significantly reduces scan time compared to the conventional approach in both healthy subjects and patients with congenital heart disease without significantly compromising image quality. This is likely due to the stricter requirement of the dNAV approach that both the systolic and diastolic navigators be in a narrow 5 mm gating window for each cardiac cycle. This is due to the condition for both systolic and diastolic 3D WH bSSFP acquisition to progress at the same rate, leading to a lower total scan efficiency compared to a similar single-phase 3D WH bSSFP with the dNAV technique. In contrast, the iNAV technique with CRUISE gating uses independent gating windows for systole and diastole, and the nominal scan efficiency of 50% is

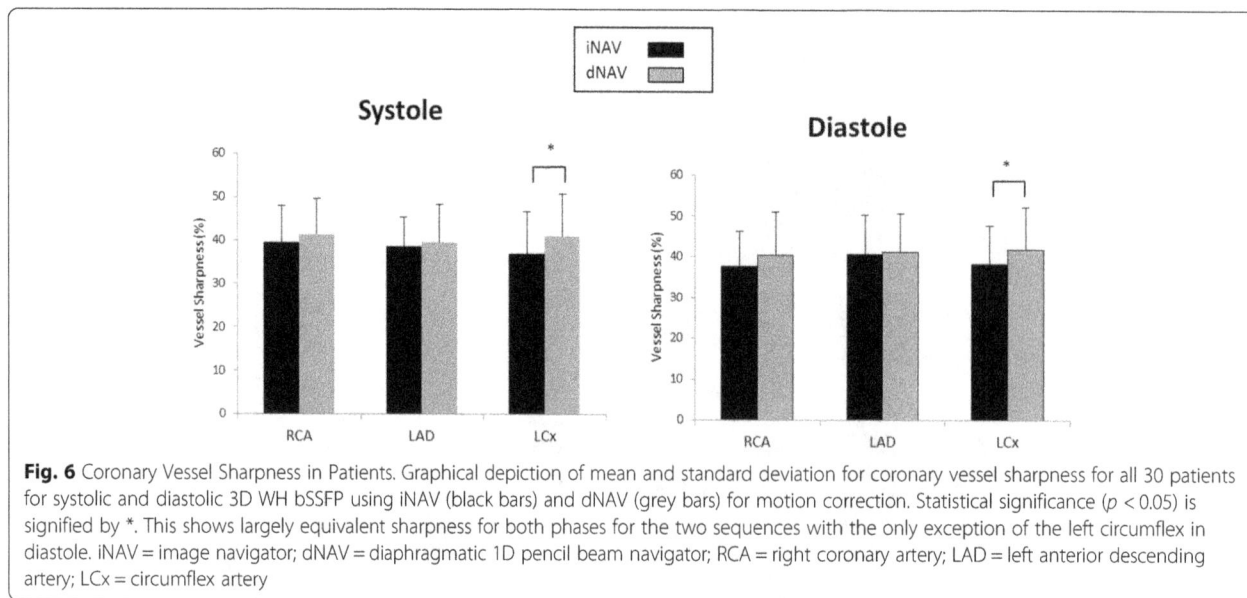

Fig. 6 Coronary Vessel Sharpness in Patients. Graphical depiction of mean and standard deviation for coronary vessel sharpness for all 30 patients for systolic and diastolic 3D WH bSSFP using iNAV (black bars) and dNAV (grey bars) for motion correction. Statistical significance ($p < 0.05$) is signified by *. This shows largely equivalent sharpness for both phases for the two sequences with the only exception of the left circumflex in diastole. iNAV = image navigator; dNAV = diaphragmatic 1D pencil beam navigator; RCA = right coronary artery; LAD = left anterior descending artery; LCx = circumflex artery

therefore also the true scan efficiency and the same as a single-phase 3D WH bSSFP scan. A potential drawback of using independent navigators is that the systolic and diastolic CMRA may be slightly misregistered, although in practice that is of minor importance as the two phases are analyzed separately.

Compared to previous studies using dNAV and iNAV for single-phase 3D WH bSSFP [10, 15], there was no improvement in coronary vessel sharpness using iNAV. This is likely related to the stricter gating criteria for the dNAV technique, as previously mentioned. As cardiac cycles only partially inside the gating window (either systolic or diastolic dNAV navigator) are rejected, these acquisitions tend to be on the periphery of the gating window, leading to a narrower distribution of motion values at the center of the gating window. This may subsequently lead to an improvement in image quality due to the narrower range of motion values in the final image. In comparison, for iNAV using independent systolic and diastolic navigators, the gating efficiency is the same for both single and dual phase 3D WH bSSFP and no change in distribution of motion values is expected. As the iNAV approach failed to yield diagnostic image quality in a few cases, imposing stricter gating criteria should be considered. Conversely, the dNAV approach had to be aborted in two patients due to extremely low gating efficiency while a further three cases yielded non-diagnostic image quality. Further work is required to devise a gating strategy which allows dual

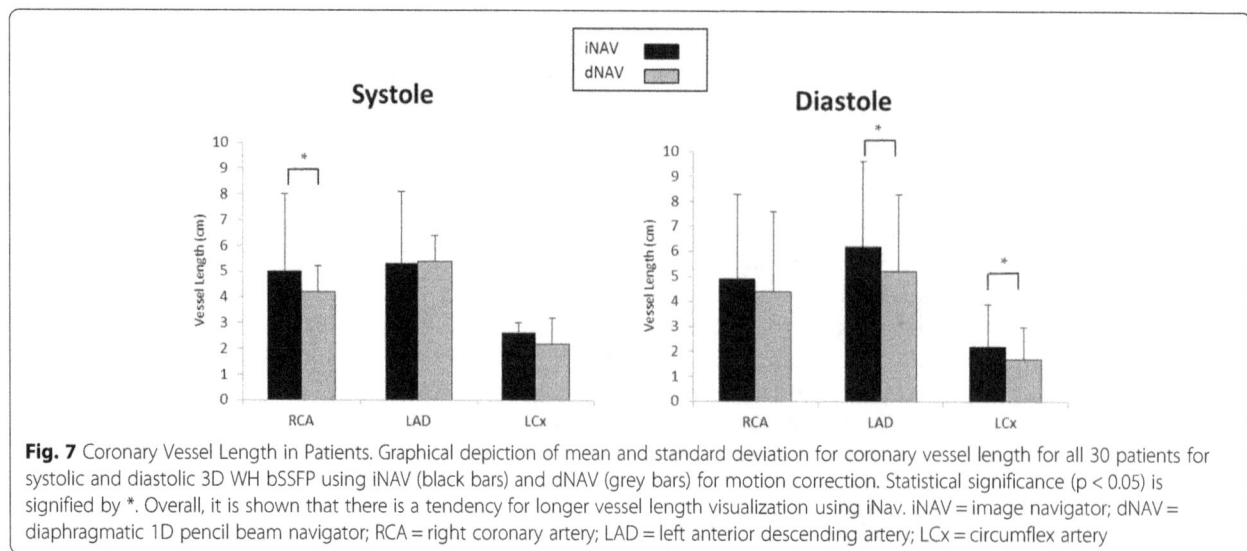

Fig. 7 Coronary Vessel Length in Patients. Graphical depiction of mean and standard deviation for coronary vessel length for all 30 patients for systolic and diastolic 3D WH bSSFP using iNAV (black bars) and dNAV (grey bars) for motion correction. Statistical significance ($p < 0.05$) is signified by *. Overall, it is shown that there is a tendency for longer vessel length visualization using iNav. iNAV = image navigator; dNAV = diaphragmatic 1D pencil beam navigator; RCA = right coronary artery; LAD = left anterior descending artery; LCx = circumflex artery

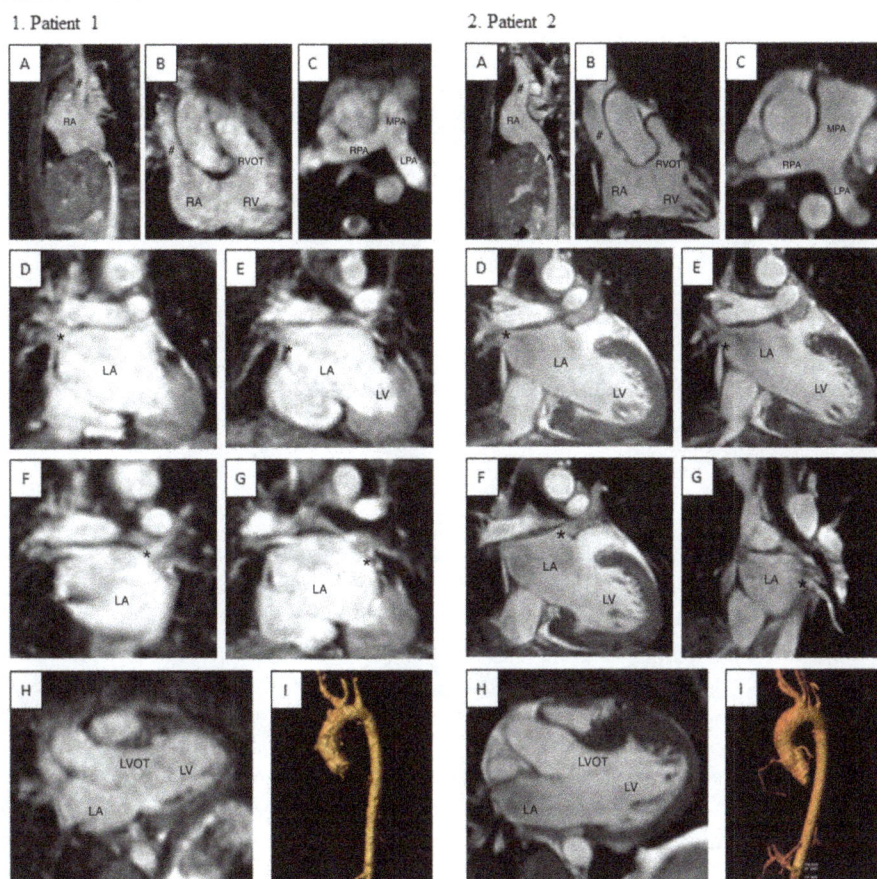

Fig. 8 Representative 3D WH bSSFP images from two patients obtained with iNAV. This figure shows the range of image quality that still allowed complete morphological diagnosis (ie. all structures identified without severe blurring [18]) 1. Collection of pictures from one patient with lower quality. Patient presented with chest pain and bicuspid aortic on echocardiogram with a suspected abnormal left coronary artery origin. Complete morphological diagnosis was possible; however, this collection is a representative of patients with slightly lower quality. 1A. SVC and IVC enter into the RA normally. 1B. SVC entering RA normally, RA to RV connection with RVOT visualized. 1C. Normal branch pulmonary arteries. 1D. Right upper pulmonary vein (*) entering into the LA. 1E. Right lower pulmonary vein (*) entering the LA. 1F. Left upper pulmonary vein (*) entering the LA. 1G. Left lower pulmonary vein (*) entering the LA. 1H. LA to LV connection with LVOT visualized. 1I. Ascending aorta, arch, head and neck vessels and descending aorta. The left carotid artery arises from the trunk of the innominate artery. 2. Higher quality pictures from another patient with hypertrophic cardiomyopathy. Complete morphological diagnosis was also possible in this patient. 2A. SVC and IVC enter into the RA normally. 2B. SVC entering RA normally, RA to RV connection with RVOT visualized. 2C. Normal branch pulmonary arteries. 2D. Right upper pulmonary vein (*) entering the LA. 2E. Right lower pulmonary vein (*) entering the LA. 2F. Left upper pulmonary vein (*) entering the LA. 2G. Left lower pulmonary vein (*) entering the LA. 2H. LA to LV connection with LVOT visualized. 2I. Ascending aorta, aortic arch, head and neck vessels and descending aorta. The left carotid artery and innominate artery arise from a common trunk from the arch. There is also a vertebral artery arising directly from the arch. iNAV = image navigator; SVC = superior vena cava (#); IVC = inferior vena cava (^); RA = right atrium; RV = right ventricle; RVOT = right ventricular outflow tract; MPA = main pulmonary artery; RPA = right pulmonary artery; LPA = left pulmonary artery; pulmonary veins labeled with asterisk (*); LA = left atrium; LV = left ventricle; LVOT = left ventricular outflow tract

phase 3D WH bSSFP with high gating efficiency but adaptable to patient breathing pattern or image quality parameters.

Using the proposed technique of independent navigator references, image quality between iNAV and dNAV was similar overall in both healthy volunteers and in patients with congenital heart disease, with a tendency towards being able to image more of the distal vessel with iNAV. The time needed for dual-phase 3D WH bSSFP image acquisition using iNAV, however, was significantly shorter. A complete cardiac morphological diagnosis was possible in the vast majority of cases. In the three cases in which complete morphological diagnosis was not possible, two failures were due to the missing structure being located outside the shim box.

Our findings further illustrate that 3D whole-heart dual phase imaging is adequate for diagnostic ability in patients with congenital heart disease and although both navigation methods (dNAV and iNAV) produce images similar in quality, the time needed to acquire such images is significantly reduced with iNAV. This

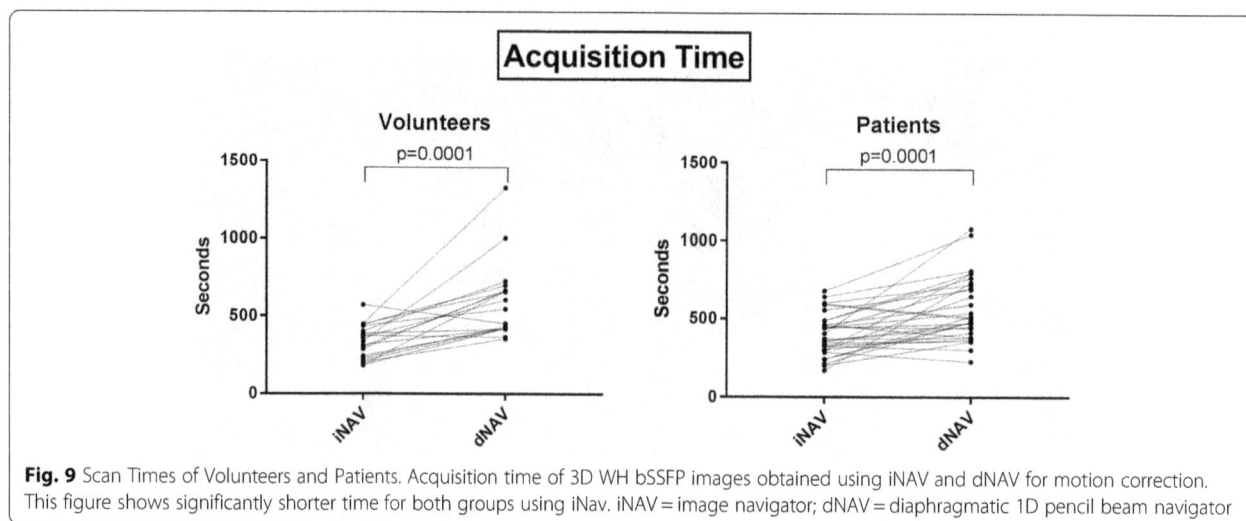

Fig. 9 Scan Times of Volunteers and Patients. Acquisition time of 3D WH bSSFP images obtained using iNAV and dNAV for motion correction. This figure shows significantly shorter time for both groups using iNav. iNAV = image navigator; dNAV = diaphragmatic 1D pencil beam navigator

shortened acquisition time will significantly improve clinical applicability and patient comfort.

In addition to the conventional approach of using a 1-dimensional diaphragmatic navigator (dNAV) and the image-based navigation (iNAV) proposed in our study, there are other strategies to correct for respiratory motion [9]. Another respiratory navigation tool is the so-called "self-navigation". This navigator, like iNAV, measures respiratory-induced motion of the heart directly which obviates the need for a motion model, however, images are acquired as 1-dimensional projections of the FOV, therefore static structures are also included in the navigator image and may reduce the motion estimation performance of the navigator. Self-navigation was recently evaluated for single-phase 3D WH bSSFP in patients with congenital heart disease [19]. Similar to this study, the self-navigation provided diagnostic image quality in 90% of patients, with a mean scan time of close to 10 min. In this study, a head--to-head comparison between self-navigation and dNAV was performed which primarily demonstrated the value of advanced motion compensation to reduce scan time.

Although in our study, the quality of images obtained with iNAV did not reach a statistically significant difference when comparing against those obtained with dNAV, there were multiple subjects with subjectively improved quality and there was a trend to better distal vessel visualization with iNAV. Further work will investigate the reproducibility of this technique.

A limitation of this study is that iNAV used a different correction and gating approach to dNAV. Therefore, it is not possible to assess the relative contribution of correction or gating when comparing iNAV to dNAV. This is due to a technical limitation, which renders iNAV incompatible with the use of a conventional gating window strategy, and the dNAV navigator is similarly incompatible with CRUISE gating.

As previously mentioned [4, 5], a theoretical limitation of dual-phase imaging is the possible reduction of signal to noise ratio because of the acquisition of two cardiac phases during a single cardiac cycle when compared with the signal-to-noise ratio obtained with a single-phase whole-heart sequence. However, if the scan is performed after contrast administration, as is commonly done, then this signal-to-noise ratio penalty is negligible.

Conclusions

In conclusion, we have implemented and evaluated a new approach for dual-phase 3D WH bSSFP using image-based navigation. This approach maintains a high accuracy of respiratory motion tracking, despite the different cardiac motion states of the data acquisition, by employing two independent navigator references. It compares favorably to the conventional dNAV approach in both healthy subjects and patients with congenital heart disease, by providing similar vessel sharpness and allowing complete morphological diagnosis for congenital and pediatric heart disease, while significantly reducing scan time.

Abbreviations

2D: Two-dimensional; 3D WH bSSFP: 3D whole heart balanced steady-state free precession; 3D: Three-dimensional; AVCD: Atrioventricular canal defect; bSSFP: Balanced steady-state free precession; CRUISE: Constant Respiratory efficiency Using Single End-expiratory threshold; dNAV: Diaphragmatic 1D pencil beam navigator; DORV: Double outlet right ventricle; ECG: Electrocardiographic; FH: Foot-head; FOV: Field of view; iNAV: Image-based navigator; LAD: Left anterior descending artery; LCx: Left circumflex artery; LR: Left-right; MRI: Magnetic resonance imaging; RCA: Right coronary artery; ROI: Region of interest; TGA: Transposition of the great arteries; VSD: Ventricular septal defect

Acknowledgements
The authors would like to specifically thank and acknowledge Amanda Potersnak, lead MRI tech, for all of her assistance with study image acquisition and Dr. Song Zhang for his statistical support at UT Southwestern Medical Center Dallas.

Funding
This research has been supported by the British Heart Foundation (PG/15/104/ 31913 and RG/12/1/29262). The Division of Imaging Sciences additionally receives support from the Centre of Excellence in Medical Engineering (funded by the Welcome Trust and EPSRC; grant number WT 088641/Z/09/Z) and the Department of Health through the National Institute for Health Research (NIHR) Biomedical Research Centre award to Guy's and St Thomas' NHS Foundation Trust in partnership with King's College London, and by the NIHR Healthcare Technology Co-operative for Cardiovascular Disease at Guy's and St Thomas' NHS Foundation Trust. The views expressed are those of the author(s) and not necessarily those of the NHS, the NIHR or the Department of Health.

Authors' contributions
TH, MH, GFG and RMB made substantial contributions to conception and design. DM, AD, TH and AT made substantial contributions to acquisition of, analysis and interpretation of data. DM, TH and MH were involved in drafting the manuscript. All authors were involved in the revising of the manuscript critically for important intellectual content. All authors read and approved the final manuscript.

Competing interests
The authors declare that they have no competing interests.

Author details
[1]Department of Pediatrics, Division of Cardiology, UT Southwestern Medical Center Dallas, Dallas, TX, USA. [2]Department of Pediatrics, Division of Cardiology, Children's Health, Children's Medical Center Dallas, Dallas, TX, USA. [3]Departments of Radiology and Biomedical Engineering, University of Texas Southwestern Medical Center, Dallas, TX, USA. [4]Division of Imaging Sciences, King's College London, London, UK. [5]Pontificia Universidad Católica de Chile, Escuela de Ingeniería, Santiago, Chile. [6]Pediatric Cardiology, Children's Health Children's Medical Center of Dallas, 1935 Medical District Drive, Dallas, TX 75235, USA.

References
1. OM W, Martin AJ, Higgins CB. Whole-heart steady-state free precession coronary artery magnetic resonance angiography. Magn Reson Med. 2003; 50(6):1223–8.
2. Greil G, Tandon AA, Silva Vieira M, Hussain T. 3D whole heart imaging for congenital heart disease. Front Pediatr. 2017;5:36.
3. Sorensen TS, Korperich H, Greil GF, et al. Operator-independent isotropic three-dimensional magnetic resonance imaging for morphology in congenital heart disease: a validation study. Circulation. 2004;110(2):163–9.
4. Uribe S, Hussain T, Valverde I, et al. Congenital heart disease in children: coronary MR angiography during systole and diastole with dual cardiac phase whole-heart imaging. Radiology. 2011;260(1):232–40.
5. Hussain T, Lossnitzer D, Bellsham-Revell H, et al. Three-dimensional dual-phase whole-heart MR imaging: clinical implications for congenital heart disease. Radiology. 2012;263(2):547–54.
6. Brittain JH, Hu BS, Wright GA, Meyer CH, Macovski A, Nishimura DG. Coronary angiography with magnetization-prepared T2 contrast. Magn Reson Med. 1995;33(5):689–96.
7. McConnell MV, Khasgiwala VC, Savord BJ, et al. Comparison of respiratory suppression methods and navigator locations for MR coronary angiography. AJR Am J Roentgenol. 1997;168(5):1369–75.
8. Uribe S, Tangchaoren T, Parish V, et al. Volumetric cardiac quantification by using 3D dual-phase whole-heart MR imaging. Radiology. 2008;248(2):606–14.
9. Henningsson M, Botnar RM. Advanced respiratory motion compensation for coronary MR angiography. Sensors (Basel). 2013;13(6):6882–99.
10. Henningsson M, Koken P, Stehning C, Razavi R, Prieto C, Botnar RM. Whole-heart coronary MR angiography with 2D self-navigated image reconstruction. Magn Reson Med. 2012;67(2):437–45.
11. Henningsson M, Smink J, Razavi R, Botnar RM. Prospective respiratory motion correction for coronary MR angiography using a 2D image navigator. Magn Reson Med. 2013;69(2):486–94.
12. Scott AD, Keegan J, Firmin DN. Beat-to-beat respiratory motion correction with near 100% efficiency: a quantitative assessment using high-resolution coronary artery imaging. J Magn Reson Imaging. 2011;29(4):568–8.
13. Wu HH, Gurney PT, Hu BS, Nishimura DG, McConnell MV. Free-breathing multiphase whole-heart coronary MR angiography using image-based navigators and three-dimensional cones imaging. Magn Reson Med. 2013; 69(4):1083–93.
14. Henningsson M, Hussain T, Vieira MS, et al. Whole-heart coronary MR angiography using image-based navigation for the detection of coronary anomalies in adult patients with congenital heart disease. J Magn Reson Imaging. 2016;43(4):947–55.
15. Henningsson M, Smink J, van Ensbergen G, Botnar R. Coronary MR angiography using image-based respiratory motion compensation with inline correction and fixed gating efficiency. Magn Reson Med. 2018;79(1):416–22.
16. Botnar RM, Stuber M, Danias PG, Kissinger KV, Manning WJ. Improved coronary artery definition with T2-weighted, free-breathing, three-dimensional coronary MRA. Circulation. 1999;99:3139–48.
17. Etienne A, Botnar RM, Van Muiswinkel AM, Boesiger P, Manning WJ, Stuber M. "soap-bubble" visualization and quantitative analysis of 3D coronary magnetic resonance angiograms. Magn Reson Med. 2002;48(4):658–66.
18. Makowski MR, Wiethoff AJ, Uribe S, et al. Congenital heart disease: cardiovascular MR imaging by using an intravascular blood pool contrast agent. Radiology. 2011;260(3):680–8.
19. Monney P, Piccini D, Rutz T, et al. Single Centre experience of the application of self navigated 3D whole heart cardiovascular magnetic resonance for the assessment of cardiac anatomy in congenital heart disease. J Cardiovasc Magn Reson. 2015;17:55.

26

Differentiation of orbital lymphoma and idiopathic orbital inflammatory pseudotumor: combined diagnostic value of conventional MRI and histogram analysis of ADC maps

Jiliang Ren[†], Ying Yuan[†], Yingwei Wu and Xiaofeng Tao[*] [ID]

Abstract

Background: The overlap of morphological feature and mean ADC value restricted clinical application of MRI in the differential diagnosis of orbital lymphoma and idiopathic orbital inflammatory pseudotumor (IOIP). In this paper, we aimed to retrospectively evaluate the combined diagnostic value of conventional magnetic resonance imaging (MRI) and whole-tumor histogram analysis of apparent diffusion coefficient (ADC) maps in the differentiation of the two lesions.

Methods: In total, 18 patients with orbital lymphoma and 22 patients with IOIP were included, who underwent both conventional MRI and diffusion weighted imaging before treatment. Conventional MRI features and histogram parameters derived from ADC maps, including mean ADC (ADC_{mean}), median ADC (ADC_{median}), skewness, kurtosis, 10th, 25th, 75th and 90th percentiles of ADC (ADC_{10}, ADC_{25}, ADC_{75}, ADC_{90}) were evaluated and compared between orbital lymphoma and IOIP. Multivariate logistic regression analysis was used to identify the most valuable variables for discriminating. Differential model was built upon the selected variables and receiver operating characteristic (ROC) analysis was also performed to determine the differential ability of the model.

Results: Multivariate logistic regression showed ADC_{10} ($P = 0.023$) and involvement of orbit preseptal space ($P = 0.029$) were the most promising indexes in the discrimination of orbital lymphoma and IOIP. The logistic model defined by ADC_{10} and involvement of orbit preseptal space was built, which achieved an AUC of 0.939, with sensitivity of 77.30% and specificity of 94.40%.

Conclusions: Conventional MRI feature of involvement of orbit preseptal space and ADC histogram parameter of ADC_{10} are valuable in differential diagnosis of orbital lymphoma and IOIP.

Keywords: Orbit, Lymphoma, Inflammatory pseudotumor, Diffusion weighted imaging, Histogram

* Correspondence: cjr.taoxiaofeng@vip.163.com
[†]Equal contributors
Department of Radiology, Shanghai Ninth People's Hospital, Shanghai Jiao Tong University School of Medicine, Shanghai, China

Background

Orbital lymphoma and idiopathic orbital inflammatory pseudotumor (IOIP) represent the most common lympho-proliferative disorders affecting the orbit [1], accounting nearly 20% of all orbital mass lesions [1–3]. Most orbital lymphomas are low-grade neoplastic lesions, and the most frequently observed subtype is mucosa-associated lymphoid tissue (MALT) lymphoma [4]. IOIP is a non-infective inflammatory condition, which often manifests borderline morphological characters [1]. Lymphoma is amenable to radiation therapy, and combined chemotherapy for high-grade and disseminated lesions, whereas IOIP responds to steroid therapy or immune-suppressive therapy [3, 4]. Therefore, the discrimination of lymphoma and IOIP is essential for clinical treatment. However, dacryoadenitis and diffuse inflammation subtypes of IOIPs are easily misdiagnosed as lymphoma because of similar clinical and imaging findings [5]. Although fine-needle aspiration is the gold standard for diagnosis, it is often limited in technically challenge in the lesions located in the far posterior orbit [6]. In addition, diffuse lymphocytic infiltrative IOIP, as the most common pathological subtype, could not be easily differentiated pathologically from orbital lymphoma [6].

Previous studies have indicated some MRI features, such as signal intensity on T2W sequence, presence of flow void sign, and degree of contrast enhancement, have the potential to discriminate between lymphoma and IOIP [5, 7, 8]. Nevertheless, overall diagnostic efficacy of morphological features was still limited [9]. In addition, the qualitative assessment of MRI features may be observer-dependent. Diffusion weighted imaging (DWI), with the apparent diffusion coefficient (ADC) value, has been used increasingly in the quantitative discrimination of lymphoma and IOIP [8, 10]. Orbital lymphoma showed lower mean ADC value than IOIP, although the overlap of mean ADC value still existed and restricted clinical application. Additionally, the mean ADC value was usually obtained from manually drawing regions of interest (ROI), with potential measurement sampling error and subjective bias. Furthermore, the mean ADC value could not represent the heterogeneity of the whole tumor. Whole-tumor histogram analysis of the ADC maps could generate several diffusion parameters, which have been shown superior efficacy than mean ADC value in discriminating and grading tumors [11–13]. By selecting volume of interest (VOI) covering the whole tumor, the histogram analysis can decrease the sampling errors [14]. Recently, whole-tumor histogram analysis of ADC maps has been demonstrated to accurately diagnose orbital masses [15, 16]. However these studies included a variety of malignant orbital tumors, such as lymphoma, adenoid cystic carcinoma, and metastases.

Therefore, the purpose of this study was to investigate the independent and combined value of conventional MRI features and whole-tumor histogram parameters derived from ADC maps in the differentiation of orbital lymphoma from IOIP.

Methods

Patients

The Institutional Review Board of Shanghai Ninth People's Hospital approved this retrospective study and the requirement for informed consent was waived. The following criteria were adopted for patient selection: 1) The mass was primary orbital tumor; 2) The patients underwent both conventional MRI and DWI scan before treatment; 3) Masses with short axis ≥ 10 mm; 4) The MR images could be acquired and interpreted. Through a comprehensive search of our institutional medical report database from January 2012 to September 2016, we identified 18 patients with orbital lymphoma (mean age, 67 years; range, 45–94 years) and 22 patients with IOIP (mean age, 54 years; range, 8–76 years). The final diagnoses were made upon histopathological results in 36 patients, and upon response to corticosteroid treatment and minimum 1-year follow-up in 4 patients with presumed IOIPs. 16 cases of lymphomas were MALT lymphomas, and the other 2 cases were diffuse large B-cell lymphomas. Myositis and optic perineuritis subtypes of IOIPs were not included in the present study because they demonstrated characteristic findings on conventional MRI, which were easy to be differentiated from lymphoma. In the current study, the patients with IOIPs included dacryoadenitis subtype ($n = 17$), tumor subtype ($n = 3$), and diffuse inflammation subtypes ($n = 2$).

MRI examination

All MRI examinations were performed on a 3.0 T scanner (Magnetom Verio 3.0 T; Siemens, Erlangen, Germany) with a 12-channel head coil. The conventional MRI protocol for orbital lesions include axial T1-weigthed images (repetition time [TR]/echo time [TE], 620/9 ms), axial fat-saturated T2-weighted images (TR/TE, 4000/75 ms), coronal T2-weighted images (TR/TE, 4000/108 ms), as well as axial, coronal and sagittal contrast enhanced fat-saturated T1-weighted images (TR/TE, 550/9 ms). For contrast-enhanced T1-weighted image, a standard dosage of 0.1 mmol/kg of gadopentetate dimeglumine (Magnevist; Schering, Berlin, Germany) was administrated.

Before contrast medium administration, diffusion-weighted images in the axial plane were acquired using a single-shot spin echo echo-planar imaging (SS-SE-EPI) sequence. The parameters were used as followings: TR/TE, 4000/100 ms; section thickness, 3 mm; flip angle (FA), 90°; field of view (FOV), 200 × 200 mm; matrix, 384 × 384; b, 0 and 700 s/mm^2.

Image analysis

Qualitative MRI analysis was performed by two radiologists with 3 and 7 years of experience in head and neck imaging, who were blinded to the clinical information and diagnosis. Consensus between the 2 readers was reached by virtue of an additional reading session. The following characteristics were evaluated and recorded from conventional MR images: 1) laterality (unilateral or bilateral), 2) margin (well-defined or ill-defined), 3) location (intraconal, extraconal, intra and extraconal), 4) signal intensity on T2-weighted image (iso- or hypointense; relative to cerebral cortex), 5) degree of contrast enhancement (moderate or significant; relative to normal ocular muscle), 6) involvement of orbit preseptal space (the mass located in or extending to orbit preseptal space) 7) presence of "flow void sign" on T2-weighted image (referring to a signal void of a vessel within the lesions), 8) findings indicative of sinusitis (thickness of paranasal mucosal exceeds 4 mm or fluid level or the presence of a retention cyst at paranasal cavity [17]).

Quantitative evaluation of DWI was performed with FireVoxel software (CAI^{2}R, New York University, NY, USA) by two radiologists independently. For each case, volume of interest (VOI) was outlined on all sections where the tumor can be visualized. T2-weighted and contrast-enhanced images were used for reference to avoid necrotic components and surrounding tissues. In addition, it should be noted that ADC measurements might be affected by image distortions due to susceptibility artifacts. Therefore the marginal part of tumor was left out to avoid the influence of these artifacts. In patient with bilateral lesions, the larger lesion was analyzed. After the VOI of the lesion was determined, voxel-based ADC map was calculated with standard monoexponential fit $S = S_0 \cdot exp.(-b \cdot ADC)$, in which S refers to the signal intensity with motion probing gradients applied and S_0 refers to the signal intensity with $b = 0$ s/mm^2. Then a histogram of ADC values with a bin width of 10^{-3} mm^2/s was generated, and concurrently the following histogram parameters were obtained including ADC_{mean}, ADC_{median}, skewness, and kurtosis. In addition, four cumulative histogram parameters were calculated including the 10th (ADC_{10}), 25th (ADC_{25}), 75th (ADC_{75}), 90th (ADC_{90}) percentiles of ADC values. To ensure intra-reader reproducibility, the DWI data was analyzed again with a minimum interval of 1 month. The average of the two measurement results was adopted for statistical analysis.

Statistical analysis

Univariate analysis was performed for each qualitative and quantitative variable in an attempt to elucidate the ability of each variable for discriminating between lymphoma and IOIP. The x^2 testing (the Fisher exact testing where appropriate) was used to compare the frequency distribution of each qualitative MRI feature. Mann–Whitney U test was used to compare all ADC histogram parameters. Multivariate logistic regression analysis was used to identify significant independent variables in the differentiation of lymphoma and IOIP. Receiver operating characteristic (ROC) curves were used to assess the diagnostic utility of identified variables and diagnostic models. Intra- and inter-observer variability of ADC histogram analysis was tested by calculating intraclass correlation coefficients (ICC). Intra-observer reproducibility was computed from the two measurements of the first reader. Inter-reader reproducibility was computed from the first measurement of reader 1 and the measurement of reader 2. Agreement was interpreted according to ICC as: < 0.40, poor; 0.41–0.60, moderate; 0.61–0.80, good; ≥0.81, excellent [18]. A P level of less than 0.05 was considered as a statistical significance. Statistical analysis was performed using SPSS (SPSS Version 19.0, Chicago, IL, USA) and MedCalc (MedClac Version 11.4, Mariakerke, Belgium).

Results

Four qualitative variables were found significant in the univariate analysis for differentiating orbital lymphoma from IOIP, including tumor margin, degree of contrast enhancement, involvement of orbit preseptal space and findings suggestive of sinusitis. The characteristics of well-defined margin ($P = 0.003$), moderate degree of contrast enhancement ($P = 0.007$) and involvement of orbit preseptal space ($P = 0.01$) were more frequently seen in orbital lymphomas. Findings suggestive of sinusitis ($P = 0.031$) were more common in IOIPs. The qualitative MRI features of lymphoma and IOIP are listed and compared in Table 1.

Based on the intraclass correlation coefficient (ICC), assessment of intra- and interobserver variability in ADC measurements demonstrated good to excellent agreement with intraobserver ICC values ranging from 0.774 to 0.854 and interobserver ICC values ranging from 0.782 to 0.870, respectively. The comparison of the ADC histogram parameters between lymphoma and IOIP is shown in Table 2. The ADC_{mean}, ADC_{median}, ADC_{10}, ADC_{25}, ADC_{75}, and ADC_{90} were significantly lower in orbital lymphoma ($P < 0.001$), whereas kurtosis was significantly higher in lymphoma ($P = 0.023$), when compared to IOIP. There was no significant difference in the skewness between the two groups. The representative cases are shown in Figs. 1 and 2. By generating and comparing the ROC curve of each histogram parameter, we found that ADC_{10} achieved the highest area under the curve (AUC) of 0.899 in the differentiation of orbital lymphoma from IOIP. Considering of collinearity between the ADC histogram parameters, only the

Table 1 Frequency Distribution of Qualitative MRI Features

Qualitative Feature	Orbital Lymphoma ($n = 18$)	IOIP ($n = 22$)	P value
Laterality			0.090
Unilateral	15	12	
Bilateral	3	10	
Margin			0.003
Well-defined	16	9	
Ill-defined	2	13	
Location			0.464
Extraconal	12	17	
Intra and extraconal	6	4	
Intraconal	0	1	
Signal intensity on T2WI			0.125
Iso	12	9	
Hypo	6	13	
Degree of contrast enhancement			0.007
Moderate	10	3	
Significant	8	19	
Involvement of orbit preseptal space			0.01
Yes	13	6	
No	5	16	
Presence of flow void sign on T2WI			0.761
Yes	8	11	
No	10	11	
Findings suggestive of sinusitis			0.031
Yes	5	14	
No	13	8	

The signal intensity on T2WI was compared with that of cerebral cortex. On contrast enhanced T1WI, the similar enhancement to normal ocular muscle was viewed as significant contrast enhancement

Table 2 Differences of Histogram Parameters between Lymphomas and IOIPs

Histogram parameter	Orbital lymphoma	IOIP	P value
Mean	0.719 ± 0.216	1.131 ± 0.317	< 0.001
Median	0.686 ± 0.202	1.099 ± 0.332	< 0.001
ADC_{10}	0.463 ± 0.150	0.794 ± 0.244	< 0.001
ADC_{25}	0.562 ± 0.163	0.923 ± 0.275	< 0.001
ADC_{75}	0.832 ± 0.269	1.305 ± 0.384	< 0.001
ADC_{90}	1.005 ± 0.336	1.519 ± 0.430	< 0.001
Skewness	1.314 ± 1.042	0.820 ± 0.737	0.135
Kurtosis	4.959 ± 6.208	1.829 ± 2.923	0.024

Data are presented as mean ± standard deviation. Unit for ADC value is 10^{-3} mm^2/s. ADC_n, nth percentile value of cumulative ADC histogram

parameter with the best differential performance was adopted for further multivariate logistic regression analysis. The diagnostic performance of histogram parameters is shown in Table 3.

Histogram and conventional MR parameters, including ADC_{10}, margin, degree of contrast enhancement, involvement of orbit preseptal space and findings suggestive of sinusitis, were entered into a multivariate logistic regression model. Multivariate logistic regression identified ADC_{10} ($P = 0.023$) and involvement of orbit preseptal space ($P = 0.029$) as significant independent variables for discrimination. By performing the ROC analysis, we found the combined model (AUC, 0.939; sensitivity, 77.30%; specificity, 94.40%) defined by these two parameters achieved a significantly higher AUC ($P = 0.0017$)

than morphological feature of involvement of orbit preseptal space alone (AUC, 0.725; sensitivity, 72.70%; specificity, 72.20%). However, no significant difference of AUC was detected between combined model and ADC_{10} ($P = 0.294$). ROC curves of ADC_{10}, involvement of orbit preseptal space and combined model are shown in Fig. 3.

Discussion

Our primary results demonstrated that involvement of orbit preseptal space and ADC_{10} were the most significant independent variables for discriminating orbital lymphoma from IOIP. To our knowledge, our study was the first to evaluate the combined diagnostic value of conventional MRI and ADC histogram for the differentiation of the two entities.

With respect to conventional MRI features, we found involvement of orbit preseptal space was more frequently observed in orbital lymphomas (13/18) than IOIPs (6/22). Akansel et al. [5] reported nearly half of orbit lymphomas were located in conjunctiva and Giovanni et al. [4] detected that eyelid was involved in 35% of orbital lymphomas. Generally orbital lymphomas are originated from lymphoid tissues, which are confined in eyelid, conjunctiva and lcarimal gland, while IOIPs are in nature inflammatory condition which could arise from elsewhere without lymphoid tissues, such as ocular muscle, orbit fat and optic nerve, without anterior preseptal involvement [3]. Previous studies have shown an extension of inflammatory changes to the mucosa of paranasal cavities in benign orbital lymphoproliferative disorders [8, 9, 19]. We also found that imaging findings indicative of sinusitis were more commonly seen in IOIP (14/22) than orbital lymphoma (5/18). We speculated that both of IOIP and paranasal sinusitis could be the clinical manifestation of idiopathic inflammation involving different structures. In addition, significant enhancement was observed more frequently in IOIP in the current study. Haradome et al. [8] reported that contrast

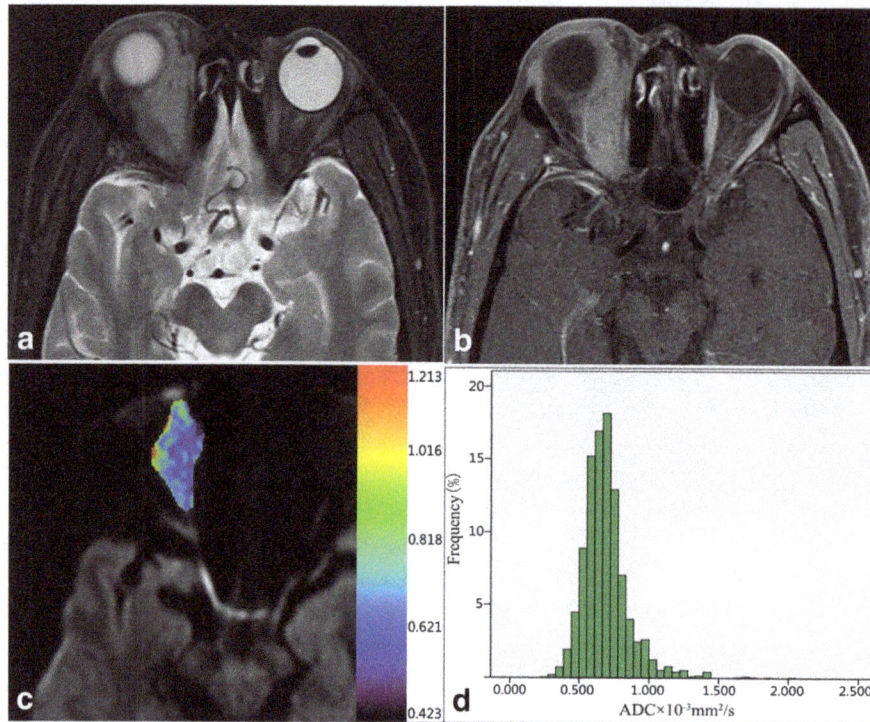

Fig. 1 A male patient with MALT lymphoma. Axial fat-saturated T2W image **a** shows a well-defined isointense mass involving intra and extraconal space and extending to the orbit preseptal space. Axial contrast enhanced T1W image **b** demonstrates homogenous moderate enhancement, lower than that of extraocular muscles. Pixel-by-pixel colored ADC map **c** was obtained and then embedded with the axial DWI. The corresponding ADC histogram from VOI **d** shows a top peak and a slight tail on the right. Whole-tumor mean ADC was 0.692×10^{-3} mm^2/s, ADC_{10} was 0.520×10^{-3} mm^2/s, skewness was 1.81, and kurtosis was 7.51

enhancement ratio of IOIP was significantly higher than that of orbital lymphoma, suggesting the hypervascular nature of the former. These qualitative characteristics could provide valuable information for the differentiation of orbital lymphoma and IOIP. Previously some investigators revealed that the presence of flow void sign on T2WI was more easily observed in IOIP than lymphoma [8]. However, we found no significant difference in the presence of a vessel signal void on T2WI between the two entities, which might be attributed to the sample difference and low reproducibility of qualitative MRI evaluation.

Besides morphological MR findings, significantly lower mean ADC value in orbital lymphoma than IOIP has been demonstrated in prior investigations [8, 10, 20]. High cellularity and enlarged nuclei of orbital lymphoma lead to the relative reduction in extracellular and intracellular diffusion spaces and corresponding decreases ADC value. On the other hand, interstitial edematous change in IOIP gives rise to increase ADC, promoting a significant difference in the ADC value than lymphoma. However, mean ADC value ignored the heterogeneity of the tumors. In fact, overlap exists between average ADC value of orbital lymphoma and IOIP [9, 20].

Being capable to measure the distribution frequency of ADC values as a marker of structural heterogeneity and complexity, ADC histogram analysis has been gaining increasing clinical adoption for differential diagnosis of benign and malignant abnormalities [16, 21], and assessment of tumor grade [11, 22, 23]. In the current study, we observed ADC_{10} had a better performance than ADC_{mean} in the differentiation. Previous studies have reported low percentiles of ADC performed better in classification and grading of tumor than high percentiles [21, 24]. Rozenberg et al. [22] suggested that ADC_{0-10} metric achieved greatly superior performance in the differentiation of low- from high-Gleason score prostate tumors. Kierans et al. [24] revealed ADC_{10} allowed for the accurate prediction of malignant endometrial lesions, while ADC_{mean} did not. Recently, Xu et al. [15, 16] reported ADC_{10} could predict malignant orbital tumors with a higher AUC than ADC_{mean}. Given our similar results in the differentiation of orbital lymphoma and IOIP, it is possible that low percentiles of ADC truly better reflect the presence of densely packed solid components within tumor tissues. The high percentile of ADC value may be easily vulnerable to the cystic or necrotic components. In clinical, small areas of microcystic changes

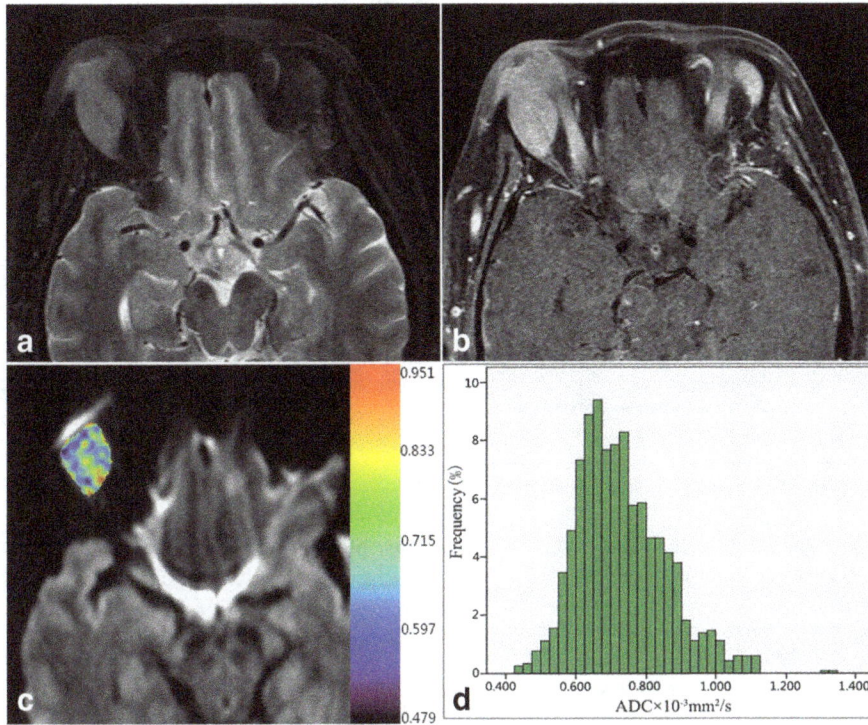

Fig. 2 A female patient with idiopathic orbital inflammatory pseudotumor. Axial fat-saturated T2W image **a** shows a well-defined isointense mass in lacrimal fossa. Axial contrast enhanced T1W image **b** demonstrates significant enhancement, similar to that of extraocular muscles. Pixel-by-pixel colored ADC map **c** was obtained and then embedded with the axial DWI. The corresponding ADC histogram from VOI **d** a relatively flat peak and a slight tail on the right. Whole-tumor ADC_{mean} was 0.730×10^{-3} mm^2/s, ADC_{10} was 0.590×10^{-3} mm^2/s, skewness was 0.73, and kurtosis was 0.80

are usually failed to be excluded from region of interests because of limitation of visual detection, which may affect the accuracy of ADC measurement. Therefore, low percentiles of ADC seemed to be more effective in discriminating the two lesions with distinct compactness.

In addition, we found significantly greater kurtosis in orbital lymphomas than IOIPs. This might be attributed to the homogeneity of orbital lymphomas. Pathologically, orbital lymphoma consists of monomorphous sheets of lymphocyte, which would appear as a steep peak in histogram [7]. In contrast, IOIP often shows polymorphous inflammatory reaction comprising mature lymphocytes,

plasma cells, eosinophils and varying amounts of fibrous stroma [7]. However, there was no significant difference in skewness between orbital lymphomas and IOIPs. Both showed positive skewness. Skewness reflects the asymmetry of the histogram distribution. Positive skewness indicates the majority of voxel values accumulating toward the lower end of the histogram [24, 25]. The visual necrotic and cystic areas with relatively higher ADC values were excluded from VOIs, which could interpret positive skewness in both groups.

With the combined qualitative MRI variable and ADC_{10}, diagnostic model achieved a higher AUC and

Table 3 Diagnostic Performance of Each Histogram parameter

Histogram parameter	Cutoff value	Sensitivity	Specitivity	AUC
Mean	0.879	72.70%	94.40%	0.871(0.727–0.956)
Median	0.834	72.70%	94.40%	0.872(0.729–0.957)
ADC_{10}	0.535	86.40%	83.30%	0.899(0.762–0.972)
ADC_{25}	0.718	72.70%	94.40%	0.895(0.757–0.970)
ADC_{75}	1.097	72.70%	94.40%	0.872 (0.729–0.957)
ADC_{90}	1.280	68.40%	93.70%	0.851(0.703–0.944)
Kurtosis	1.976	72.70%	72.20%	0.710(0.545–0.842)

Data in parentheses indicate 95% confidence intervals. Unit for ADC value is 10^{-3} mm^2/s. ADC_n, nth percentile value of cumulative ADC histogram; AUC, area under the ROC curve

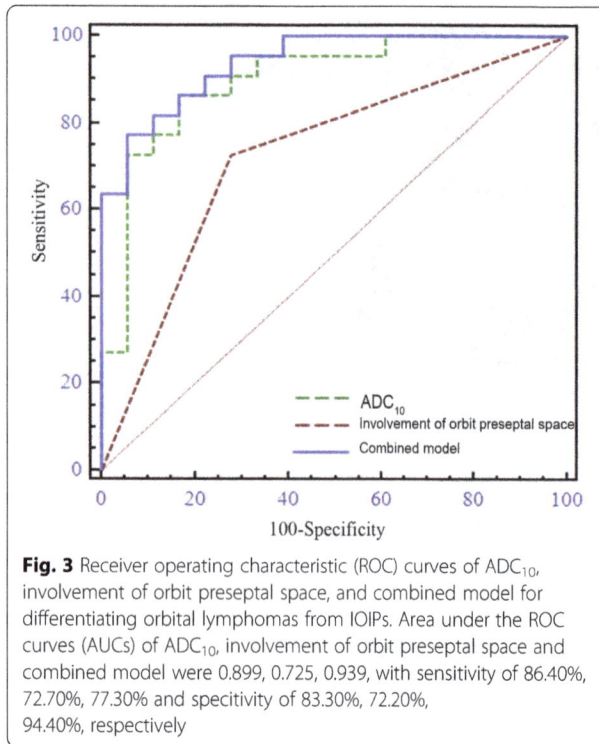

Fig. 3 Receiver operating characteristic (ROC) curves of ADC_{10}, involvement of orbit preseptal space, and combined model for differentiating orbital lymphomas from IOIPs. Area under the ROC curves (AUCs) of ADC_{10}, involvement of orbit preseptal space and combined model were 0.899, 0.725, 0.939, with sensitivity of 86.40%, 72.70%, 77.30% and specivity of 83.30%, 72.20%, 94.40%, respectively

specificity than using either alone in the differentiation. The optimal specificity would enhance our diagnostic confidence, which is necessary for the prompt determination of a therapy plan and doctor-patient communication. However, significant difference of AUC between combined model and ADC_{10} was not observed. Further studies with a larger sample size would be needed to validate our results.

Most quantitative DWI studies of orbital tumors have been based on 2-dimensional region of interest (ROI) placed on a representative slice of the tumor [20, 26]. In the present study, we used VOIs that covered the whole lesions. This method could allow comprehensive measurement, avoiding sample bias from selection of a localized area of the tumor [22]. Given that the histogram parameters, such as skewness and kurtosis, reflect the cumulative distribution of the ADC values, it would be rational to use whole-tumor VOIs rather than localized ROIs for analysis. Furthermore, the good to excellent intra and inter-observer reliabilities based on intraclass correlation coefficients indicated the reproducibility of this measurement method, which will facilitate further clinical application of histogram analysis of ADC maps.

Our study had several limitations. First, it was a retrospective study with relatively small amount of patients, which may contribute to the inconspicuous difference in the differential utility between combined model and ADC_{10}. Secondly, although cases with severe susceptibility artifacts have been excluded, slight image distortion

might still exists in some images imperceptible with naked eye. Further improvement of the imaging quality of DWI would be essential for the study of orbital lesions. Turbo field echo with diffusion-sensitised driven-equilibrium preparation (DSDE-TFE) technique and half-Fourier acquired single-shot turbo spin-echo (HASTE) DWI sequence would be feasible to reduce these artifacts [27, 28]. Thirdly, we adopted b value of 700 s/mm^2 for DWI. In fact, b values of 800 or 1000s/mm^2 was more commonly used in previous orbit studies. The threshold values of ADC histogram parameters obtained in the present study might not be applicable for other studies that used b = 800 or 1000s/mm^2. Moreover, we did not discuss dynamic contrast enhanced magnetic resonance imaging (DCE-MRI) in the current study, which is approved to be helpful for differential diagnosis of orbital lesions [9]. Only conventional contrast enhanced MR images were available in the present study. Further study combining histogram parameters derived from DWI and DCE-MRI would be worth to conduct.

Conclusion

ADC_{10} and involvement of orbit preseptal space were significant independent variables for differentiating orbital lymphoma from IOIP. Histogram analysis of ADC maps demonstrates the heterogeneity of the lesions, which can provide additional and valuable information for the diagnosis of the two entities.

Abbreviations
ADC: Apparent diffusion coefficient; AUC: Area under the ROC curve; DWI: Diffusion weighted imaging; ICC: Intraclass correlation coefficient; IOIP: Idiopathic orbital inflammatory pseudotumor; MALT: Mucosa-associated lymphoid tissue; MRI: Magnetic resonance imaging; ROC: Receiver operating characteristic; ROI: Region of interest; VOI: Volume of interest

Acknowledgements
Not Applicable.

Funding
Not Applicable.

Authors' contributions
XT and JR conceived and designed the study. JR, YY and YW collected the data. JR and YY analyzed the data and wrote the paper. All authors read and approved the final manuscript for publication.

Competing interests
The authors declare that they have no competing interests.

References

1. Li EY, Yuen HK, Cheuk W. Lymphoproliferative Disease of the orbit. Asia Pac J Ophthalmol (Phila). 2015;4(2):106–11.
2. Watkins LM, Carter KD, Nerad JA. Ocular adnexal lymphoma of the extraocular muscles: case series from the University of Iowa and review of the literature. Ophthalmic Plast Reconstr Surg. 2011;27(6):471–6.
3. Ding ZX, Lip G, Chong V. Idiopathic orbital pseudotumour. Clin Radiol. 2011; 66(9):886–92.
4. Gerbino G, Boffano P, Benech R, Baietto F, Gallesio C, Arcuri F, et al. Orbital lymphomas: clinical and radiological features. J Craniomaxillofac Surg. 2014; 42(5):508–12.
5. Akansel G, Hendrix L, Erickson BA, Demirci A, Papke A, Arslan A, et al. MRI patterns in orbital malignant lymphoma and atypical lymphocytic infiltrates. Eur J Radiol. 2005;53(2):175–81.
6. Yan J, Wu Z, Li Y. The differentiation of idiopathic inflammatory pseudotumor from lymphoid tumors of orbit: analysis of 319 cases. Orbit. 2004;23(4):245–54.
7. Cytryn AS, Putterman AM, Schneck GL, Beckman E, Valvassori GE. Predictability of magnetic resonance imaging in differentiation of orbital lymphoma from orbital inflammatory syndrome. Ophthal Plast Reconstr Surg. 1997;13(2):129–34.
8. Haradome K, Haradome H, Usui Y, Ueda S, Kwee TC, Saito K, et al. Orbital lymphoproliferative disorders (OLPDs): value of MR imaging for differentiating orbital lymphoma from benign OPLDs. AJNR Am J Neuroradiol. 2014;35(10):1976–82.
9. Xu XQ, Hu H, Liu H, Wu JF, Cao P, Shi HB, et al. Benign and malignant orbital lymphoproliferative disorders: differentiating using multiparametric MRI at 3.0T. J Magn Reson Imaging. 2017;45(1):167–76.
10. Politi LS, Forghani R, Godi C, Resti AG, Ponzoni M, Bianchi S, et al. Ocular adnexal lymphoma: diffusion-weighted mr imaging for differential diagnosis and therapeutic monitoring. Radiology. 2010;256(2):565–74.
11. Woo S, Cho JY, Kim SY, Kim SH. Histogram analysis of apparent diffusion coefficient map of diffusion-weighted MRI in endometrial cancer: a preliminary correlation study with histological grade. Acta Radiol. 2013; 55(10):1270–7.
12. Brendle C, Martirosian P, Schwenzer NF, Kaufmann S, Kruck S, Kramer U, et al. Diffusion-weighted imaging in the assessment of prostate cancer: comparison of zoomed imaging and conventional technique. Eur J Radiol. 2016;85(5):893–900.
13. Just N. Improving tumour heterogeneity MRI assessment with histograms. Br J Cancer. 2014;111(12):2205–13.
14. Ryu YJ, Choi SH, Park SJ, Yun TJ, Kim JH, Sohn CH. Glioma: application of whole-tumor texture analysis of diffusion-weighted imaging for the evaluation of tumor heterogeneity. PLoS One. 2014;9(9):e108335.
15. Xu XQ, Hu H, Su GY, Liu H, Hong XN, Shi HB, et al. Utility of histogram analysis of ADC maps for differentiating orbital tumors. Diagn Interv Radiol. 2016;22(2):161–7.
16. Xu XQ, Hu H, Su GY, Zhang L, Liu H, Hong XN, et al. Orbital indeterminate lesions in adults: Combined Magnetic Resonance Morphometry and Histogram Analysis of Apparent Diffusion Coefficient Maps for Predicting Malignancy. Acad Radiol. 2016;23(2):200–8.
17. Bhattacharyya N. The role of CT and MRI in the diagnosis of chronic rhinosinusitis. Curr Allergy Asthma Rep. 2010;10(3):171–4.
18. Crewson PE. Reader agreement studies. AJR Am J Roentgenol. 2005;184(5): 1391–7.
19. Li J, Ge X, Ma JM. Relationship between dacryoadenitis subtype of idiopathic orbital inflammatory pseudotumor and paranasal sinusitis. Int J Ophthalmol. 2016;9(3):444–7.
20. Fatima Z, Ichikawa T, Ishigame K, Motosugi U, Waqar AB, Hori M, et al. Orbital masses: the usefulness of diffusion-weighted imaging in lesion categorization. Clin Neuroradiol. 2014;24(2):129–34.
21. Takahashi M, Kozawa E, Tanisaka M, Hasegawa K, Yasuda M, Sakai F. Utility of histogram analysis of apparent diffusion coefficient maps obtained using 3.0T MRI for distinguishing uterine carcinosarcoma from endometrial carcinoma. J Magn Reson Imaging. 2016;43(6):1301–7.
22. Rozenberg R, Thornhill RE, Flood TA, Hakim SW, Lim C, Schieda N. Whole-tumor quantitative apparent diffusion coefficient histogram and texture analysis to predict Gleason score upgrading in intermediate-risk 3 + 4 = 7 prostate cancer. AJR Am J Roentgenol. 2016;206(4):775–82.
23. Kang Y, Choi SH, Kim YJ, Kim KG, Sohn CH, Kim JH, et al. Gliomas: histogram analysis of apparent diffusion coefficient maps with standard- or high-b-value diffusion-weighted MR imaging–correlation with tumor grade. Radiology. 2011;261(3):882–90.
24. Kierans AS, Doshi AM, Dunst D, Popiolek D, Blank SV, Rosenkrantz AB. Retrospective assessment of histogram-based diffusion metrics for differentiating benign and malignant endometrial lesions. J Comput Assist Tomogr. 2016;40(5):723–9.
25. Suo ST, Chen XX, Fan Y, Wu LM, Yao QY, Cao MQ, et al. Histogram Analysis of Apparent Diffusion Coefficient at 3.0 T in Urinary Bladder Lesions. Acad Radiol. 2014;21(8):1027–34.
26. Sepahdari AR, Politi LS, Aakalu VK, Kim HJ, Razek AA. Diffusion-weighted imaging of orbital masses: multi-institutional data support a 2-ADC threshold model to categorize lesions as benign, malignant, or indeterminate. AJNR Am J Neuroradiol. 2014;35(1):170–5.
27. Hiwatashi A, Yoshiura T, Togao O, Yamashita K, Kikuchi K, Fujita Y, et al. Diffusivity of intraorbital lymphoma vs. IgG4-related DISEASE: 3D turbo field echo with diffusion-sensitised driven-equilibrium preparation technique. Eur Radiol. 2014;24(3):581–6.
28. De Graaf P, Pouwels PJ, Rodjan F, Moll AC, Imhof SM, Knol DL, et al. Single-shot turbo spin-echo diffusion-weighted imaging for retinoblastoma: initial experience. AJNR Am J Neuroradiol. 2012;33(1):110–8.

27

The value of ^{99m}Tc-methylene diphosphonate single photon emission computed tomography/computed tomography in diagnosis of fibrous dysplasia

Linqi Zhang[1†], Qiao He[2†], Wei Li[1] and Rusen Zhang[1*]

Abstract

Background: Fibrous dysplasia (FD) is a rare benign bone disorder in which the normal bone is replaced by immature fibro-osseous tissue. However, some case reports have reported that FD showed significantly increased ^{99m}Tc-methylene diphosphonate (^{99m}Tc-MDP) uptake on whole-body bone scintigraphy (WBS), which may mimic bone metastasis or skeletal involvement of the patients with known cancer. Thus, the purpose of present study is to observe the reliable characteristics and usefulness of single photon emission computed tomography/computed tomography (SPECT/CT) for the diagnosis of FD.

Methods: This was a retrospective review of 21 patients with FD (14 males and 7 females, mean age 51.2 ± 12.5 years) who were referred to have WBS to determine whether there was any osseous metastasis. WBS and SPECT/CT images were independently interpreted by two experienced nuclear medicine physician together with a diagnostic radiologist. In cases of discrepancy, consensus was obtained by a joint reading. The final diagnosis was based on biopsy proof and radiologic follow-up over at least 1 year.

Results: The lesions of FD were most frequently found in craniofacial region (15/21). Eighteen of the 21 (85.7%) cases showed moderate and high metabolism on WBS (compared to sternum). On CT imaging, GGO and expansion were the most common finding, were noted in 90.5% and 85.7% of the patients. Lytic lesions were present in 61.9% of the patients, and sclerosis was present in 38.1% of the patients. Cortical disruption was not seen in any patient.

Conclusions: FD has certain characteristic appearance on SPECT/CT. It should be enrolled in the differential diagnoses when lesions show elevated ^{99m}Tc-MDP uptake on WBS. For SPECT/CT, the CT features of GGO and expansion in the areas of abnormal radiotracer uptake are helpful for the diagnosis of FD.

Keywords: Fibrous dysplasia, ^{99m}Tc-MDP, Single photon emission computed tomography, Computed tomography

* Correspondence: zhangrusen2015@163.com
†Equal contributors
[1]Department of Nuclear Medicine, Affiliated Cancer Hospital&Institute of Guangzhou Medical University, 78 Hengzhigang Road, Guangzhou 510095, Guangdong province, People's Republic of China
Full list of author information is available at the end of the article

Background

Fibrous dysplasia (FD) is a rare benign bone disorder in which the normal bone is replaced by immature fibro-osseous tissue. The actual prevalence of FD is difficult to estimate, but it may affect about 1/30,000 persons with a similar distribution around the world. The disease may involve single bone (monostotic FD, 70%) or multiple bones (polyostotic FD, 30%) with a predilection for the craniofacial bones and ribs. Patients are usually asymptomatic and detected incidentally on imaging studies that are performed for other purposes. In rare symptomatic cases, FD can present as bone pain, deformity, or pathologic fracture [1, 2]. ^{99m}Tc-MDP (^{99m}Tc-labeled methylene diphosphonate) whole-body bone scans (WBS) has been widely used for detection of metastasis for various malignant diseases. However, some case reports have reported that FD showed significantly increased ^{99m}Tc-MDP uptake, which may mimic bone metastasis or skeletal involvement of the patients with known cancer [3–5]. Therefore, active diagnosis and radiological familiarity of FD are thought to be essential for distinguishing bone metastasis and preventing unnecessary examinations or therapy. Single photon emission computed tomography/computed tomography (SPECT/CT) offers the opportunity to obtain diagnostic-quality CT and SPECT images, hence enabling more accurate localization and characterization of SPECT lesions using the CT component. However, the SPECT/CT features of FD have not been summarized. In present study, we wished to observe the reliable characteristics and usefulness of SPECT/CT in a larger cohort of patients with FD.

Methods

Patients

A total of 27,859 patients underwent ^{99m}Tc-MDP WBS from March 2009 to January 2017 at Department of Nuclear Medicine. Among which, there were 8517 patients had SPECT/CT for further evaluation. Of these patients, twenty one patients (fourteen males and seven females, mean age 51.2 ± 12.5 years, age range 23 ~ 70 years) found to have FD were recruited in the study. In 13 cases, the clinician performed biopsies to determine whether there was any osseous metastasis, because the anatomic site of the lesion was easily accessible. Pathologic analysis confirmed the diagnosis of FD. In 8 cases, the patients had been diagnosed based on radiologic investigations (SPECT/CT and/or MRI) and follow up at least one year.

Table 1 Clinical data and SPECT/CT findings of FD in 21 patients with known cancer

Pat. No.	Localization	Known cancer	Diagnostic Method	GGO	Expansion	Lytic	Sclerosis	Cortical Disruption
1	Mandible	Lung cancer	Biopsy	+	+	−	−	−
2	Sphenoid	Gastric lymphoma	radiologic follow-up	+	+	−	−	−
3	Maxillary	Lung cancer	Biopsy	+	+	+	−	−
4	Sphenoid	HCC	radiologic follow-up	+	+	+	−	−
5	conjoint sphenoid and ethmoid	HCC	Biopsy	+	+	−	+	−
6	L. Rib	NPC	Biopsy	−	+	+	+	−
7	L. Frontal bone	Lung cancer	Biopsy	+	+	+	−	−
8	R. Parietal bone	ESCC	Biopsy	+	+	−	+	−
9	R. Frontal bone	LSCC	Biopsy	+	+	+	−	−
10	R. Ischium	Breast cancer	Biopsy	−	−	+	−	−
11	R. Occipital bone	NPC	Biopsy	+	−	+	−	−
12	L. Tibia	NPC	Biopsy	+	−	−	+	−
13	Maxillary	ESCC	radiologic follow-up	+	+	−	+	−
14	Rib, vertebra	HCC	radiologic follow-up	+	+	+	−	−
15	R. Frontal bone	ESCC	Biopsy	+	+	+	−	−
16	R. Rib	NPC	radiologic follow-up	+	+	+	−	−
17	Maxillary	Lung cancer	Biopsy	+	+	+	+	−
18	Maxillary	NPC	radiologic follow-up	+	+	−	−	−
19	Mandible	Cervical cancer	radiologic follow-up	+	+	−	−	−
20	Sphenoid	LSCC	radiologic follow-up	+	+	+	+	−
21	R. Rib	ESCC	Biopsy	+	+	+	+	−

Pat. No patient number, *R* right, *L* left, *HCC* hepatocellular carcinoma, *NPC* nasopharyngeal carcinoma, *ESCC* esophageal squamous carcinoma, *LSCC* laryngeal squamous carcinoma, *GGO* ground-glass opacity, + positive, − negative.

Table 2 Summary SPECT/CT features of 21 patients with FD

SPECT/CT findings	No. Patients(n)	Percentage (%)
Moderate and high metabolism	18	85.7%
GGO	19	90.5%
Expansion	18	85.7%
Lytic	13	61.9%
Sclerosis	8	38.1%
Cortical disruption	0	0

GGO ground-glass opacity

SPETCT/CT scanning

All examinations were carried out using a SPECT/CT scanner (Philips, Netherlands,16-slice diagnostic CT). The whole-body scan was performed 3 h after intravenous injection of 15 ~ 25 mCi ^{99m}Tc-MDP. The images were immediately reviewed by a nuclear medicine radiologist after image acquisition. If areas of abnormal radiotracer uptake were detected, the patient then proceeded directly for SPECT/CT for anatomic location and attenuation correction of the areas. The acquisition parameters for CT were as following: 140KeV, window width 15%, pitch 1.25, and slice thickness 5.0 mm. Directly after CT imaging, the SPECT acquisition protocol was started. The SPECT/CT imaging was integrated and analyzed by using Philips Jet Steam Workspace integrated program. The coronal, sagittal and transverse plane of SPECT, CT and SPECT/CT was evaluated, respectively.

Imaging analysis

The WBS and SPECT/CT images were independently interpreted by two experienced nuclear medicine physician together with a diagnostic radiologist. In cases of discrepancy, consensus was obtained by a joint reading. It was considered high metabolism if the lesion showing uptake of ^{99m}Tc-MDP higher than that of sternum on WBS images, equal to that of sternum was considered moderate metabolism, and lower than that of sternum was considered low metabolism. The following radiologic features were evaluated on CT images: ground-glass opacity (GGO), expansion, lytic lesions, sclerosis, and cortical disruption (presence or absence).

Statistical analysis

Categorical data are expressed as numbers and frequency (%). Continuous data are expressed as means

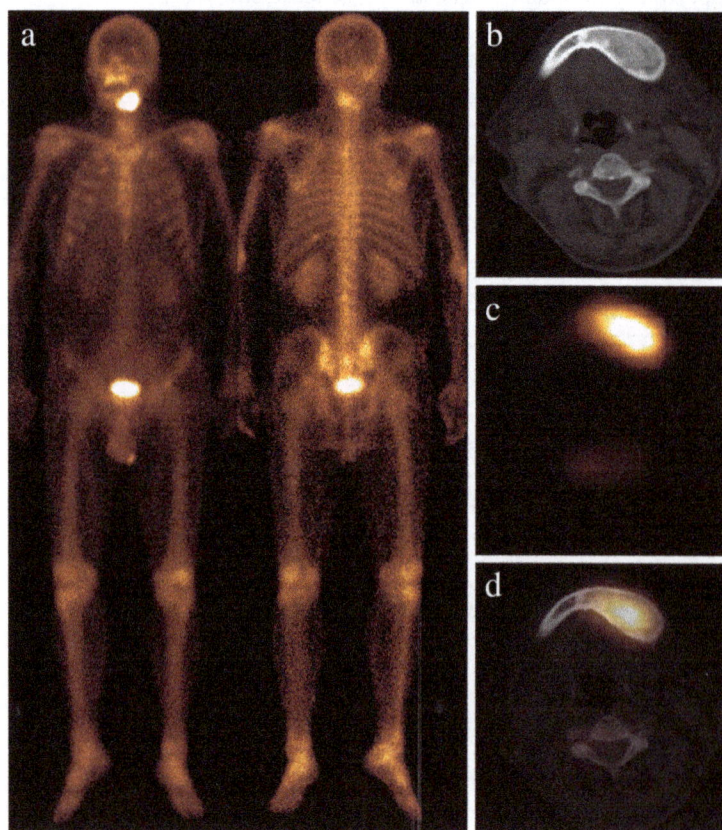

Fig. 1 Patient 1 presented with newly diagnosed lung cancer. The WBS (**a**) demonstrated markedly increasing ^{99m}Tc-MDP uptake in the left facial bone. Axial CT (**b**), SPECT (**c**), and hybrid SPECT/spiral CT imaging (**d**) demonstrated increasing ^{99m}Tc-MDP uptake corresponding to expansion and ground glass density on mandible. A biopsy was subsequently performed and pathologic analysis confirmed the diagnosis of FD

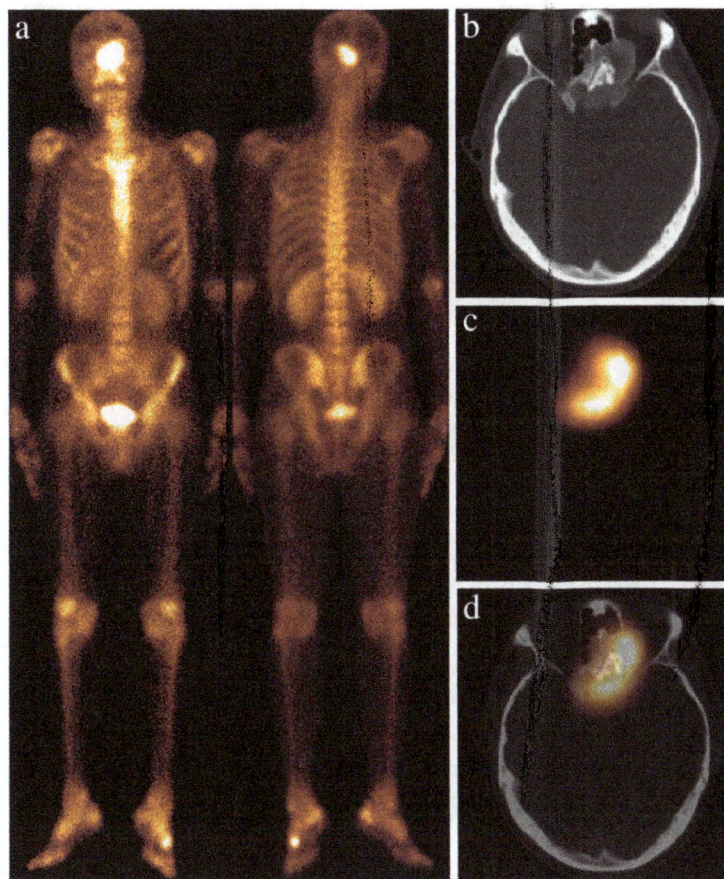

Fig. 2 Patient 5 presented with HCC. The WBS (**a**) demonstrated markedly increasing ^{99m}Tc-MDP uptake in the base of skull. Axial CT (**b**), SPECT (**c**), and hybrid SPECT/spiral CT imaging (**d**) showed an expansile lesion, which presented with GGO and ill-defined borders in the conjoint sphenoid and ethmoid. The clinician decided immediately to perform a biopsy, because the anatomic site of the lesion was easily accessible by endoscopic sinus. Pathologic analysis confirmed the diagnosis of FD

and standard deviations. All the statistical tests were performed using SPSS Statistics 17.0 (SPSS Inc., Chicago, IL, USA) software.

Result

Patient population

A summary of clinical characteristics (including age, gender, known malignancy and diagnostic method), WBS and SPECT/CT findings (including location and CT features) of all 21 patients with FD were given in Table 1. Nineteen of 21 patients (90.5%) were asymptomatic and detected incidentally on WBS. The remaining 2 patients (9.5%) presented with aspecific symptoms: one (patient 5) with nasal obstruction, and another (patient 12) with dull pain in left tibia. Only one patient (patient 14) (4.8%) was polyostotic and other 20 patients (95.2%) were monostotic. Lesions were most frequently found in craniofacial region, accounting for 71.4% (15/21) of patients, five of the patients in the skull, three in the maxillary, three in the mandible, three in sphenoid, and one patient showed conjoint sphenoid and ethmoid involvement. The remaining 6

patients, one patient with polyostotic lesion involvement of rib and vertebra, other 5 patients with solitary lesion in rib ($n = 3$), ischium ($n = 1$), and long bone ($n = 1$).

WBS and SPECT/CT findings

Summary SPECT/CT features of 21 patients with FD were shown in Table 2. On WBS, all the lesions showed increased uptake of ^{99m}Tc-MDP. Among which, there were 18 of the 21 (85.7%) cases showed moderate and high metabolism (compared to sternum). Both GGO and Expansion were noted in vast majority of patients. GGO was present in 90.5% of patients (19/21, Figs. 1, 2, 3 and 4). Expansion was present in 85.7% of patients (18/21, Figs. 1, 2, 4). Lytic lesions were present in 13 patients (13/21, 61.9%, Fig. 4) with FD. Sclerosis was noted in only 8 patients (38.1%, Figs. 2, 3) with FD. Cortical disruption was not seen in any patients.

Discussion

WBS using ^{99m}Tc-MDP is one of the most frequently performed radionuclide procedures. Its excellent

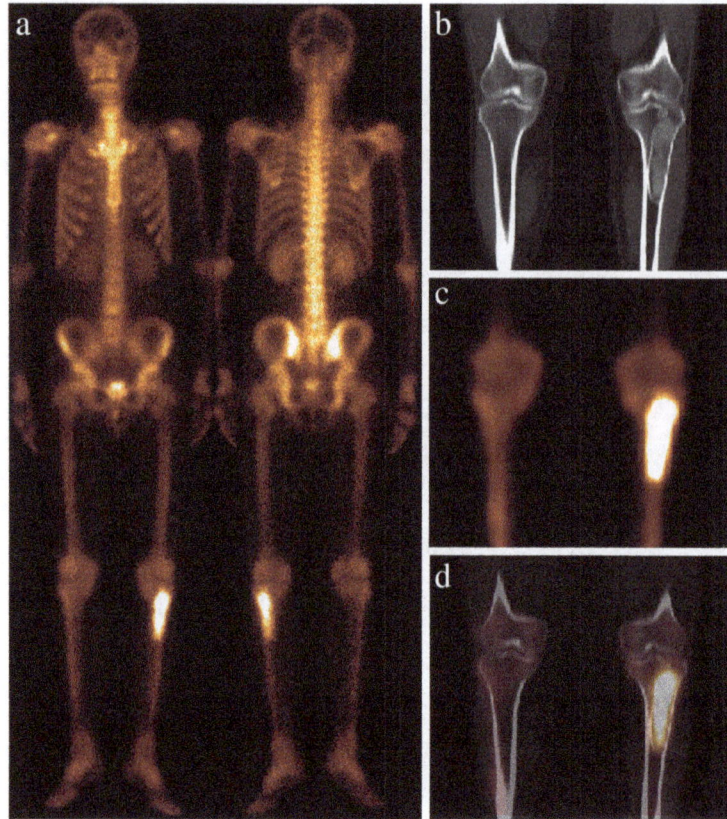

Fig. 3 Patient 12 presented with NPC. On the WBS (**a**), there is an area of abnormal ^{99m}Tc-MDP uptake seen in the left upper tibia, which may mimic bone metastasis. No additional area of abnormal ^{99m}Tc-MDP uptake was identified on the remainder of the skeleton. Axial CT (**b**), SPECT (**c**), and hybrid SPECT/spiral CT imaging (**d**) depicted show increasing ^{99m}Tc-MDP uptake corresponding to a sclerotic lesion with GGO localized in the left tibia. Based on the imaging finding which was suspicious for primary bone malignancy. A biopsy was subsequently performed and pathologic analysis confirmed the diagnosis of FD

sensitivity makes it useful in screening for generalized bone abnormalities, but with lower specificity due to trauma, inflammation, and other malignant or benign bone diseases [6–8]. In some previous case reports, it has been recognized as being metabolically active on WBS [3–5]. However, the diagnosis of FD could not always be established only by WBS, which often needs to combine with an anatomical imaging (such as X-ray, CT, or MRI). Hybrid SPECT/spiral CT offers the opportunity to obtain diagnostic-quality CT and SPECT images, which provides a clear view of the anatomic sites of the lesions showed elevated ^{99m}Tc-MDP uptake [9, 10].

Of the cases examined in present study, all the patients showed increased uptake of ^{99m}Tc-MDP on WBS. Eighteen of the 21 (85.7%) cases showed moderate and high metabolism. The mechanism of different degree of ^{99m}Tc-MDP metabolism of FD is unclear. One reason can be accounted for that. As we known, FD is a developmental failure in the remodeling of primitive bone to mature lamellar bone. Fibroblasts are the predominant proliferating cells in FD lesions, and the different degree of ^{99m}Tc-MDP metabolism among FD may be due to the difference in the amount of proliferating fibroblasts or their metabolic turnover [11].Tracers uptake of FD have also been found in PET/CT, including radionuclide of ^{68}Ga, ^{18}F–fluorodeoxyglucose and ^{11}C–choline [12–14].

On SPECT/CT imaging, GGO and expansion were the most common findings, noted in 90.5% and 85.7% of the cases. Lytic lesions were present in 61.9% of the cases, and sclerosis was present in 38.1% of the cases. Cortical disruption was not seen in any patients. Some previous studies have reported that the typical CT features of FD are ground-glass opacity (GGO) and expansion of the bone, due to the simultaneous presence of bone trabeculae and fibrous tissue [15–17]. Given these result, GGO and expansion appear to be reliable CT feature for diagnosis of fibro-osseous lesions. The differential diagnosis should include the other fibro-osseous diseases (ossifying fibroma and osseous dysplasia) and Paget disease [18].

The management of FD is not surgical unless it causes progressive deformity, cranial nerve compromise, pain, or malignant transformation. A

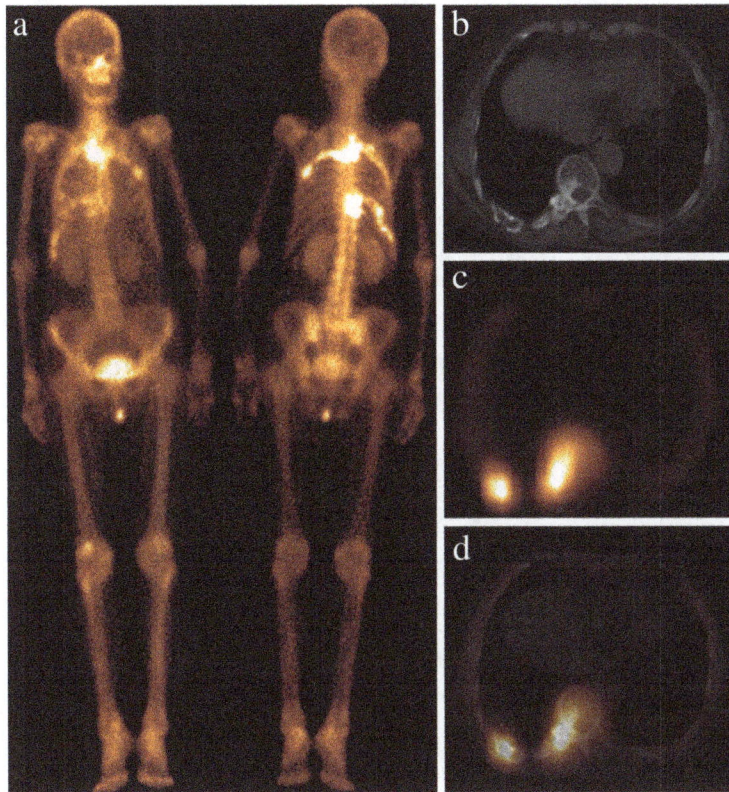

Fig. 4 Patient 14 presented with HCC. On the WBS (**a**), there were multiple areas of abnormal ^{99m}Tc-MDP uptake seen in the bilateral ribs and thoracic vertebra, which may mimic multiple bone metastasise. Axial CT (**b**), SPECT (**c**), and hybrid SPECT/spiral CT imaging (**d**) depicted increasing ^{99m}Tc-MDP uptake corresponding to an expansile and lytic lesion with GGO in the lesion of bilateral ribs and thoracic vertebra. During the 2-year follow-up, no difference was detected in the WBS and CT image. The diagnosis of FD was established by a combined assessment of clinical and radiologic follow-up

malignant transformation of FD is rare, which occurs less than 1% of cases [19, 20]. In present study, the clinicians performed biopsy or surgery for 13 of the patients. All pathological results were reported as fibrous dysplasia, and no malignancy changes were detected. Some previous studies have reported that a history of radiotherapy may result in malignant transformation of FD [21]. Long-term medical imaging monitoring of FD is essential, especially in patient with a history of radiotherapy.

Conclusions

In conclusion, FD has certain characteristic appearance on SPECT/CT. It should be enrolled in the differential diagnoses when lesions show elevated ^{99m}Tc-MDP uptake on WBS image. On SPECT/CT image, the CT features of GGO and expansion in the areas of abnormal radiotracer uptake are helpful for the diagnosis of FD.

Abbreviations
^{99m}Tc-MDP: ^{99m}Tc-methylene diphosphonate; FD: Fibrous dysplasia; SPECT/CT: Single photon emission computed tomography/computed tomography.; WBS: whole-body bone scintigraphy

Acknowledgements
The authors thank Dr.Xi Zhong for his help of SPECT/CT images interpretation.

Funding
This work was supported by the Youth Foundation of Guangzhou Medical University (No.2016A24).

Authors' contributions
LQZ and QH participated in design of the study, collected the patients' data, and drafted the manuscript. WL processed the figures, helped draft the manuscript, and performed critical revision of the manuscript. RSZ conceived and designed the study, supervised the project. All authors read and approved the final version of the manuscript.

Competing interests
The authors declare that they have no competing interests.

Author details
[1]Department of Nuclear Medicine, Affiliated Cancer Hospital&Institute of Guangzhou Medical University, 78 Hengzhigang Road, Guangzhou 510095, Guangdong province, People's Republic of China. [2]Department of Nuclear Medicine, the First Affiliated Hospital of Sun Yat-Sen University, 58 Zhongshan Er Road, Guangzhou 510080, Guangdong province, People's Republic of China.

References

1.   Benhamou J, Gensburger D, Messiaen C, Chapurlat R. Prognostic factors from an epidemiologic evaluation of fibrous dysplasia of bone in a modern cohort: the FRANCEDYS study. J Bone Miner Res. 2016;31(12):2167–72.

2.   DiCaprio MR, Enneking WF. Fibrous dysplasia. Pathophysiology, evaluation, and treatment. J Bone Joint Surg Am. 2005;87(8):1848–64.

3.   Nakahara T, Fujii H, Hashimoto J, Kubo A. Use of bone SPECT in the evaluation of fibrous dysplasia of the skull. Clin Nucl Med. 2004;29(9):554–9.

4.   Rambalde E, Parra A, Santapau A, Tardin L, Freile E, Banzo J. SPECT/CT with (9)(9)mTc-MDP in a patient with monostotic fibrous dysplasia of the rib. Rev Esp Med Nucl Imagen Mol. 2013;32(2):126–7.

5.   Tuncel M, Kiratli PO, Gedikoglu G. SPECT-CT imaging of poliostotic fibrous dysplasia. Rev Esp Med Nucl Imagen Mol. 2012;31(1):47–8.

6.   Gnanasegaran G, Ballinger JR. Molecular imaging agents for SPECT (and SPECT/CT). Eur J Nucl Med Mol Imaging. 2014;41(Suppl 1):S26–35.

7.   Huellner MW, Strobel K. Clinical applications of SPECT/CT in imaging the extremities. Eur J Nucl Med Mol Imaging. 2014;41(Suppl 1):S50–8.

8.   Helyar V, Mohan HK, Barwick T, Livieratos L, Gnanasegaran G, Clarke SE, Fogelman I. The added value of multislice SPECT/CT in patients with equivocal bony metastasis from carcinoma of the prostate. Eur J Nucl Med Mol Imaging. 2010;37(4):706–13.

9.   Palmedo H, Marx C, Ebert A, Kreft B, Ko Y, Turler A, Vorreuther R, Gohring U, Schild HH, Gerhardt T, et al. Whole-body SPECT/CT for bone scintigraphy: diagnostic value and effect on patient management in oncological patients. Eur J Nucl Med Mol Imaging. 2014;41(1):59–67.

10. Abikhzer G, Srour S, Keidar Z, Bar-Shalom R, Kagna O, Israel O, Militianu D. Added value of SPECT/CT in the evaluation of benign bone diseases of the Appendicular skeleton. Clin Nucl Med. 2016;41(4):e195–9.

11. Zhao Z, Li L, Li FL. Radiography, bone scintigraphy, SPECT/CT and MRI of fibrous dysplasia of the third lumbar vertebra. Clin Nucl Med. 2009;34(12):898–901.

12. Papadakis GZ, Millo C, Sadowski SM, Karantanas AH, Bagci U, Patronas NJ. Fibrous dysplasia mimicking malignancy on 68Ga-DOTATATE PET/CT. Clin Nucl Med. 2017;42(3):209–10.

13. Gu CN, Hunt CH, Lehman VT, Johnson GB, Diehn FE, Schwartz KM, Eckel LJ. Benign fibrous dysplasia on [(11)C]choline PET: a potential mimicker of disease in patients with biochemical recurrence of prostate cancer. Ann Nucl Med. 2012;26(7):599–602.

14. Strobel K, Bode B, Lardinois D, Exner U. PET-positive fibrous dysplasia–a potentially misleading incidental finding in a patient with intimal sarcoma of the pulmonary artery. Skelet Radiol. 2007;36(Suppl 1):S24–8.

15. Sirvanci M, Karaman K, Onat L, Duran C, Ulusoy OL. Monostotic fibrous dysplasia of the clivus: MRI and CT findings. Neuroradiology. 2002;44(10):847–50.

16. Unal Erzurumlu Z, Celenk P, Bulut E, Baris YS. CT imaging of craniofacial fibrous dysplasia. Case Rep Dent. 2015;2015:134123.

17. Park SK, Lee IS, Choi JY, Cho KH, Suh KJ, Lee JW, Song JW. CT and MRI of fibrous dysplasia of the spine. Br J Radiol. 2012;85(1015):996–1001.

18. Fusconi M, Conte M, Pagliarella M, De Vincentiis C, De Virgilio A, Benincasa AT, Alessi S, Gallo A. Fibrous dysplasia of the maxilla: diagnostic reliability of the study image. Literature review. J Neurol Surg B Skull Base. 2013;74(6):364–8.

19. Qu N, Yao W, Cui X, Zhang H. Malignant transformation in monostotic fibrous dysplasia: clinical features, imaging features, outcomes in 10 patients, and review. Medicine (Baltimore). 2015;94(3):e369.

20. Mardekian SK, Tuluc M. Malignant sarcomatous transformation of fibrous dysplasia. Head Neck Pathol. 2015;9(1):100–3.

21. Mock D, Rosen IB. Osteosarcoma in irradiated fibrous dysplasia. J Oral Pathol. 1986;15(1):1–4.

28

High-definition neural visualization of rodent brain using micro-CT scanning and non-local-means processing

Ko-Chin Chen[1,3,4*] (iD), Alon Arad[2,3], Zan-Ming Song[4] and David Croaker[1,4]

Abstract

Background: Micro-CT holds promising potential for phenotyping and histological purposes. However, few have clarified the difference in the neuroimaging quality between ex vivo and in vivo micro-CT scanners. In addition, no direct comparison has been made between micro-CT scans and standard microscopy. Furthermore, while the efficacy of various stains for yielding soft-tissue contrast in CT scans have been compared in other studies for embryos, staining protocols for larger samples have yet to be clarified. Lastly, post-acquisition processing for image enhancements have not been addressed.

Methods: Comparisons of postnatal rat brain micro-CT scans obtained through custom-built ex vivo and commercially available in vivo micro-CT scanners were made. Subsequently, the scanned rat brains were then H&E stained for microscopy. Neuroanatomy on micro-CT scanning and 4x microscopy of rat brain were compared. Diffusion and perfusion staining using iodine or PTA were trialled on adult and neonatal encapsulated rat brains. Different combinations of stain concentration and staining time were trialled.
Post-acquisition denoising with NLM filter was completed using a modern General-Purpose Graphic Processing Unit (GPGPU) and custom code for prompt processing.

Results: Ex vivo micro-CT scans of iodine-stained postnatal rat brains yields 3D images with details comparable to 4x H&E light micrographs. Neural features shown on ex vivo micro-CT scans were significantly more distinctive than those on in vivo micro-CT scans.
Both ex vivo and in vivo micro-CT scans required diffusion staining through small craniotomy. Perfusion staining is ineffective. Iodine staining was more efficient than PTA in terms of time.
Consistently, enhancement made by NLM denoising on in vivo micro-CT images were more pronounced than that on ex vivo micro-CT scans due to their difference in image signal-to-noise indexes.

Conclusions: Micro-CT scanning is a powerful and versatile visualization tool available for qualitative and potential quantitative anatomical analysis. Simple diffusion staining via craniotomy with 1.5% iodine is an effective and minimal structural-invasive method for both in vivo and ex vivo micro-CT scanning for studying the microscopic morphology of neonatal and adult rat brains. Post-acquisition NLM filtering is an effective enhancement technique for in vivo micro-CT brain scans.

Keywords: Micro-CT, Neuroimaging, NLM image processing

---

* Correspondence: ckochin@gmail.com
[1]The Canberra Hospital, Yamba Drive, Garran, ACT 2605, Australia
[3]Automated Analytics, Sugar Land, TX 77479, USA
Full list of author information is available at the end of the article

Background

Non-destructive whole-volumetric phenotyping studies through three-dimensional (3D) image reconstruction have gained increasing popularity among biomedical researchers over recent decades, especially with recent advancements in imaging acquisition and processing techniques. Three-dimensional visualization techniques may be divided into two categories: serial sectional image reconstruction and whole-volume imaging. The former includes confocal microscopy, episcopic microscopy [1], and the latter includes optical projection tomography (OPT) [2], micro-magnetic resonance imaging (micro-MRI) [3, 4], and micro-computed tomography (micro-CT) [5].

Whole-volumetric imaging is superior to serial imaging in many aspects. Serial imaging reconstructions such as confocal microscopy or confocal laser scanning microscopy (CLSM) can provide detailed and fluorescence-labelled representations of the sample, but of only limited thickness, typically <2–300 μm due to the need for optical transparency [6]. Although image reconstruction may be employed to obtain the entire 3D view of the sample, the process is laborious and often with operator-dependent results. Episcopic microscopy overcomes this shortfall by adopting automatic serial slice alignment, and reconstructs relatively well-preserved images; however, such a process destroys the tissue sample post-imaging and prohibits further sample use [1, 7]. Whole-volumetric imaging, on the other hand, does not have the above restrictions. For example, optical projection tomography (OPT) can be used to localize and measure structures within a whole organ, but only for restricted sample thicknesses [8]. Micro-MRI can offer great soft-tissue contrast with adequate resolution images, but its use is limited by its restricted availability, high cost and extended scanning time [4, 9, 10]. Micro-CT is now a widely accessible imaging modality, offering a mean for accurate visualization of three-dimensional structures, quantitative volumetric measurements, and tissue characterizations such as bone stress and vascular density [11–15]. Although many are still unaware of this versatile tool, micro-CT has gradually becoming a popular whole-volume scanning research method, in large part due to its versatility for volume exploration, ease of tissue preparation, and quantitative analysis potentials.

Although many recent papers have published various staining techniques for successful micro-CT scanning of biological samples, including chicken embryo, *Xenopus* embryo, mouse embryo, tumour angiogenesis, and other animal internal organs [5, 16, 17], few study have clarified the scanning protocols for micro-CT scans on postnatal model animals or made direct comparisons between the ex vivo micro-CT, in vivo micro-CT, and histology scans of rat neuroanatomy. Furthermore, even though prior study has suggested staining with iodine or phosphotungstic acid

(PTA) were efficient and effective for embryos, no comments have been made on their staining power for postnatal animals [5]. In addition, the effect of iodine and PTA staining on subsequent microscopy processing has not been illustrated in the past. Lastly, we are also not aware of studies trialling image processing protocols on the rat brain micro-CT scans, which may facilitate future quantitative analysis.

Our study aims to complement previous studies by illustrating the following:

1. Simple, safe, and effective staining method for successful micro-CT scans of both small and large rat brains.
2. The potential neuroanatomical details of rat brain and image magnification and resolution achievable by micro-CT scanning using one of the most high-powered ex vivo micro-CT scanners available currently.
3. Validate neuroanatomical information of micro-CT scan by direct comparison with H&E light microscopy.
4. The difference in image quality between in vivo and ex vivo micro-CT scans of rat brain.
5. Effectively improve image clarity and potentiate organs of interest through non-local means (NLM) denoising algorithms.

Methods

Compliance with ethical practice

All tissues and animals used in this study were handled with strict adherence to the requirements of the ACT Health Human Research Ethics Committee (ACTH-H-REC) and Australian National University Animal Experimentation Ethics Committee (ANU-AEEC), project number A2011/67.

Differences between the principles of ex vivo and in vivo micro-CT setups

We have chosen the Caliper Quantum FX machine (Fig. 1a) as representative of in vivo micro-CT setup and a custom-built micro-CT system by ANU Applied Mathematical Department as representative of ex vivo micro-CT setup (Fig. 1b).

The in vivo micro-CT system is set up as a mini-medical CT system. It incorporates an X-ray source and detectors rotating around a stationary sample, achieving a spatial resolution of 10–100 μm/voxel, which is restricted by the fixed distance between X-ray source and detector. In the Caliper Quantum FX, the tissue specimen was placed in a stationary loading dock positioned between the rotating system of X-ray source plus detector. The scanning time was pre-set between 17 s and 4.5 min, depending on the field of view (FOV; ranging

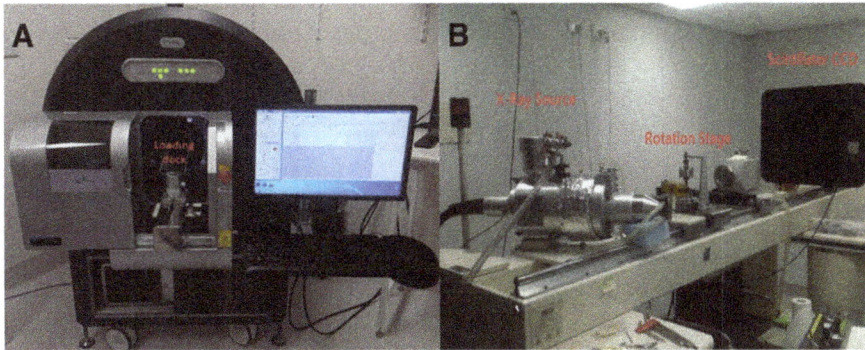

Fig. 1 In vivo and ex vivo micro-CT machines utilized in this study. **a** The Caliper Quantum FX machine representing in vivo micro-CT setup, with loading dock labelled and situated in between the rotating X-ray source and detectors; X-ray source and detector are hidden within the casing. **b** The custom-built ex vivo micro-CT scanner by ANU applied mathematical department. The rotational sample stage is placed in-between the adjustable X-ray source and scintillator/detector for maximal magnification

from 5 to 75 mm in diameter) and imaging quality selected (ranging from "standard" to "fine"). The advantages of in vivo micro-CT scanners including a shorter scanning time and lower radiation exposure, both of which were essential for live animal study. The resultant images were stored as DICOM series and visualized with FIJI and Drishti, both of which were open-source software [18, 19].

In contrast, the ex vivo micro-CT system involves a specimen placed on a rotating stage between a stationary but adjustable system of X-ray source and detector. Its main focus is to achieve high spatial resolution, up to 1 μm/voxel, with high signal-to-noise ratio images. These benefits are achieved at the expense of longer scanning time and hence higher radiation dose. It is therefore mainly used for tissue study. The custom-built micro-CT system at the ANU Department of Applied Mathematics requires the sample to be fixed within an aluminium tube before being placed on the rotational sample stage between the adjustable X-ray source and scintillator-coupled-CCD, at a position that depends on the resolution desired. All samples were allocated at least 15 h of scanning time, with a subsequent 8 h of image-processing time required at the National Computational Infrastructure (NCI). The maximal achievable resolution is 1 μm/voxel, limited by the physical size of the sample. The resultant images were stored as netCDF files and visualized with Drishti. Segmentation for organs of interest was performed semi-automatically using Drishti paint, a component of Drishti open-source software [18].

As a side note, because the adjustable X-ray source can be brought much closer to the sample (limited by the sample size) with ex vivo than in vivo micro-CT setup, higher resolution is achievable. The same cannot be achieved with in vivo micro-CT setup due to current constructional challenges of fitting X-ray source and sufficient number of detectors onto a small rotational stand.

Tissue samples and staining preparations for micro-CT scanning

Adult rats and neonatal rat culling

Five fully-grown rats (>21 and 27 days) and thirteen 24- and 48-h old rats were over-anaesthetized with 5% isoflurane and then culled via abdominal aortotomy. Each rat was weighed. One adult rat was prepared through the perfusion protocol and the remaining rats were prepared via the diffusion protocol, as described below.

Perfusion protocol for adult rat brains

To test the staining potential of perfusion protocols, we culled one 27-days-old rat via cardiotomy with a 22G cannula. The rat was then perfused with 200 mL of 0.1 M phosphate-buffered saline (PBS) solution and subsequently 200 mL of 4% formalin for successful fixation, indicated by tail rigidity; each stage took about 45 min. The perfusate existed the vascular system through inferior vena cava venotomy. Next, the rat was perfused with a series of progressively concentrated ethanol solutions (20%, 50%, 70%, 90%) over 1 h at each concentration to replace intravascular formalin, for subsequent staining. Staining was then attempted by perfusing the animal with 1.5% iodine (in 90% ethanol) through left ventricles for 2.5 h in a lab basin.

Diffusion staining protocols for encapsulated adult and neonatal rat brains and isolated rat brains

To explore the alternative staining techniques, we attempted diffusion staining by the following. Four adult rats' heads (average age 25 days) were isolated from the neck and up following culling. A diamond-shaped craniotomy of 20-mm in diameter on parietal bones was created for staining. The craniotomy was completed firstly by a superficial cross-incision of 20 mm in diameter (through the thickness of the skull) using a dissection scalpel followed by diagonal excisions of skull using iris scissors. Superficial dissection was carefully performed to avoid brain tissue damage. Minimal damage of the brain was confirmed by the absence of brain tissue destruction in the following micro-CT scans.

Four-percent formalin was first used to fixate the rat head for 24 h followed by washout with graded ethanol in the following steps. Each fixed tissue was immersed in progressive concentrated ethanol (EtOH) series: 20, 50, 70, and 90% for 1 day each to replace formalin solution. Each sample was then stained in 1.5% iodine (with 90% EtOH) or 0.5% phosphotungstic acid (PTA) or 1% PTA in 70% EtOH for various durations (listed in Additional file 1: Table S1) as attempts to find the most effective staining time for successful CT scanning. Contrast concentration was decided based on the successful results of previous studies on embryo staining [5, 16].

Similarly, diffusion staining on 13 neonatal rat brains was achieved through similar processes: isolation of upper body from the level of diaphragm, creation of a 5-mm in diameter diamond-shaped craniotomy on parietal bones, 4% formalin-fixation for storage, progressive ethanol washout prior to staining, and diffusion staining with 1.5% iodine, 0.5% PTA, or 1.0% PTA for various periods (listed in Additional file 1: Table S1).

Lastly, three 24-h-old rat brains were dissected and fixed as described above prior to staining with 1.5% iodine and 1.5% PTA, respectively. Macroscopic views of PTA- and iodine-stained brains are shown by Additional file 2: Figure S1 and Additional file 3: Figure S2.

Hematoxylin and eosin (H&E) histology preparations for comparison with micro-CT scans

To confirm the neuroanatomical details of the micro-CT scan and assess the potential tissue distortion created by the iodine or PTA staining process, as shown by the macroscopic brown-discoloration of brain tissues due to iodine staining (Additional file 2: Figure S1 and Additional file 3: Figure S2), we processed the stained rat samples with standard H&E protocols [20].

H&E processing were conducted in the following steps. The iodine- or PTA-stained tissues were first sectioned sagittally into blocks of 4 mm in thickness to fit in cassettes. These tissue-blocks were then transferred to 90% EtOH for 48 h for contrast washout and dehydration. Next, the alcohol was cleared by xylol prior to paraffin embedding at 60 °C. Following embedment, samples were sliced into tissue-sheets of 4 μm in thickness using a microtome. These tissue-sheets were then laid in water-bath of 5–6 °C to minimize wrinkles while being positioned onto labelled-glass slides. These slides were dried overnight at 37 °C.

H&E staining was completed by progressive staining. The slides were placed in alum-haematoxylin solutions until dark red colour was visualized. This was followed by washing and then 'bluing' with lithium carbonate solution. The slides were then washed before counter-stained with 0.5% eosin alcoholic solution.

All of the H&E slides were then examined with an Olympus IX71 Microscope with 4×, 20×, and 40× magnification.

Post-acquisition image processing: non-local means (NLM) denoising

To improve the micro-CT image clarity, we denoised the acquired images to enhance image signal-to-noise ratios using NLM algorithm, which was first developed by Buades et al. [21]. The algorithm was based on the premises that similarity exists between different regions of an image as long as these region sizes were kept relatively small. Using these similarity characteristics, image noise could be removed through averaging the similar parts of the image. For more accurate removal of the image noise, we used standard NLM with locally adaptive estimates for both types of micro-CT scans. Traditionally, this process was time-consuming due to the high demand on computational power thus making its computer-processing-unit (CPU) runtime unacceptably high for all but the smaller 2-dimentional (2D) images. However, we adopted parallel processing using a General-Purpose Graphic Processing Unit (GPGPU) and shortened the processing time to 1-min and thirsty seconds for a 512^3 sample, rendering this process effective and efficient for regular research use.

This code was implemented on an Intel (R) Core ™ i7-4770 K CPU @3.5GHz with 32G of RAM and Nvidia GeForce GTX Titan Black Kepler GK110 architecture running Linux. The processed CT data were then reviewed using Fiji [22].

Implementation of the NLM algorithm

A brief description of our NLM implementation is provided as follow. The vast majority of the NLM runtime is spent computing the sum of squared differences (ssd). The ssd computation for adjacent voxels is highly similar. We can exploit this similarity by using a pseudo moving average filter (MAF) to perform the ssd from one pixel/voxel to the next. For 2D, the square area of intensities used for one voxel's ssd search neighbourhood differs from an adjacent voxel's search neighbourhood only in the end rows or columns. The same principle applies in 3D, adjacent cubes differ only in two end slices.

In 3D, if M is the number of voxels of the inner ssd cube and N is the total number of cubes that we performed the ssd on, then the total number of difference operations: with no MAF, we performed $N \times M^3$ difference operations; with the MAF, we performed $M^3 + (N - 1) \times 2 \times M^2$ difference operations. For a large N, this becomes a significant reduction in computation. As a simple example, if M is 100 voxels and N is a billion, the second operation is then a two-orders of magnitude less operation.

Most implementations of the NLM require the user to specify at least three parameters: an estimate of the image noise standard deviation, an outer search window size, and an inner search neighbourhood size. All these factors influence the quality of the de-noise operation. An accurate estimate of the noise, the size of the search window and neighbourhood is generally impossible and often the user has not even the vaguest notion of what the optimized values may be. This leads to tedious and time-consuming testing and retesting of the de-noising operation with different parameters until acceptable results are obtained. Our implementation does not require these unknown and often arbitrarily chosen parameters to be specified. Our implementation automatically computes an estimate of the noise in the local area of the pixel/voxel being de-noised. Each local noise estimate is combined with internally computed parameters determined from various image properties such as the number of intensity values i.e. 256 or 65 K, to compute the final smoothing parameter of the NLM algorithm automatically.

The computation of the smoothing parameter and estimation of the image noise is adapted from Coupe et al. [23]. Our implementation differs from theirs in the computation of a unique noise estimate for local sub blocks of the image, as opposed to a single value for the entire image. We also consider the gray scale value (gsv) intensity range in the calculation of the smoothing parameter. The inclusion of the gsv intensity range was found empirically to be a significant factor in the success of the automatic de-noising over a range of different image types i.e. CT, scanning electron microscopy (SEM), ultrasound etc. Our implementation of NLM follows the original model of Additive Gaussian White Noise (AGWN) but also allows for some adjustment of shape of the Gaussian kernel to better approximate the real noise distribution for images with non-AGWN.

As with Coupe et al. [23], we also concluded that the best de-noising quality is achieved with a local estimate of the noise, the correction factor for non-AGWN images, and fixed window sizes. Little, if any, gain in quality was obtained with larger search window sizes. It is obvious that in many cases, image quality degrades with larger search window sizes as the statistics of the similarity between these regions degrades.

Results
Simple tissue preparation for successful micro-CT scanning
In the first part of study, we proceeded to elaborate the simple staining process for postnatal rat samples required to achieve successful micro-CT scanning of the brains. The results of various combinations of contrasting agent, stain concentration, and contrast types were summarized in Additional file 1: Tables S1.

Staining of encapsulated postnatal rat brains for successful micro-CT neural imaging
We first attempted 1.5% iodine perfusion staining on an adult rat of 27 days but with little success, as shown by Fig. 2a. Intracranial neural tissue exhibits little X-ray attenuation and minimal neuroanatomy was observed. The same rat's head with intact skull was re-scanned following 14-days of 1.5% iodine diffusion-staining with no improvement in image quality (Figures not shown). Subsequently, 44-days of iodine-diffusion-staining through craniotomy was trialled with a 25-days-old rat's head; micro-CT scan demonstrated differentiated intracranial details as shown by Fig. 2b: neural tissue differentiation became apparent. Consistently, same staining techniques also worked for neonatal rat brains but required only a staining period of 16 days; the resultant micro-CT scans yielded good neural anatomical information, as shown by Fig. 2c.

As an attempt to find an alternative contrast agent, we explored PTA diffusion staining using both 0.5 and 1.0% concentration solutions. Figure 2d and e are micro-CT scans of adult rat brains (25-days-old) derived from 2.5 years of PTA staining; both showed only peripheral brain of 2–4 mm in thickness. Similarly, as shown by Fig. 2f and g, incomplete neuroanatomy visualization was observed on micro-CT scans of neonatal rat's head despite prolonged staining of 148 days. Interestingly, lower concentrations of PTA seemed to achieve more pervasive staining than higher, Fig. 2f vs g, although neither performed well.

Staining of dissected neonatal rat brains for successful micro-CT neural imaging
As the PTA staining was found to have suboptimal staining with encapsulated post-natal rat brain, we further evaluated its usefulness in staining small dissected rat brains, namely 1 cm^3 in size. The result showed that PTA staining, although slow, did achieve full-staining and yield neural micro-CT scan quality similar to that derived from iodine staining. The comparison between the temporal series of iodine stained (Fig. 2i–k) and PTA stained (Fig. 2l–n) rat brains demonstrated the efficiency of iodine contrast. As Fig. 2j demonstrated, iodine staining was completed within 6 h; further staining did not improve image quality and tissue differentiation, Fig. 2k. On the other hand, only modest staining progress was made from 3-h PTA staining, Fig. 2l, and staining completion required 6 days, Fig. 2n. There were no significant image quality difference between the micro-CT scans derived from iodine-stained and PTA-stained rat brains.

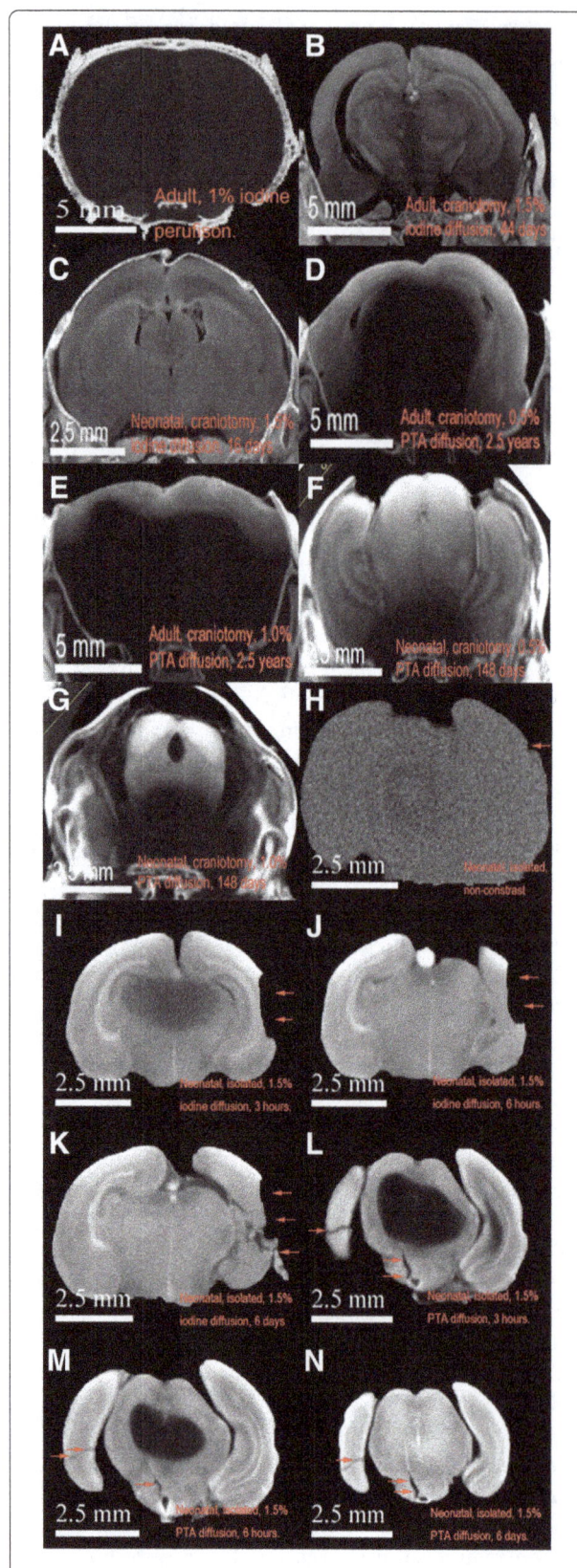

Fig. 2 Successful tissue differentiation on micro-CT scanning demonstrate iodine diffusion staining technique is practical for both large (age of 25 days) and small (age of 36 h) postnatal encapsulated rat brain, Figure (**a**–**g**). (**a**) demonstrates unsuccessful neural-tissue scanning using 1.0% iodine perfusion staining for adult rat, whereas (**b**) and (**c**) show 1.5% iodine diffusion staining yielded good neural tissue contrast with adult and neonatal rat brains after 44 and 16 days, respectively. However, the same staining techniques using 0.5 and 1.0% PTA yielded little success on adult rat brains, (**d**) and (**e**), even after 2.5 years. Similarly, (**f**) and (**g**) show incomplete tissue differentiation of neonatal rat brains despite prolonged staining of 148 days using 0.5 and 1.0% PTA staining, respectively. Because PTA staining was non-uniform, selected coronal views were chosen to illustrate regions of incomplete tissue differentiation: (**a**–**d**) are anterior coronal views while (**e**–**g**) are posterior coronal views. Figure (**h**–**n**) illustrate iodine diffusion staining is equally effective but more efficient temporally to PTA staining for micro-CT scanning of small and isolated neural tissues. (**h**) shows lack of tissue contrast with no staining. (**i**–**k**) illustrate progressive improvement of tissue details on micro-CT scans with 1.5% iodine staining over time: 3, 6 h, and 6 days, respectively. Similarly, (**l**–**n**) show the same with 1.5% PTA staining over the same respective durations. Iodine staining was significantly faster

In both cases, tissue differentiation as a result of staining was faster than when brain material was encapsulated in the skull, Fig. 2c. However, all scans revealed microscopic tissue damages of the rat brains indicated by arrows across Fig. 2h–n from dissection and handling despite macroscopically intact, as shown by Additional file 3: Figure S2. These brain damages were not seen on micro-CT scans of encapsulated brains, Fig. 2b and c.

Image quality of micro-CT scans

In the second part of the study, we explored the image details and 3D-visualization capability of rat brain micro-CT scans.

High display versatility of micro-CT scan data using 3D-volume rendering

In this study, we demonstrated the investigatory power of micro-CT scanning by providing examples of the full visualization capability of current ex vivo micro-CT scanning through 3D-volume rendering. Figure 3s show the 3D-volume rendering of neonatal rat brain in high definition, 2048*2048*2048 voxels, with a resolution of 10.7 μm/voxel. Through manipulations of visual planes, one can identify and analyse organs of interest. For instance, the dorsal and ventral external features of the neonatal rats are illustrated in Fig. 3a and b, respectively. In addition, Fig. 3c–e show internal organs visualized in parasagittal and sagittal views, ranging from salivary glands, musculatures, nasal cavity, oral cavity, and neuroanatomy. Figure 3c and d show high-definition progressive views of the brain and identified organs such as olfactory bulb, cerebral cortex, cerebellum, and cochlea in structural-preserved manner. Similarly, progressive anterior to posterior axial views, Fig. 3f–h, provide alternative visualizations of

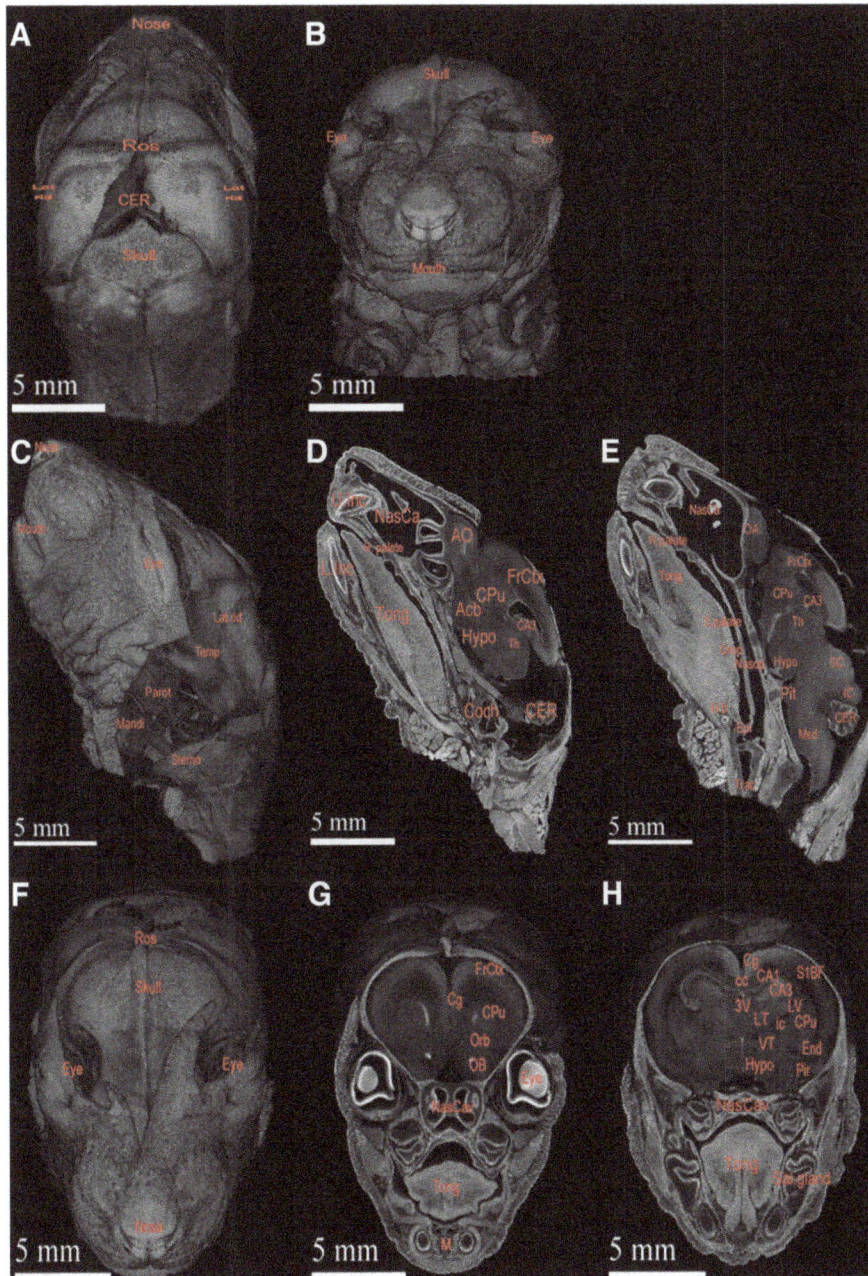

Fig. 3 Volumetric rendering of ex vivo micro-CT scan of neonatal rat's head enables detailed visualization and potential high-powered quantitative analysis. (**a** and **b**) illustrate respective anterior and posterior views of external features of rat's head and neck, including mouth, nose, and muscle distributions. (**c**, **d**, and **e**) are respective external, parasagittal, and sagittal views of rat's head and neck. (**f**, **g**, and **h**) are progressive coronal explorations of the same rat. These different views demonstrate the high-resolution power and flexibility of micro-CT scans. These exploration images show blood vessels, parotid glands, nasal anatomy, oral anatomy, and intracranial anatomy along with obvious muscular features throughout the head. Anatomical structures are labelled as follow: *Acb = accumbens nucleus; AO = anterior olfactory bulb; apons = anterior pons; ATh = anterior thalamus; CA1 = CA1 field of hippocampus; CA3 = CA3 field of hippocampus; cc = corpus callosum; CER = cerebellum; Cg = cingulate gyrus; Coch = cochlea; CPu = caudate putamen; End = Endopiriform nucleus; Epi = epiglottis; EPi = external plexiform layer; FrCtx = frontal cortex; H. b = hyoid bone; H. palate = hard palate; Hypo = hypothalamus; IC = inferior colliculus; ic = internal capsule; Lat rid = lateral ridge of skull; L. Inc = lower incisor; LT = lateral thalamus; LV = lateral ventricle; M = mandible; Mandi = mandibular gland; Med = medulla; NasCa = nasal cavity; Nasop = nasopharynx; OB = olfactory bulb; Orb = orbital cortex; OV = olfactory ventricle; Parot = parotid gland; Pir = piriform cortex; Pit = pituitary gland; PTh = posterior thalamus; ROS = rostral ridge of skull; Sal. Gland = salivary gland; SC = superior colliculus; S. palate = soft palate; S1BF = Somatosensory 1 Barrel Field; Sterno = sternomastoideus; Temp = temporalis; 3 V = 3rd ventricle; Th = thalamus; Tong = tongue; Trac = trachea; U. Inc = upper incisor; VT = ventral thalamus*

cross-sectional rat brain anatomy that are difficult to appreciate in other views, such as cingulate gyrus, lateral thalamus and ventral thalamus. Overall, Fig. 3a–h demonstrate that through different visual-planes exploration, various external and internal features of buccal, nasal, and intracranial organs can be visualized with excellent tissue contrast. Additionally, simple quantitative size measurement can be made with reference to the scale bar listed.

Validating neuroanatomical information offered by micro-CT scans with H&E histology

To validate micro-CT scanning method and explore potential microscopic tissue distortion as a result of the staining preparations for micro-CT scanning, we compared the ex vivo micro-CT scan, Fig. 4a, to H&E microscopy, Fig. 4b, both of which derived from the same iodine-stained rat brain. This comparison demonstrates that 3D rendering of the rat brain micro-CT scans offered neuroanatomical information comparable to that shown in 4× H&E microscopy. The grayscale distribution of micro-CT scans correlated strongly to the H&E distribution and therefore enabled successful neural structure distinguishment including olfactory bulb, caudate putamen, frontal cortex, thalamus, medulla, and cerebellum. Furthermore, the tissue integrity was well preserved in micro-CT scans when comparing to H&E light microscopy, Fig. 4b–d, which demonstrated micro-tears as a result of sectioning and H&E staining process. Moreover, successful light microscopy of iodine-stained rat brain demonstrated macroscopic discoloration by iodine,

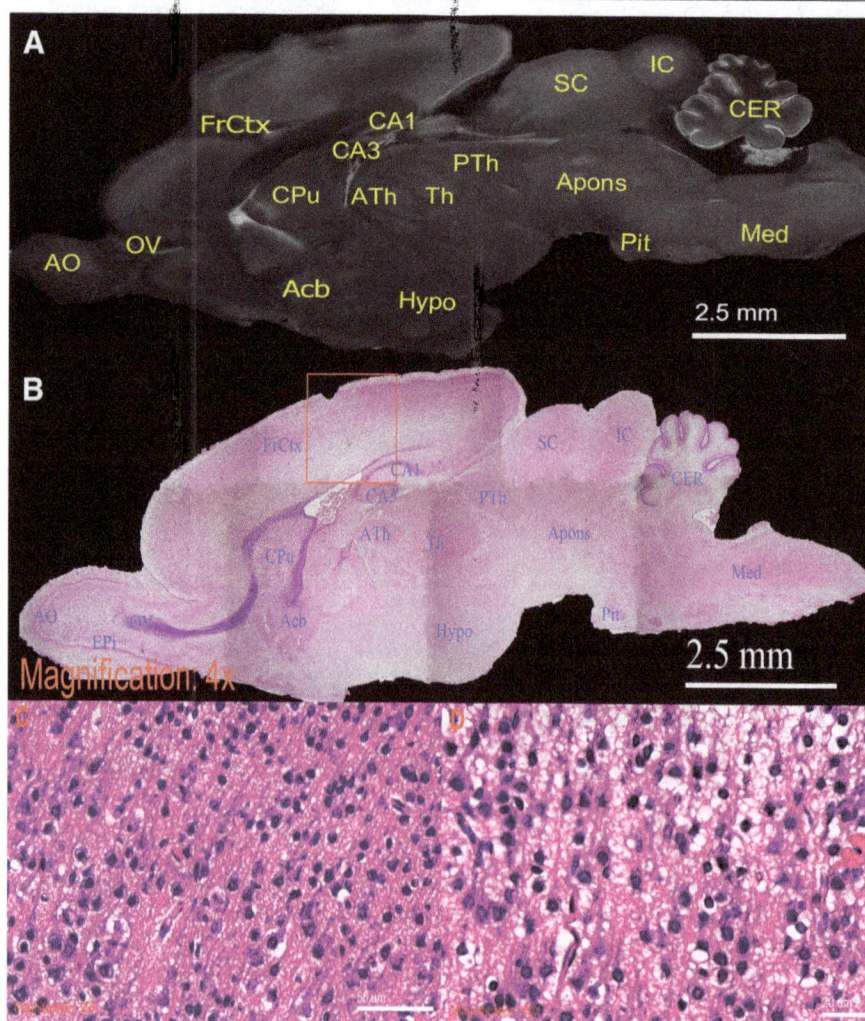

Fig. 4 High-powered demonstration of rat brain by ex vivo micro-CT scan. Direct comparison between the sagittal section of rat brain in (**a**), micro-CT slice, and (**b**), H&E stained 4× light micrograph. Similar structural details are seen in these two imaging. (**c** and **d**) are respective 20× and 40× light micrographs of selected FrCtX region, demonstrating neuronal cell bodies. Anatomical structures of comparable visibility are labelled as follows: *Acb* = accumbens nucleus; *AO* = anterior olfactory bulb; *apons* = anterior pons; *ATh* = anterior thalamus; *CA1* = CA1 field of hippocampus; *CA3* = CA3 field of hippocampus; *CER* = cerebellum; *CPu* = caudate putamen; *EPi* = external plexiform layer; *FrCtx* = frontal cortex; *Hypo* = hypothalamus; *IC* = inferior colliculus; *Med* = medulla; *OV* = olfactory ventricle; *Pit* = pituitary gland; *PTh* = posterior thalamus; *SC* = superior colliculus; *Th* = thalamus

Additional file 2: Figure S1B, did not prohibit tissue from histology processing and higher magnifications of microscopy can still be achieved, Fig. 4c (20× magnification) and Fig. 4d (40× magnification), where nuclei can be visualized clearly.

Direct comparison of image quality of in vivo and ex vivo micro-CT scanning

We illustrated the image difference between the in vivo and ex vivo micro-CT scans of the same iodine-stained rat-brain through direct comparison, as shown by Fig. 5. This comparison demonstrated the in vivo micro-CT scan's imaging limitations.

Both types of scans offered gross anatomical information; however, ex vivo micro-CT scans provided significantly more detailed neuroanatomy and sharper outlines than those of in vivo micro-CT scans. By comparing Fig. 5Aa and Ba, the respective ex vivo and in vivo micro-CT scans of a 24-h-old rat brain, one can clearly appreciate the frontal cortex, caudate putamen, superior and inferior colliculus, and trabeculae of the skull; all of which are well-defined in Fig. 5Aa. Higher magnification of the distinctive morphology in and around the cerebellum was chosen to further demonstrate how this difference can impact potential qualitative and quantitative analysis, as shown by Fig. 5Ab (ex vivo micro-CT scan) and Fig. 5Bb (in vivo micro-CT scan). While the rough outline of cerebellar fissures and vermis are still discernible in the in vivo micro-CT scan (Fig. 5Bb), intrinsic noise and oversaturation of the scan render boundaries much less crisply resolved than in the ex vivo micro-CT scan (Fig. 5Ab). Hence, one can easily define the ten cerebellar vermis and their respective sizes in Fig. 5Ab but not in Fig. 5Bb. This demonstrated the analytic limitations of in vivo micro-CT scans. In addition, volumetric measurements of brain based on segmentations of in vivo micro-CT scans differs slightly to that of ex vivo micro-CT scans, 424.75 mm^3 vs 395.54 mm^3. Although small, this discrepancy is due to the image quality difference resulting less precise segmentation from in vivo micro-CT scans.

Post-acquisition image processing: non-local means (NLM) denoising

Post-acquisition image processing using NLM algorithm was incorporated into this study as attempts to improve CT image quality for better visualization of neural differentiation through denoising, which is particularly useful for in vivo micro-CT scans due to the high intrinsic images noise. Pre- and post-processing of

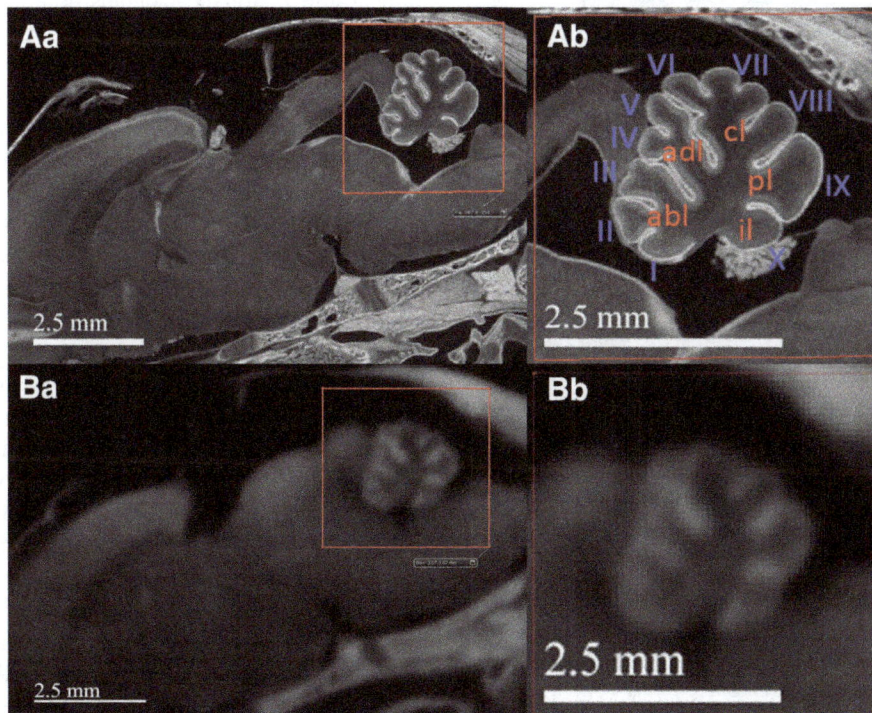

Fig. 5 Direct comparison of ex vivo (spatial resolution of 10.7 μm/voxel) and in vivo (spatial resolution of 20 μm/voxel) micro-CT scans of the same 24-h-old rat's head shows the image-quality difference between the two. (**Aa**) and (**Ba**) are sagittal illustrations of ex vivo and in vivo micro-CT scans, respectively. Gross neuroanatomy can be visualized in both scans with subtle difference appreciated by close-viewing, (**Ab**) and (**Bb**). Detailed cerebellar fissures, vermis (I–X), and lobes, can only be appreciated on ex vivo scans: *abl = anterobasal lobe; adl = anterodorsal lobe; cl = central lobe; pl = posterior lobe; il = inferior lobe*

ex vivo micro-CT scans, Fig. 6Aa and Ba, show organ boundaries are subtly enhanced by NLM processing. This is more evident in their respective magnified views, namely the bordering of caudate putamen and external capsule, as

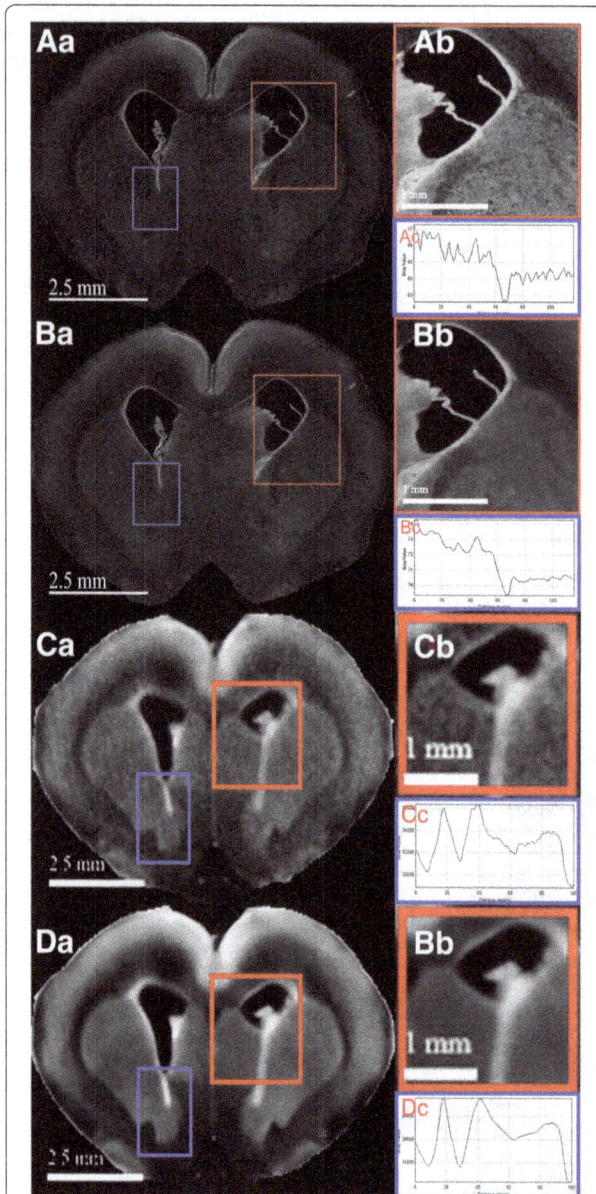

Fig. 6 Neuroanatomical differentiation of both ex vivo and in vivo micro-CT scan are enhanced by NLM denoising. The original (**Aa**) and denoised (**Ba**) ex vivo scans illustrate sharper periventricular edges seen in (**Ba**) while gross neuroanatomical details are preserved in both. The difference in image noises is more obvious when comparing the respective magnified views, (**Ab**) and (**Bb**). Similar but more prominent edge enhancements is shown by the comparison of (**Ca**) and (**Da**), original and denoised in vivo micro-CT scans, respectively. The markedly improved signal-to-noise ratio is easily appreciated in the magnified denoised (**Db**) from the original (**Cb**) views. The respective grayscale line profile of each scan revealed reductions in intensity variability in denoised group, (**Bc**) and (**Dc**), in comparison to the originals, (**Ac**) and (**Cc**)

demonstrated by Fig. 6Ab and Bb. In addition, their respective grayscale line profiles illustrate reductions in intensity spread, Fig. 6Ac and Bc, demonstrating noise reduction following processing. Similarly, the same but more prominent effect can be seen from the processing of in vivo micro-CT scans, as shown by Fig. 6Ca and Da, demonstrating edge enhancements of caudate putamen, lateral ventricles, and external capsules; these difference are obvious in their respective magnified views, Fig. 6Cb and Db. The comparison of their respective grayscale line profiles also demonstrated decreases in intensity variability, Fig. 6Cc and Dc.

Discussion

Through proper micro-CT setup, sample preparation, and image processing, informative neural micro-CT scans can be generated with postnatal animals. These scans enable internal visualization and potential quantitative analyses including volumetric and dimensional measurements by providing images with neural-tissue differentiation comparable, if not better, to micro-MRI brain scans, as illustrated Denic et al. [24]. Furthermore, micro-CT scans has a maximal spatial resolution of 1 μm/voxel with 16-h scanning time, significantly higher than 20 μm/voxel of micro-MRI achieved by 24 h of high-magnetic-fields scanning [4, 25]. Consistently, this high-magnification power of micro-CT provides anatomical and histological details comparable to those of 4× H&E light-microscopy, Fig. 4b. As a result of these characteristics, 3D rendering of the ex vivo micro-CT scans can show detailed and refined micro-neuroanatomy, Fig. 3. This function can therefore be applied to morphological study on genetic-disease model animals or cancer studies. Moreover, because tissue sample can be preserved following micro-CT scanning for H&E processing, Fig. 4c and d, micro-CT scan can serve as a screening tool for area of interest in the brain for further histology analysis. Although high-resolution micro-CT has the drawback of large dataset size, >4.6 GB/dataset, the high demand in computational and storage power for image analysis are met by the recent advancement in computing hardware, rendering this a practical research modality.

Although the difference between ex vivo and in vivo micro-CT has been addressed in previous studies, few have made direct comparisons of the quality difference of postnatal neural scans using these two modalities [26, 27]. In this study, we demonstrated the difference in magnification and resolution potentials of micro-CT scans using a custom-built ex vivo micro-CT scanner versus a commercial in vivo micro-CT scanner, as shown by Fig. 5. Consistent with expectations, our results have shown that ex vivo micro-CT scans offer finer detailed scans than in vivo micro-CT scans, due to the higher magnification achieved by having the X-ray source closer to the sample (i.e., a short source-sample distance, *SSD*). In theory, reducing the *SSD* increases the image noises and blurs edges, an effect clearly shown in Fig. 5Ba and Bb. However, image degradation can be minimized by using a low source current and careful focusing to minimize source spot size to obtain a best resolution of <2–3 μm/voxel while extending the scanning time to over 15 h to achieve high signal-to-noise ratio images. In comparison, commercial in vivo micro-CT scanners have limited magnifications and thus lower resolution due to the preset values of SSD. Furthermore, higher image noise in in vivo micro-CT scans is due to the shorter scanning time required to minimize the radiation exposure in live-animal scanning. In general, the best image quality needs the longest possible scanning time in either ex or in vivo micro-CT setups.

Based on the prior success of embryo study, we compared two contrast agents, iodine and PTA, for postnatal neural tissue staining [16]. The contrasts were chosen for their safety, ease of handling, and the likely effectiveness based on prior studies. Perfusion was first trialled in the hope of preserving rat skull integrity. Unfortunately, iodine staining was ineffective when introduced this way, likely due to poor penetration through the blood brain barrier and slow diffusion rate through capillary walls to end-organs [28, 29]. Contrary to prior embryo studies, simple diffusion staining with intact skull was also trialled with little success, suggesting contrast penetration through calcified skull was not possible [16]. Hence, diffusion-staining through a small craniotomy was subsequently adopted and found effective using iodine staining on all tested tissues. However, PTA was less effective as a stain using the same protocols on partially encapsulated tissues, especially on large adult rat brains; staining remained incomplete after 2.5 years, Fig. 2d and e, rendering this method impractical.

Due to concerns of prolonged staining may cause potential structural damage and prohibit tissues from future histology uses, as shown in Additional file 2: Figure S1, we tested PTA and iodine staining on dissected rat brains of small sizes with hope, Additional file 3: Figure S2. The result showed both stains yield similar quality of rat brain micro-CT images, as demonstrated by Fig. 2k and n. However, iodine was able to complete tissue staining faster than PTA due to its much higher penetration. In addition, iodine was better in staining poorly vascularized tissues such as the central nervous system, where PTA had little success in staining tissues with size greater than 1 cm^3. This is likely due to the size and polarity difference of the two contrast agents: iodine is a non-polar molecule that is about 20 times smaller than the polytungstate anion of PTA [30–33]. Nevertheless, we found staining times to be significantly longer than previously described [5, 16]. To compensate for the lower penetration of PTA, limiting tissue volume to 1 cm^3 and complete organ isolation through dissection may be required for successful

staining. While these modifications to the method have proven effective, adopting such an approach defeats the purpose of using micro-CT, since dissection and excessive handling increase the risks of structural damage, even by experienced dissectors, as illustrated by the micro-tears shown by micro-CT scans, Fig. 2h through n. Based on our findings and the known difference in the properties of iodine and PTA, we recommend diffusion-iodine staining with partial craniotomy as the method of choice for micro-CT scans of postnatal rat brains. Additionally, successful H&E processing on both iodine- and PTA-stained brain tissues confirmed that prolonged contrast staining for micro-CT scanning compromises little, if any, tissue integrity and neuronal cell bodies can be visualized in higher magnification light micrographs, Fig. 4c and d. This suggests micro-CT scans may serve as a targeting tool for regions of interest and reduce unnecessary histopathology processing in pathology study, thus reduce labour and time.

Post-acquisition image processing through NLM filtering was performed to enhance image clarity and structural boundaries. NLM algorithm was chosen for its property of spatial detail preservation [21]. Although denoising only modestly improved ex vivo micro-CT scans, Fig. 6Aa and Ba, due to the scan's high intrinsic signal-to-noise ratio, it has proven useful for in vivo micro-CT scans, which has high intrinsic image-noises, Fig. 6Ca. This image-noise was significantly reduced after processing, Fig. 6Da. These improvements are obvious in selected magnified views of caudate putamen, Fig. 6Cb and Db. We appreciate that commercially available in vivo micro-CT scanners are more widely available than custom ex vivo micro-CT scanners. By demonstrating the quality of in vivo micro-CT scans can be effectively improved through NLM algorithms, we support in vivo micro-CT data can also offer anatomical visualizations and accurate quantitative analysis. Lastly, denoising reduces the image noise, as demonstrated by the reduction in the variability of intensity profiles, Fig. 6Bc and Dc; this is an important step for the future developments of accurate automated segmentation for organs of interests.

Conclusions

Micro-CT scanning, using either ex vivo or in vivo micro-CT scanners, is a powerful and effective neuro-anatomy visualization modality for lab animals. Furthermore, micro-CT digital data is easy to store and manipulate. The anatomical details and accuracy offered by micro-CT scanning have been validated with the traditional H&E stained light micrograph. Moreover, the safety, simplicity, and tissue-preserving characteristic of the iodine-diffusion staining through craniotomy render micro-CT scanning a very easy-to-use study modality. Lastly, we appreciate that in vivo micro-CT scanners are more widely accessible and have a faster image processing time than ex vivo micro-CT scanners, the low signal-to-noise ratio due to the physical data acquisition restraints of in vivo micro-CT scans has been addressed. The improvement made by simple and efficient post-acquisition NLM processing reduces image degradation and enhances anatomical clarity, particularly with in vivo micro-CT scans, thus promoting versatile structural segmentation for quantitative analysis of animal morphology, including volumetric measurements. Based on described imaging methods, future studies may include: 1. internal organ visualization and quantitative analysis on animal models of genetic disease, e.g. Hirschsprung's disease; 2. cancer treatment response studies on animal models; 3. identifying areas of interest for histological processing in pathology studies.

Abbreviations

3V: 3rd ventricle; ACTH-HREC: ACT Health Human Research Ethics Committee; AGWN: Additive Gaussian White Noise; ANU-AEEC: Australian National University Animal Experimentation Ethics Committee; CA1: CA1 field of hippocampus; CA3: CA3 field of hippocampus;; cc: corpus callosum; CCD: X-ray coupled-charged device.; Cg: Cingulate gyrus; CLSM: Confocal laser scanning microscopy; Coch: Cochlea; DICOM: Digital imaging and communications in medicine; DSD: Detector-sample distance; End: Endopiriform nucleus; Epi: Epiglottis; EtOH: Ethanol; FOV: Field of view; gsv: gray scale value; H&E: Hematoxylin and Eosin stain; H. b: Hyoid bone; H. palate: Hard palate; ic: internal capsule; L. Inc.: Lower incisor; Lat rid: Lateral ridge of skull; LT: Lateral thalamus; LV: Lateral ventricle; M: Mandible; MAF: Moving average filter; Mandi: Mandibular gland; Micro-CT: Micro-computed tomography; Micro-MRI: Micro-magnetic resonance imaging; NasCa: Nasal cavity; Nasop: Nasopharynx; NCI: National Computational Infrastructure; NetCDF: Network Common Data Form; NLM: Non-local-means processing; OB: Olfactory bulb; OPT: Optical projection tomography; Orb: Orbital cortex; Parot: Parotid gland; PBS: Phosphate-buffered saline; Pir: Piriform cortex; Pit: Pituitary gland; PS: Pixel size; PSNR: Peak signal to noise ratio; PTA: Phosphotungstic acid; ROS: Rostral ridge of skull; S. palate: Soft palate; S1BF: Somatosensory 1 Barrel Field; Sal. Gland: Salivary gland; SDD: Source-detector distance; SEM: Scanning electron microscopy; SSD: Sample-source distance; ssd: sum of squared differences; Sterno: Sternomastoideus; Temp: Temporalis; Tong: Tongue; Trac: Trachea; U. Inc.: Upper incisor; VT: Ventral thalamus

Acknowledgements

The authors gratefully acknowledge the staff of Australian National University Applied Mathematic Department for their technical support of this project.

Funding

None declared.

Authors' contributions

Conceived the study: KC, AA, ZMS, GDH. Developed the methodology, performed the experiment and analysis: KC, AA, ZMS, GDH. Performed the post-acquisition image processing: KC, AA. Wrote the paper: KC, AA, ZMS, GDH. All authors read and approved the final manuscript.

Competing interests

The authors declare that they have no competing interests.

Author details

[1]The Canberra Hospital, Yamba Drive, Garran, ACT 2605, Australia. [2]Massachusetts Institute of Technology, Cambridge, MA 02139, USA. [3]Automated Analytics, Sugar Land, TX 77479, USA. [4]Medical School, Australian National University, Canberra, ACT 2601, Australia.

References

1. Weninger WJ, Geyer SH, Mohun TJ, Rasskin-Gutman D, Matsui T, Ribeiro I, et al. High-resolution episcopic microscopy: a rapid technique for high detailed 3D analysis of gene activity in the context of tissue architecture and morphology. Anat Embryol. 2006;211(3):213–21.
2. Sharpe J, Ahlgren U, Perry P, Hill B, Ross A, Hecksher-Sørensen J, et al. Optical projection tomography as a tool for 3D microscopy and gene expression studies. Science. 2002;296(5567):541–5.
3. Dhenain M, Ruffins SW, Jacobs RE. Three-dimensional digital mouse atlas using high-resolution MRI. Dev Biol. 2001;232(2):458–70.
4. Turnbull DH, Mori S. MRI in mouse developmental biology. NMR Biomed. 2007;20(3):265–74.
5. Metscher BD. MicroCT for developmental biology: a versatile tool for high-contrast 3D imaging at histological resolutions. Dev Dyn. 2009;238(3):632–40.
6. Smithpeter CL, Dunn AK, Welch AJ, Richards-Kortum R. Penetration depth limits of in vivo confocal reflectance imaging. Appl Opt. 1998;37(13):2749–54.
7. Weninger WJ, Geyer SH. Episcopic 3D imaging methods: tools for researching gene function. Curr Genomics. 2008;9(4):282–9.
8. Alanentalo T, Loren CE, Larefalk A, Sharpe J, Holmberg D, Ahlgren U. High-resolution three-dimensional imaging of islet-infiltrate interactions based on optical projection tomography assessments of the intact adult mouse pancreas. J Biomed Opt. 2008;13(5):054070.
9. Ruffins SW, Martin M, Keough L, Truong S, Fraser SE, Jacobs RE, et al. Digital three-dimensional atlas of quail development using high-resolution MRI. TheScientificWorldJOURNAL. 2007;7:592–604.
10. Wong MD, Spring S, Henkelman RM. Structural stabilization of tissue for embryo phenotyping using micro-CT with iodine staining. PLoS One. 2013; 8(12):e84321.
11. Burghardt AJ, Link TM, Majumdar S. High-resolution computed tomography for clinical imaging of bone microarchitecture. Clin Orthop Relat Res. 2011; 469(8):2179–93.
12. Mather ML, Morgan SP, White LJ, Tai H, Kockenberger W, Howdle SM, et al. Image-based characterization of foamed polymeric tissue scaffolds. Biomed Mater. 2008;3(1):015011.
13. Missbach-Guentner J, Hunia J, Alves F. Tumor blood vessel visualization. Int J Dev Biol. 2011;55(4–5):535–46.
14. Nakagaki S, Iijima M, Handa K, Koike T, Yasuda Y, Saito T, et al. Micro-CT and histologic analyses of bone surrounding immediately loaded miniscrew implants: comparing compression and tension loading. Dent Mater J. 2014; 33(2):196–202.
15. Peyrin F. Evaluation of bone scaffolds by micro-CT. Osteoporos int. 2011; 22(6):2043–8.
16. Metscher BD. MicroCT for comparative morphology: simple staining methods allow high-contrast 3D imaging of diverse non-mineralized animal tissues. BMC Physiol. 2009;9:11.
17. Pauwels E, Van Loo D, Cornillie P, Brabant L, Van Hoorebeke L. An exploratory study of contrast agents for soft tissue visualization by means of high resolution X-ray computed tomography imaging. J Microsc. 2013; 250(1):21–31.
18. Limaye A. Drishti, A Volume Exploration and Presentation Tool. In: Developments in X-Ray Tomography Viii, vol. 8506; 2012.
19. Schindelin J, Rueden CT, Hiner MC, Eliceiri KW. The ImageJ ecosystem: An open platform for biomedical image analysis. Mol Reprod Dev. 2015;82(7-8): 518–29.
20. Kiernan JA. Histological and histochemical methods : theory and practice. 3rd ed. Oxford: Butterworth-Heinemann; 1999. p. 502.

21. Buades A, Coll B, Morel JM, editors. A non-local algorithm for image denoising. 2005 IEEE Computer Society Conference on Computer Vision and Pattern Recognition (CVPR'05); 2005.

22. Schindelin J, Arganda-Carreras I, Frise E, Kaynig V, Longair M, Pietzsch T, et al. Fiji: an open-source platform for biological-image analysis. Nat Methods. 2012;9(7):676–82.

23. Coupé P, Yger P, Prima S, Hellier P, Kervrann C, Barillot C. An optimized blockwise nonlocal means denoising filter for 3-D magnetic resonance images. IEEE Trans Med Imaging. 2008;27(4):425–41.

24. Denic A, Macura SI, Mishra P, Gamez JD, Rodriguez M, Pirko I. MRI in rodent models of brain disorders. Neurotherapeutics : the journal of the American Society for Experimental NeuroTherapeutics. 2011;8(1):3–18.

25. Gabbay-Benziv R, Reece EA, Wang F, Bar-Shir A, Harman C, Turan OM, et al. A step-wise approach for analysis of the mouse embryonic heart using 17.6 tesla MRI. Magn Reson Imaging. 2017;35:46–53.

26. Schambach SJ, Bag S, Schilling L, Groden C, Brockmann MA. Application of micro-CT in small animal imaging. Methods. 2010;50(1):2–13.

27. Stauber M, Muller R. Micro-computed tomography: a method for the non-destructive evaluation of the three-dimensional structure of biological specimens. Methods Mol Biol. 2008;455:273–92.

28. Pardridge WM. Introduction to the blood-brain barrier methodology, biology, and pathology. Cambridge: Cambridge University Press; 1998. p. XIV, 486 S.

29. Neuwelt EA. Mechanisms of disease: the blood-brain barrier. Neurosurgery. 2004;54(1):131–40 discussion 41-2.

30. Cotton FA, Cotton FA. Advanced inorganic chemistry. 6th ed. New York: Wiley; 1999. p. xv, 1355.

31. Everett M, Miller W. The role of phosphotungstic and phosphomolybdic acids in connective tissue staining I. Histochemical studies. Histochem J. 1974;6(1):25–34.

32. Gignac PM, Kley NJ. Iodine-enhanced micro-CT imaging: methodological refinements for the study of the soft-tissue anatomy of post-embryonic vertebrates. J Exp Zool B Mol Dev Evol. 2014;322(3):166–76.

33. Wells AF. Structural inorganic chemistry. 5th ed. Oxford: Clarendon Press; 1984. p. 1.

Permissions

The contributors of this book come from diverse backgrounds, making this book a truly international effort. This book will bring forth new frontiers with its revolutionizing research information and detailed analysis of the nascent developments around the world.

We would like to thank all the contributing authors for lending their expertise to make the book truly unique. They have played a crucial role in the development of this book. Without their invaluable contributions this book wouldn't have been possible. They have made vital efforts to compile up to date information on the varied aspects of this subject to make this book a valuable addition to the collection of many professionals and students.

This book was conceptualized with the vision of imparting up-to-date information and advanced data in this field. To ensure the same, a matchless editorial board was set up. Every individual on the board went through rigorous rounds of assessment to prove their worth. After which they invested a large part of their time researching and compiling the most relevant data for our readers.

The editorial board has been involved in producing this book since its inception. They have spent rigorous hours researching and exploring the diverse topics which have resulted in the successful publishing of this book. They have passed on their knowledge of decades through this book. To expedite this challenging task, the publisher supported the team at every step. A small team of assistant editors was also appointed to further simplify the editing procedure and attain best results for the readers.

Apart from the editorial board, the designing team has also invested a significant amount of their time in understanding the subject and creating the most relevant covers. They scrutinized every image to scout for the most suitable representation of the subject and create an appropriate cover for the book.

The publishing team has been an ardent support to the editorial, designing and production team. Their endless efforts to recruit the best for this project, has resulted in the accomplishment of this book. They are a veteran in the field of academics and their pool of knowledge is as vast as their experience in printing. Their expertise and guidance has proved useful at every step. Their uncompromising quality standards have made this book an exceptional effort. Their encouragement from time to time has been an inspiration for everyone.

The publisher and the editorial board hope that this book will prove to be a valuable piece of knowledge for researchers, students, practitioners and scholars across the globe.

List of Contributors

Frederikke P. Fliedner, Jesper T. Jørgensen and Andreas Kjær
Department of Clinical Physiology, Nuclear Medicine & PET and Cluster for Molecular Imaging, Rigshospitalet and University of Copenhagen, Blegdamsvej 9, 2100 Copenhagen, Denmark

Anders E. Hansen
Department of Clinical Physiology, Nuclear Medicine & PET and Cluster for Molecular Imaging, Rigshospitalet and University of Copenhagen, Blegdamsvej 9, 2100 Copenhagen, Denmark
Department of Micro- and Nanotechnology, Center for Nanomedicine and Theranostics, DTU Nanotech, Technical University of Denmark, Building 423, 2800 Lyngby, Denmark

Ewa Zmysłowska-Polakowska, Mateusz Radwański, Michał Łęski and Sławomir Ledzion
Department of Endodontics, Medical University of Lodz, ul. Pomorska 251, Łódź 92-213, Poland

Monika Łukomska-Szymańska
Department of General Dentistry, Medical University of Lodz, ul. Pomorska 251, Łódź 92-213, Poland

Michał Polguj
Department of Angiology, Interfaculty Chair of Anatomy and Histology, Medical University of Lodz, ul. Narutowicza 60, Łódź 90-136, Poland

Brian Quinn and Zak Dauer
Department of Medical Physics, Memorial Sloan Kettering Cancer Center, 1275 York Avenue, New York, NY 10065, USA

Lawrence T. Dauer
Department of Medical Physics, Memorial Sloan Kettering Cancer Center, 1275 York Avenue, New York, NY 10065, USA
Department of Radiology, Memorial Sloan Kettering Cancer Center, New York, USA

Neeta Pandit-Taskar and Heiko Schoder
Department of Radiology, Memorial Sloan Kettering Cancer Center, New York, USA

Zebin Xiao, Jian Li, Yuyang Zhang, Dejun She and Dairong Cao
Department of Radiology, First Affiliated Hospital of Fujian Medical University, 20 Cha-Zhong Road, Fuzhou, Fujian 350005, China

Chengqi Li
Department of Radiology, Sanming Hospital of Integrated Traditional and Western, Sanming, Fujian 365000, China

Lei chen, Kai Zhou, Jiandong Yuan, Guangjian Jing, Xiaojing Huang and Chun Chen
Department of Orthopaedics, the First Affiliated Hospital, Wenzhou Medical University, Nan baixiang Road, Shangcai Village, Wenzhou 325000, Zhejiang, People's Republic of China

Raoying Xie
Department of Orthopaedics, the First Affiliated Hospital, Wenzhou Medical University, Nan baixiang Road, Shangcai Village, Wenzhou 325000, Zhejiang, People's Republic of China
Department of Radiation and chemotherapy division, the First Affiliated Hospital, Wenzhou Medical University, Wenzhou, Zhejiang, People's Republic of China

linhui Ruan
Department of Neurosurgery, the First Affiliated Hospital of Wenzhou Medical University, Wenzhou, Zhejiang, People's Republic of China

Wei Ji
Department of Orthopaedics, Navy General Hospital, Beijing, People's Republic of China

Qinglei Shi
Siemens Ltd, China Healthcare Sector MR Business Group, Beijing, People's Republic of China

Caroline De Coninck, Jean-Christophe Noël, Rachel Boutemy and Philippe Simon
Erasme Hospital, 808 route de Lennik, 1070 Anderlecht, Belgium

Ulrika Pahlm, Håkan Arheden, Marcus Carlsson and Ellen Ostenfeld
Department of Clinical Physiology, Lund University, Skane University Hospital, Lund, Sweden

Einar Heiberg
Department of Clinical Physiology, Lund University, Skane University Hospital, Lund, Sweden
Department of Biomedical Engineering, Faculty of Engineering, Lund University, Lund, Sweden

Felicia Seemann
Department of Clinical Physiology, Lund University, Skane University Hospital, Lund, Sweden
Department of Numerical Analysis, Faculty of Engineering, Lund University, Lund, Sweden
Department of Biomedical Engineering, Faculty of Engineering, Lund University, Lund, Sweden

Katarina Steding-Ehrenborg
Department of Clinical Physiology, Lund University, Skane University Hospital, Lund, Sweden
Department of Health Sciences, Physiotherapy, Lund University, Lund, Sweden

David Erlinge
Department of Cardiology, Clinical Sciences, Lund University, Lund, Sweden

Jean-Luc Dubois-Rande
Assistance Publique Hôpitaux de Paris, Hôpital Henri Mondor, Créteil, France

Svend Eggert Jensen
Department of Cardiology, Aalborg University Hospital, Aalborg, Denmark

Dan Atar
Department of Cardiology B, Oslo University Hospital Ullevål and Faculty of Medicine, University of Oslo, Oslo, Norway

Jihang Sun, Tong Yu, Xiaomin Duan, Di Hu, Yong liu and Yun Peng
Imaging Center, Beijing Children's Hospital, Capital Medical University, No.56, Nanlishi Road, Xicheng District, Beijing 100045, People's Republic of China

Jinrong Liu
Department of respiratory, Beijing Children's Hospital, Capital Medical University, Beijing 100045, People's Republic of China

Sebastian F. Baumbach, Jakob Binder and Ekkehard Euler
Department of General, Trauma and Reconstructive Surgery, University Hospital LMU Munich, Nussbaumstr. 20, Munich 80336, Germany

Alexander Synek
Institute of Lightweight Design and Structural Biomechanics, Vienna University of Technology, Getreidemarkt 9, Vienna 1060, Austria

Fabian G. Mück
Department of Clinical Radiology, University Hospital LMU Munich, Nussbaumstr. 20, Munich 80336, Germany

Yan Chevalier
Department of Orthopaedic Surgery, Physical Medicine and Rehabilitation, University Hospital LMU Munich, Campus Grosshadern, Marchioninistraße 15, Munich 81377, Germany

Georg Langs
Computational Imaging Research Laboratory, Department of Biomedical Imaging and Image-guided Therapy, Medical University of Vienna, Waehringer Guertel 18-20, Vienna 1090, Austria

Lukas Fischer
Computational Imaging Research Laboratory, Department of Biomedical Imaging and Image-guided Therapy, Medical University of Vienna, Waehringer Guertel 18-20, Vienna 1090, Austria
Software Competence Center Hagenberg GmbH, Softwarepark 21, Hagenberg 4232, Austria

Sven Weum and James B. Mercer
Medical Imaging Research Group, Department of Clinical Medicine, UiT The Arctic University of Norway, 9037 Tromsø, Norway
Department of Radiology, University Hospital of North Norway, Sykehusveien 38, 9038 Tromsø, Norway

Louis de Weerd
Medical Imaging Research Group, Department of Clinical Medicine, UiT The Arctic University of Norway, 9037 Tromsø, Norway
Department of Plastic Surgery and Hand Surgery, University Hospital of North Norway, 9038 Tromsø, Norway

Ryousuke Kawai, Jiro Hata, Noriaki Manabe, Hiroshi Imamura and Ai Iida
Department of Clinical Pathology and Laboratory Medicine, Kawasaki Medical School, 577 Matsushima, Kurashiki, Okayama 701-0192, Japan

Nobuko Koyama
Department of Hepatology and Pancreatology, Kawasaki Medical School, 577 Matsushima, Kurashiki, Okayama 701-0192, Japan

Hiroaki Kusunoki
Department of General Medicine, Kawasaki Medical School, 577 Matsushima, Kurashiki, Okayama 701-0192, Japan

Ayşegül Altunkeser
Department of Radiology, Konya Education and Research Hospital, Konya, Turkey
Konya Eğitim ve Araştırma Hastanesi, Radyoloji Bölümü, Hacı Şaban Mah, Meram Yeni Yol Caddesi, No: 97, PK: 42090 Meram, Konya, Turkey

M. Kazım Körez
Department of Statistics, Faculty of Science, Selcuk University, Konya, Turkey

Mie Holm Vilstrup and Eivind Antonsen Segtnan
Department of Nuclear Medicine, Odense University Hospital, Sdr. Boulevard 29, 5000 Odense C, Denmark

Oke Gerke
Department of Nuclear Medicine, Odense University Hospital, Sdr. Boulevard 29, 5000 Odense C, Denmark
Centre of Health Economics Research, University of Southern Denmark, Campusvej 55, 5230 Odense M, Denmark

Poul Flemming Høilund-Carlsen
Department of Nuclear Medicine, Odense University Hospital, Sdr. Boulevard 29, 5000 Odense C, Denmark
Department of Clinical Research, University of Southern Denmark, Winsløwparken 19, 5000 Odense C, Denmark

Ulrich Halekoh
Epidemiology, Biostatistics and Biodemography, University of Southern Denmark, J. B. Winsløws Vej 9b, 5000 Odense C, Denmark

Suzanne L. Duce, Shona Z. Matthew, Deirdre B. Cassidy, Lynne McCormick, Jill J. F. Belch and Allan D. Struthers
Division of Cardiovascular and Diabetes Medicine, Medical Research Institute, University of Dundee, DD1 9SY, UK

J. Graeme Houston
Division of Cardiovascular and Diabetes Medicine, Medical Research Institute, University of Dundee, DD1 9SY, UK
NHS Tayside Clinical Radiology, Ninewells Hospital, Dundee DD1 9SY, UK

Jonathan R. Weir-McCall
Division of Cardiovascular and Diabetes Medicine, Medical Research Institute, University of Dundee, DD1 9SY, UK
NHS Tayside Clinical Radiology, Ninewells Hospital, Dundee DD1 9SY, UK
Division of Cardiovascular and Diabetic Medicine, Level 7, Ninewells Hospital, Dundee DD1 9SY, UK

Stephen J. Gandy
NHS Tayside Clinical Radiology, Ninewells Hospital, Dundee DD1 9SY, UK
NHS Tayside Medical Physics, Ninewells Hospital, Dundee DD1 9SY, UK

Patricia Martin
NHS Tayside Clinical Radiology, Ninewells Hospital, Dundee DD1 9SY, UK

Helen M. Colhoun
Division of Population Health Sciences, Medical Research Institute, The Mackenzie Building, University of Dundee, DD2 4BF, UK

Xiang-ke Niu, Yan Xiong, Chao-bing Yang and Tao Peng
Department of Radiology, Affiliated Hospital of Chengdu University, Chengdu 610081, China

Jun Li
Department of General Surgery, Affiliated Hospital of Chengdu University, No. 82 2nd North Section of Second Ring Road, Chengdu, Sichuan 610081, China

Susant Kumar Das
Department of Intervention Radiology, Tenth People's Hospital of Tongji University, Shanghai 200072, China

Tino Ebbers
Center for Medical Image Science and Visualization, Linkoping University, SE-581 83 Linkoping, Sweden

Charlotta Andersson
Center for Medical Image Science and Visualization, Linkoping University, SE-581 83 Linkoping, Sweden
Department of Clinical Physiology, Linkoping University, SE-603 79 Norrkoping, Sweden

Johan Kihlberg
Center for Medical Image Science and Visualization, Linkoping University, SE-581 83 Linkoping, Sweden
Department of Diagnostic Radiology, Linkoping University, SE-581 85 Linkoping, Sweden

Carl-Johan Carlhäll and Jan E. Engvall
Center for Medical Image Science and Visualization, Linkoping University, SE-581 83 Linkoping, Sweden
Department of Medical and Health Sciences, Linkoping University, SE-581 83 Linkoping, Sweden
Department of Clinical Physiology, Linkoping University, SE-581 85 Linkoping, Sweden

Lena Lindström
Department of Clinical Physiology, Linkoping University, SE-603 79 Norrkoping, Sweden

Faik Afifi
Department of Orthopaedic Surgery and Traumatology, Kantonsspital Baselland Bruderholz, Liestal, Laufen, Switzerland

Emilienne Barthassat and Michael T. Hirschmann
Department of Orthopaedic Surgery and Traumatology, Kantonsspital Baselland Bruderholz, Liestal, Laufen, Switzerland
Basel University, Basel, Switzerland

Praveen Konala
Fellow- Musculoskeletal Radiology, The Robert Jones and Agnes Hunt Orthopaedic Hospital NHS Foundation Trust, Oswestry, UK

Helmut Rasch
Institute for Radiology and Nuclear Medicine, Kantonsspital Baselland-Bruderholz, Bruderholz, Switzerland

Maliheh Kadivar, Ziba Mosayebi, Reza Shervin Badoo, Raziyeh Sangesari, Saeed Jedari Attari, Maryam Saeedi and Elahe Movahedi Moghadam
Neonatal Health Research Center, Research Institute for Children Health, Shahid Beheshti University of Medical Sciences, Tehran, Iran

Anu Bhattarai, Yusri Dwi Heryanto, Tetsuya Higuchi and Yoshito Tsushima
Department of Diagnostic Radiology and Nuclear Medicine, Gunma University Graduate School of Medicine, 3-39-22 Showa-machi, Maebashi, Gunma 371-8511, Japan

Arifudin Achmad
Department of Diagnostic Radiology and Nuclear Medicine, Gunma University Graduate School of Medicine, 3-39-22 Showa-machi, Maebashi, Gunma 371-8511, Japan
Department of Nuclear Medicine and Molecular Imaging, Faculty of Medicine, Padjadjaran University, Jl. Professor Eyckman No.38, Bandung, West Java 40161, Indonesia

Ryan Yudistiro
Department of Diagnostic Radiology and Nuclear Medicine, Gunma University Graduate School of Medicine, 3-39-22 Showa-machi, Maebashi, Gunma 371-8511, Japan
Department of Nuclear Medicine, Mochtar Riady Comprehensive Cancer Center, Jl. Garnisun Dalam No. 2–3, Semanggi, Jakarta 12930, Indonesia

Mariana Reza, Per Wollmer and Elin Trägårdh
Department of Clinical Physiology and Nuclear Medicine, Skåne University Hospital, Inga Marie Nilssons gata 49, SE-205 02 Malmö, Sweden
Department of Translational Medicine, Lund University, Malmö, Sweden

Anders Bjartell
Department of Translational Medicine, Lund University, Malmö, Sweden
Department of Urology, Skåne University Hospital, Malmö, Sweden

Reza Kaboteh and May Sadik
Department of Molecular and Clinical Medicine, Sahlgrenska University Hospital, Gothenburg, Sweden

Ru Yu Tan, Suh Chien Pang, Kian Guan Lee and Chieh Suai Tan
Department of Renal Medicine, Singapore General Hospital, Singapore, Singapore

Tze Tec Chong
Department of Vascular Surgery, Singapore General Hospital, Singapore, Singapore

Fu Chieh Tsai and Apoorva Gogna
Department of Vascular and Interventional Radiology, Singapore General Hospital, Singapore, Singapore

Alicia Huiying Ong
Duke-NUS Medical School, Singapore, Singapore

Stefan Baumann, Michael Behnes, Benjamin Sartorius, Tobias Becher, Ibrahim El-Battrawy, Christian Fastner, Uzair Ansari, Dirk Loßnitzer, Martin Borggrefe and Ibrahim Akin
First Department of Medicine, University Medical Centre Mannheim, Theodor-Kutzer-Ufer 1-3, 68167 Mannheim, Germany

Kambis Mashayekhi
Division of Cardiology and Angiology II, University Heart Center Freiburg-Bad Krozingen, Bad Krozingen, Germany

Thomas Henzler and Stefan O. Schoenberg
Institute of Clinical Radiology and Nuclear Medicine, University Medical Center Mannheim, Medical Faculty Mannheim, Heidelberg University, Mannheim, Germany

Kai Liu, Zenglin Ma and Lili Feng
Department of Radiology, The Third Affiliated Hospital of Beijing University of Chinese Medicine, No. 51 Xiaoguan Street, Andingmenwai, Chaoyang District, Beijing, People's Republic of China

Inger Havsteen, Janus Damm Nybing and Anders Christensen
Department of Radiology, Copenhagen University Hospital Bispebjerg, Bispebjerg Bakke 23, 2400 Copenhagen, NV, Denmark

Lasse Willer, Christian Ovesen, Karen Ægidius, Jacob Marstrand, Per Meden, Sverre Rosenbaum, Marie Norsker Folke and Hanne Christensen
Department of Neurology, Copenhagen University Hospital Bispebjerg, Bispebjerg Bakke 23, 2400 Copenhagen, NV, Denmark

Adrian K. Dyer
Department of Pediatrics, Division of Cardiology, UT Southwestern Medical Center Dallas, Dallas, TX, USA
Department of Pediatrics, Division of Cardiology, Children's Health, Children's Medical Center Dallas, Dallas, TX, USA

Danielle M. Moyé
Department of Pediatrics, Division of Cardiology, UT Southwestern Medical Center Dallas, Dallas, TX, USA
Department of Pediatrics, Division of Cardiology, Children's Health, Children's Medical Center Dallas, Dallas, TX, USA
Pediatric Cardiology, Children's Health Children's Medical Center of Dallas, 1935 Medical District Drive, Dallas, TX 75235, USA

Tarique Hussain, Animesh Tandon and Gerald F. Greil
Department of Pediatrics, Division of Cardiology, UT Southwestern Medical Center Dallas, Dallas, TX, USA
Department of Pediatrics, Division of Cardiology, Children's Health, Children's Medical Center Dallas, Dallas, TX, USA
Departments of Radiology and Biomedical Engineering, University of Texas Southwestern Medical Center, Dallas, TX, USA

Rene M. Botnar
Division of Imaging Sciences, King's College London, London, UK
Pontificia Universidad Católica de Chile, Escuela de Ingeniería, Santiago, Chile

Markus Henningsson
Division of Imaging Sciences, King's College London, London, UK

Jiliang Ren, Ying Yuan, Yingwei Wu and Xiaofeng Tao
Department of Radiology, Shanghai Ninth People's Hospital, Shanghai Jiao Tong University School of Medicine, Shanghai, China

Linqi Zhang, Wei Li and Rusen Zhang
Department of Nuclear Medicine, Affiliated Cancer Hospital&Institute of Guangzhou Medical University, 78 Hengzhigang Road, Guangzhou 510095, Guangdong province, People's Republic of China

Qiao He
Department of Nuclear Medicine, the First Affiliated Hospital of Sun Yat-Sen University, 58 Zhongshan Er Road, Guangzhou 510080, Guangdong province, People's Republic of China

Ko-Chin Chen
The Canberra Hospital, Yamba Drive, Garran, ACT 2605, Australia
Automated Analytics, Sugar Land, TX 77479, USA
Medical School Australian National University, Canberra, ACT 2601, Australia

David Croaker
The Canberra Hospital, Yamba Drive, Garran, ACT 2605, Australia
Medical School Australian National University, Canberra, ACT 2601, Australia

Alon Arad
Massachusetts Institute of Technology, Cambridge, MA 02139, USA
Automated Analytics, Sugar Land, TX 77479, USA

Zan-Ming Song
Medical School Australian National University, Canberra, ACT 2601, Australia

Index